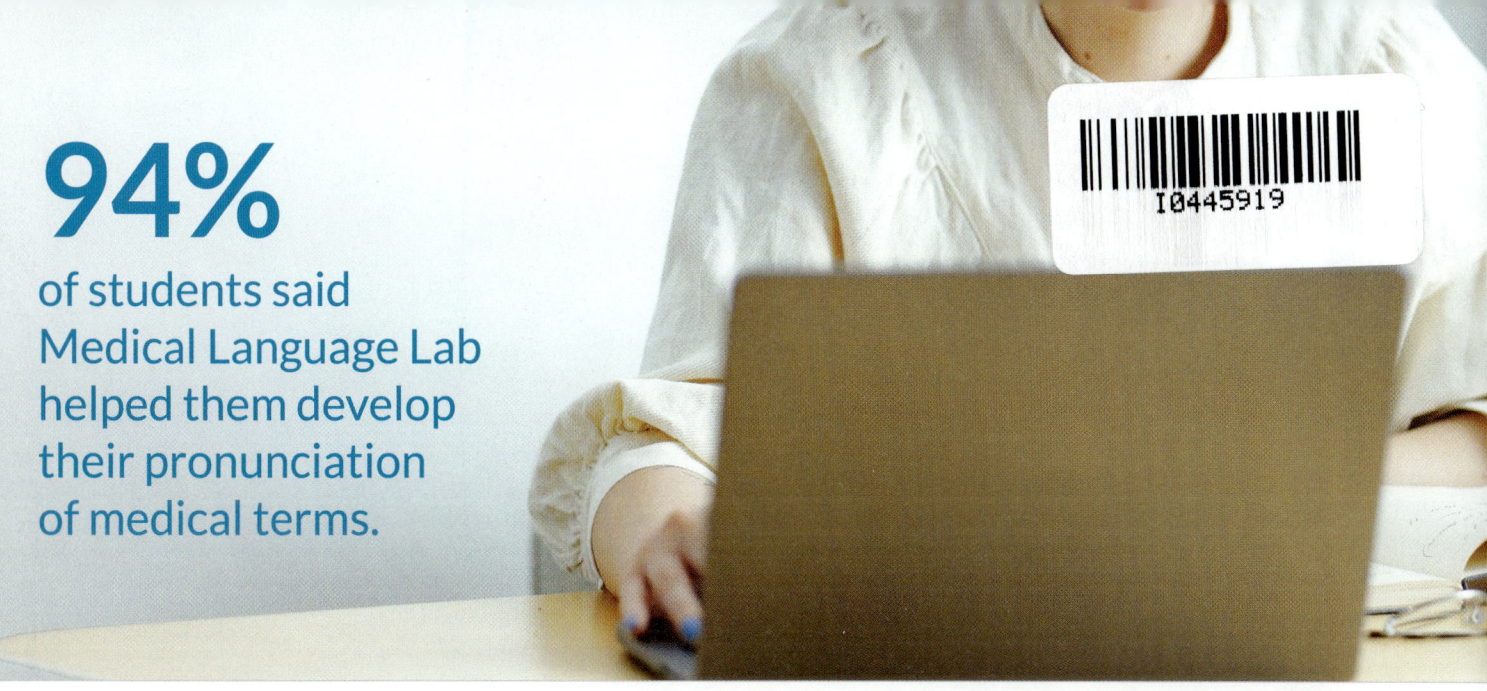

94%

of students said Medical Language Lab helped them develop their pronunciation of medical terms.

Medical Language Lab

Progress from basic through advanced levels of writing and speaking proficiency until you've mastered the language of medicine and are ready to apply it in class and in practice.

- **Pretest & Study Plans**
  Create your personalized Study Plan and identify the areas where you need to focus your study time.

- **Lecture Videos**
  Master the must-know concepts that connect anatomy and physiology to terminology to develop your word-building skills.

- **Pronunciation Exercises & Pronunciation Guides**
  Practice your speaking skills by listening to audio files of important terms and assess your progress with speaking exercises that provide immediate feedback.

- **Audio Clinical Scenarios**
  Listen to recordings of simulated clinical situations and answer questions that prepare you for professional practice.

- **Electronic Medical Record Workout**
  Learn essential documentation skills with questions based on EMR content.

- **Word-Building Practice Exercises**
  Apply your skills as you develop your knowledge of medical terminology.

- **Practice & Review**
  Complete additional practice activities based on your strengths and weaknesses as you master more challenging topics.

- **Personalized Gradebook**
  Track your progress and performance in real time, including what modules you've completed and your grades for each exercise and activity.

eBook

Reference your text anywhere, anytime to complete readings and study for exams. Add notes, highlights, and bookmarks.

READY TO GET STARTED?

Scan the code below for step-by-step instructions

FOR INSTRUCTORS

Medical Terminology Systems

A **BODY SYSTEMS** APPROACH

NINTH EDITION

Medical Terminology Systems

A **BODY SYSTEMS** APPROACH

NINTH EDITION

Regina M. Masters, MEd, BSN, RN, CMA
Toledo, Ohio

Barbara A. Gylys, MEd, CMA-A (AAMA)
Professor Emerita
University of Toledo
Toledo, Ohio

Mary Ellen Wedding, MEd, MT(ASCP), CMA (AAMA), CPC (AAPC)
Professor Emerita
University of Toledo
Toledo, Ohio

F.A. DAVIS

Philadelphia

F. A. Davis Company
1915 Arch Street
Philadelphia, PA 19103
www.fadavis.com

Copyright © 2026 by F. A. Davis Company

Printed in the United States of America

Last digit indicates print number: 10 9 8 7 6 5 4 3 2 1

Editor-in-Chief: Jean Rodenberger
Publisher: T. Quincy McDonald
Director of Content Development: George W. Lang
Content Project Manager: Julie Chase
Senior Developmental Editor, Digital Products: Amy R. Gibbons
Senior Manager of Art and Design: Carolyn O'Brien

As new scientific information becomes available through basic and clinical research, recommended treatments and drug therapies undergo changes. The author(s) and publisher have done everything possible to make this book accurate, up to date, and in accord with accepted standards at the time of publication. The author(s), editors, and publisher are not responsible for errors or omissions or for consequences from application of the book, and make no warranty, expressed or implied, in regard to the contents of the book. Any practice described in this book should be applied by the reader in accordance with professional standards of care used in regard to the unique circumstances that may apply in each situation. The reader is advised always to check product information (package inserts) for changes and new information regarding dose and contraindications before administering any drug. Caution is especially urged when using new or infrequently ordered drugs.

Library of Congress Cataloging-in-Publication Data

Names: Masters, Regina M., 1959- author | Gylys, Barbara A. author |
    Wedding, Mary Ellen author
Title: Medical terminology systems : a body systems approach / Regina M.
    Masters, BSN, MEd, RN, CMA, Toledo, OH, Barbara A. Gylys, MEd, CMA-A
    (AAMA), Professor Emerita University of Toledo, Toledo, OH, Mary Ellen
    Wedding, MEd, MT(ASCP), CMA (AAMA), CPC (AAPC), Professor Emerita
    University of Toledo, Toledo, OH.
Description: Ninth edition. | Philadelphia : F.A. Davis Company, [2026] |
    Includes index.
Identifiers: LCCN 2025020309 (print) | LCCN 2025020310 (ebook) | ISBN
    9781719651059 paperback | ISBN 9781719654784 epub
Subjects: LCSH: Medicine—Terminology
Classification: LCC R123 .G94 2026 (print) | LCC R123 (ebook) | DDC
    610.1/4—dc23/eng/20250707
LC record available at https://lccn.loc.gov/2025020309
LC ebook record available at https://lccn.loc.gov/2025020310

Dedication

Barbara's lifelong passion for language and medicine has left an indelible mark on education. Through her exceptional contributions, she has illuminated the path for hundreds of thousands of students, creating interactive activities and resources that have transformed the learning and teaching of medical terminology.

Barbara's unique ability to see through the lens of her students has inspired the creation of innovative educational features, designed to embrace diverse learning styles. She also has a way of simplifying complex topics, which empowers beginners to confidently master medical terminology. Her dedication to excellence has set a benchmark in the field, exemplified by the groundbreaking interactive activities and learning tools she has developed—setting a new standard in medical terminology education. Her development of a variety of tools has simplified and enhanced the effectiveness of teaching medical terminology for instructors.

Her collaborative spirit, rooted in a desire to grow and evolve alongside others, has not only enriched her work but also has deeply inspired her family. Her legacy thrives through her children and grandchildren, many of whom have followed her into the fields of medicine and writing.

Now, she enjoys a well-earned retirement in Florida with her devoted husband of 68 years, who has always been her greatest supporter and steadfast believer in contributing to her publishing journey. Barbara entrusts her enduring legacy to the next generation. Her daughter, Regina Masters, a coauthor of several published books at F.A. Davis Company, and her granddaughter, Julia Halm, a practicing physician, carry forward her mission of shaping the future of medical education. Together, they honor Barbara's vision, ensuring her contributions continue to inspire and educate for years to come.

Acknowledgments

The authors would like to acknowledge the valuable contributions of F.A. Davis's editorial and production team who were responsible for this project:

- **Quincy McDonald, Publisher,** who provided the overall design and layout for the ninth edition. His vision and guidance focused the authors at the onset of the project, and his support throughout this endeavor provided cohesiveness.
- **Julie Chase, Content Project Manager,** who meticulously guided the manuscript through the developmental and production phases of the textbook.
- **Former Editor-in-Chief Margaret Biblis,** once again provided her support and efforts to ensure the quality of the finished product.

In addition, we wish to acknowledge the many exceptionally dedicated publishing partners that helped in this publication:

- George W. Lang, Director of Content Development
- Amy Gibbons, Senior Developmental Editor, Digital Products
- Kate Margeson, Senior Illustration Coordinator
- Maria Everitt, Production Manager
- Carolyn O'Brien, Senior Manager of Design and Illustration
- Jacque Ginn, Project Manager

Preface

I am Regina M. Masters, and it is both an honor and a privilege to step into the role of author for this ninth edition of *Medical Terminology Systems,* a work that has long served as a cornerstone in the field. I am deeply grateful to the previous authors, whose dedication and expertise have shaped this book's reputation for academic excellence over the years. A current author of two other medical terminology books published by F.A. Davis with Barbara A. Gylys, my experience allows me to deliver the high-quality content that users have come to expect. While this edition retains the foundational principles established by its predecessors, it also incorporates the latest advances in the medical field to ensure its relevance in today's ever evolving health care environment. I look forward to continuing the legacy of this trusted resource for students, educators, and professionals.

The ninth edition of *Medical Terminology Systems: A Body Systems Approach* sets a new standard in mastering the language of medicine. New and updated content throughout integrates seamlessly with figures to accommodate diverse learning styles and bring a better understanding of medical terms related to diseases and conditions and diagnostic, surgical, and therapeutic procedures. Tables and flow charts have been added to simplify complex physiology.

Building on the success of previous editions, the ninth edition continues its well-established record of presenting medical word building principles based on competency-based curricula. Leveraging the pedagogical success of previous editions, it continues its structural design as a combined textbook and workbook, making it adaptable to various teaching methods, including traditional lectures, online courses, and self-paced study. The popular core features of the previous edition have been updated and enhanced. The body systems chapters provide a more inclusive range of diseases, conditions, procedures, and treatments. The disease focus and oncology sections of the chapter have been expanded to include current developments for a better understanding of the most encountered medical conditions, their presentations, and treatments. The textbook continues to incorporate authentic medical records with activities aimed at strengthening the application of medical terminology in clinical practice. Additional questions have been added to the learning activities to include the new content. This approach equips students of various learning levels with the essential skills and tools needed to retain medical terminology,

enabling them to communicate effectively in the health care setting.

Every chapter contains entirely new anatomical artwork that brings the human body to life on the page. With vibrant, full color, three-dimensional illustrations, students can examine each body system with exceptional clarity and detail. These new figures improve the learning of anatomy while creating a more engaging and impactful experience for students. There are over 200 newly created anatomical illustrations. As in earlier editions, illustrations and photos to enrich written text are integrated throughout the chapters. This ninth edition includes over 300 new illustrations specifically designed to portray course content in new and interesting ways and to help clarify difficult concepts. Unique to this edition are photographs and innovative illustrations created for Chapters 1 through 3 to help students understand the various applications of suffixes and prefixes in word building.

This edition continues to present eponyms without showing the possessive form, such as Bowman capsule, Cushing syndrome, and Parkinson disease. Medical dictionaries as well as the American Association for Medical Transcription (AAMT) and the American Medical Association support these changes. In addition, ICD-10-PCS replacement terms for discontinued eponyms are summarized in Appendix H.

We remain committed to incorporating valuable suggestions from instructors and students and greatly appreciate their contributions to improving this book. Undoubtedly, the recommendations have helped to make *Medical Terminology Systems: A Body Systems Approach* a leading textbook in educational institutions and one that continues to be well received by instructors and students. Here is a brief summary of chapter content:

- Chapter 1 explains the techniques of medical word building using basic word elements.
- Chapter 2 categorizes major surgical, diagnostic, symptomatic, and grammatical suffixes.
- Chapter 3 presents major prefixes of position, number and measurement, direction, and other parameters.
- Chapter 4 introduces anatomical, physiological, and pathological terms. It also presents combining forms denoting cellular and body structures, body position and direction, and regions of the body, in addition to combining forms related to diagnostic methods and pathology.

General diagnostic and therapeutic terms are described and provide a solid foundation for specific terms addressed in the body systems chapters that follow.

- Chapters 5 through 16 are organized according to specific body systems and may be taught in any sequence. These chapters include key anatomical and physiological terms, basic anatomy and physiology, a body systems connections table, and a comprehensive table of word elements, including combining forms, suffixes, and prefixes. The remaining chapter material consists of a disease focus section, followed by tables that include updated diseases and conditions; diagnostic, surgical, and therapeutic procedures; pharmacology; and abbreviations. Each body systems chapter concludes with several learning activities that assess comprehension of material and medical record activities that illustrate various clinical applications and reinforce medical record documentation.
- Chapter 15 has been significantly expanded to include mental disorders and their most recently developed therapeutic treatments. A new table in the anatomy and physiology section contains common neurotransmitters of the nervous system with a description of their function and clinical significance.
- Appendix A: Answer Key contains answers to each learning activity to validate proficiency and provide immediate feedback for student assessment. Although the answer key for the terminology section of each Documenting Health-Care Activities is not included in this appendix, it is available to adopters in the Instructor's Guide.
- Appendix B: Common Abbreviations and Symbols includes an updated, comprehensive list of medical abbreviations and their meanings and an updated summary of common symbols.
- Appendix C: Glossary of Medical Word Elements contains alphabetical lists of medical word elements and their meanings. This appendix presents two methods for word-element indexing—first by medical word element, then by English term.
- Appendix D: Index of Genetic Disorders lists genetic disorders presented in the textbook.
- Appendix E: Index of Clinical, Laboratory, and Imaging Procedures lists radiographic and other diagnostic imaging procedures presented in the textbook.
- Appendix F: Index of Pharmacology lists drug classifications presented in the textbook.

- Appendix G: Index of Oncological Terms lists oncological diseases presented in the textbook.
- Appendix H: Index of Discontinued Abbreviations and Eponyms summarizes abbreviations discontinued in medical charts. It also contains discontinued eponyms along with their replacement terms for coding purposes.

Medical Language Lab (MLL)

Included in every new copy of *Medical Terminology Systems: A Body Systems Approach*, Ninth Edition, is access to the ultimate online medical terminology resource for students. The Medical Language Lab (MLL) is a rich learning environment utilizing proven language development methods to help students become effective users of medical language. To access the MLL, students visit *www.fadavis.com* and redeem the access code provided in their new copies of *Medical Terminology Systems: A Body Systems Approach*, Ninth Edition.

Each lesson in the MLL teaches students how to listen critically for important terms, respond to terms using medical terminology, and generate their own terminology-rich writing and speaking skills. By following the activities in each lesson, students graduate from simple memorization to becoming stronger users of medical language, including the correct pronunciations.

In addition, the MLL provides students with a wide variety of practice activities that help them to solidify their recall of key terms from the chapter. It also contains an audio glossary in which students can hear words pronounced and used properly in context.

Designed to work in conjunction with *Medical Terminology Systems: A Body Systems Approach*, Ninth Edition, each activity in the MLL has been crafted with content specific to the textbook. Every chapter in *Medical Terminology Systems: A Body Systems Approach*, Ninth Edition, contains a corresponding lesson in the MLL that is relevant and useful in helping students develop medical terminology skills.

Instructors benefit from an instructor's page that is powerful yet easy to understand and allows them to decide which chapters and activities will be available to their students, as well as set grading options.

F.A. Davis Online Resources

Although the study of medical terminology demands hard work and discipline, various self-paced activities offer interest and variety to the learning process. Many activities and resources are available to adopters of the textbook at *www.fadavis.com* to help teachers teach and students learn medical terminology in an exciting, challenging, effective fashion.

Instructor Online Resources

The F.A. Davis Instructor Online Resource Center provides many updated, innovative instructional activities. These activities make teaching medical terminology easier and more effective. Teachers can use the supplemental activities in various educational settings—traditional classroom, distance learning, or independent or self-paced studies. The many ancillaries help instructors maximize the benefits of the textbook and include the following:

• Electronic test bank
• PowerPoint presentations for each chapter
• Searchable image bank
• Printable Instructor's Guide

Electronic Test Bank

This edition offers a powerful updated test-generating program that allows instructors to create custom-made or randomly generated tests in a printable or online format from a test bank of more than 2,600 test items, with the addition of nearly 100 new questions.

PowerPoint Lecture Notes

The lecture notes provide a unique and reinforcing dimension to the learning process.

Over 1,400 slides are carefully designed to supplement and augment the material covered in the textbook. The PowerPoint presentations suggest various teaching techniques to make learning and teaching profoundly effective. Notes at the bottom of various slides offer faculty suggestions to tailor or expand the presentations to suit their individual academic needs.

Each chapter has an outline-based presentation, consisting of a chapter overview, main functions of the body system, and selected pathology, vocabulary, and procedures. Included are interactive, clinically related exercises that highlight real-life situations. Full-color illustrations reinforce many of the clinically related exercises.

Image Bank

The image bank contains all illustrations from the textbook. It is fully searchable and allows users to zoom in and out and display a JPG image of an illustration that can be copied into a Microsoft Word document or PowerPoint presentation.

Instructor's Guide

The printable Instructor's Guide is a resource full of instructional activities that have been updated to meet today's instructional needs. It is available in PDF format among the instructor resources on *www.fadavis.com* and includes the following elements:

• Suggested Course Outlines. Course outlines of various lengths, providing effective methods of covering material presented in the textbook.
• Chapter Teaching Guides. These sections provide guidance on how to integrate the many resources available for each chapter, including Instructor's Guide and textbook activities, into a lesson plan.
• Student- and Instructor-Directed Activities. These comprehensive teaching aids are updated and extended for this edition. They offer an assortment of activities for each body systems chapter that are easily incorporated as course requirements, supplemental activities, or collaborative projects. Included are peer evaluation forms and numerous community and internet resources, including technical journals, community organizations, and websites that complement course content.
• Supplemental Documenting Health-Care Activities. The supplemental medical record activities have been updated to parallel the new Documenting Health-Care Activities sections presented in each of the body systems chapters. As in the textbook, these activities use actual medical records to show how medical terminology is used to document patient care. Terminology and analysis exercises reinforce the medical vocabulary in the report to help students develop critical thinking skills. Instructors can use the answer key for grading purposes or give it to the students for self-evaluation. In addition, they can use these medical records for various activities, including oral reports, medical coding, medical transcribing, or individual assignments.
• Pronunciations and Answer Keys. Answer keys are provided in the Instructor's Guide for the activities in the Medical Word Elements tables and Documenting Health-Care Activities Terminology tables in the textbook. These keys should prove helpful for grading or for class presentations.

Student Online Resources

In addition to the Medical Language Lab (MLL) access provided with new copies of *Medical Terminology Systems: A Body Systems Approach,* Ninth Edition, students will find a link to resources for the previous edition, including animations of medical processes and pathologies, audio pronunciation guides, and interactive medical record activities.

Taber's Cyclopedic Medical Dictionary

The world-famous *Taber's Cyclopedic Medical Dictionary* is the recommended companion reference for this book. Virtually all terms in Systems may be found in *Taber's.* In addition, *Taber's* contains etymologies for nearly all main entries presented in this textbook.

Discontinued Eponyms with ICD-10-PCS Replacement Terms

ICD-10-CM contains the use of eponyms when assigning certain codes for diagnoses and procedures. However, all surgical eponyms have been removed from ICD-10-PCS. In their place are root terms that describe the objective of the procedure and other parameters to assign the proper code(s). The ICD-10-PCS procedural codes are more specific, more clinically accurate, and use a more logical structure than the previous coding systems. There are still some diagnostic eponyms in ICD-10-PCS, but most have been replaced by a constructed term that identifies the disease or condition. A summary of eponyms found in this textbook along with the ICD-10-PCS 2015 term(s) that replace the eponym are provided in Appendix H.

I hope you enjoy using this new edition I'm confident it will be the best edition yet!

Regina M. Masters

Contributors

Julia M. Halm, DO
Attending Psychiatrist
Perrysburg, Ohio

I want to acknowledge Julia M. Halm, DO, who has done an impeccable job of reviewing and editing the chapters of this latest edition. As a respected and knowledgeable physician in the field of psychiatry, she has given meticulous attention to detail in recommending edits, making this ninth edition accurate and up to date. She has exceptional professional qualifications, and it has been a personal pleasure to collaborate with my daughter and to mentor her as a future third-generation author, a tradition that began with Barabara A. Gylys, her grandmother and my mother.

Reviewers

The authors extend a special thanks to the clinical reviewers who read and edited the manuscript and provided detailed evaluations and ideas for improving the textbook.

Contents at a Glance

Contents

Basic Elements of a Medical Word

Objectives

Upon completion of this chapter, you will be able to:

- Identify the four word elements used to build medical words.
- Divide medical words into their component parts.
- Apply the basic rules to define and build medical words.
- Locate the pronunciation guidelines chart and interpret pronunciation marks.
- Pronounce medical terms presented in this chapter.
- Demonstrate your knowledge of this chapter by completing the learning activities.

Medical Word Elements

The language of medicine is a specialized vocabulary used by health-care providers. Many current medical word elements originated as early as the 4th century B.C., when Hippocrates practiced medicine. With technological and scientific advancements in medicine, new terms have evolved to reflect these innovations. For example, radiographic terms, such as magnetic resonance imaging (MRI) and ultrasound (US), are now commonly used to describe current diagnostic procedures.

A medical word consists of some or all of the following elements:

- word root
- combining form
- suffix
- prefix

How these elements are combined and whether all or some of them are present in a medical term determines the meaning of a word. To understand the meaning of medical words, it is important to learn how to divide them into their basic elements. The purpose of this chapter is to cover the basic principles of medical word building and learn how to pronounce the terms correctly. Thus, pronunciations of medical terms are provided throughout the textbook. In addition, pronunciation guidelines are located on the inside back cover of this book. They can be used as a convenient reference to help pronounce terms correctly.

Word Roots

A **word root** is the foundation of a medical term and contains its primary meaning. All medical terms have at least one word root. Most word roots are derived from the Greek or Latin language; therefore, two different roots may have the same meaning. For example, the Greek word *dermatos* and the Latin word *cutane* both refer to the skin. As a general rule, Greek roots describe a disease, condition, treatment, or diagnosis. Latin roots describe anatomical structures. Consequently, the Greek root *dermat* describes a disease, condition, treatment, or diagnosis of the skin; the Latin root *cutane* describes an anatomical structure (see Table 1-1).

TABLE 1-1 **Examples of Word Roots**			
This table lists examples of English terms with their Greek and Latin origins as well as word analyses of corresponding medical terms. Phonetic pronunciations are provided to help you practice pronouncing the medical terms.			
English Term	**Greek or Latin Term***	**Word Root**	**Word Analysis**
skin	dermatos (Gr)	dermat	**dermat**/itis (dĕr-mă-TĪ-tĭs): inflammation of the skin
			Dermatitis is a general term used to describe an inflammatory condition of the skin.
	cutis (L)	cutane	**cutane**/ous (kū-TĀ-nē-ŭs): pertaining to the skin
			Cutaneous is a term that identifies an anatomical structure.
kidney	nephros (Gr)	nephr	**nephr**/oma (nĕ-FRŌ-mă): tumor of the kidney
			Nephroma is a tumor (benign or malignant) of kidney tissue.
	renes (L)	ren	**ren**/al (RĒ-năl): pertains to the kidney
			Renal is a term that identifies an anatomical structure.

TABLE 1-1 Examples of Word Roots—cont'd

English Term	Greek or Latin Term*	Word Root	Word Analysis
mouth	stomatos (Gr)	stomat	**stomat**/itis (stō -mă-TĪ-tĭs): inflammation of the mouth *The word root stomat is commonly confused with the English term stomach. However, stomat is derived from the Greek word for mouth. The word root for the stomach is gastr, derived from the Greek word gastros.*
	oris (L)	or	**or**/al (OR-ăl): pertaining to the mouth *Oral is a term that identifies an anatomical structure.*

*It is not important to know the origin of a medical word. This information is provided here to clarify and illustrate that there may be two different word roots for a single term.

Combining Forms

A **combining form** is created when a word root is combined with a vowel. The vowel, known as a **combining vowel,** is usually an *o* but is sometimes an *i*. The combining vowel has no meaning of its own but enables the connection of two or more word elements. Like a word root, a combining form is the basic foundation to which other word elements are added to build a complete medical word. In this text, a combining form will be listed as *word root/vowel* (such as *gastr/o*), as illustrated in Table 1-2.

TABLE 1-2 Examples of Combining Forms

*This table illustrates how word roots and vowels create combining forms. Learning combining forms rather than word roots makes pronunciations easier because of the terminal vowel. For example, in this table, the word roots **gastr** and **nephr** are difficult to pronounce, whereas their combining forms **gastr/o** and **nephr/o** are easier to pronounce.*

Word Root	+	Vowel	=	Combining Form	Meaning
erythr/	+	o	=	erythr/o	red
gastr/	+	o	=	gastr/o	stomach
hepat/	+	o	=	hepat/o	liver
immun/	+	o	=	immun/o	immune, immunity, safe
nephr/	+	o	=	nephr/o	kidney
oste/	+	o	=	oste/o	bone

Suffixes

A **suffix** is a word element placed at the end of a word that alters its meaning. All medical terms have a suffix. In the terms *pancreat/itis* (inflammation of the pancreas) and *pancreat/o/pathy* (disease of the pancreas), the suffixes are **-itis** (inflammation) and **-pathy** (disease). In medical terminology, a suffix usually describes a pathology (disease or abnormality), symptom, surgical or diagnostic procedure, or part of speech.

To link a suffix that begins with a vowel, use a word root. To link a suffix that begins with a consonant, use a combining form. Review Table 1-3, which illustrates this principle.

TABLE I-3 Examples of Suffixes

This table lists examples of pathological suffixes linked with a word root (WR) and a combining form (CF). Phonetic pronunciations are provided to help you practice pronouncing the medical terms.

Suffix	=	Medical Word	Meaning	Rationale
-itis (inflammation)	=	gastr/itis găs-TRĪ-tĭs	inflammation of the stomach*	The suffix -itis begins with a vowel and requires a WR.
-megaly (enlargement)	=	gastr/o/megaly găs-trō-MĔG-ă-lē	enlargement of the stomach	The suffix -megaly begins with a consonant and requires a CF.
-oma (tumor)	=	hepat/oma hĕp-ă-TŌ-mă	tumor of the liver	The suffix -oma begins with a vowel and requires a WR.
-cyte (cell)	=	hepat/o/cytes HĔP-ă-tō-sīts	cells in the liver	The suffix -cytes begins with a consonant and requires a CF.

*To define a medical term, first define the suffix and then the first part of the word.

Prefixes

A **prefix** is a word element attached to the beginning of a word or word root. However, not all medical terms have a prefix. Adding or changing a prefix changes the meaning of the word. Prefixes usually indicate a number, time, position, direction, or negation. Many of the same prefixes used in medical terminology are also used in the English language. Review Table 1-4 to reinforce the principles of linking a prefix to other word elements.

TABLE I-4 Examples of Prefixes

This table lists examples of prefixes linked to a word root and a suffix. Note that the suffixes begin with a vowel and are linked to a word root. Phonetic pronunciations of the constructed medical words are provided to help you practice pronouncing the medical terms.

Prefix	+	Word Root	+	Suffix	=	Medical Word	Meaning
an- (without, not)	+	esthes (feeling)	+	-ia (condition)	=	an/esthes/ia ăn-ĕs-THĒ-zē-ă	condition of not feeling
hyper- (excessive, above normal)	+	therm (heat)	+	-ia (condition)	=	hyper/therm/ia hī-pĕr-THĔR-mē-ă	condition of excessive heat
intra- (in, within)	+	muscul (muscle)	+	-ar (pertaining to)	=	intra/muscul/ar ĭn-tră-MŬS-kū-lăr	pertaining to within the muscle
para- (near, beside; beyond)	+	nas (nose)	+	-al (pertaining to)	=	para/nas/al păr-ă-NĀ-săl	pertaining to (area) near the nose
poly (many, much)	+	ur (urine)	+	-ia (condition)	=	poly/ur/ia pŏl-ē-Ū-rē-ă	condition of much urine
pre- (before)	+	nat (birth)	+	-al (pertaining to)	=	pre/nat/al prē-NĀ-tăl	pertaining to before birth

Basic Guidelines

Defining and building medical words are crucial skills in understanding the meaning of a medical word. Following the basic guidelines will help you develop these skills.

Defining Medical Words

Here are three steps for defining medical words using *gastr/o/enter/itis* as an example.

- **Step 1.** Define the **suffix,** or last part of the word. In this case, the suffix *–itis* means *inflammation.*
- **Step 2.** Define the **first part of the word** (which may be a word root, combining form, or prefix). In this case, the combining form *gastr/o* means *stomach.*
- **Step 3.** Define the **middle parts of the word.** In this case, the word root *enter* means *intestine.*

When you analyze *gastr/o/enter/itis* following the three steps, the meaning is:

1. inflammation (of)
2. stomach (and)
3. intestine

The meaning of **gastr/o/enter/itis** is *inflammation (of) stomach (and) intestine.* Table 1-5 further illustrates this process.

TABLE 1-5 Defining Gastroenteritis

This table illustrates the three steps of defining a medical word using the example gastroenteritis.

Combining Form	Middle	Suffix
gastr/o	enter/	-itis
stomach	intestine	inflammation
(step 2)	(step 3)	(step 1)

Building Medical Words

There are three basic rules for building medical words.

Rule 1

A word root links a suffix that begins with a vowel.

Word Root	+	Suffix	=	Medical Word	Meaning
hepat	+	-itis	=	hepatitis	inflammation of the liver
(liver)		(inflammation)		hĕp-ă-TĪ-tĭs	

Rule 2

A combining form (root + o) links a suffix that begins with a consonant.

Combining Form	+	Suffix	=	Medical Word	Meaning
hepat/o (liver)	+	-cyte (cell)	=	hepatocyte HĔP-ă-tō-sīt	liver cell

Rule 3

A combining form links one root to another root to form a compound word. This rule holds true even if the second root begins with a vowel, as in **oste/o/arthr/itis.** Keep in mind that the rules for linking multiple roots to each other are slightly different from the rules for linking roots and combining forms to suffixes.

Combining Form	+	Word Root	+	Suffix	=	Medical Word	Meaning
oste/o (bone)	+	chondr (cartilage)	+	-itis (inflammation)	=	osteochondritis ŏs-tē-ō-kŏn-DRĪ-tĭs	inflammation of bone and cartilage
	+	arthr (joint)	+	-itis (inflammation)	=	osteoarthritis ŏs-tē-ō-ăr-THRĪ-tĭs	inflammation of bone and joint

 It is time to review medical word elements by completing Learning Activities 1-1 and 1-2 on pages 8-9.

Pronunciation Guidelines

Although pronunciation of medical words usually follows the same rules that govern pronunciations of English words, some medical words may be difficult to pronounce when first encountered. Therefore, selected terms in this book include the phonetic pronunciation. Also, pronunciation guidelines can be found on the inside back cover of this book and at the end of selected tables. Use them whenever you need help with pronunciation of medical words.

 It is time to review pronunciations, analysis of word elements, and defining medical terms by completing Learning Activities 1-3, 1-4, and 1-5 on pages 10-12.

Medical Word Building Summary

The illustration that follows demonstrates medical word building. Building a medical word that means *enlargement of the stomach* requires knowledge of the word element for *stomach* (**gastr** or **gastr/o**) and the suffix for *enlargement* (**-megaly**). The medical word for *enlargement of the stomach* is **gastromegaly**. To develop medical word building skills, study the combinations of word building elements in the digestive system illustration that follows.

Food bolus

Liver
(hepat + itis)

Gallbladder
(cholecyst + itis)

Pancreas
(pancreat + itis)

Appendix
(append + ectomy)

Stomach
(gastr/o + megaly)

Spleen
(splen/o + megaly)

Colon
(colon/o + scopy)

 It is time to practice building medical words by completing Learning Activity 1–6 on page 13.

LEARNING ACTIVITIES

The learning activities that follow provide a review of the basic medical word elements introduced in this chapter. Complete each activity and review your answers to evaluate your understanding of this chapter.

Learning Activity 1-1
Understanding Medical Word Elements

Fill in the blanks to complete the sentences correctly.

1. The four elements used to form words are _____.

2. A root is the main part or foundation of a word. In the words *arthritis, arthrectomy,* and *arthroscope,* the root is _____.

Identify the statements as true or false. If false, rewrite the statement correctly on the line provided.

3. A combining vowel is usually an e.   True   False
   _____

4. A word root links a suffix that begins with a vowel.   True   False
   _____

5. A combining form links multiple roots to each other.   True   False
   _____

6. A combining form links a suffix that begins with a consonant.   True   False
   _____

7. To define a medical word, first define the prefix.   True   False
   _____

8. In the term *intramuscular, intra* is the prefix.   True   False
   _____

Underline the word root in each of the combining forms.

9. splen/o (spleen)

10. hyster/o (uterus)

11. enter/o (intestine)

12. neur/o (nerve)

13. ot/o (ear)

14. dermat/o (skin)

15. immun/o (immune, immunity, safe)

✓ *Check your answers in Appendix A. Review material that you did not answer correctly.*

Correct Answers _____ X 6.67 = _____ % Score

Identifying Word Roots and Combining Forms

Underline the word roots in the medical words that follow.

Medical Word	Meaning
1. nephritis	inflammation of the kidney
2. arthrodesis	fixation of a joint
3. cutaneous	pertaining to the skin
4. dentist	specialist in teeth
5. gastrectomy	excision of the stomach
6. chondritis	inflammation of cartilage
7. hepatoma	tumor of the liver
8. muscular	pertaining to muscle
9. gastric	pertaining to the stomach
10. osteoma	tumor of the bone

Underline the combining forms.

11. erythr	red
12. hepat/o	liver
13. arthr	joint
14. oste/o/arthr	bone, joint
15. cholangi/o	bile vessel

✓ *Check your answers in Appendix A. Review material that you did not answer correctly.*

Correct Answers _____ **X 6.67 =** _____ **% Score**

Learning Activity 1-3

Understanding Pronunciations

Review the pronunciation guidelines (located on the inside back cover of this book) and then underline the correct answer in each of the statements.

1. The diacritical mark - is called a (breve, macron).

2. The diacritical mark ˘ is called a (breve, macron).

3. The - indicates the (short, long) sound of vowels.

4. The ˘ indicates the (short, long) sound of vowels.

5. The combination *ch* is sometimes pronounced like (k, chiy). Examples are *cholesterol, cholemia.*

6. When *pn* is at the beginning of a word, it is pronounced only with the sound of (p, n). Examples are *pneumonia, pneumotoxin.*

7. When *pn* is in the middle of a word, the *p* (is, is not) pronounced. Examples are ortho*pnea*, hyper*pnea.*

8. When *i* is at the end of a word, it is pronounced like (eye, ee). Examples are bronch*i*, fung*i*, nucle*i.*

9. For *ae* and *oe*, only the (first, second) vowel is pronounced. Examples are burs*ae*, pleur*ae*, roentgen.

10. When *e* and *es* form the final letter or letters of a word, they are commonly pronounced as (combined, separate) syllables. Examples are syncope, systole, nares.

✓ *Check your answers in Appendix A. Review material that you did not answer correctly.*

Correct Answers _____ X 10 = _____ % Score

Learning Activity 1-4
Identifying Suffixes and Prefixes

Pronounce the medical terms that follow. Then analyze each term and write the suffix in the right-hand column. The first suffix is completed for you.

Term   Suffix

1. thoracotomy   *-tomy*
   thōr-ă-KŎT-ō-mē

2. gastroscope   _____
   GĂS-trō-skōp

3. tonsillitis   _____
   tŏn-sĭl-Ī-tĭs

4. gastric   _____
   GĂS-trĭk

5. hepatocyte   _____
   HĔP-ă-tō-sīt

Pronunciation Help	Long Sound	ā — rate	ē — rebirth	ī — isle	ō — over	ū — unite
	Short Sound	ă — alone	ĕ — ever	ĭ — it	ŏ — not	ŭ — cut

Pronounce the medical terms that follow. Then analyze each term and write the element that is a prefix in the right-hand column. The first prefix is completed for you.

Term   Prefix

6. anesthesia   *an-*
   ăn-ĕs-THĒ-zē-ă

7. prenatal   _____
   prē-NĀ-tăl

8. intramuscular   _____
   ĭn-tră-MŬS-kū-lăr

9. paranasal   _____
   păr-ă-NĀ-săl

10. polyuria   _____
    pŏl-ē-Ū-rē-ă

✓ *Check your answers in Appendix A. Review material that you did not answer correctly.*

Correct Answers _____ X 10 = _____ % Score

Learning Activity I-5

Defining Medical Words

The three steps for defining medical words are:

1. Define the last part of the word, or suffix.
2. Define the first part of the word, or prefix, word root, or combining form.
3. Define the middle of the word.

First, pronounce the term aloud. Then apply the three steps to define the terms in the table that follows. If you are not certain of a definition, refer to Appendix C, Part 1, of this textbook, which provides an alphabetical list of word elements and their meanings.

Term	Definition
1. gastritis găs-TRĪ-tĭs	_____
2. nephritis nĕf-RĪ-tĭs	_____
3. gastrectomy găs-TRĔK-tō-mē	_____
4. osteoma ŏs-tē-Ō-mă	_____
5. hepatoma hĕp-ă-TŌ-mă	_____
6. hepatitis hĕp-ă-TĪ-tĭs	_____

Refer to the section "Building Medical Words" on pages 5–6 to complete this activity. Write the number for the rule that applies to each listed term and give a short summary of the rule. Use the abbreviation WR to designate *word root*, and use CF to designate *combining form*. The first one is completed for you.

Term	Rule	Summary of the Rule
7. arthr/itis ăr-THRĪ-tĭs	*I*	*A WR links a suffix that begins with a vowel.*
8. scler/osis sklĕ-RŌ-sĭs	_____	_____
9. arthr/o/centesis ăr-thrō-sĕn-TĒ-sĭs	_____	_____
10. colon/o/scope kō-LŎN-ō-skōp	_____	_____
11. chondr/itis kŏn-DRĪ-tĭs	_____	_____
12. chondr/oma kŏn-DRŌ-mă	_____	_____

13. oste/o/chondr/itis   _____   _____
    os-tē-ō-kŏn-DRĪ-tĭs

14. muscul/ar   _____   _____
    MŬS-kū-lăr

15. oste/o/arthr/itis   _____   _____
    ŏs-tē-ō-ăr-THRĪ-tĭs

✓ *Check your answers in Appendix A. Review material that you did not answer correctly.*

Correct Answers _____ X 6.67 = _____ % Score

Learning Activity 1-6
Building Medical Words

Refer to the figure on page 7 to complete this activity.
Use *–ectomy* (excision) to build medical words that mean *excision of the:*

1. spleen: _____
2. appendix: _____
3. pancreas: _____
4. gallbladder: _____
5. kidney: _____
6. stomach: _____

Use *–itis* (inflammation) to build medical words that mean *inflammation of the:*

7. spleen: _____
8. liver: _____
9. pancreas: _____
10. gallbladder: _____
11. colon: _____
12. ear: _____

Use *–megaly* (enlargement) to build medical words that mean *enlargement of the:*

13. liver: _____
14. spleen: _____
15. stomach: _____

✓ *Check your answers in Appendix A. Review material that you did not answer correctly.*

Correct Answers _____ X 6.67 = _____ % Score

Suffixes

Chapter Outline

Objectives

Upon completion of this chapter, you will be able to:

- Identify examples of surgical, diagnostic, pathological, and related suffixes.
- Link combining forms and word roots to suffixes.
- Define and provide surgical, diagnostic, pathological, and related suffixes.
- Define and provide adjective, noun, and diminutive suffixes.
- Locate and apply guidelines for pluralizing terms.
- Pronounce medical terms presented in this chapter.
- Demonstrate your knowledge of the chapter by completing the learning activities.

Suffix Linking

In medical words, a suffix is added to the end of a word root or combining form to change its meaning. Recall Rule 1 and Rule 2 on page 5–6 for linking suffixes. When a suffix begins with a vowel, use the root word for linking the two word elements. When the suffix begins with a consonant, use the combining form for linking the two word elements. For example, the word root **hemat** means *blood*. The suffix **-emesis** means *vomiting,* and **-logy** means *study of.* Hemat/**emesis** means *vomiting blood;* hemat/o/**logy** is the *study of blood.* Review Table 2-1, which illustrates examples of word roots linked with suffixes that begin with a vowel and combining forms linked with suffixes that begin with a consonant.

TABLE 2-1 Word Roots and Combining Forms With Suffixes

This table provides examples of word roots linking a suffix that begins with a vowel. It also provides examples of combining forms (root + o) linking a suffix that begins with a consonant.

Element	+	Suffix	=	Medical Word	Meaning
Word Roots					
hemat (blood)	+	-emesis (vomiting)	=	hemat/emesis hĕm-ăt-ĔM-ĕ-sĭs	vomiting blood
arthr (joint)	+	-itis (inflammation)	=	arthr/itis ăr-THRĪ-tĭs	inflammation of a joint
oste (bone)	+	-oma (tumor)	=	oste/oma ŏs-tē-Ō-mă	tumor of bone
Combining Forms					
hemat/o (blood)	+	-logy (study of)	=	hemat/o/logy hē-mă-TŎL-ō-jē	study of blood
arthr/o (joint)	+	-centesis (surgical puncture)	=	arthr/o/centesis ăr-thrō-sĕn-TĒ-sĭs	surgical puncture of a joint
oste/o (bone)	+	-dynia (pain)	=	oste/o/dynia ŏs-tē-ō-DĬN-ē-ă	pain in bone

Words that contain more than one word root are known as **compound words.** Multiple roots within a compound word are joined together with a vowel, regardless of whether the second root begins with a vowel or a consonant. Notice that a vowel is used in Table 2-2 between *oste* and *arthr,* even though the second root, *arthr,* begins with a vowel.

TABLE 2-2 Compound Words With Suffixes

This table provides examples of medical terms with more than one word root, also known as compound words. The table lists suffixes linked with roots when the suffix begins with a vowel, and it lists combining forms when the suffix begins with a consonant.

Combining Form	+	Word Root	+	Suffix	=	Medical Word	Meaning
oste/o (bone)	+	arthr (joint)	+	-itis (inflammation)	=	oste/o/arthr/itis ŏs-tē-ō-ăr-THRĪ-tĭs	inflammation of the bone and joint
encephal/o (brain)	+	mening (meninges)	+	-itis (inflammation)	=	encephal/o/mening/itis ĕn-sĕf-ă-lō-mĕn-ĭn-JĪ-tĭs	inflammation of the brain and meninges
oste/o (bone)	+	arthr/o (joint)	+	-pathy (disease)	=	oste/o/arthr/o/pathy ŏs-tē-ō-ăr-THRŎP-ă-thē	disease of the bone and joint
encephal/o (brain)	+	mening/o (meninges)	+	-pathy (disease)	=	encephal/o/mening/o/pathy ĕn-sĕf-ă-lō-m ĕn-ĭn-GŎP-ă-thē	disease of the brain and meninges

Keep in mind that the rule for linking multiple roots is slightly different from the rules for linking roots to suffixes. To reinforce your understanding of building compound words, refer to Rule 3 on page 6 of this textbook. Use the steps when in doubt about building a medical word.

Suffix Types

An effective method in mastering medical terminology is to learn the major types of suffixes in categories. Grouping the surgical, diagnostic, pathological, related, and grammatical suffixes makes them easier to remember.

Surgical, Diagnostic, Pathological, and Related Suffixes

Surgical suffixes describe a type of invasive procedure performed on a body part (see Table 2-3). Diagnostic suffixes describe a procedure performed to identify the cause and nature of an illness. Pathological suffixes describe an abnormal condition or disease (see Table 2-4).

TABLE 2-3 Surgical Suffixes

This table lists commonly used surgical suffixes along with their meanings and word analyses.

Suffix	Meaning	Word Analysis
-centesis	surgical puncture	arthr/o/**centesis** (ăr-thrō-sĕn-TĒ-sĭs): surgical puncture of a joint *arthr/o*: joint *Arthrocentesis is a surgical puncture to remove fluid in a joint by using a needle inserted into the joint space. It may also help to obtain samples of synovial fluid for diagnostic purposes and to instill medications (see Fig. 2-1).*

Patella

Figure 2-1 Arthrocentesis of the knee.

(continued)

TABLE 2-3 Surgical Suffixes—cont'd

Suffix	Meaning	Word Analysis
-clasis	to break; surgical fracture	oste/o/**clasis** (ŏs-tē-ŎK-lă-sĭs): surgical fracture of a bone *oste/o:* bone *Osteoclasis is performed to correct a deformity of a bone.*
-desis	binding, fixation (of a bone or joint)	arthr/o/**desis** (ăr-thrō-DĒ-sĭs): binding or fixation of a joint *arthr/o:* joint *Arthrodesis fuses bones across the joint space in a degenerated, unstable joint.*
-ectomy	excision, removal	append/**ectomy** (ăp-ĕn-DĔK-tō-mē): excision of the appendix *append:* appendix
-lysis	separation; destruction; loosening	thromb/o/**lysis** (thrŏm-BŎL-ĭ-sĭs): destruction or separation of a blood clot *thromb/o:* blood clot *Drug therapy is usually used to dissolve a blood clot.*
-pexy	fixation (of an organ)	mast/o/**pexy** (MĂS-tō-pĕks-ē): fixation of the breast(s) *mast/o:* breast *Mastopexy, an elective surgery, affixes sagging breasts in a more elevated position, commonly improving their shape.*
-plasty	surgical repair	rhin/o/**plasty** (RĪ-nō-plăs-tē): surgical repair of the nose *rhin/o:* nose *Rhinoplasty is a type of surgery that changes the size or shape of the nose.*
-rrhaphy	suture	my/o/**rrhaphy** (mī-OR-ă-fē): suture of a muscle *my/o:* muscle
-stomy	forming an opening (mouth)	trache/o/**stomy** (trā-kē-ŎS-tō-mē): forming an opening (mouth) into the trachea *trache/o:* trachea (windpipe) *A tracheostomy is an artificial opening created to bypass an obstructed upper airway.*
-tome	instrument to cut	oste/o/**tome** (ŎS-tē-ō-tōm): instrument to cut bone *oste/o:* bone *An osteotome is a surgical chisel used to cut through bone.*
-tomy	incision	trache/o/**tomy** (trā-kē-ŎT-ō-mē): incision of the trachea *trache/o:* trachea (windpipe) *Tracheotomy opens a direct airway through the neck and into the trachea (the windpipe).*

TABLE 2-3 **Surgical Suffixes—cont'd**

Suffix	Meaning	Word Analysis
-tripsy	crushing	lith/o/**tripsy** (LĬTH-ō-trĭp-sē): crushing a stone
		lith/o: stone, calculus
		Lithotripsy is a surgical procedure to remove a stone or calculus in the kidney, ureter, bladder, or gallbladder (see Fig. 2-2).

Figure 2-2 Kidney stone pieces from shock wave lithotripsy that crushed a large kidney stone into small pieces, which then left the body through the urinary tract upon urination.

TABLE 2-4 Diagnostic, Pathological, and Related Suffixes

This table lists commonly used diagnostic, pathological, and related suffixes, along with their meanings and word analyses.

Suffix	Meaning	Word Analysis
Diagnostic		
-gram	record, writing	electr/o/cardi/o/**gram** (ē-lĕk-trō-KĂR-dē-ō-grăm): record of electrical activity of the heart *electr/o:* electricity *cardi/o:* heart
-graph	instrument for recording	electr/o/cardi/o/**graph** (ē-lĕk-trō-KĂR-dē-ō-grăf): instrument for recording electrical activity of the heart *electr/o:* electricity *cardi/o:* heart
-graphy	process of recording	electr/o/cardi/o/**graphy** (ē-lĕk-trō-kăr-dē-ŎG-ră-fē): process of recording electrical activity of the heart (see Fig. 2-3) *electr/o:* electricity *cardi/o:* heart

Figure 2-3 Electrocardio**graphy** (ECG) is the ***process of recording*** electrical activity of the heart. Electrodes are attached to the chest, upper arm, and leg. The electrocardio**graph** is the ***instrument for recording*** the heart rhythm to produce a paper strip ***record*** of the electrical activity of the heart called an electrocardio**gram**.

-scope	instrument for examining	endo/**scope** (ĔN-dō-skōp): instrument for examining within *endo-:* in, within *An endoscope is a flexible or rigid instrument consisting of a tube and optical system for observing the inside of a hollow organ or cavity.*
-scopy	visual examination	endo/**scopy** (ĕn-DŎS-kō-pē): visual examination within *endo-:* in, within *Endoscopy is performed to visualize a body cavity or canal using a specialized lighted instrument called an endoscope.*

TABLE 2-4 Diagnostic, Pathological, and Related Suffixes—cont'd

Suffix	Meaning	Word Analysis
Pathological and Related		
-algia	pain	neur/**algia** (nū-RĂL-jē-ă): pain of a nerve *neur:* nerve *Neuralgic pain usually occurs along the path of a nerve.*
-dynia		ot/o/**dynia** (ō-tō-DĬN-ē-ă): pain in the ear *ot/o:* ear *Otodynia, also called otalgia, is commonly known as an earache.*
-cele	hernia, swelling	hepat/o/**cele** (hĕ-PĀT-ō-sēl): hernia or swelling of the liver *hepat/o:* liver
-ectasis	dilation, expansion	bronchi/**ectasis** (brŏng-kē-ĔK-tă-sĭs): dilation or expansion of the bronchi *bronchi:* bronchus (plural, *bronchi*)
-emesis	vomiting	hyper/**emesis** (hī-pĕr-ĔM-ē-sĭs): excessive vomiting *hyper-:* excessive, above normal
-emia	blood condition	leuk/**emia** (loo-KĒ-mē-ă): white blood *leuk:* white *Leukemia is a cancer of the white blood cells (leukocytes).*
-gen	forming, producing, origin	carcin/o/**gen** (kăr-SĬN-ō-jĕn): forming, producing, or origin of cancer *carcin/o:* cancer *A carcinogen is a substance or agent, such as a cigarette, that causes the development or increases the incidence of cancer.*
-genesis		carcin/o/**genesis** (kăr-sĭ-nō-JĔN-ē-sĭs): forming, producing, or origin of cancer *carcin/o:* cancer *Carcinogenesis is the transformation of normal cells into cancer cells, commonly as a result of chemical, viral, or radioactive damage to genes.*
-itis	inflammation	gastr/**itis** (găs-TRĪ-tĭs): inflammation of the stomach *gastr:* stomach
-malacia	softening	chondr/o/**malacia** (kŏn-drō-măl-Ā-shē-ă): softening of cartilage *chondr/o:* cartilage
-megaly	enlargement	cardi/o/**megaly** (kăr-dē-ō-MĔG-ă-lē): enlargement of the heart *cardi/o:* heart
-oma	tumor	neur/**oma** (nū-RŌ-mă): tumor of a nerve *neur:* nerve *A neuroma is a benign tumor composed of nerve tissue.*

(continued)

TABLE 2-4 Diagnostic, Pathological, and Related Suffixes—cont'd

Suffix	Meaning	Word Analysis
-osis	abnormal condition; increase (used primarily with blood cells)	cyan/**osis** (sī-ă-NŌ-sĭs): dark blue or purple discoloration of the skin and mucous membrane *cyan:* blue *Cyanosis is a bluish discoloration of the skin that indicates a deficiency of oxygen in the blood (see Fig. 2-4).*

Figure 2-4 Cyanosis of the hands caused by lack of circulation of blood and low oxygen in the fingertips.

Suffix	Meaning	Word Analysis
-pathy	disease	my/o/**pathy** (mī-ŎP-ă-thē): disease of muscle *my/o:* muscle
-penia	decrease, deficiency	oste/o/**penia** (ŏs-tē-ō-PĒ-nē-ă): decrease in bone mass *oste/o:* bone *Osteopenia is characterized by bone loss that is not as severe as that in osteoporosis.*
-phobia	fear	hem/o/**phobia** (hē-mō-FŌ-bē-ă): fear of blood *hem/o:* blood *Hemophobia is an abnormal aversion to the sight of blood.*

TABLE 2-4 **Diagnostic, Pathological, and Related Suffixes—cont'd**

Suffix	Meaning	Word Analysis
-plegia	paralysis	quadri/**plegia** (kwŏd-rĭ-PLĒ-jē-ă): paralysis of four *quadri*: four *Quadriplegia is a paralysis of four extremities, both arms and legs (see Fig. 2-5).*

Figure 2-5 Quadriplegia as a result of cervical injuries.

(continued)

TABLE 2-4 Diagnostic, Pathological, and Related Suffixes—cont'd

Suffix	Meaning	Word Analysis
-ptosis	prolapse, downward displacement	blephar/o/**ptosis** (blĕf-ă-rō-TŌ-sĭs): prolapse or downward displacement of the eyelid *blephar/o:* eyelid *Blepharoptosis is a drooping of the upper eyelid(s) (see Fig. 2-6).*

Figure 2-6 (A) Blepharoptosis of the right eye that was surgically fixed with (B) blepharoplasty by a plastic surgeon.

Suffix	Meaning	Word Analysis
-rrhea	discharge, flow	dia/**rrhea** (dī-ă-RĒ-ă): discharge or flow through *dia-:* through, across *Diarrhea is an abnormally frequent discharge or flow of fluid fecal matter from the bowel.*
-rrhexis	rupture	arteri/o/**rrhexis** (ăr-tē-rē-ō-RĔK-sĭs): rupture of an artery *arteri/o:* artery
-sclerosis	abnormal condition of hardening	arteri/o/**sclerosis** (ăr-tē-rē-ō-sklĕ-RŌ-sĭs): abnormal condition of hardening of an artery *arteri/o:* artery
-spasm	involuntary contraction, twitching	blephar/o/**spasm** (BLĔF-ă-rō-spăsm): involuntary contraction or twitching of the eyelid *blephar/o:* eyelid
-stenosis	narrowing, stricture	arteri/o/**stenosis** (ăr-tē-rē-ō-stĕ-NŌ-sĭs): abnormal narrowing or stricture of an artery *arteri/o:* artery
-toxic	poison	hepat/o/**toxic** (HĔP-ă-tō-tŏk-sĭk): pertaining to poison in the liver *hepat/o:* liver *Alcohol and drugs are examples of agents that have destructive effects on the liver.*

🎯 *It is time to review surgical suffixes by completing Learning Activities 2-1, 2-2, and 2-3. It is time to review diagnostic, pathological, and related suffixes by completing Learning Activities 2-4 and 2-5.*

Grammatical Suffixes

Short grammatical suffixes are attached to word roots to form parts of speech, such as adjectives and nouns. Many of these same suffixes are used in the English language (see Table 2-5).

TABLE 2-5 Adjective and Noun Suffixes

This table lists adjective and noun suffixes that are attached to word roots in a medical term, along with their meanings and word analyses.

Suffix	Meaning	Word Analysis
Adjective		
-ac	pertaining to	cardi/**ac** (KĂR-dē-ăk): pertaining to the heart *cardi:* heart
-al		neur/**al** (NŪ-răl): pertaining to a nerve *neur:* nerve
-ar		muscul/**ar** (MŬS-kū-lăr): pertaining to muscle *muscul:* muscle
-ary		pulmon/**ary** (PŬL-mō-nĕr-ē): pertaining to the lungs *pulmon:* lung
-eal		esophag/**eal** (ē-sŏf-ă-JĒ-ăl): pertaining to the esophagus *esophag:* esophagus
-ic		thorac/**ic** (thō-RĂS-ĭk): pertaining to the chest *thorac:* chest
-ior		poster/**ior** (pŏs-TĒ-rē-or): pertaining to the back (of the body) *poster:* back (of body), behind, posterior
-ous		cutane/**ous** (kū-TĀ-nē-ŭs): pertaining to the skin *cutane:* skin
-tic		acous/**tic** (ă-KOOS-tĭk): pertaining to hearing *acous:* hearing

(continued)

TABLE 2-5 Adjective and Noun Suffixes—cont'd

Suffix	Meaning	Word Analysis
Noun		
-ia	condition	pneumon/**ia** (nū-MŌ-nē-ă): condition of the lung(s) *pneumon:* air; lung *Pneumonia is an infection of the lung, usually caused by bacteria, viruses, or diseases (see Fig. 2-7).*

Figure 2-7 (A) Chest x-ray of a healthy lung. (B) Pneumonia of the right lung.

-ism		thyroid/**ism** (THĪ-royd-ĭzm): condition of the thyroid gland *thyroid:* thyroid gland
-iatry	medicine; treatment	psych/**iatry** (sī-KĪ-ă-trē): treatment of the mind *psych/o:* mind *Psychiatry is the medical specialty concerned with treatment of mental illness, emotional disturbance, and abnormal behavior.*
-ist	specialist	hemat/o/log/**ist** (hē-mă-TŎL-ō-jĭst): specialist in the study of blood *hemat/o:* blood *log:* study of

TABLE 2-5 **Adjective and Noun Suffixes—cont'd**

Suffix	Meaning	Word Analysis
-y	condition; process	neur/o/path/y (nū-RŎP-ă-thē): condition of nerve diseases *neur/o:* nerve *path:* disease *Neuropathy is the study of disorders of the nerves.*
Diminutive		
-icle	small, minute	ventr/**icle** (VĔN-trĭ-kl): small cavity, as of the brain or heart *ventr:* belly, belly side
-ole		arteri/**ole** (ăr-TĒ-rē-ōl): small or minute artery *arteri:* artery *Arteries narrow to form arterioles (minute arteries), which branch into capillaries (microscopic blood vessels).*
-ule		ven/**ule** (VĔN-ūl): small or minute vein *ven:* vein *A venule is a small vein that is continuous with a capillary.*

 It is time to review grammatical suffixes by completing Learning Activity 2-6.

Plural Suffixes

Suffixes are also used to denote singular and plural forms of a word. English endings have also been adopted for commonly used medical terms. When a word changes from a singular to a plural form, the suffix of the word is the part that changes. A summary of the rules for changing a singular word into its plural form is located on the inside back cover of this textbook. Use it to complete Learning Activity 2-7 and whenever you need help forming plural words.

 It is time to review the rules for forming plural words by completing Learning Activity 2-7.

LEARNING ACTIVITIES

These activities provide review of the suffixes introduced in this chapter. Complete each activity and review your answers to evaluate your understanding of the chapter.

Learning Activity 2-1

Building Surgical Words

Use the meanings in the right column to complete the surgical words in the left column. The first one is completed for you. Note: The word roots are underlined in the left column.

Incomplete Word	Meaning
1. <u>episi</u>/o/ <u>t o m y</u>	incision of the perineum
2. <u>col</u> _ _ _ _ _ _	excision (of all or part)* of the colon
3. <u>arthr</u>/o/ _ _ _ _ _ _ _ _	surgical puncture of a joint (to remove fluid)
4. <u>my</u>/o/ _ _ _ _ _ _ _	suture of a muscle
5. <u>col</u>/o/ _ _ _ _ _	forming an opening (mouth) into the colon
6. <u>oste</u>/o/ _ _ _ _	instrument to cut bone
7. <u>tympan</u>/o/ _ _ _ _	incision of the tympanic membrane
8. <u>trache</u>/o/ _ _ _ _ _	forming an opening (mouth) into the trachea
9. <u>thromb</u>/o/ _ _ _ _ _	destruction or separation of a blood clot
10. <u>lith</u>/o/ _ _ _ _	incision to remove a stone or calculus
11. <u>hemorrhoid</u> _ _ _ _ _ _	excision of hemorrhoids

Build a surgical word that means:

12. forming an opening (mouth) into the colon: _____

13. surgical refracture of a bone: _____

14. instrument to cut bone: _____

15. surgical puncture of a joint: _____

16. incision to remove a stone: _____

17. excision of a breast: _____

18. incision of the tympanic membrane: _____

19. forming an opening (mouth) into the trachea: _____

20. excision of the spleen: _____

✔ *Check your answers in Appendix A. Review any material that you did not answer correctly.*

Correct Answers _____ X 5 = _____ % Score

---

*Information in parentheses is used to clarify the meaning of the word but not to build the medical term.

Learning Activity 2-2
Building More Surgical Words

Use the meanings in the right column to complete the surgical words in the left column.
The word roots are underlined in the left column.

Incomplete Word   Meaning

1. <u>arthr</u>/o/ _ _ _ _ _   fixation or binding of a joint
2. <u>rhin</u>/o/ _ _ _ _ _ _   surgical repair of the nose
3. <u>ten</u>/o/ _ _ _ _ _ _   surgical repair of tendons
4. <u>my</u>/o/ _ _ _ _ _ _ _   suture of a muscle
5. <u>mast</u>/o/ _ _ _ _   fixation of a (pendulous)* breast
6. <u>cyst</u>/o/ _ _ _ _ _ _ _   suture of the bladder
7. <u>oste</u>/o/ _ _ _ _ _ _   surgical fracture of a bone
8. <u>neur</u>/o/ _ _ _ _ _ _   crushing of a nerve
9. <u>enter</u>/o/ _ _ _ _ _   separation of intestinal (adhesions)
10. <u>lith</u>/o/ _ _ _ _ _ _   crushing a stone

Build a surgical word that means:

11. surgical repair of the nose: _____
12. surgical puncture of a joint: _____
13. suture of an eyelid: _____
14. fixation of a (pendulous) breast: _____
15. suture of the bladder: _____
16. surgical repair of tendons: _____
17. excision of the appendix: _____
18. crushing of stones: _____
19. separation of intestinal (adhesions): _____
20. crushing of a nerve: _____

✔ *Check your answers in Appendix A. Review any material that you did not answer correctly.*

Correct Answers _____ X 5 = _____ % Score

_____
*Information in parentheses is used to clarify the meaning of the word but not to build the medical term.

Learning Activity 2-3
Selecting a Surgical Suffix

Use the list of suffixes to build surgical words in the right column that reflect the meanings in the left column. Information in parentheses is used to clarify the meaning of the word but not to build the medical term. You may use the same suffix more than one time.

-centesis	-ectomy	-plasty	-tome
-clasis	-lysis	-rrhaphy	-tomy
-desis	-pexy	-stomy	-tripsy

1. forming an opening (mouth) into the colon: col/o/ _____
2. puncture of a joint (to remove fluid):*   arthr/o/ _____
3. excision of the spleen: splen/ _____
4. crushing of a stone: lith/o _____
5. instrument to cut skin: derma/ _____
6. forming an opening (mouth) into the trachea: trache/o/ _____
7. incision to remove a stone or calculus: lith/ _____ / _____
8. excision of a breast: mast/ _____
9. loosening of nerve (tissue):   neur/ _____ / _____
10. incision of the thyroid gland: thyroid/o/ _____
11. fixation of a breast: mast/ _____ / _____
12. excision of the colon: col/ _____
13. suture of the stomach (wall):   gastr/ _____ / _____
14. fixation of the uterus: hyster/ _____ / _____
15. surgical repair of the nose: rhin/ _____ / _____
16. fixation or binding of a joint: arthr/ _____ / _____
17. to break or surgically fracture a bone: oste/ _____ / _____
18. excision of hemorrhoids: hemorrhoid/ _____
19. suture of muscle: my/o/ _____
20. incision of the tympanic membrane: tympan/ _____ / _____

✓ *Check your answers in Appendix A. Review any material that you did not answer correctly.*

Correct Answers _____ X 5 = _____ % Score

_____

*Information in parentheses is used to clarify the meaning of the word but not to build the medical term.

Learning Activity 2-4

Selecting Diagnostic, Pathological, and Related Suffixes

Use the suffixes in this list to build diagnostic, pathological, and related words in the right column that reflect the meanings in the left column.

-algia	-emia	-osis	-rrhexis
-cele	-graph	-pathy	-spasm
-ectasis	-malacia	-penia	-toxic
-emesis	-megaly	-rrhea	

1. pertaining to poison in the liver: hepat/o/ _____
2. pain (along the course) of a nerve: neur/ _____
3. white blood condition: leuk/ _____
4. abnormal condition of the skin: dermat/ _____
5. enlargement of the kidney: nephr/o/_____
6. discharge or flow from the ear: ot/ _____ / _____
7. twitching of the eyelid: blephar/ _____ / _____
8. rupture of the uterus: hyster/ _____ / _____
9. herniation of the bladder: cyst/ _____ / _____
10. excessive vomiting: hyper/ _____
11. disease of muscle (tissue):   my/ _____ / _____
12. softening of the bones: oste/ _____ / _____
13. dilation of a bronchus: bronchi/ _____
14. decrease in bone (mineral density):   oste/ _____ / _____
15. instrument for recording (electrical activity) of the heart: cardi/o/ _____

 Check your answers in Appendix A. Review any material that you did not answer correctly.

Correct Answers _____ X 6.67 = _____ % Score

Learning Activity 2-5

Building Pathological and Related Words

Use the meanings in the right column to complete the pathological and related words in the left column.

Incomplete Word   Meaning

1. neur/o/ _____   disease of the nerves

2. chole/ _____   gallstone

3. carcin/o/ _____   forming or producing cancer

4. oste/ _____ / _____   softening of bone

5. hem/ _____ / _____   fear of blood

6. neur/ _____   tumor composed of nervous tissue

7. hepat/ _____ / _____   herniation of the liver

8. bronchi/_____   dilation of a bronchus

9. dermat/ _____   abnormal condition of the skin

10. chondr/o/ _____   softening of cartilage

11. blephar/ _____ / _____   prolapse of the eyelid

12. arteri/o/ _____   abnormal condition of arterial hardening

13. cephal/o/ _____   pain in the head; headache

14. blephar/ _____ / _____   twitching of the eyelid

15. hepat/ _____ / _____   enlargement of the liver

Check your answers in Appendix A. Review any material that you did not answer correctly.

Correct Answers _____ X 6.67 = _____ % Score

Learning Activity 2-6

Selecting Adjective, Noun, and Diminutive Suffixes

Use the adjective suffixes in the list to create medical terms. The first one is completed for you. Note: When in doubt about the validity of a word, refer to a medical dictionary.

-ac	-ary	-ic	-tic
-al	-eal	-ous	-tix

Element	Medical Term	Meaning
1. aqua/	_aquatic_	pertaining to water
2. bacteri/		pertaining to bacteria
3. gastr/		pertaining to the stomach
4. axill/		pertaining to the armpit
5. cardi/		pertaining to the heart
6. membran/		pertaining to a membrane
7. spin/		pertaining to the spine

Use the noun suffixes in the list to create medical terms.

-er	-is	-ole
-ia	-ism	-ule
-iatry	-ist	-y

Element	Medical Term	Meaning
8. man/		condition of madness
9. psych/		treatment of the mind
10. sigmoid/o/scop/		visual examination of the sigmoid colon
11. alcohol/		condition of (excessive) alcohol
12. allerg/		specialist in treating allergic disorders
13. intern/		specialist in internal medicine
14. arteri/		minute artery
15. ven/		small vein

✓ *Check your answers in Appendix A. Review any material that you did not answer correctly.*

Correct Answers _____ X 6.67 = _____ % Score

Learning Activity 2-7
Forming Plural Words

Review the guidelines for plural suffixes (located on the inside back cover of this book).
Then write the plural form for each of the singular terms and briefly state the rule that
applies. The first one is completed for you.

Singular	Plural	Rule
1. diagnosis	*diagnoses*	*Drop the* is *and add* es.
2. testis		
3. vertebra		
4. keratosis		
5. prognosis		
6. spermatozoon		
7. appendix		
8. coccus		
9. ganglion		
10. bronchus		
11. thrombus		
12. septum		
13. bacterium		
14. fornix		
15. nevus		

✔ *Check your answers in Appendix A. Review any material that you did not answer correctly.*

Correct Answers _____ X 6.67 = _____ % Score

Medical Language Lab
Turning terminology into language

Visit the Medical Language Laboratory at the website *medicallanguagelab.com*.
Use it to enhance your study and for reinforcement of suffixes with the flash
card activity related to suffixes. We recommend that you complete the flash
card activity before moving on to Chapter 3.

Prefixes

Objectives

Upon completion of this chapter, you will be able to:

- Define common prefixes used in medical terminology.
- Describe how a prefix changes the meaning of a medical word.
- Recognize and define prefixes of position, number and measurement, and direction.
- Pronounce medical terms presented in this chapter.
- Demonstrate your knowledge of this chapter by completing the learning activities.

Prefix Linking

Most medical words contain a root or combining form with a suffix. Some of them also contain prefixes. A prefix is a word element located at the beginning of a word. Substituting one prefix for another alters the meaning of the word. For example, in the term **macro/cyte**, **macro-** is a prefix meaning *large;* **-cyte** is a suffix meaning *cell.* A **macr/o/cyte** is a *large cell.* Changing the prefix **macro-** (large) to **micro-** (small) changes the meaning of the word. A **micr/o/cyte** is a *small cell.* See Table 3-1 for other examples of how a prefix changes the meaning of a word.

TABLE 3-1 Changing Prefixes and Meanings

In this table, each word has the same root, nat *(birth), and suffix,* -al *(pertaining to). By substituting different prefixes, new words with different meanings are formed.*

Prefix	+	Word Root	+	Suffix	=	Medical Word	Meaning
pre- (before)	+	nat (birth)	+	-al (pertaining to)	=	pre/nat/al prē-NĀ-tăl	pertaining to (the period) before birth
peri- (around)	+	nat (birth)	+	-al (pertaining to)		peri/nat/al pĕr-ĭ-NĀ-tăl	pertaining to (the period) around birth
post- (after)	+	nat (birth)	+	-al (pertaining to)		post/nat/al pōst-NĀ-tăl	pertaining to (the period) after birth

Prefix Types

Learning the major types of prefixes, such as prefixes of position, number and measurement, and direction, as well as some others, will help you master medical terminology.

Prefixes of Position, Number, Measurement, and Direction

Prefixes used in medical terms denote position, number and measurement, and direction. Prefixes of position describe a place or location (see Table 3-2). Prefixes of number and measurement describe an amount, size, or degree of involvement (see Table 3-3). Prefixes of direction indicate a pathway or route (see Table 3-4).

TABLE 3-2 Prefixes of Position

This table lists commonly used prefixes of position, along with their meanings and word analyses.

Prefix	Meaning	Word Analysis
endo-	in, within	**endo**/crine (ĔN-dō-krĭn): secrete within *-crine:* secrete *Endocrine describes a gland that secretes directly into the bloodstream.*

intra-		**intra**/muscul/ar (ĭn-tră-MŬS-kū-lăr): within the muscle
		  muscul: muscle
		  -ar: pertaining to

epi-	above, upon	**epi**/derm/is (ĕp-ĭ-DĔR-mĭs): upon the skin
		  derm: skin
		  -is: noun ending
		The epidermis is the outer layer of the skin.

TABLE 3-2 Prefixes of Position—cont'd

Prefix	Meaning	Word Analysis
hypo-	under, below; deficient	**hypo**/derm/ic (hī-pō-DĔR-mĭk): pertaining to under the skin *derm:* skin *-ic:* pertaining to *Hypodermic needles are used for subcutaneous injections and to take fluid samples from the body, for example, taking blood from a vein in venipuncture (see Fig. 3-1).*

Subcutaneous

Intramuscular

Intradermal

Epidermis

Dermis

Subcutaneous tissue

Muscle

Figure 3-1 Hypodermic needles inserted within the skin (**intra**dermal), under the skin (**sub**cutaneous), or in between the muscular layers (**intra**muscular).

Prefix	Meaning	Word Analysis
infra-	under, below	**infra**/cost/al (ĭn-fră-KŎS-tăl): below the ribs *cost:* ribs *-al:* pertaining to
sub-		**sub**/cutane/ous (sŭb-kū-TĀ-nē-ŭs): pertaining to under the skin *cutane:* skin *-ous:* pertaining to *The subcutaneous tissue is the deepest layer of skin. It binds the dermis to underlying structures.*
inter-	between	**inter**/cost/al (ĭn-tĕr-KŎS-tăl): between the ribs *cost:* ribs *-al:* pertaining to
retro-	backward, behind	**retro**/version (rĕt-rō-VĔR-shŭn): turning backward *-version:* turning *Retroversion refers to tipping backward of an organ (such as the uterus) from its normal position.*

TABLE 3-3 **Prefixes of Number and Measurement**

This table lists commonly used prefixes of number and measurement, along with their meanings and word analyses.

Prefix	Meaning	Word Analysis
bi-	two	**bi**/later/al (bī-LĂT-ĕr-ăl): pertaining to two sides *later:* side *-al:* pertaining to
dipl-	double	**dipl**/opia (dĭp-L Ō-pē-ă): double vision *-opia:* vision
diplo-		**diplo**/bacteri/al (dĭp-lō-băk-TĒR-ē-ăl): bacteria linked together in pairs *bacteri:* bacteria *-al:* pertaining to *Diplobacteria reproduce in such a manner that they are joined together in pairs (see Fig. 3-2).*

Figure 3-2 A stained slide under the microscope showing gram-negative diplobacteria that cause sexually transmitted gonorrhea infection.

TABLE 3-3 Prefixes of Number and Measurement—cont'd

Prefix	Meaning	Word Analysis
hemi-	one-half	**hemi**/plegia (hĕm-ē-PLĒ-jē-ă): paralysis of one half -*plegia:* paralysis *Hemiplegia is a paralysis of one-half of the body, either the right side or the left side.*
hyper-	excessive, above normal	**hyper**/calc/emia (hī-pĕr-kăl-SĒ-mē-ă): excessive calcium in the blood *calc:* calcium -*emia:* blood condition
macro-	large	**macro**/cyte (MĂK-rō-sīt): large cell -*cyte:* cell
micro-	small	**micro**/scope (MĪ-krō-skōp): instrument for examining small (objects) -*scope:* instrument for examining *A microscope is an optical instrument that greatly magnifies minute objects.*
mono-	one	**mono**/therapy (MŎN-ō-thĕr-ă-pē): one treatment -*therapy:* treatment *An example of monotherapy is treatment using only a single drug or a single treatment modality.*
uni-		**uni**/nucle/ar (ū-nĭ-N Ū-klē-ăr): pertaining to one nucleus *nucle:* nucleus -*ar:* pertaining to
multi-	many, much	**multi**/gravida (mŭl-tĭ-GRĂV-ĭ-dă): woman who has been pregnant more than once -*gravida:* pregnant woman
poly		**poly**/phobia (pŏl-ē-F Ō-bē-ă): fear of many things -*phobia:* fear
quadri-	four	**quadri**/plegia (kwŏd-rĭ-PLĒ-jē-ă): paralysis of four -*plegia:* paralysis *Quadriplegia is a paralysis of all four extremities, usually caused by an injury to or disease of the cervical spinal cord.*
tri-	three	**tri**/ceps (TRĪ-cĕps): three heads -*ceps:* head *Triceps describes a muscle having three heads or points of origin.*

TABLE 3-4 **Prefixes of Direction**

This table lists commonly used prefixes of direction as well as their meanings and word analyses.

Prefix	Meaning	Word Analysis
ab-	from, away from	**ab**/duction (ăb-DŬK-shun): movement of a limb away from (the body) *-duction:* act of leading, bringing, conducting *Abduction is a body movement away from the midline or axis of the body (see Fig. 3-3).*
ad-	toward	**ad**/duction (ăb-DŬK-shŭn): movement of a limb toward (the body) *-duction:* act of leading, bringing, conducting *Adduction is a body movement toward the midline or axis of the body (see Fig. 3-3).*

Adduction   **Ab**duction

Figure 3-3 Adduction and **Ab**duction.

circum-	around	**circum**/ren/al (sĕr-kŭm-RĒ-năl): pertaining to around the kidney
		  ren: kidney
		  -al: pertaining to

peri-		**peri**/odont/al (pĕr-ē-ō-DŎN-tăl): pertaining to around a tooth
		  odont: teeth
		  -al: pertaining to

dia-	through, across	**dia**/rrhea (dī-ă-RĒ-ă): flow through *-rrhea:* discharge, flow *Diarrhea is a condition of abnormally frequent discharge or flow of fluid fecal matter through the bowel.*

trans-		**trans**/vagin/al (trăns-VĂJ-ĭn-ăl): pertaining to across or through the vagina
		  vagin: vagina
		  -al: pertaining to

TABLE 3-4 **Prefixes of Direction—cont'd**

Prefix	Meaning	Word Analysis

ecto-	outside, outward	**ecto**/gen/ous (ĕk-TŎJ-ĕ-nŭs): forming outside (the body or structure)
		   gen: forming, producing, origin
		   -ous: pertaining to
		An ectogenous infection is one that originates outside of the body.

exo-		**exo**/tropia (ĕks-ō-TRŌ-pē-ă): turning outward *-tropia:* turning *Exotropia refers to the turning outward of the eyes (see Fig. 3-4).*

extra-		**extra**/crani/al (ĕks-tră-KRĀ-nē-ăl): pertaining to outside the skull
		   crani: cranium (skull)
		   -al: pertaining to

Figure 3-4 Exotropia of the eye where the eye deviates and turns outward.

Prefix	Meaning	Word Analysis

para-*	near, beside; beyond	**para**/nas/al (păr-ă-NĀ-săl): beside the nose
		   nas: nose
		   -al: pertaining to

super-	upper, above	**super**/ior (soo-PĒ-rē-or): pertaining to above or the upper part of a structure *-ior:* pertaining to

supra-	above; excessive; superior	**supra**/ren/al (soo-pră-RĒ-năl): pertaining to above the kidney
		   ren: kidney
		   -al: pertaining to

ultra-	excess, beyond	**ultra**/son/ic (ŭl-tră-SŎN-ĭk): pertaining to sound beyond (that which can be heard by the human ear)
		   son: sound
		   -ic: pertaining to

Para- may also be used as a suffix meaning *to bear (offspring).*

Other Common Prefixes

Many other common prefixes may also change the meaning of a word. See Table 3-5 for a list of other common prefixes.

TABLE 3-5 **Other Common Prefixes**

This table lists other commonly used prefixes, along with their meanings and word analyses.

Prefix	Meaning	Word Analysis
a-*	without, not	**a**/mast/ia (ă-MĂS-tē-ă): without a breast *mast:* breast *-ia:* condition *Amastia may be the result of a congenital defect, an endocrine disorder, or mastectomy.*
an-**		**an**/esthesia (ăn-ĕs-THĒ-zē-ă): without feeling *-esthesia:* feeling *Anesthesia may be a partial or complete loss of sensation with or without loss of consciousness.*
anti-	against	**anti**/bacteri/al (ăn-tĭ-băk-TĒR-ē-ăl): against bacteria *bacteri:* bacteria *-al:* pertaining to *Antibacterials are substances that kill bacteria or inhibit their growth or replication.*
contra-		**contra**/ception (kŏn-tră-SĔP-shŭn): against conceiving *-ception:* conceiving *Contraceptive techniques prevent pregnancy by means of medication, a device, or a method that blocks or alters one or more of the processes of reproduction.*
auto-	self, own	**auto**/graft (AW-tō-grăft): transplantation to self *-graft:* transplantation *An autograft is tissue transplanted from one site and grafted to another site of the same person (see Fig. 3-5).*

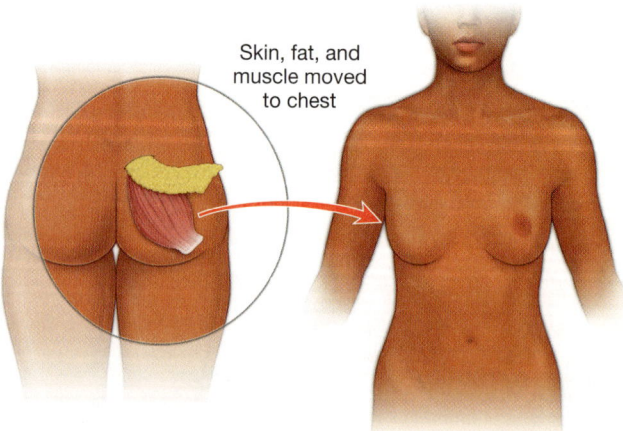

Skin, fat, and muscle moved to chest

Figure 3-5 Autograft in which tissue from the patient's buttocks is transplanted to her breast.

---

*The prefix *a-* is usually used before a consonant.

**The prefix *an-* is usually used before a vowel.

TABLE 3-5 Other Common Prefixes—cont'd

Prefix	Meaning	Word Analysis
brady-	slow	**brady**/cardia (brăd-ē-KĂR-dē-ă): slow heart rate *-cardia:* heart
dys-	bad; painful; difficult	**dys**/tocia (dĭs-TŌ-sē-ă): difficult childbirth *-tocia:* childbirth, labor
eu-	good, normal	**eu**/pnea (ūp-NĒ-ă): normal breathing *-pnea:* breathing
hetero-	different	**hetero**/graft (HĔT-ĕ-rō-grăft): different transplantation; also called *xenograft* *-graft:* transplantation *A heterograft is a transplant from one species to another (see Fig. 3-6).*

Heart valve

Figure 3-6 Heterograft in which tissue (heart valve) from one species (pig) is transplanted to another species (human).

(continued)

TABLE 3-5 Other Common Prefixes—cont'd

Prefix	Meaning	Word Analysis
homo-	same	**homo**/graft (HŌ-mō-grăft): same transplantation *-graft:* transplantation *A homograft, also called an allograft, is a graft of tissue or an organ taken from a donor of the same species as the recipient. Commonly transplanted organs include the kidneys, lungs, and heart (see Fig. 3-7).*
homeo-		**homeo**/plasia (hō-mē-ō-PLĀ-zē-ă): formation or growth of same (or similar tissue) *-plasia:* formation, growth

Muscles
Blood vessels
Bone plates
Skin flap
Donor hand
Skin flap
Tendon
Recipient arm

Figure 3-7 Homograft of an arm taken from a human donor and transplanted to another human.

| tachy- | rapid | **tachy**/pnea (tăk-ĭp-NĒ-ă): rapid breathing
-pnea: breathing |

It is time to review prefixes by completing Learning Activities 3-1, 3-2, and 3-3.

LEARNING ACTIVITIES

The activities that follow provide review of the prefixes introduced in this chapter. Complete each activity and review your answers to evaluate your understanding of the chapter.

Learning Activity 3-1
Identifying and Defining Prefixes

Place a slash after each of the prefixes and then define the prefix. The first one is completed for you.

Word	Definition of Prefix
1. inter/dental	*between*
2. hypodermic	
3. abduction	
4. multigravida	
5. sublingual	
6. quadriplegia	
7. antibacterial	
8. triceps	
9. anesthesia	
10. intramuscular	
11. suprapelvic	
12. bilateral	
13. transvaginal	
14. bradycardia	
15. tachypnea	
16. dystocia	
17. eupnea	
18. heterograft	
19. ultrasonic	
20. circumrenal	

Check your answers in Appendix A. Review any material that you did not answer correctly.

Correct Answers _____ X 5 = _____ % Score

Learning Activity 3-2

Matching Prefixes of Position, Number and Measurement, and Direction

Match the terms with the definitions in the numbered list.

adduction	hypodermic	polyphobia
circumrenal	intercostal	postoperative
diplopia	macrocyte	retroversion
epigastric	monotherapy	subnasal
hemiplegia	periodontal	suprarenal

1. _____ tipping back of an organ
2. _____ pertaining to under the skin
3. _____ movement of a limb toward the body
4. _____ pertaining to under the nose
5. _____ after surgery
6. _____ pertaining to between the ribs
7. _____ pertaining to (the area) above the stomach
8. _____ pertaining to around the teeth
9. _____ double vision
10. _____ one treatment
11. _____ above the kidney
12. _____ paralysis of one-half (of the body)
13. _____ pertaining to around the kidney
14. _____ (abnormally) large blood cell
15. _____ many fears

Check your answers in Appendix A. Review any material that you did not answer correctly.

Correct Answers _____ X 6.67 = _____ % Score

Learning Activity 3-3
Matching Other Prefixes

Match the terms with the definitions in the numbered list.

amastia   dyspepsia   homograft
anticonvulsant   dystocia   hypercalcemia
bradycardia   eupnea   infracostal
bradypnea   heterograft   paranasal
contraception   homeoplasia   tachycardia

1. _____ difficult digestion
2. _____ tissue transplant from a different species
3. _____ slow breathing
4. _____ excessive calcium in the blood
5. _____ slow heartbeat
6. _____ prevents or relieves convulsions
7. _____ without a breast
8. _____ below the ribs
9. _____ good or normal breathing
10. _____ beside the nose
11. _____ rapid heartbeat
12. _____ against conceiving
13. _____ tissue transplant from the same species
14. _____ difficult childbirth
15. _____ formation of the same tissue

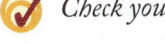 *Check your answers in Appendix A. Review any material that you did not answer correctly.*

Correct Answers _____ X 6.67 = _____ % Score

Medical Language Lab
Turning terminology into language

Visit the Medical Language Laboratory at the website medicallanguagelab.com. Use it to enhance your study and for reinforcement of prefixes with the flash card activity related to prefixes. We recommend that you complete the flash card activity before moving on to Chapter 4.

Body Structure

Chapter Outline

Objectives

Upon completion of this chapter, you will be able to:

- List the levels of organization of the body.
- Define and identify three planes of the body.
- Identify the cavities, quadrants, and regions of the body.
- List and identify terms related to direction, position, and planes of the body.
- Recognize, pronounce, spell, and build words related to body structure.
- Describe diseases, conditions, and procedures related to body structure.
- Demonstrate your knowledge of this chapter by completing the learning and documenting health-care activities.

Introduction

This chapter provides an orientation to the body as a whole and contains general terms that are relevant to all body systems. Learning these terms and how they are used to locate and describe structures within the body helps to master the material presented in subsequent chapters of this book. Included are terms associated with diseases, abnormal conditions, and diagnostic and medical procedures used in the clinical setting. Also, case studies provide prototypes for documenting health-care services in a patient's electronic medical record.

Body Structure Key Terms

This section introduces important terms associated with body structure, along with their definitions and pronunciations. The key terms are highlighted in color throughout the introduction. Word analyses are also provided for selected terms.

Term	Definition
chromatin ☐ KRŌ-mă-tĭn	Structural component of the nucleus, composed of nucleic acids and proteins *Chromatin condenses to form chromosomes during cell division.*
chromosome ☐ KRŌ-mō-sōm	Threadlike structures within the nucleus composed of deoxyribonucleic acid (DNA) that carries hereditary information encoded in genes *Each sperm or egg has 23 unpaired chromosomes. After fertilization, each cell of the embryo then has 46 chromosomes (23 pairs). In each pair of chromosomes, one chromosome is provided by the father and the other by the mother.*
deoxyribonucleic acid (DNA) ☐ dē-ŏk-sē-rī-bō-noo-KLĀ-ĭk ĂS-ĭd	Molecule that holds genetic information capable of replicating and producing an exact copy whenever the cell divides
metabolism ☐ mĕ-TĂB-ō-lĭzm	Sum of all physical and chemical changes that take place in a cell or an organism *Metabolism includes the building up (anabolism) and breaking down (catabolism) of body constituents.*
organelle ☐ or-găn-ĔL	Cellular structure that provides a specialized function, such as the nucleus (reproduction), ribosomes (protein synthesis), Golgi apparatus (removal of material from the cell), and lysosomes (digestion) *The membranes of many organelles act as sites of chemical reactions.*

Pronunciation Help	Long Sound	ā — rate	ē — rebirth	ī — isle	ō — over	ū — unite
	Short Sound	ă — apple	ĕ — ever	ĭ — it	ŏ — not	ŭ — cut

Levels of Organization

The human body contains several levels of structure and function. Each of these levels builds on the previous level and contributes to the structure and function of the entire organism. Five levels of organization are relevant to understanding anatomy, physiology, and pathology: the cells, tissues, organs, systems, and organism (see Fig. 4-1).

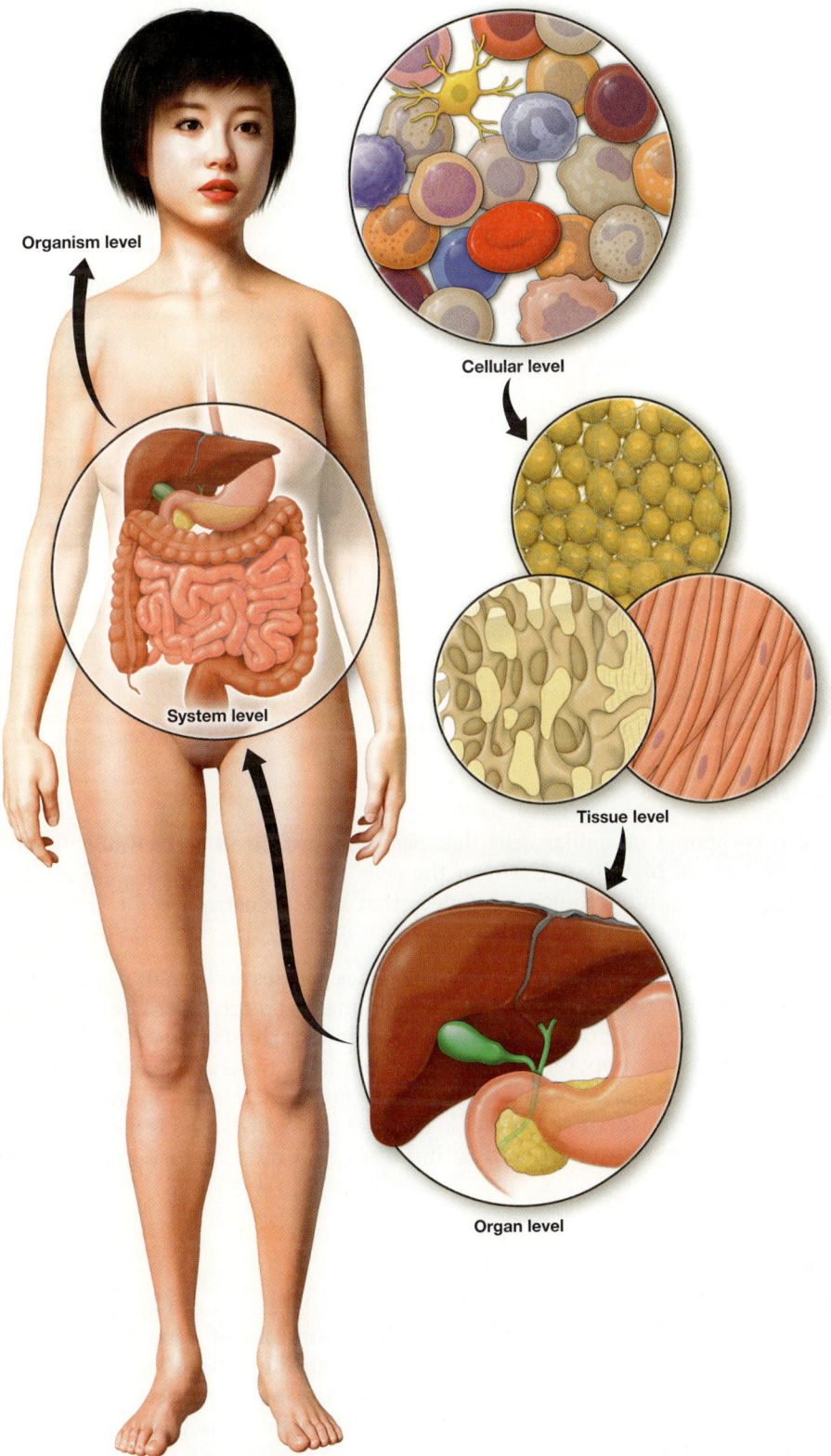

Figure 4-1 Levels of organization of the human body.

Cells

The cell is the smallest structural and functional unit of life. Body cells perform all activities associated with life, including utilizing food, facilitating reproduction, and eliminating waste products. Cells have many shapes and sizes, but they share three main structures: **cell membrane**, **cytoplasm**, and **nucleus**. The study of the body at the cellular level is called **cytology**.

Cell Membrane and Cytoplasm

The cell membrane acts as a barrier that supports and protects the intracellular contents. Within the cell membrane is a jellylike matrix of proteins, salts, water, dissolved gases, and nutrients called **cytoplasm.** Inside the cytoplasm are specialized structures called **organelles.** These organelles perform specific functions of the cell, such as reproduction and digestion. The largest cell organelle is the nucleus, which directs the cell's activities and contains **chromosomes**.

Nucleus

The nucleus is responsible for **metabolism,** growth, and reproduction. It also carries the genetic blueprint of the organism. This blueprint is found in a complex molecule called **deoxyribonu- cleic acid (DNA)** that is organized into a threadlike structure called **chromatin.** When the cell is ready to divide, chromatin forms **chromosomes,** which carry thousands of genes that make up our genetic blueprint. Each body cell, with the exception of the female ovum and the male spermatozoa, contains 23 pairs of chromosomes that determine its genetic makeup. In each of the 23 pairs, one of the chromosomes was inherited from the mother and the other from the father. About 20,000 to 25,000 genes in the body determine unique human characteristics. Genes pass biological information from one generation to the next. This biological information includes such traits as hair color, body structure, and metabolic activity.

Tissues

Tissue is composed of similar cells that perform specialized or common functions. The study of tissues is called **histology.** Between the cells that make up tissues are varying amounts and types of nonliving, intercellular substances that provide pathways for cellular interaction. The body contains four types of tissues:

- **Epithelial tissue** covers surfaces of organs, lines cavities and canals, forms tubes and ducts, provides the secreting portions of glands, and makes up the outer layer **(epidermis)** of the skin. It is composed of cells arranged in a continuous sheet consisting of one or more layers.
- **Connective tissue** supports and connects other body tissues. There are various types of connective tissue, including cartilage, adipose (fat), bone, elastic fibrous, and blood.
- **Muscle tissue** provides the contractile tissue of the body, which is responsible for movement.
- **Nervous tissue** transmits electrical impulses as it relays information throughout the entire body.

Organs

Organs are body structures that perform specialized functions. They are composed of two or more tissue types. For example, the stomach is made up of connective tissue, muscle tissue, epithelial tissue, and nervous tissue. Muscle and connective tissue form the wall of the stomach. Epithelial and connective tissue cover the inner and outer surfaces of the stomach. Nervous tissue penetrates the epithelial lining of the stomach and its muscular wall to stimulate the release of chemicals for digestion.

Systems

A body system is composed of varying numbers of organs and accessory structures that have similar or related functions. For example, organs of the gastrointestinal system include the esophagus, stomach, small intestine, and colon. Some of its accessory structures include the liver, gallbladder, and pancreas. The main function of the digestive system is to digest food, remove and absorb its nutrients, and expel waste products.

Organism

The highest level of organization is the organism. An organism is a complete living entity capable of independent existence. All complex organisms, including humans, are made up of several body systems that work together to sustain life.

Anatomical Position

Anatomical position is a body posture used among anatomists and clinicians as a position of reference to ensure uniformity and consistency in locating anatomical parts or divisions of the human body. In the anatomical position, the person stands erect, facing forward, and the arms are at the sides of the body, with the palms of the hands turned forward and the feet parallel to each another. No matter how the body is actually positioned—standing or lying down, facing forward or backward—or how the limbs are actually placed, the positions and relationships of a structure are always described as if the body were in the anatomical position.

Body Planes

A **plane** is an imaginary flat surface that divides the body into two sections. When the body is in the anatomical position, the planes serve as points of reference to identify the different sections of the body. The most commonly used planes are coronal (frontal), transverse (horizontal), and midsagittal (median). The section is named for the plane along which it is cut. A **coronal (frontal) plane** divides the body into an anterior and posterior section; a **transverse (horizontal) plane** divides the body into top and bottom sections. The **midsagittal plane** runs through the center of the body, dividing the body into right and left halves (see Fig. 4-2).

Before the development of modern imaging techniques, standard x-ray images showed only a single plane, and many body abnormalities were difficult, if not impossible, to see. Current imaging procedures, such as magnetic resonance imaging (MRI) and computed tomography (CT), produce three-dimensional images on more than one plane. Thus, structural abnormalities and body masses that were previously not found using a standard single plane x-ray are now detected with scanning devices that show images taken in several body planes.

Directional Terms

Directional terms help indicate the position of structures, surfaces, and regions of the body. These terms are always identified relative to the anatomical position. For example, the knee is *superior* to the ankle; the legs are *inferior* to the trunk. Refer to Figure 4-3 to locate the directional terms *superior* and *inferior*. Physicians commonly use directional terms in medical reports and in communications with other health-care providers and patients. Directional terms identify the location of diseases, injuries, and surgical sites. In a clinical setting, health-care providers may describe the location of a heart attack to the patient as occurring in the front, or *anterior*, part of the heart. A tumor on the back of the kidney may be described as being located on the *posterior* surface of the kidney (see Table 4-1).

Body Cavities

Body cavities are spaces within the body that hold, protect, separate, and support internal organs. Clinicians refer to these cavities to locate internal organs and identify abnormalities within the cavities. The body has two main cavities: the **dorsal cavity**, located on the back of the body **(posterior)**, and the **ventral cavity**, located on the front of the body **(anterior)** (see Fig. 4-4).

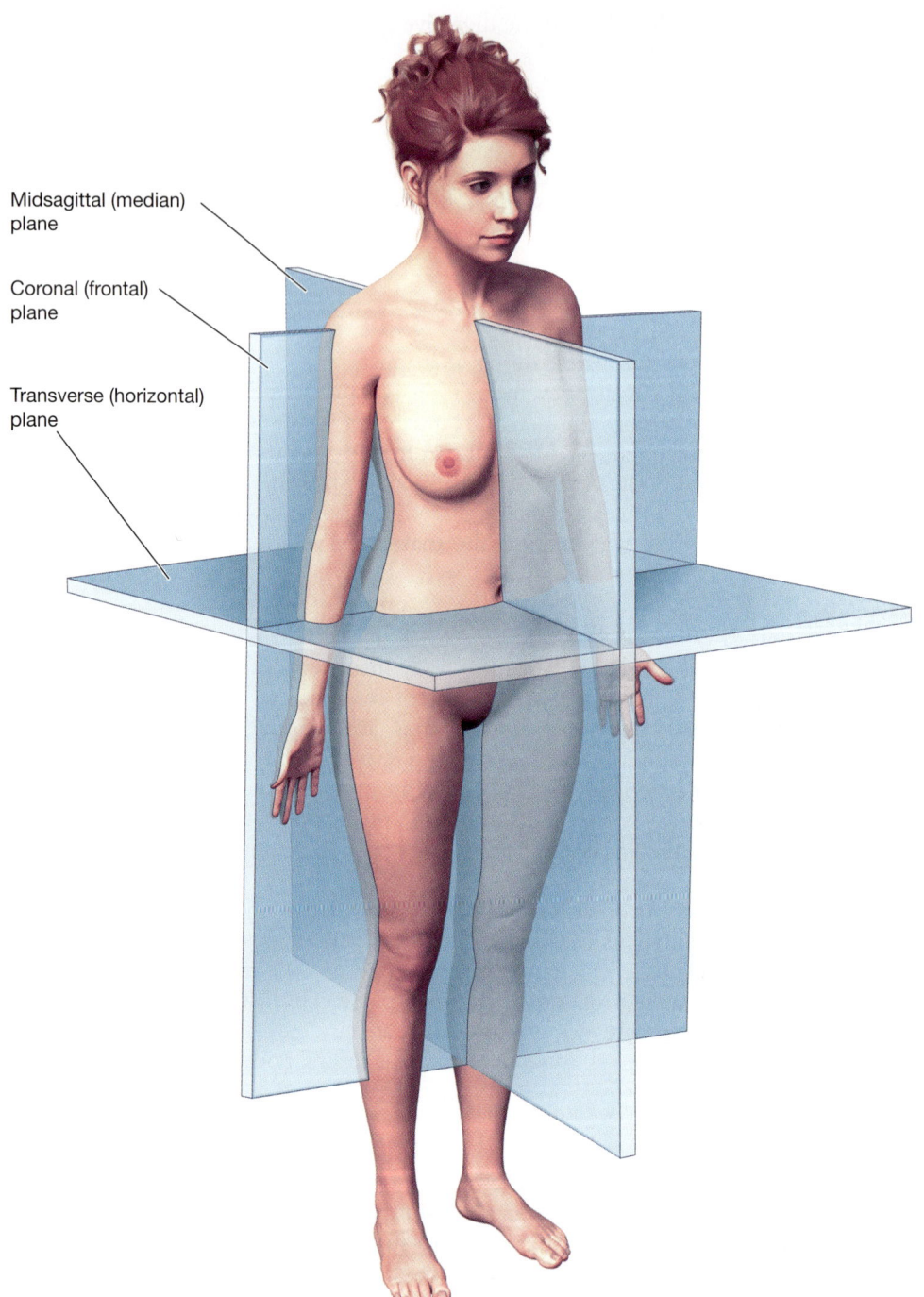

Midsagittal (median) plane

Coronal (frontal) plane

Transverse (horizontal) plane

Figure 4-2 Body planes. (Note that the body is in anatomical position.)

Figure 4-3 Directional terms.

TABLE 4-1 Directional Terms

This table provides a comprehensive summary of directional terms, along with their definitions. Opposing terms are presented consecutively to aid memorization.

Term	Definition
Abduction	Movement away from the midsagittal (median) plane of the body or one of its parts
Adduction	Movement toward the midsagittal (median) plane of the body
Medial	Pertaining to the midline of the body or structure
Lateral	Pertaining to a side
Superior (cephalad)	Toward the head or upper portion of a structure
Inferior (caudal)	Away from the head, or toward the tail or lower part of a structure
Proximal	Nearer to the center (trunk of the body) or to the point of attachment to the body
Distal	Further from the center (trunk of the body) or from the point of attachment to the body
Anterior (ventral)	Front of the body
Posterior (dorsal)	Back of the body
Parietal	Pertaining to the outer wall of the body cavity
Visceral	Pertaining to the viscera, or internal organs, especially the abdominal organs
Prone	Lying on the abdomen, face down
Supine	Lying horizontally on the back, face up
Inversion	Turning inward or inside out
Eversion	Turning outward
Palmar	Pertaining to the palm of the hand
Plantar	Pertaining to the sole of the foot
Superficial	Toward the surface of the body (external)
Deep	Away from the surface of the body (internal)

Dorsal Cavity

The **dorsal cavity** is divided into the *cranial cavity* and the *spinal cavity*. The **cranial cavity**, formed by the skull, contains the brain; the **spinal cavity**, formed by the **backbone** (spine), contains the spinal cord. The **meninges** are the membranes that line these cavities and also cover the brain and spinal cord. The dorsal cavity is continuous; no wall or structure separates the cranial cavity from the spinal cavity.

Ventral Cavity

The **ventral cavity** is divided into the *thoracic cavity* and *abdominopelvic cavity*. The thoracic cavity is separated from the abdominopelvic cavity by a muscular wall called the **diaphragm**. The **thoracic cavity** contains the lungs and heart. The **abdominal pelvic cavity** is further divided into the *abdominal cavity* and *pelvic cavity*. The **abdominal cavity** contains the liver, stomach, intestines, and kidneys. The **pelvic cavity**, positioned inferior to the abdominal cavity, contains the urinary bladder and reproductive organs, such as the uterus in women and the prostate gland in men. Examine the divisions of the ventral cavity in Figure 4-4.

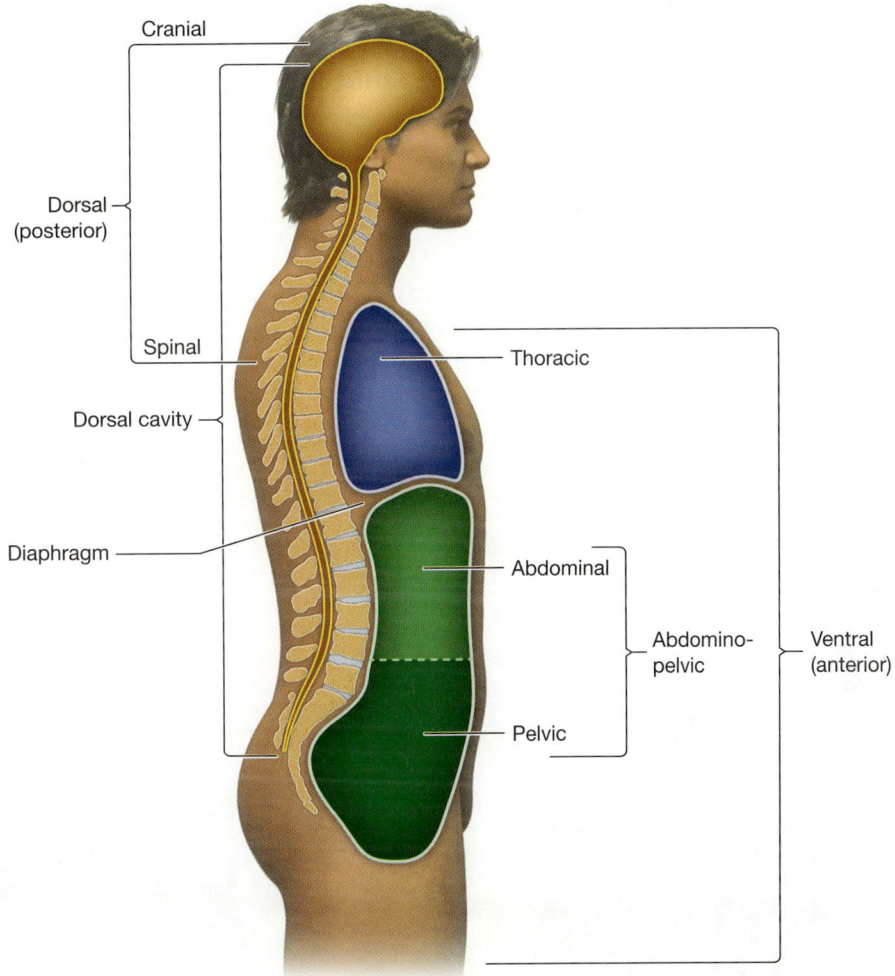

Figure 4-4 Body cavities.

Abdominopelvic Quadrants and Regions

To describe the location of the many abdominal and pelvic organs more easily, anatomists and clinicians use two methods of dividing the abdominopelvic cavity into smaller areas. These two divisions are known as **quadrants** and **regions**.

Quadrants

The abdominopelvic cavity is divided into four **quadrants** with two imaginary lines that form a cross in the midsection of the lower torso. The quadrants provide a means of locating specific sites of the abdomen for descriptive and diagnostic purposes (see Table 4-2). They also provide a point of reference in clinical examinations and medical reports. Clinicians will commonly describe pain, lesions, abrasions, punctures, and burns as located in a specific quadrant. They will also identify incision sites by using body quadrants (see Fig. 4-5).

Regions

Anatomists and clinicians divide the abdominopelvic cavity into nine **abdominopelvic regions**. They use these regions primarily to identify the location of underlying body structures and visceral organs (see Table 4-3). For example, the stomach is located in the left hypochondriac and epigastric region; the appendix is located in the right inguinal region.

TABLE 4-2 Abdominopelvic Quadrants

Quadrant	Abbreviation	Major Structures
Right upper	RUQ	Right lobe of the liver, the gallbladder, part of the pancreas, and part of the small and large intestines
Left upper	LUQ	Left lobe of the liver, the stomach, the spleen, part of the pancreas, and part of the small and large intestines
Right lower	RLQ	Part of the small and large intestines, the appendix, the right ovary, the right fallopian tube, and the right ureter
Left lower	LLQ	Part of the small and large intestines, the left ovary, the left fallopian tube, and the left ureter

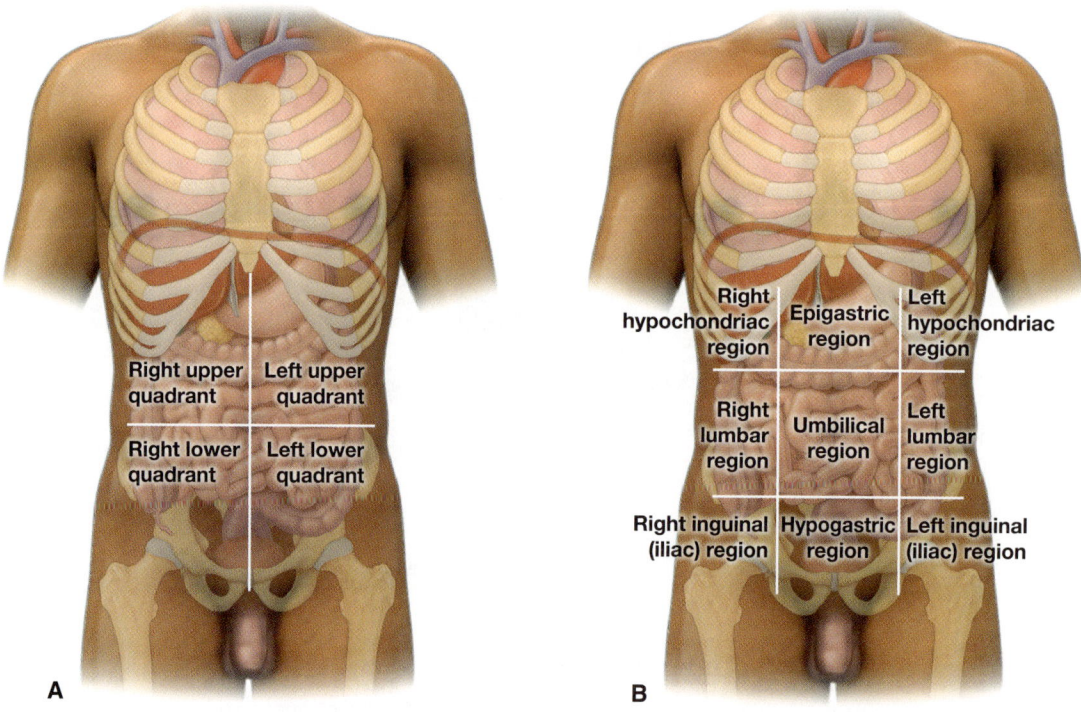

Figure 4-5 Quadrants and regions. (A) Four quadrants of the abdomen. (B) Nine regions of the abdomen.

TABLE 4-3 Abdominopelvic Regions

Region	Location
Right hypochondriac	Upper right lateral region beneath the ribs
Epigastric	Upper middle region
Left hypochondriac	Upper left lateral region beneath the ribs
Right lumbar	Middle right lateral region
Umbilical	Region of the navel
Left lumbar	Middle left lateral region
Right inguinal (iliac)	Lower right lateral region
Hypogastric	Lower middle region
Left inguinal (iliac)	Lower left lateral region

Anatomy Review: Body Planes

To review the body planes and directional terms, label the illustration using the terms that follow.

anterior

coronal (frontal) plane

inferior

lateral

medial

midsagittal (median) plane

posterior

superior

transverse (horizontal) plane

Check your answers by referring to Figure 4–2 on page 54. Review material that you did not answer correctly.

Anatomy Review: Quadrants and Regions

To review quadrants and regions, label the quadrants in Figure A and the regions in Figure B using the terms that follow.

epigastric region

hypogastric region

left hypochondriac region

left iliac region

left lower quadrant

left lumbar region

left upper quadrant

right hypochondriac region

right iliac region

right lower quadrant

right lumbar region

right upper quadrant

umbilical region

A

B

  Check your answers by referring to Figures 4–5A and 4–5B on page 58. Review material that you did not answer correctly.

Spine

The spine (**vertebral column** or **backbone**) is composed of a series of bones that extend from the base of the skull to the pelvis. It is formed from 26 irregular bones (**vertebrae**, singular: **vertebra**) and connective tissue in such a way that a flexible, curved structure results. The spine is divided into sections corresponding to the vertebrae located in the spinal column. These divisions are as follows:

- Cervical (neck)
- Thoracic (chest)
- Lumbar (loin)
- Sacral (lower back)
- Coccyx (tailbone)

  It is time to review body cavities, the spine, and directional terms by completing Learning Activity 4–1.

Medical Word Elements

This section introduces combining forms, suffixes, and prefixes related to body structure. Word analyses are also provided. From the information provided, complete the meaning of the medical words in the right-hand column. The first one is completed for you.

Element	Meaning	Word Analysis and Meaning
Combining Forms		
Cellular Structure		
cyt/o	cell	**cyt/o**/logist (sī-TŎL-ō-jĭst): *specialist in the study of cells* *-logist:* specialist in the study of *Cytologists study the formation, structure, and function of cells.*
hist/o	tissue	**hist/o**/logy (hĭs-TŎL-ō-jē): _____ *-logy:* study of *Histology is the branch of science that investigates the microscopic structures and functions of tissues.*
kary/o	nucleus	**kary/o**/lysis (kăr-ē-ŎL-ĭ-sĭs): _____ *-lysis:* separation; destruction; loosening *Karyolysis results in death of the cell.*
nucle/o		**nucle**/ar (NŪ-klē-ăr): _____ *-ar:* pertaining to
Position and Direction		
anter/o	anterior, front	**anter**/ior (ăn-TĒR-ē-or): _____ *-ior:* pertaining to
caud/o	tail	**caud**/ad (KAW-dăd): _____ *-ad:* toward
cephal/o	head	**cephal**/ad (SĔF-ă-lăd) *-ad:* toward
dist/o	far, farthest	**dist**/al (DĬS-tăl): _____ *-al:* pertaining to
dors/o	back (of body)	**dors**/al (DOR-săl): _____ *-al:* pertaining to
infer/o	lower, below	**infer**/ior (ĭn-FĒR-rē-or): _____ *-ior:* pertaining to
later/o	side, to one side	**later**/al (LĂT-ĕr-ăl): _____ *-al:* pertaining to
medi/o	middle	**medi**/ad (MĒ-dē-ăd): _____ *-ad:* toward

Continued

Medical Word Elements—cont'd

Element	Meaning	Word Analysis and Meaning
poster/o	back (of body), behind, posterior	**poster/**ior (pōs-TĔR-ē-or): _____ -_ior:_ pertaining to
proxim/o	near, nearest	**proxim/**al (PRŎK-sĭm-ăl): _____
ventr/o	belly, belly side	**ventr/**al (VĔN-trăl): _____ -_al:_ pertaining to
Color		
albin/o	white	**albin/**ism (ĂL-bĭn-ĭzm): _____ -_ism:_ condition *Albinism is characterized by a partial or total lack of pigment in the skin, hair, and eyes.*
leuk/o		**leuk/o/**cyte (LOO-kō-sīt): _____ -_cyte:_ cell *A leukocyte is a white blood cell.*
chrom/o	color	hetero/**chrom/**ic (hĕt-ĕr-ō-KRŌ-mĭk): _____ _hetero-:_ different -_ic:_ pertaining to *Heterochromia is associated with the iris or sections of the iris of the eyes. Thus, the individual with heterochromia may have one brown iris and one blue iris.*
cirrh/o	yellow	**cirrh/**osis (sĭr-RŌ-sĭs): _____ -_osis:_ abnormal condition; increase (used primarily with blood cells) *In cirrhosis, the skin, sclera of the eyes, and mucous membranes take on a yellow color.*
jaund/o		**jaund/**ice (JAWN-dĭs): _____ -_ice:_ noun ending *Jaundice is the yellowing of the skin, mucous membranes, and sclera caused by excessive bilirubin in the blood.*
xanth/o		**xanth/**oma (ZĂN-thō-sĭs): _____ -_oma:_ tumor *A xanthoma is a nodule or patch composed of lipoid material commonly associated with disturbances in lipid metabolism.*
cyan/o	blue	**cyan/o/**tic (sī-ăn-ŎT-ĭk): _____ -_tic:_ pertaining to *Cyanosis is associated with lack of oxygen in the blood and a bluish discoloration of the skin.*
erythr/o	red	**erythr/o/**cyte (ĕ-RĬTH-rō-sīt): _____ -_cyte:_ cell *An erythrocyte is a red blood cell.*
melan/o	black	**melan/**oma (mĕl-ă-NŌ-mă): _____ -_oma:_ tumor *Melanoma is a malignancy that arises from melanocytes.*

Medical Word Elements—cont'd

Element	Meaning	Word Analysis and Meaning
poli/o	gray; gray matter (of the brain or spinal cord)	**poli/o**/myel/itis (pō-lē-ō-mī-ĕ-LĪ-tĭs): _____ *myel:* bone marrow; spinal cord *-itis:* inflammation

Other

Element	Meaning	Word Analysis and Meaning
radi/o	radiation, x-ray; radius (lower arm bone on thumb side)	**radi/o**/logist (rā-dē-ŎL-ŏ-jĭst): _____ *-logist:* specialist in the study of *Radiologists are physicians who employ imaging techniques to help medical doctors diagnose and treat diseases.*
tom/o	to cut	**tom/o**/graphy (tō-MŎG-ră-fē): _____ *-graphy:* process of recording *Tomography is an imaging procedure that employs a computer to produce images that appear as cuts (or slices) of an organ or structure.*
viscer/o	internal organs	**viscer**/al (VĬS-ĕr-ăl): _____ *-al:* pertaining to

Suffixes

Element	Meaning	Word Analysis and Meaning
-ar	pertaining to	lumb/**ar** (LŬM-băr): _____ *lumb/o:* loins (lower back)
-ic	pertaining to	gastr/**ic** (ĕp-ĭ-GĂS-trĭk): _____ *gastr/o:* stomach
-graphy	process of recording	son/o/**graphy** (sō-NŎG-ră-fē): _____ *son/o:* sound *Sonography is a diagnostic imaging procedure using sound in the inaudible range (ultrasound) to visualize internal structures.*

Prefixes

Element	Meaning	Word Analysis and Meaning
infra-	below, under	**infra**/cost/al (ĭn-fră-KŎS-tăl): _____ *cost:* ribs *-al:* pertaining to
peri-	around	**peri**/umbilic/al (pĕr-ē-ŭm-BĬL-ĭ-kăl): _____ *umbilic:* umbilicus, navel *-al:* pertaining to
super-	upper, above	**super**/ior (soo-PĒ-rē-or): _____ *-ior:* pertaining to *Superior is a directional term meaning toward the head or upper portion of a structure.*
ultra-	excess, beyond	**ultra**/son/ic (ŭl-tră-SŎN-ĭk): _____ *son:* sound *-ic:* pertaining to *Ultrasound includes sound frequencies too high to be perceived by the human ear.*

⊕ *It is time to review medical word elements by completing Learning Activities 4–2 and 4–3.*

Disease Focus

All body cells require oxygen and nutrients for survival. They also need a stable internal environment (**homeostasis**) that provides a narrow range of temperature, water, acidity, and salt concentration. When homeostasis is disrupted and cells, tissues, organs, or systems are unable to function effectively, the condition is called **disease**. From a clinical point of view, disease is a **pathological**, or **morbid**, condition that presents a group of signs, symptoms, and clinical findings. **Signs** are objective indicators that are observable. A rash, tissue redness, and swelling are examples of signs. In Figure 4-6, the rash is a sign of rubella (German measles), which is an acute infectious disease.

Figure 4-6 Skin rash (a sign of disease).

A **symptom (Sx)** is a subjective indicator of disease. As such, only the patient can experience it. Dizziness, pain, and nausea are examples of symptoms. Clinical findings are the results of radiological, laboratory, and other medical procedures performed on the patient or the patient's specimens (see Fig. 4-6).

Establishing a **diagnosis (Dx)**, the cause and nature of a disease, helps in the selection of a **treatment (Tx)**. A **prognosis** is the prediction of the course of a disease and its probable outcome. An **idiopathic disease** is one whose cause is unknown or exists without any connection with a known cause. Some diseases, injuries, or treatments cause complications. For example, a head injury may cause paralysis, and treatment with a toxic drug may cause deafness.

A variety of diagnostic and therapeutic procedures can help identify and treat diseases. These procedures are categorized as clinical, surgical, endoscopic, laboratory, and imaging procedures. Many diagnostic and therapeutic procedures include more than one testing modality. For example, many surgical procedures are undertaken using radiological methods to guide the surgeon during the procedure.

Each of the various types of imaging modalities produces a unique type of image. Physicians select the type of imaging procedure that provides the information that is relevant to a particular diagnosis or treatment (see Fig. 4-7).

Figure 4-7 Medical imaging. (A) Chest radiograph of the mediastinum. (B) Ultrasonography of blood flow with colors indicating direction. (C) Nuclear scan of the liver and spleen. (D) Computed tomography (CT) scan of the eye in lateral view showing a tumor (arrows). (E) Magnetic resonance imaging (MRI) scan of the midsagittal section of the head. (F) Positron emission tomography (PET) scan of the brain in transverse section (frontal lobes at top).

Diseases and Conditions

This section introduces diseases and conditions, along with their meanings and their pronunciations. These terms are applicable to the body system chapters that follow. Word analyses for selected terms are also provided.

Term	Definition
adhesion ăd-HĒ-zhŭn	Abnormal fibrous band that holds or binds together tissues that are normally separated *Adhesions may occur within body cavities as a result of surgery (see Fig. 4-8).*

Figure 4-8 Abdominal adhesions

edema ĕ-DĒ-mă	Abnormal accumulation of fluid within tissue spaces as a result of systemic disease or failure of the lymphatic system to drain tissue fluid from the site (see Fig. 4-9A) *After applying pressure to a small area, if the indentation persists after the release of pressure, the condition is known as pitting edema (see Fig. 4-9B).*

A   B

Figure 4-9 Edema. (A) Right normal foot and left foot with edema. (B) Pitting edema of the foot.

Diseases and Conditions—cont'd

Term	Definition
febrile FĒ-brĭl	Having or showing symptoms of a fever
gangrene GĂNG-grēn	Death and decay of soft tissue, usually caused by circulatory obstruction or infection *Risk of developing gangrene of the extremities is associated with diabetes and atherosclerosis as a result of poor circulation.*
hernia HĔR-nē-ă	Protrusion of any organ through the structure that normally contains it
inflammation ĭn-flă-MĀ-shŭn	Body defense against injury, infection, or allergy marked by redness, swelling, heat, and pain, sometimes with loss of function *Inflammation is a mechanism used by the body to protect against invasion by foreign organisms and to repair injured tissue.*
mycosis mī-KŌ-sĭs *myc:* fungus (plural, *fungi*) *-osis:* abnormal condition; increase (used primarily with blood cells)	Any fungal infection in or on the body *Mycotic infections can be superficial, affecting the skin, or deep seated, affecting structures beneath the skin, especially the brain, bone marrow, or other internal organs.*
perforation pĕr-fō-RĀ-shŭn	Hole that completely penetrates a structure *A perforation in the gastrointestinal tract is a medical emergency because gastrointestinal contents may flow into the abdominal cavity and infect the peritoneum.*
peritonitis pĕr-ĭ-tō-NĪ-tĭs *periton:* peritoneum *-I:* inflammation	Inflammation of the peritoneum, the serous membrane that surrounds the abdominal cavity and covers its organs, usually caused by bacteria or fungi *Peritonitis requires prompt medical attention to fight the infection and, if necessary, to treat any underlying medical conditions.*
rupture RŬP-chūr	Sudden breaking or bursting of a structure or organ
septicemia sĕp-tĭ-SĒ-mē-ă	Severe bacterial infection of the tissues that spreads to the blood; also called *sepsis* or *blood poisoning* *In septicemia, bacteria and their endotoxins cause severe systemic symptoms.*
suppuration sŭp-ū-RĀ-shŭn	Process of forming pus *Suppuration occurs when the agent that provoked the inflammation is difficult to eliminate.*

It is time to review diseases and conditions by completing Learning Activity 4–4.

Diagnostic and Surgical Procedures

This section introduces surgical and diagnostic procedures that are applicable in the body systems chapters. Descriptions are provided, along with pronunciations and word analyses for selected terms.

Procedure	Description
Diagnostic	
Clinical	
assessment techniques	Sequence of procedures designed to evaluate the health status of a patient
auscultation aws-kŭl-TĀ-shŭn	Listening to the heart, bowel, and lungs with or without a stethoscope to assess the presence and quality of sounds
inspection	General observation of the patient as a whole, progressing to specific body areas
palpation păl-PĀ-shŭn	Gentle application of the hands to a specific structure or body area to determine size, consistency, texture, symmetry, and tenderness of underlying structures
percussion pĕr-KŬSH-ŭn	Tapping a body structure with the hand or fingers to assess consistency and the presence or absence of fluids within the underlying structure *Percussion is especially helpful in assessing the thorax and abdomen.*

Diagnostic and Surgical Procedures—cont'd

Procedure	Description
Endoscopic	
endoscopy ĕn-DŎS-kō-pē *endo-:* in, within *-scopy:* visual examination	Visual examination of a body cavity or canal using a specialized lighted instrument called an endoscope *Endoscopy is used for biopsy, surgery, aspiration of fluids, and coagulation of bleeding areas. The endoscope is usually named for the organ, cavity, or canal being examined, such as gastroscope and sigmoidoscope. A camera and video recorder are used during the procedure to provide a permanent digital record (see Fig. 4–10).*

Figure 4-10 Endoscopy (gastroscopy). Doctor directing the endoscope through the oral cavity and throat into the stomach while performing gastroscopy on the patient.

Laboratory	
blood chemistry analysis ă-NĂL-ĭ-sĭs	Laboratory test, usually performed on serum, to determine biochemical imbalances, abnormalities, and nutritional conditions *An example of a blood chemistry analysis is the cholesterol test. The results will identify the patient's cholesterol value and where it falls in the normal or abnormal range.*

Continued

Diagnostic and Surgical Procedures—cont'd

Procedure	Description
complete blood count (CBC)	Broad screening test used to evaluate red blood cells, white blood cells, and platelets to determine anemias, infections, and other diseases *The CBC is usually included as part of routine physical examinations to determine general health status.*
culture and sensitivity (C&S)	Laboratory test of a body fluid placed on a culture medium to identify the cause of an infection (usually a bacterium) and a sensitivity test that determines which antibiotic drug works best to treat the infection *A C&S test may be done on many different body fluids, such as urine, mucus, blood, pus, saliva, spinal fluid, or discharge from the vagina or the penis (see Fig. 4–11).*

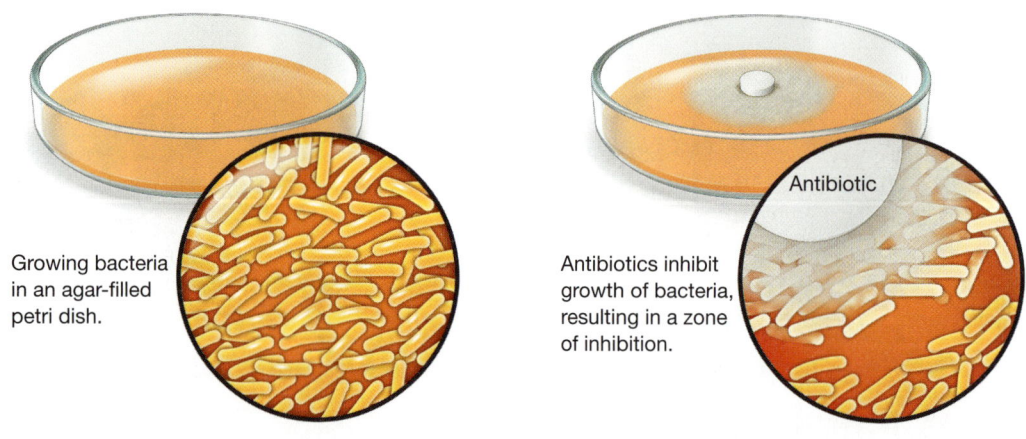

Growing bacteria in an agar-filled petri dish.

Antibiotic

Antibiotics inhibit growth of bacteria, resulting in a zone of inhibition.

Figure 4-11 Culture and sensitivity (C&S) laboratory test.

Imaging

computed tomography (CT) kŏm-PŪ-tĕd tō-MŎG-ră-fē *tom/o:* to cut *-graphy:* process of recording	Imaging technique that rotates an x-ray emitter around the area to be evaluated and measures the intensity of transmitted rays from different angles to generate a detailed cross-sectional image that appears as a three-dimensional slice of the body area (see Fig. 4-7D) *CT shows all types of tissues and makes soft tissue images clear. It may detect tumor masses, bone displacement, and fluid accumulation. This technique may be used with or without a contrast medium (see Fig. 4-12).*

Figure 4-12 Computed tomography (CT). (A) Patient entering the x-ray scanner. (B) Control panel and screen of a CT scanner.

Diagnostic and Surgical Procedures—cont'd

Procedure	Description
fluoroscopy floo-or-ŎS-kō-pē *fluor/o:* luminous, fluorescent *-scopy:* visual examination	Technique in which x-rays are directed through the body to a fluorescent screen that displays internal structures in continuous motion *Fluoroscopy helps to view the motion of organs and follow the movement of contrast dye during a cardiac catheterization, an angiography, or an upper gastrointestinal series (barium swallow) and to aid in the placement of catheters or other devices.*
magnetic resonance imaging (MRI) RĔZ-ĕn-ăns ĬM-ăj-ĭng	Technique that uses radio waves and a strong magnetic field, rather than an x-ray beam, to produce highly detailed, multiplanar, cross-sectional views of soft tissues (see Fig. 4-7E) *MRI helps diagnose a growing number of diseases because it provides superior soft tissue contrast. It commonly proves superior to CT scan for most central nervous system images, musculoskeletal images, and images of the pelvic areas. The procedure usually does not require a contrast medium.*
nuclear scan NŪ-klē-ăr	Technique in which a radioactive material (radiopharmaceutical) called a tracer is introduced into the body (inhaled, ingested, or injected), and a specialized camera (gamma camera) produces images of organs and structures (see Fig. 4-7C) *A nuclear scan is the reverse of a conventional radiograph. Rather than being directed into the body, radiation comes from inside the body and is then detected by a specialized camera to produce an image.*
positron emission tomography (PET) PŎZ-ĭ-trŏn ē-MĬSH-ŭn tō-MŎG-ră-fē	CT records the positrons (positively charged particles) emitted from a radiopharmaceutical to produce a cross-sectional image of the metabolic activity of body tissues to determine the presence of disease (see Fig. 4-7F) *PET is particularly useful in scanning the brain and nervous system to diagnose disorders that involve abnormal tissue metabolism, such as schizophrenia, brain tumors, epilepsy, stroke, Alzheimer disease, and pulmonary disorders.*
radiography rā-dē-ŎG-ră-fē *radi/o:* radiation, x-ray; radius (lower arm bone on thumb side) *-graphy:* process of recording	Technique in which x-rays are passed through the body or area and captured on a film to generate an image; also called x-ray (see Fig. 4-7A) *Radiography of soft tissue usually requires the use of a contrast medium to enhance images. Commonly used x-ray contrast media are barium and iodine compounds.*
single-photon emission computed tomography (SPECT) FŌ-tŏn ē-MĬ-shŭn tō-MŎG-ră-fē *tom/o:* to cut *-graphy:* process of recording	Radiological technique that integrates CT and a radioactive material (tracer) injected into the bloodstream to visualize blood flow to tissues and organs *SPECT differs from a PET scan in that the tracer remains in the bloodstream rather than being absorbed by surrounding tissue. It is especially useful to visualize blood flow through arteries and veins in the brain.*
ultrasonography (US) ŭl-tră-sŏn-ŎG-ră-fē *ultra-:* excess, beyond *son/o:* sound *-graphy:* process of recording	High-frequency sound waves (ultrasound) are directed at soft tissue and reflected as "echoes" to produce an image on a monitor of an internal body structure; also called ultrasound, sonography, and echo (see Fig. 4-7B) *US, unlike most other imaging methods, creates real-time moving images, allowing the visualization of organs and functions of organs in motion. A computer analyzes the reflected echoes and converts them into an image on a video monitor. Because this procedure does not utilize ionizing radiation (x-ray), it is used during pregnancy to observe fetal growth and also to study other internal organs for possible pathologies or lesions.*

Continued

Diagnostic and Surgical Procedures—cont'd

Procedure	Description
Surgical	
biopsy (bx) BĪ-ŏp-sē	Removal of a representative tissue sample from a body site for microscopic examination, usually to establish a diagnosis
excisional ĕk-SĬ-zhŭn-ăl	Biopsy in which the entire lesion is removed
incisional ĭn-SĬZH-ŭn-ăl	Biopsy in which only a small sample of the lesion is removed
Surgical	
ablation ăb-LĀ-shŭn	Removal of a body part, pathway, or function by surgery, chemical destruction, electrocautery, freezing, or radio frequency (RF) *Ablation procedures are common for treating atrial fibrillation and varicose veins and destroying abnormal tissues found in various organs, including the lungs, liver, kidneys, and uterus.*
anastomosis ă-năs-tō-MŌ-sĭs	Surgical joining of two ducts, vessels, or bowel segments to allow flow from one to another (see Fig. 4-13) End-to-end anastomosis End-to-side anastomosis Side-to-side anastomosis **Figure 4-13** Anastomoses.
curettage kū-rĕ-TĂZH	Scraping of a body cavity with a spoon-shaped instrument called a *curette* (curet)
electrocauterization ē-lĕk-trō-KAW-tĕr-ĭ-ZĀ-shŭn *electr/o:* electricity *cauter:* heat, burn *-ization:* process (of)	Use of an electrically activated instrument to burn and destroy diseased tissue *Electrocauterization is used to prevent or stop bleeding after an injury or during surgery, destroy abnormal tissue, remove skin growths, and treat chronic nosebleeds.*
incision and drainage (I&D) ĭn-SĬZH-ŭn, DRĀN-ĭj	Incision made to allow the free flow of fluids and pus from a wound, abscess, or body cavity

Diagnostic and Surgical Procedures—cont'd

Procedure	Description
laser surgery LĂ-zĕr SŬR-jĕr-ē	Use of a high-intensity laser light beam to remove diseased tissues, to stop bleeding, or for cosmetic purposes *Laser surgery is used in a wide variety of noninvasive and minimally invasive procedures, including removal of lesions, scars, tattoos, wrinkles, sunspots, or birthmarks.*
revision	Surgical procedure used to replace or compensate for a previously implanted device or correct an undesirable result or effect of a previous surgery
robotic-assisted surgery (RAS)	Minimally invasive surgery technique performed through small incisions, or no incisions, that employs the use of robotic arms for holding instruments, a camera, and magnifying screen that are controlled by the doctor sitting at a computer console manipulating the instruments attached to the robotic arms to perform the operation (see Fig. 4-14) *Robotic surgery has a greater range of motion and dexterity with fewer resulting complications during surgery. Other advantages include less blood loss, lower rate of infection, fewer complications, less pain, and faster recovery. Doctors must be successfully trained in the robotic surgical system utilized at their facility.*

Figure 4-14 Robotic-assisted surgery (RAS). The surgeon sits at a computer console to direct robotic arms above the patient on the surgery table as nurses and other members of the surgical team facilitate the operation.

Abbreviations

This section introduces body structure abbreviations and their meanings.

Abbreviation	Meaning	Abbreviation	Meaning
AP	anteroposterior	LUQ	left upper quadrant
Bx, bx	biopsy	MRI	magnetic resonance imaging
CBC	complete blood count	PET	positron emission tomography
C&S	culture and sensitivity	RLQ	right lower quadrant
CT	computed tomography	RUQ	right upper quadrant
DNA	deoxyribonucleic acid	SPECT	single-photon emission computed tomography
Dx	diagnosis	Sx	symptom
I&D	incision and drainage	Tx	treatment
LAT, lat	lateral	U&L, U/L	upper and lower
LLQ	left lower quadrant	US	ultrasound, ultrasonography

It is time to review procedures and abbreviations by completing Learning Activity 4–5.

LEARNING ACTIVITIES

The activities that follow provide review of the body structure terms introduced in this chapter. Complete each activity and review your answers to evaluate your understanding of the chapter.

Learning Activity 4-1
Body Structures and Directional Terms

Match each term on the left with its meaning on the right.

1. _____ abdominopelvic	a. pertaining to the sole of the foot
2. _____ abduction	b. tailbone
3. _____ cervical	c. ventral cavity that contains the heart, lungs, and associated structures
4. _____ coccyx	d. movement away from the midsagittal plane of the body
5. _____ adduction	e. lying horizontal with face downward
6. _____ eversion	f. turning outward
7. _____ inferior (caudal)	g. nearer to the center (trunk of the body)
8. _____ inversion	h. ventral cavity that contains digestive, reproductive, and excretory structures
9. _____ lumbar	i. turning inward or inside out
10. _____ plantar	j. part of the spine known as the *neck*
11. _____ posterior (dorsal)	k. movement toward the median plane
12. _____ prone	l. away from the head; toward the tail or lower part of a structure
13. _____ proximal	m. pertaining to the outer wall of a body cavity
14. _____ parietal	n. part of the spine known as the *loin*
15. _____ thoracic	o. near the back of the body

 Check your answers in Appendix A. Review any material that you did not answer correctly.

Correct Answers _____ **X 6.67 =** _____ **% Score**

Medical Language Lab
Turning terminology into language

Visit the Medical Language Laboratory at the website medicallanguagelab.com. Use it to enhance your study and for reinforcement of this chapter with the flash card activity. We recommend that you complete the flash card activity before starting Learning Activities 4-2 and 4-3.

Learning Activity 4-2
Basic Word Elements

Select the word element that matches the definition in the numbered list.

Combining Forms		Suffixes	Prefixes
anter/o	leuk/o	-ar	endo-
caud/o	melan/o	-graphy	peri-
cyan/o	poli/o		super-
dist/o	proxim/o		ultra-
dors/o	tom/o		
hist/o	ventr/o		
later/o	xanth/o		

1. black _____
2. far, farthest _____
3. pertaining to _____
4. anterior, front _____
5. white _____
6. blue _____
7. yellow _____
8. back (of body) _____
9. gray; gray matter (of the brain or spinal cord) _____
10. around _____
11. side, to one side _____
12. tail _____
13. to cut _____
14. excess, beyond _____
15. belly, belly side _____
16. upper, above _____
17. tissue _____
18. near, nearest _____
19. process of recording _____
20. in, within _____

Check your answers in Appendix A. Review any material that you did not answer correctly.

Correct Answers _____ **X 5 =** _____ **% Score**

Learning Activity 4-3

Building Basic Terms

Read the definition in the numbered list. Then select two elements from the table to build a medical word. You may use the elements more than once. The first one is completed for you.

Combining Forms		Suffixes		Prefixes
albin/o	gastr/o	-ad	-logist	epi-
anter/o	melan/o	-al	-oma	hypo-
cephal/o	myc/o	-cyte	-osis	
chrom/o	radi/o	-ic		
cirrh/o	spin/o	-ior		
dors/o	ventr/o	-ism		
erythr/o	viscer/o	-itis		

1. pertaining to the front (of the body) anterior _____
2. toward the head _____
3. pertaining to the back (of the body) _____
4. pertaining to the belly side (front of the body) _____
5. abnormal condition of yellow (ing) _____
6. cell that is red _____
7. tumor that is black _____
8. specialist in the study of radiation or x-rays _____
9. pertaining to above the (area of the) stomach _____
10. pertaining to under or below the (area of the) stomach _____
11. pertaining to color _____
12. abnormal condition of fungus _____
13. pertaining to internal organs _____
14. condition of white (lack of pigment in the skin) _____
15. pertaining to the spine _____

✓ *Check your answers in Appendix A. Review any material that you did not answer correctly.*

Correct Answers _____ **X 6.67 =** _____ **% Score**

Learning Activity 4-4
Building Medical Words

Use *cyt/o* to build words that mean

   1. specialist in the study of cells _____

   2. study of cells _____

Use *–cyte* (cells) to build words that mean

   3. red (blood) cell _____

   4. white (blood) cell _____

   5. black cell _____

Use *–al* (pertaining to) to build words that mean *pertaining to the*

   6. belly or belly side _____

   7. nearest (point of attachment) _____

   8. middle _____

   9. farthest (point of attachment) _____

10. side, to one side _____

Use *–scopy* (visual examination) to build words that mean *visual examination*

11. using luminous or fluorescence _____

12. in, within (the body) _____

Use *–logy* to build words that mean *study of*

13. cells _____

14. the stomach _____

15. tissue _____

  ✓ *Check your answers in Appendix A. Review any material that you did not answer correctly.*

Correct Answers _____ **X 6.67 =** _____ **% Score**

Learning Activity 4-5
Diseases and Conditions

adhesion	hernia	peritonitis
diagnosis	inflammation	prognosis
edema	jaundice	septicemia
febrile	melanoma	suppuration
gangrene	perforation	symptom

Match the terms with the definitions in the numbered list.

1. characterized by an elevated body temperature _____
2. establishing the cause and nature of a disease _____
3. fibrous band that binds together tissues that are normally separated _____
4. death and decay of soft tissue _____
5. protrusion of any organ through the structure that normally contains it _____
6. inflammation of the serous membrane that surrounds the abdominal cavity _____
7. severe bacterial infection of the tissues that spreads to the blood _____
8. producing or forming pus _____
9. prediction of the course of a disease and its probable outcome _____
10. body defense against injury, infection, or allergy, marked by redness, heat, pain, and swelling _____
11. yellowing of the skin and sclera caused by excessive bilirubin in the blood _____
12. subjective indicator of a disease _____
13. abnormal accumulation of fluid in tissue spaces _____
14. malignancy that arises from melanocytes _____
15. hole that forms through a structure or a body part _____

Check your answers in Appendix A. Review any material that you did not answer correctly.

Correct Answers _____ **X 6.67 =** _____ **% Score**

Learning Activity 4-6
Procedures and Abbreviations

Match the terms with the definitions in the numbered list.

ablation	*curettage*	*MRI*
anastomosis	*electrocautery*	*nuclear scan*
CBC	*endoscopy*	*palpation*
computed tomography	*fluoroscopy*	*robotic surgery*
C&S	*I&D*	*US*

 1. technique with the advantages of less blood loss, lower rate of infection, fewer complications, less pain, and faster recovery _____

 2. scraping of a body cavity with a spoon-shaped instrument _____

 3. panel of blood tests used as a broad screening test for anemias, infections, and other diseases _____

 4. removal of a part, pathway, or function by surgery, chemical destruction, or other technique _____

 5. visual examination of a cavity or canal using a special lighted instrument _____

 6. imaging technique that directs x-rays to a fluorescent screen and displays live images on a monitor _____

 7. utilizes high-frequency sound waves to produce images of internal body structures_____

 8. use of an electrically activated instrument to burn and destroy diseased tissue _____

 9. determines which antibiotic drug will work best to treat an infection _____

10. imaging procedure that uses radio waves and a strong magnetic field to produce images _____

11. surgical joining of two ducts, vessels, or bowel segments _____

12. imaging procedure that uses a radioactive material introduced into the body to produce an image _____

13. gentle application of hands to evaluate a specific structure of the body _____

14. incision that allows a free flow of fluids or pus from a wound _____

15. imaging procedure that generates detailed cross-sectional images that appear as slices _____

✔ *Check your answers in Appendix A. Review any material that you did not answer correctly.*

Correct Answers _____ **X 6.67 =** _____ **% Score**

DOCUMENTING HEALTH CARE

The electronic medical record (EMR) is a systematic collection in digital format of a patient's health history. In other words, it is an electronic version of a paper medical chart. The EMR contains a history of the patient's medical care, including diagnoses, treatments, and other vital health information. The digital version allows practitioners to electronically monitor and track the health status, preventive health services, treatments, and care planning of patients and serves as a more efficient method of documenting patient care. The electronic connection provides a platform to share medical documents between providers who are caring for the same patient so that there is continuity of treatment without duplication of effort.

Besides ease of access, this method of documentation decreases errors associated with poor penmanship, lost pages, and misfiled records. It also provides documentation of health-care information that will be needed if legal issues arise. In addition, it is the basis for reimbursement of medical services. Therefore, it is important that all information entered into the medical record be complete, current, correct, and maintained in confidentiality.

Currently, increasing numbers of physician offices, clinics, hospitals, and other medical settings are providing patients with access to their individual EMRs. In this way, the EMR is available instantly and securely for patients and other authorized users. The Documenting Health-Care Activities in this chapter and throughout the book are designed to familiarize you with the appearance and terminology of various medical records and to develop the critical thinking skills necessary to interpret these records in a medical setting.

DOCUMENTING HEALTH-CARE ACTIVITIES

This section provides practical application activities in the form of exercises to help students develop skills in documenting patient care. First, read the medical report. Then complete the activities and exercises that follow.

Documenting Health-Care Activity 4-1
Emergency Department Report: Spider Bite

General Hospital and Medical Center
2422 Rodeo Drive ■ ■ Sun City, USA 12345 ■ ■ (555) 333–2427

Date of Visit: 07/05/20XX
Patient Name: Albert Wild   **Patient ID:** 955-78-21
Birth Date: 05/14/20XX   **Room Number:** ER

CHIEF COMPLAINT: Spider bite, left thigh

HISTORY OF PRESENT ILLNESS: This is an 18-year-old male who comes to the emergency department complaining of a spider bite to his left thigh. The spider bite has been there for several weeks. The area on his left thigh is red and very painful. He denies any fever. He says it hurts when he stands and walks. Pain is 7/10. Nursing notes reviewed.

REVIEW OF SYSTEMS: He denies weakness, numbness, or tingling. Review of systems otherwise negative.

PAST MEDICAL HISTORY: None.

ALLERGIES: None.

CURRENT MEDICATIONS: None.

IMMUNIZATIONS: Up to date.

SOCIAL HISTORY: He does smoke one pack of cigarettes a day.

PHYSICAL EXAMINATION:

VITAL SIGNS: Temperature 98.8, pulse 72, respirations 16, blood pressure 110/70, oxygen saturation on room air 98%.
GENERAL: Well-appearing, nontoxic 18-year-old male. He is alert. He is oriented x3. He is calm and cooperative during examination.
EXTREMITIES: Round, erythematous, fluctuant mass over the anterior, proximal portion of the left thigh. The area of induration measures 4 cm × 4 cm. The lesion and surrounding area of cellulitis are tender to palpation and warm to the touch. No drainage or ulceration noted. Full range of motion of the leg with very minimal pain over the medial and lateral aspects of the thigh. No lower extremity edema is noted. No lymphadenopathy noted.

DIAGNOSTICS: Culture sent to laboratory.

PROCEDURE: Incision and drainage. The area was prepped with Betadine, infiltrated with total of 9 mL bupivacaine without epinephrine with good results. The area was opened with an 11 blade. Hemostats were inserted in the wound to break up loculated fluid and debride this area. Unfortunately, this was not able to be packed. The area was bandaged.

IMPRESSION:
1. Left thigh abscess.

DISCHARGE INSTRUCTIONS:
1. Follow up with medicine on call in 2 days for wound check.
2. Return for pain, redness, and swelling.
3. Wound care instructions.
4. Bactrim DS morning and bedtime × 10 days.
5. Acetaminophen for pain prn.

Adrian Jones, MD
Adrian Jones, MD

aj:bg

D: 07/05/20XX

T: 07/05/20XX

Terminology

The terms listed in the table that follows are taken from *Emergency Room Report: Spider Bite.*
Use a medical dictionary such as *Taber's Cyclopedic Medical Dictionary,* the appendices of this
book, or other resources to define each term. Then review the pronunciations for each term
and practice by reading the medical record aloud.

Term	Definition
acetaminophen ă-sē-tă-MĬN-ŭh-fĭn	
Bactrim DS BĂK-trĭm	
bupivacaine bū-PĬV-ă-cān	
edema ĕ-DĒ-mă	
epinephrine ĕp-ĕ-NĔF-rĕn	
fluctuant mass FLŬK-chū-ănt	
erythematous ĕr-ĭ-THĔM-ă-tŭs	
lymphadenopathy lĭm-făd-ĕ- NŎP-ă-thē	

Visit the Medical Terminology Systems online resource center at FADavis.com
to practice pronunciation and reinforce the meanings of the terms in this
medical report.

Critical Thinking

Review *Emergency Room: Spider Bite* to answer the questions.

1. What was the presenting problem?

2. How did the lesion affect the patient's leg movement?

3. What procedure was performed on the affected area?

4. What finding by the doctor led to performing this procedure?

5. Why was a culture performed on the wound?

6. What medication was prescribed to treat the infection?

Documenting Health-Care Activity 4-2

Radiology Report: Injury of Left Wrist, Elbow, and Humerus

General Hospital
1511 Ninth Avenue ■ ■ Sun City, USA 12345 ■ ■ (555) 802–1887

RADIOLOGY REPORT

Date:	June 5, 20xx	Patient:	Hill, Joan
Physician:	Adrian Jones, MD	DOB:	5/25/19xx
Examination:	Left wrist, left elbow, and left humerus	x-ray No.:	43201

Left Wrist: Images obtained with the patient's arm taped to an arm board. There are fractures through the distal shafts of the radius and ulna. The radial fracture fragments show approximately 8-mm overlap with dorsal displacement of the distal radial fracture fragment. The distal ulnar shaft fracture shows ventral-lateral angulation at the fracture apex. There is no over-riding at this fracture. No additional fracture is seen. Soft tissue deformity is present, correlating with the fracture sites.

Left Elbow and Left Humerus: Single view of the left elbow was obtained in the lateral projection. AP view of the humerus was obtained to include a portion of the elbow. A third radiograph was obtained but is not currently available for review. There is lucency through the distal humerus on the AP view along its medial aspect. It would be difficult to exclude fracture just above the medial epicondyle. On the lateral view, there is elevation of the anterior and posterior fat pad. These findings are of some concern. Repeat elbow study is recommended.

Adrian Jones, MD
Adrian Jones, MD

JS: bg

D: 6–05–20xx
T: 6–05–20xx

Terminology

The terms listed in the table that follows are taken from *Radiology Report: Injury of Left Wrist, Elbow, and Humerus.* Use a medical dictionary such as *Taber's Cyclopedic Medical Dictionary,* the appendices of this book, or other resources to define each term. Then review the pronunciations for each term and practice by reading the medical record aloud.

Term	Definition
AP	
anterior ăn-TĬR-ē-or	
distal DĬS-tăl	
dorsal DOR-săl	
epicondyle ĕp-ĭ-KŎN-dĭl	
humerus HŪ-mĕr-ŭs	
lucency LOO-sĕnt-sē	
medial MĒ-dē-ăl	
mm	
posterior	
radius RĀ-dē-ŭs	
ulna ŬL-nă	
ventral-lateral VĔN-trăl-LĂT-ĕr-ăl	

Visit the Medical Terminology Systems online resource center at FADavis.com to practice pronunciation and reinforce the meanings of the terms in this medical report.

Critical Thinking

Review *Radiology Report: Injury of Left Wrist, Elbow, and Humerus* to answer the questions.

1. Where are the fractures located?

_____

_____

_____

2. What caused the soft tissue deformity?

_____

_____

_____

3. Did the radiologist take any side views of the left elbow?

_____

_____

_____

4. In the AP view of the humerus, what structure was also visualized?

_____

_____

_____

5. What findings are causes of concern for the radiologist?

_____

_____

_____

Integumentary System

Chapter Outline

Objectives

Upon completion of this chapter, you will be able to:

- Locate the major organs of the integumentary system and describe their structure and function.
- Describe the functional relationship between the integumentary system and other body systems.
- Pronounce, spell, and build words related to the integumentary system.
- Describe diseases, conditions, and procedures related to the integumentary system.
- Explain pharmacology associated with the treatment of skin disorders.
- Demonstrate your knowledge of this chapter by completing the learning and documenting health-care activities.

Anatomy and Physiology

The skin, also called the **integument**, is the largest organ in the body. Together with its accessory organs (hair, nails, and glands), the skin makes up the **integumentary system**. This elaborate system of distinct tissues includes glands that produce several types of secretions, nerves that transmit impulses, and blood vessels that help regulate body temperature. The skin covers and protects all outer surfaces of the body and performs many vital functions, including the sense of touch.

Anatomy and Physiology Key Terms

This section introduces important terms, along with their definitions and pronunciations. The key terms are highlighted in color in the Anatomy and Physiology section. Word analyses for selected terms are also provided. Pronounce the term and place a check mark in the box after you do so.

Term	Definition
androgen ☐ ĂN-drō-jĕn	Generic term for an agent (usually a hormone, such as testosterone or androsterone) that stimulates development of male characteristics *Androgens also regulate the production of sebum.*
ductule ☐ DŬK-tūl *duct:* to lead; carry *-ule:* small, minute	Very small duct
homeostasis ☐ hō-mē-ō-STĀ-sĭs *homeo-:* same, alike *-stasis:* standing still	State of equilibrium of the internal environment of the body despite changes in the external environment *Homeostasis encompasses the regulatory mechanisms of the body that control temperature, acidity, and the concentration of salt, food, and waste products.*
synthesize ☐ SĬN-thĕ-sīz	Forming a complex substance by the union of simpler compounds or elements *Skin synthesizes vitamin D (needed by bones for calcium absorption).*

Pronunciation Help	Long Sound	ā — rate	ē — rebirth	ī — isle	ō — over	ū — unite
	Short Sound	ă — apple	ĕ — ever	ĭ — it	ŏ — not	ŭ — cut

Skin

The skin protects underlying structures from injury and provides sensory information to the brain. Beneath the skin's surface is an intricate network of nerve fibers that register sensations of temperature, pain, and pressure. Other important functions of the skin include protecting the body against ultraviolet rays, regulating body temperature, and preventing dehydration. The skin also acts as a reservoir for food and water. It also **synthesizes** vitamin D when exposed to sunlight. The skin consists of two distinct layers: the epidermis and the dermis. A subcutaneous layer of tissue binds the skin to underlying structures (see Fig. 5-1).

Epidermis

The outer layer of the skin, the (1) **epidermis**, is relatively thin over most areas but is thickest on the palms of the hands and the soles of the feet. Although the epidermis is composed of several sublayers called **strata**, the (2) **stratum corneum** and the (3) **basal layer**, which is the deepest layer, are of greatest importance.

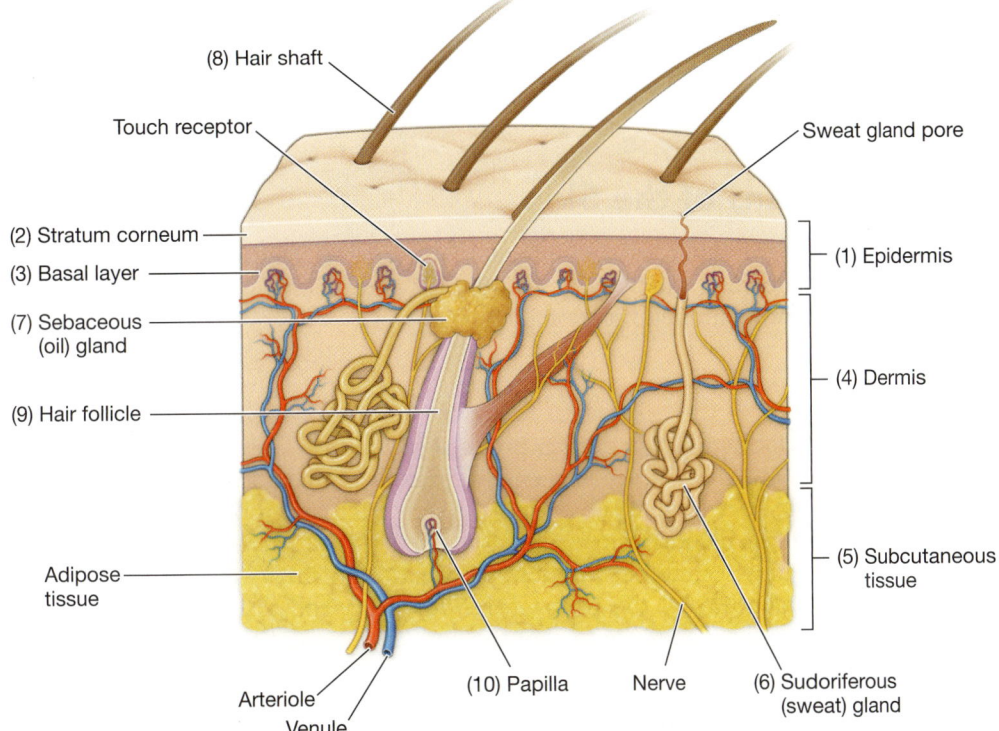

Figure 5-1 Structure of the skin and subcutaneous tissue.

The stratum corneum is composed of dead, flat cells that lack a blood supply and sensory receptors. Its thickness is related to normal wear of the area it covers. The basal layer is the only layer of the epidermis that is composed of living cells where new cells are formed. As these cells move toward the stratum corneum to replace the cells that have been sloughed off, they die and become filled with a hard protein material called **keratin**. The relatively waterproof characteristic of keratin prevents body fluids from evaporating and moisture from entering the body. The entire process by which a cell forms in the basal layer, rises to the surface, becomes keratinized, and sloughs off takes about 1 month.

In the basal layer, special cells called **melanocytes** produce a black pigment called **melanin**. Melanin provides a protective barrier from the damaging effects of the sun's ultraviolet radiation, which can cause skin cancer. Moderate sun exposure increases the rate of melanin production and results in a suntan. However, overexposure results in sunburn caused by melanin's inability to absorb sufficient ultraviolet rays to prevent the burn.

Differences in skin color are attributed to the amount of melanin in each cell. Dark-skinned people produce large amounts of melanin and are less likely to have wrinkles or skin cancer. Production of melanocytes is genetically regulated and, thus, inherited. Local accumulations of melanin are seen in pigmented moles and freckles. An absence of pigment in the skin, eyes, and hair is most likely the result of an inherited inability to produce melanin. An individual who cannot produce melanin, known as an **albino**, has a marked deficiency of pigment in the eyes, hair, and skin.

Dermis

The second layer of the skin, the (4) **dermis**, also called the **corium**, lies directly beneath the epidermis. It is composed of living tissue and contains numerous capillaries, lymphatic vessels, and nerve endings. Hair follicles, **sebaceous** (oil) glands, and **sudoriferous** (sweat) glands are also located in the dermis.

The (5) **subcutaneous layer**, also called the **hypodermis**, binds the dermis to underlying structures. It is composed primarily of loose connective tissue and **adipose** (fat) tissue interlaced with blood vessels. The subcutaneous layer stores fats, insulates and cushions the body, and regulates temperature. The amount of fat in the subcutaneous layer varies with the region of the body and sex, age, and nutritional state.

Accessory Organs of the Skin

The accessory organs of the skin consist of integumentary glands, hair, and nails. The glands play an important role in defending the body against disease and maintaining **homeostasis**, whereas the hair and nails have more limited functional roles.

Glands

Two important glands located in the dermis produce secretions: The (6) **sudoriferous (sweat) glands** produce sweat and the (7) **sebaceous (oil) glands** produce oil. These two glands are **exocrine glands** because they secrete substances through ducts to an outer surface of the body rather than directly into the bloodstream.

The sudoriferous glands secrete perspiration, or sweat, onto the surface of the skin through pores. Pores are most plentiful on the palms, soles, forehead, and **axillae** (armpits). The main functions of the sudoriferous glands are to cool the body by evaporation, excrete waste products, and moisten surface cells.

The sebaceous glands are filled with cells, the centers of which contain fatty droplets. As these cells disintegrate, they yield an oily secretion called **sebum.** The acidic nature of sebum helps destroy harmful organisms on the skin, thus preventing infection. When **ductules** of the sebaceous glands become blocked, acne may result. Congested sebum causes formation of pimples or whiteheads. If the sebum is dark, it forms blackheads. Sex hormones, particularly **androgens**, regulate the production and secretion of sebum. During adolescence, secretions increase; as the person ages, secretions diminish. The loss of sebum, which lubricates the skin, may be one of the reasons for the formation of wrinkles that accompanies old age. Sebaceous glands are present over the entire body except on the soles of the feet and the palms of the hands. They are especially prevalent on the scalp and face; around such openings as the nose, mouth, external ear, and anus; and on the upper back.

Hair

Hair is found on nearly all parts of the body except for the lips, nipples, palms of the hands, soles of the feet, and parts of the external genitalia. The visible part of the hair is the (8) **hair shaft**; the part that is embedded in the dermis is the hair root. The root, together with its coverings, forms the (9) **hair follicle**. At the bottom of the follicle is a loop of capillaries enclosed in a covering called the (10) **papilla**. The cluster of epithelial cells lying over the papilla reproduces and is responsible for the eventual formation of the hair shaft. As long as these cells remain alive, hair will regenerate even if it is cut, plucked, or otherwise removed. Alopecia (baldness) occurs when the hairs of the scalp are not replaced because of death of the papillae (singular, *papilla*).

Like skin color, hair color is related to the amount of pigment produced by epidermal melanocytes. Melanocytes are found at the base of the hair follicle. Melanin ranges in color from yellow to reddish brown to black. Varying amounts of melanin produce hair ranging in color from blond to brunette to black; the more abundant the melanin, the darker the hair. Heredity and aging affect melanin levels. A decrease or an absence of melanin causes loss of hair color.

Nails

Nails protect the tips of the fingers and toes from bruises and injuries (see Fig. 5-2). Each nail is formed in the (1) **nail root** and is composed of keratinized, stratified, squamous epithelial cells producing a very tough covering. As the nail grows, it stays attached and slides forward over the

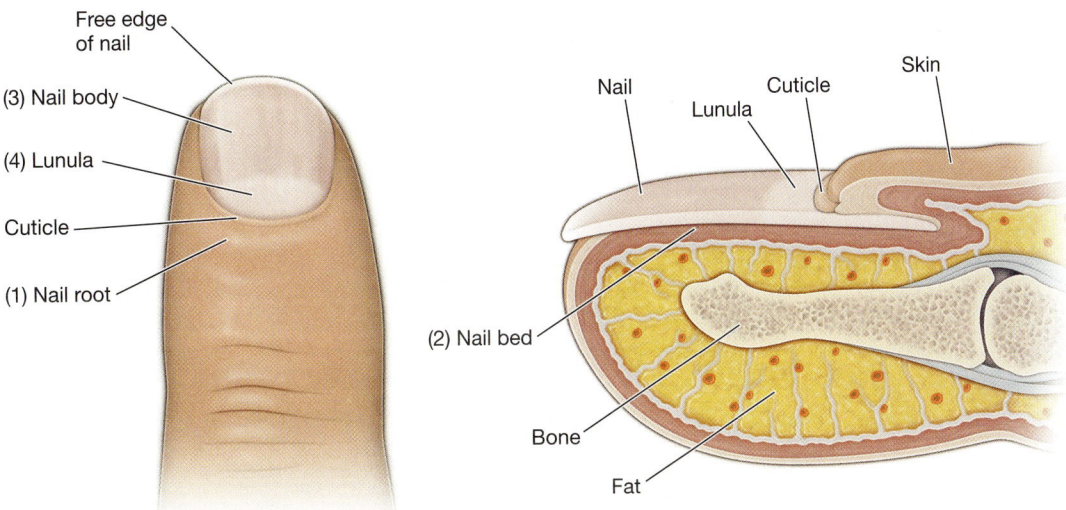

Figure 5-2 Structure of a fingernail.

layer of epithelium called the (2) **nailbed**. This epithelial layer is continuous with the epithelium of the skin. Most of the (3) **nail body** appears pink because of the underlying vascular tissue. The half-moon shaped area at the base of the nail, the (4) **lunula**, is the region where new growth occurs. The lunula has a whitish appearance because the vascular tissue underneath does not show through.

Anatomy Review: Integumentary System

To review the anatomy of the integumentary system, label the illustration using the listed terms.

basal layer

dermis

epidermis

hair follicle

hair shaft

papilla

sebaceous (oil) gland

stratum corneum

subcutaneous tissue

sudoriferous (sweat) gland

 Check your answers by referring to Figure 5–1 on page 91. Review material that you did not answer correctly.

CONNECTING BODY SYSTEMS—INTEGUMENTARY SYSTEM

The main function of the skin is to protect the entire body, including all of its organs, from the external environment. Specific functional relationships between the skin and other body systems are summarized here.

Blood, Lymphatic, and Immune
- Skin is the first line of defense against the invasion of pathogens into the body.

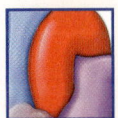

Cardiovascular
- Cutaneous blood vessels dilate and constrict to help regulate body temperature.

Digestive
- Skin absorbs vitamin D (produced when skin is exposed to sunlight), which is needed for intestinal absorption of calcium.
- Excess calories are stored as subcutaneous fat.

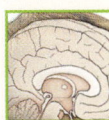

Endocrine
- The subcutaneous layer of the skin stores adipose tissue when insulin secretions cause excess carbohydrate intake to be stored as fat.

Female Reproductive
- Subcutaneous receptors provide pleasurable sensations associated with sexual behavior.
- Skin stretches to accommodate the growing fetus during pregnancy.

Male Reproductive
- Receptors in the skin respond to sexual stimuli.

Musculoskeletal
- Skin synthesizes the vitamin D needed for absorption of calcium, which is essential for muscle contraction.
- Skin also synthesizes the vitamin D needed for growth, repair, and maintenance of bones.

Nervous
- Cutaneous receptors detect stimuli related to touch, pain, pressure, and temperature.

Respiratory
- Skin temperature may influence respiratory rate. As temperature increases, respiratory rate may also increase.
- Hairs of the nasal cavity filter particles from inspired air before it reaches the lower respiratory tract.

Urinary
- Skin provides an alternative route for excreting salts and nitrogenous wastes in the form of perspiration.

Medical Word Elements

This section introduces combining forms, suffixes, and prefixes related to the integumentary system. Word analyses are also provided. From the information provided, complete the meaning of each medical word in the right–hand column. The first one is completed for you.

Element	Meaning	Word Analysis
Combining Forms		
adip/o	fat	**adip**/osis (ăd-ĭ-PŌ-sĭs): *abnormal condition of fat* *-osis:* abnormal condition; increase (used primarily with blood cells) *Adiposis is an abnormal accumulation of fatty tissue in the body.*
lip/o		**lip**/oma (lĭ-PŌ-mă): _____ *-oma:* tumor
steat/o		**steat**/itis (stē-ă-TĪ-tĭs): _____ *-itis:* inflammation
cutane/o	skin	sub/**cutane**/ous (sŭb-kū-TĀ-nē-ŭs): _____ *sub-:* under, below *-ous:* pertaining to
dermat/o		**dermat/o**/plasty (DĔR-mă-tō-plăs-tē): _____ *-plasty:* surgical repair
derm/o		hypo/**derm**/ic (hī-pō-DĔR-mĭk): _____ *hypo-:* under, below, deficient *-ic:* pertaining to *Hypodermic needles are used for subcutaneous injections.*
hidr/o	sweat	**hidr**/aden/itis (hī-drăd-ĕ-NĪ-tĭs): _____ *aden:* gland *-itis:* inflammation *Do not confuse* hidr/o *(sweat) with* hydr/o *(water).*
sudor/o		**sudor**/esis (soo-dō-RĒ-sĭs): _____ *-esis:* condition *Sudoresis is the body's physiological means to regulate body temperature.*
ichthy/o	dry, scaly	**ichthy**/osis (ĭk-thē-Ō-sĭs): _____ *-osis:* abnormal condition; increase (used primarily with blood cells) *Ichthyosis can be any of several dermatological conditions in which the skin is dry and hardened (hyperkeratotic), resembling fish scales. A mild form of ichthyosis, called* winter itch, *is commonly seen on the legs of older patients, especially during the winter months.*
kerat/o	horny tissue; hard; cornea	**kerat**/osis (kĕr-ă-TŌ-sĭs): _____ *-osis:* abnormal condition; increase (used primarily with blood cells) *Keratosis is a thickened area of the epidermis or any horny growth on the skin, such as a callus or wart.*

Medical Word Elements—cont'd

Element	Meaning	Word Analysis
melan/o	black	**melan/**oma (mĕl-ă-NŌ-mă): _____ *-oma:* tumor *Melanoma is a malignant tumor of melanocytes that commonly begins in a darkly pigmented mole and can metastasize widely.*
myc/	fungus (plural, fungi)	dermat/o/**myc/**osis (dĕr-mă-tō-mī-KŌ-sĭs): _____ *dermat/o:* skin *-osis:* abnormal condition; increase (used primarily with blood cells)
onych/o	nail	**onych/o/**malacia (ŏn-ĭ-kō-mă-LĀ-shē-ă): _____ *-malacia:* softening
ungu/o		**ungu/**al (ŬNG-gwăl): _____ *-al:* pertaining to
pil/o	hair	**pil/o/**nid/al (pī-lō-NĪ-dăl): _____ *nid:* nest *-al:* pertaining to *A pilonidal cyst commonly develops in the skin at the base of the spine. It develops as a growth of hair in a dermoid cyst.*
trich/o		**trich/o/**pathy (trĭk-ŎP-ă-thē): _____ *-pathy:* disease
scler/o	hardening; sclera (white of eye)	**scler/o/**derma (sklĕ-rō-DĔR-mă): _____ *-derma:* skin *Scleroderma is an autoimmune disorder that causes the skin and internal organs to become progressively hardened as a result of deposits of collagen. It may occur as a localized form or as a systemic disease.*
seb/o	sebum, sebaceous	**seb/o/**rrhea (sĕb-ō-RĒ-ă): _____ *-rrhea:* discharge, flow *Seborrhea is an overactivity of the sebaceous glands.*
squam/o	scale	**squam/**ous (SKWĀ-mŭs): _____ *-ous:* pertaining to
xen/o	foreign, strange	**xen/o/**graft (ZĔN-ō-grăft): _____ *-graft:* transplantation *Xenografts are used as a temporary graft to protect the patient against infection and fluid loss.*
xer/o	dry	**xer/o/**derma (zē-rō-DĔR-mă): _____ *-derma:* skin *Xeroderma is a chronic skin condition characterized by dryness and roughness and is a mild form of ichthyosis.*

Continued

Medical Word Elements—cont'd

Element	Meaning	Word Analysis
Suffixes		
-cyte	cell	lip/o/**cyte** (LĬP-ō-sīt): _____ *lip/o:* fat
-derma	skin	py/o/**derma** (pī-ō-DĔR-mă): _____ *py/o:* pus *Pyoderma is an acute, inflammatory, purulent bacterial dermatitis. It may be primary, such as impetigo, or secondary to a previous skin condition.*
-logist	specialist in the study of	dermat/o/**logist** (dĕr-mă-TŎL-ō-jĭst): _____ *dermat/o:* skin
-logy	study of	dermat/o/**logy** (dĕr-mă-TŎL-ō-jē): _____ *dermat/o:* skin
-therapy	treatment	cry/o/**therapy** (krī-ō-THĔR-ă-pē): _____ *cry/o:* cold *Cryotherapy is used to destroy tissue by freezing with liquid nitrogen. Cutaneous warts and actinic keratosis are common skin disorders that respond well to cryotherapy treatment.*
Prefixes		
an-	without, not	**an**/hidr/osis (ăn-hī-DRŌ-sĭs): _____ *hidr:* sweat *-osis:* abnormal condition; increase (used primarily with blood cells)
epi-	above, upon	**epi**/derm/is (ĕp-ĭ-DĔR-mĭs): _____ *derm:* skin *-is:* noun ending *The epidermis is the outermost layer of the skin.*
homo-	same	**homo**/graft (HŌ-mō-grăft): _____ *-graft:* transplantation

Visit the Medical Terminology Systems online resource center at FADavis.com for an audio exercise of the terms in this table. Other activities are also available to reinforce content.

It is time to review medical word elements by completing Learning Activities 5-1 and 5-2.

Disease Focus

The general appearance and condition of the skin are clinically important because they may provide clues to body conditions or dysfunctions. Pale skin may indicate shock; red, flushed, very warm skin may indicate fever and infection. A rash may indicate allergies or local infections. Even chewed fingernails may be a clue to emotional problems. For diagnosis, treatment, and management of skin disorders, the medical services of a specialist may be warranted. **Dermatology** is the medical specialty concerned with diseases that directly affect the skin and systemic diseases that manifest their effects on the skin. The physician who specializes in diagnosis and treatment of skin diseases is known as a **dermatologist**.

Skin Lesions

Lesions are areas of tissue that have been pathologically altered by injury, wound, or infection. Lesions may affect tissue over an area of a definite size **(localized)** or may be widely spread throughout the body **(systemic)**. Evaluation of skin lesions, injuries, or changes to tissue helps establish the diagnosis of skin disorders.

Lesions are described as primary or secondary. **Primary skin lesions** are the initial reaction to **pathologically** altered tissue and may be flat or elevated. **Secondary skin lesions** are changes that take place in the primary lesion as a result of infection, scratching, trauma, or various stages of a disease. Lesions are also described by their appearance, color, location, and size as measured in centimeters. Some of the major primary and secondary skin lesions are described and illustrated in Figure 5-3 on page 100.

It is time to review skin lesions by completing Learning Activity 5-3.

Primary Lesions

FLAT LESIONS
Flat, discolored, circumscribed lesions of any size

Macule
Flat, pigmented, circumscribed area less than 1 cm in diameter.
Examples: Freckle, flat mole, or rash that occurs in rubella.

ELEVATED LESIONS

Solid

Papule
Solid, elevated lesion less than 1 cm in diameter that may be the same color as the skin or pigmented.
Examples: Nevus, wart, pimple, ringworm, psoriasis, eczema.

Fluid-filled

Vesicle
Elevated, circumscribed, fluid-filled lesion less than 0.5 cm in diameter.
Examples: Poison ivy, shingles, chicken pox.

Nodule
Palpable, circumscribed lesion; larger and deeper than a papule (0.6 to 2 cm in diameter); extends into the dermal area.
Examples: Intradermal nevus, benign or malignant tumor.

Pustule
Small, raised, circumscribed lesion that contains pus; usually less than 1 cm in diameter.
Examples: Acne, furuncle, pustular psoriasis, scabies.

Tumor
Solid, elevated lesion larger than 2 cm in diameter that extends into the dermal and subcutaneous layers.
Examples: Lipoma, steatoma, dermatofibroma, hemangioma.

Bulla
A vesicle or blister larger than 1 cm in diameter.
Examples: Second-degree burns, severe poison oak, poison ivy.

Wheal
Elevated, firm, rounded lesion with localized skin edema (swelling) that varies in size, shape, and color; paler in the center than its surrounding edges; accompanied by itching.
Examples: Hives, insect bites, urticaria.

Secondary Lesions

DEPRESSED LESIONS
Depressed lesions caused by loss of skin surface

Excoriations
Linear scratch marks or traumatized abrasions of the epidermis.
Examples: Scratches, abrasions, chemical or thermal burns.

Fissure
Small slit or cracklike sore that extends into the dermal layer; could be caused by continuous inflammation and drying.

Ulcer
An open sore or lesion that extends to the dermis and usually heals with scarring.
Examples: Pressure sore, basal cell carcinoma.

Figure 5-3 Primary and secondary lesions.

Burns

Burns are tissue injuries caused by contact with thermal, chemical, electrical, or radioactive agents. Although burns generally occur on the skin, they can also affect the respiratory and digestive tract linings. Burns that have a local effect are not as serious as those that have a systemic effect. Systemic effects are life-threatening and may include dehydration, shock, and infection.

Burns are usually classified as first-, second-, or third-degree burns. The extent of injury and degree of severity determine a burn's classification. **First-degree (superficial) burns** are the least serious type of burn because they injure only the top layers of the skin, the epidermis. These burns are most commonly caused by brief contact with dry or moist heat **(thermal burn)**, spending too much time in the sun **(sunburn)**, or exposure to chemicals **(chemical burn)**. Injury is restricted to local effects, such as skin redness **(erythema)** and acute sensitivity to such sensory stimuli as touch, heat, or cold **(hyperesthesia)**. Generally, blisters do not form, and the burn heals without scar formation (see Fig. 5-4A). **Second-degree (partial-thickness)** burns are deep burns that damage the epidermis and part of the dermis. These burns may be caused by contact with flames, hot liquids, or chemicals. Symptoms mimic those of first-degree burns, but fluid-filled blisters **(vesicles** or **bullae)** form, and the burn may heal with little or no scarring (see Fig. 5-4B).

Figure 5-4 (A) Shoulder and upper back with first-degree burn from overexposure to the sun. (B) Forearm with second-degree burn from frying oil with small blisters and a large bulla. (C) Foot with third-degree burn from fire with destruction of the epidermis and damage to the subcutaneous tissue with charred and white borders.

In **third-degree (full-thickness) burns,** the epidermis and dermis are destroyed, and some of the underlying connective tissue is damaged, leaving the skin waxy and charred with insensitivity to touch (see Fig. 5-4C). The underlying bones, muscles, and tendons may also be damaged. These burns may be caused by corrosive chemicals, flames, electricity, or extremely hot objects; immersion of the body in extremely hot water; or clothing that catches fire. Because of the extensiveness of tissue destruction, ulcerating wounds develop, and the body attempts to heal itself by forming scar tissue. Skin grafting (**dermatoplasty**) is commonly required to protect the underlying tissue and assist in recovery.

A formula for estimating the percentage of adult body surface area affected by burns is to apply the rule of nines. This method assigns values of 9% or 18% of surface area to specific regions. The formula is modified in infants and children because of the proportionally larger head size (see Fig. 5-5). To determine treatment, it is important to know the amount of the burned surface area because the patient requires intravenous (IV) fluids for hydration to replace fluids lost from tissue damage.

Oncology

Neoplasms are abnormal growths of tissue that are classified as benign or malignant. **Benign neoplasms** are noncancerous growths composed of the same type of cells as the tissue in which they are growing. They harm the individual only insofar as they place pressure on or interfere with the functioning of surrounding structures. If the benign neoplasm remains small, it does not commonly require removal. When the tumor enlarges, causes pain, or interferes with other organs or structures, excision is necessary. **Malignant neoplasms,** also called **cancer,** are composed of cells that tend to become invasive and spread to remote regions of the body (**metastasis**). Once the malignant cells from the primary tumor invade surrounding tissues, they tend to enter blood and lymph vessels and travel to remote regions of the body to form secondary tumor sites. If left untreated, cancer tends to be progressive and generally fatal.

Cancer treatment includes surgery, chemotherapy, immunotherapy, and radiation therapy. **Immunotherapy,** also called **biotherapy,** is a more recent treatment that stimulates the body's own immune defenses to fight tumor cells. To provide the most effective treatment, the physician may prescribe one of the previously listed treatments or use a combination of them (**combined-modality treatment**).

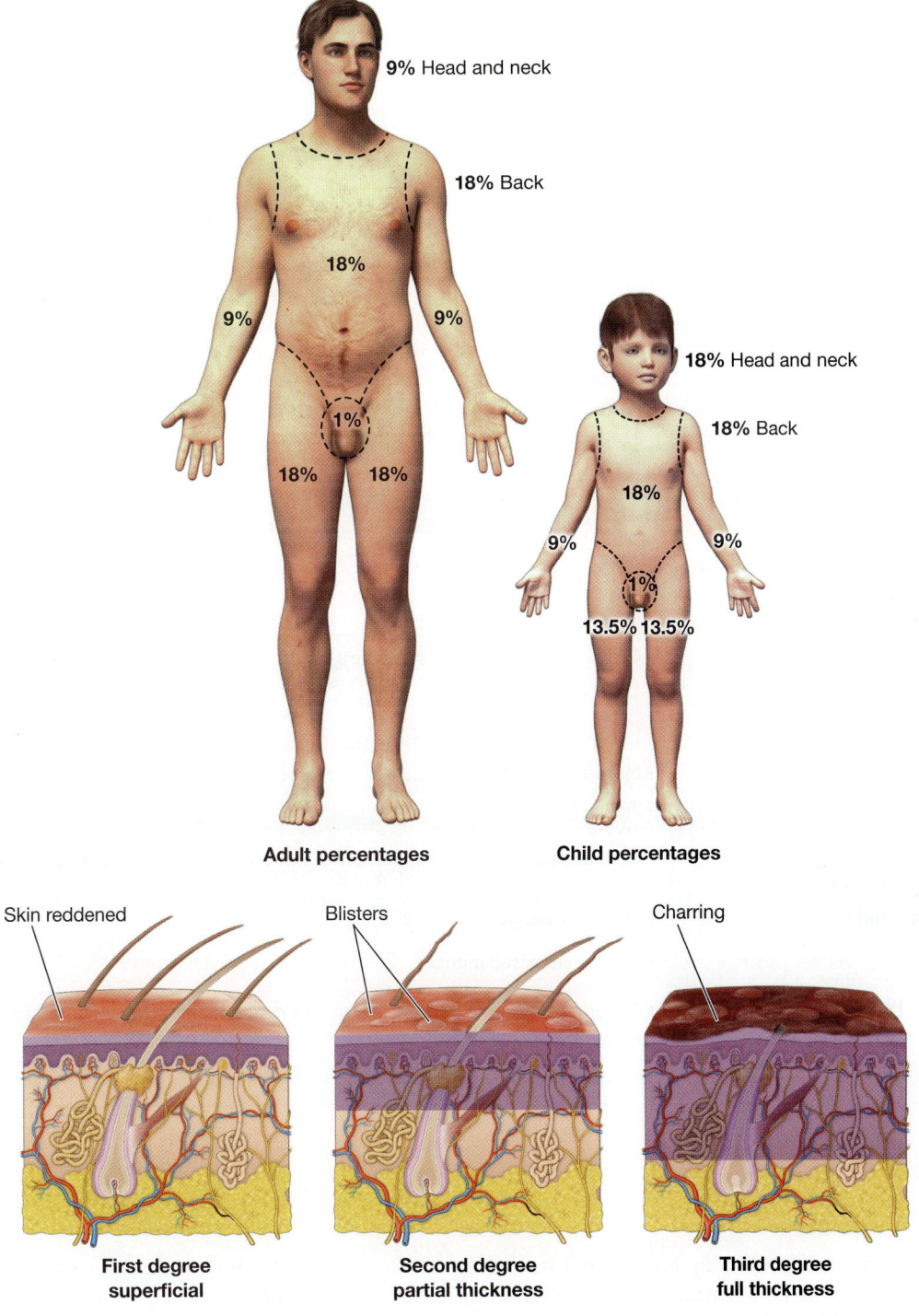

9% Head and neck

18% Back

18%

9%

9%

1%

18%   **18%**

Adult percentages

18% Head and neck

18% Back

18%

9%

9%

1%

13.5% **13.5%**

Child percentages

Skin reddened

Blisters

Charring

First degree superficial

Second degree partial thickness

Third degree full thickness

Figure 5-5 Rule of nines and burn classification.

Grading and Staging Cancer

Pathologists grade and stage tumors to help in diagnosis and treatment planning, provide a possible prognosis, and aid comparison of treatment results when different treatment methods are used.

Tumor Grading

In tumor **grading,** cells from the tumor site are evaluated to determine how closely the biopsied tissue resembles normal tissue. The greater the difference between the normal tissue and the biopsied tissue, the more serious is the grade of cancer. Pathologists commonly describe these changes using four grades of severity based on the microscopic appearance of the cells (see Table 5-1). A grade I tumor shows cells that closely resemble the tissue of origin. In other words, most of the cells are well differentiated and able to carry on the function of the tissue. A patient with a grade I tumor has a good prognosis for full recovery. On the other hand, a grade IV tumor shows cells that are very poorly differentiated and grow rapidly. These cells spread to surrounding tissue, revert back to their primitive state **(anaplasia),** and are incapable of carrying on the normal function of the tissue. A patient with a grade IV tumor has the poorest prognosis.

TABLE 5-1 Tumor Grading

This table defines the four tumor grades and their characteristics.

Grading	Tumor Characteristics
Grade I Tumor cells well differentiated	• Close resemblance to tissue of origin, retaining some specialized functions
Grade II Tumor cells moderately or poorly differentiated	• Less resemblance to tissue of origin • More variation in size and shape of tumor cells • Increased mitoses
Grade III Tumor cells poorly differentiated	• Increased abnormality in appearance, with only remote resemblance to the tissue of origin • Marked variation in shape and size of tumor cells • Greatly increased mitoses
Grade IV Tumor cells very poorly differentiated	• Abnormal appearance to the extent that recognition of the tumor's tissue origin is difficult • Extreme variation in size and shape of tumor cells

---

Tumor Staging

The most common system used for staging tumors is the **tumor, node, metastasis (TNM) system.** It is an international system that allows comparison of statistics among cancer centers. The TNM staging system classifies solid tumors by size and degree of spread according to three basic criteria:

- **T**—size and invasiveness of the primary tumor
- **N**—area lymph nodes involved
- **M**—invasiveness (metastasis) of the primary tumor

Numbers are used to indicate size or spread of the tumor. The higher the number, the greater is the extent or spread of the malignancy. For example, *T2* designates a small tumor; *M0* designates no evidence of metastasis (see Table 5-2). As with grading, staging provides valuable information to guide treatment plans.

TABLE 5-2 **TNM System of Staging**

This table outlines the tumor, node, metastasis (TNM) system of staging, including designations, stages, and degrees of tissue involvement.

Designation	Stage	Tissue Involvement
Tumor		
TX		Primary tumor that cannot be evaluated
T0		No evidence of tumor
Tis	Stage I	Carcinoma in situ, which indicates that the tumor is in a defined location and shows no invasion into surrounding tissues
T1, T2, T3, T4	Stage II	Primary tumor size and extent of local invasion, where T1 is small with minimal invasion, and T4 is large with extensive local invasion into surrounding organs and tissues
Node		
NX		Regional lymph nodes that cannot be evaluated
N0		Regional lymph nodes that show no abnormalities
N1, N2, N3, N4	Stage III	Degree of lymph node involvement and spread to regional lymph nodes, where N1 is less involvement with minimal spreading, and N4 is more involvement with extensive spreading
Metastasis		
MX		Distant metastasis that cannot be evaluated
M0		No evidence of metastasis
M1	Stage IV	Presence of metastasis

Basal Cell Carcinoma

Basal cell carcinoma, the most common type of skin cancer, is a malignancy of the basal layer of the epidermis, or hair follicles. This type of cancer is commonly caused by overexposure to sunlight. The tumors are locally invasive but rarely metastasize (see Fig. 5-6). Basal cell carcinoma is most prevalent in blond, fair-skinned men and is the most common malignant tumor affecting white people. Although these tumors grow slowly, they commonly ulcerate as they increase in size and develop crusting that is firm to the touch. Metastases are uncommon with this type of cancer; however, the disease can invade the tissue sufficiently to destroy an ear, nose, or eyelid. Depending on the location, size, and depth of the lesion, treatment may include curettage and electrodesiccation, cryosurgery, radiation therapy, topical chemotherapy, photodynamic therapy, surgical excision, or Mohs surgery.

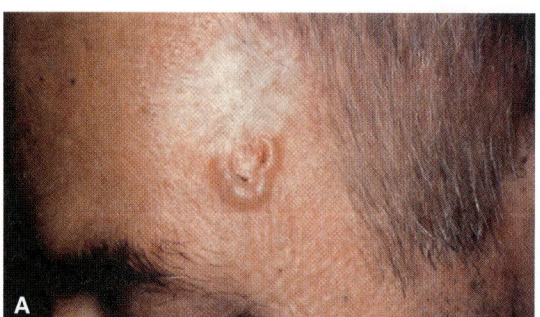

Figure 5-6 Basal cell carcinoma. (A) Basal cell carcinoma with pearly, flesh-colored papule with depressed center and rolled edge. (B) Common sites of basal cell carcinoma. From Goldsmith LA, Lazarus GS, Tharp MD: *Adult and Pediatric Dermatology: A Color Guide to Diagnosis and Treatment,* Philadelphia, 1997, F.A. Davis, p. 157, with permission.

Squamous Cell Carcinoma

Squamous cell carcinoma arises from skin that undergoes pathological hardening (**keratinizing**) of epidermal cells. It is an invasive tumor with potential for metastasis and occurs most commonly in fair-skinned white men over age 60 (see Fig. 5-7). Repeated overexposure to the sun's ultraviolet rays greatly increases the risk of squamous cell carcinoma. Other predisposing factors associated with this type of cancer include radiation therapy; chronic skin irritation and inflammation; exposure to cancer-causing agents (**carcinogens**), including tar and oil; hereditary diseases (such as **xeroderma pigmentosum** and **albinism**); and the presence of premalignant lesions (such as **actinic keratosis** or **Bowen disease**).

There are two types of squamous cell carcinoma: those that are confined to the original site (**in situ**) and those that penetrate the surrounding tissue (**invasive**). Depending on the location, size, shape, degree of invasion, and condition of the underlying tissue, treatment is removal by surgical excision, **Mohs** surgery, laser therapy, photodynamic therapy, cryotherapy, radiotherapy, or electrodesiccation and curettage. A combination of these treatment methods may be required for a deeply invasive tumor.

Figure 5-7 Squamous cell carcinoma, in which the surface is fragile and bleeds easily. From Goldsmith LA, Lazarus GS, Tharp MD: *Adult and Pediatric Dermatology: A Color Guide to Diagnosis and Treatment,* Philadelphia, 1997, F.A. Davis, p. 237, with permission.

Malignant Melanoma

Malignant melanoma, as the name implies, is a malignant growth of melanocytes (see Fig. 5-8). This tumor is highly metastatic, with a higher mortality rate than basal or squamous cell carcinomas. It is the most lethal of the skin cancers and can metastasize extensively to the liver, lungs, or brain.

Several factors may influence the development of melanoma, but persons at greatest risk have fair complexions, blue eyes, red or blond hair, and freckles. Excessive exposure to sunlight and severe sunburn during childhood are believed to increase the risk of melanoma in later life. Avoiding the sun and using sunscreen have proved effective in preventing the disease.

Melanomas are diagnosed by **biopsy** and histological examination. Treatment requires surgery to remove the primary cancer, along with adjuvant therapies to reduce the risk of metastasis. The extent of surgery depends on the size and location of the primary tumor and is determined by staging the disease.

Figure 5-8 Melanoma on a man's forehead after a biopsy.

 It is time to review burn and oncology terms by completing Learning Activity 5–4.

Diseases and Conditions

This section introduces terms related to diseases and conditions of the integumentary system, along with their meanings and pronunciations. Word analyses for selected terms are also provided.

Term	Definition
abscess ĂB-sĕs	Localized collection of pus at the site of an infection (characteristically a staphylococcal infection) *When a localized abscess originates in a hair follicle, it is called a furuncle or boil. A cluster of furuncles in the subcutaneous tissue results in the formation of a carbuncle (see Fig. 5-9).* **Figure 5-9** Dome-shaped abscess that has formed a furuncle in the hair follicles of the neck. Large furuncles with connecting channels to the skin surface form a carbuncle.
acne ĂK-nē	Inflammatory disease of the sebaceous glands and hair follicles of the skin with characteristic lesions that include blackheads (*comedos*), inflammatory papules, pustules, nodules, and cysts and are usually associated with seborrhea; also called *acne vulgaris* (see Fig. 5-10). *Acne results from thickening of the follicular opening, increased sebum production, and the presence of bacteria. It is associated with an inflammatory response. The face, neck, and shoulders are common sites for this condition.* **Figure 5-10** Acne vulgaris. From Goldsmith LA, Lazarus GS, Tharp MD: *Adult and Pediatric Dermatology: A Color Guide to Diagnosis and Treatment,* Philadelphia, 1997, F.A. Davis, p. 227, with permission.
alopecia al-ō-PĒ-shē-ă	Partial or complete loss of hair resulting from normal aging, an endocrine disorder, a drug reaction, anticancer medication, or a skin disease; commonly called *baldness*

Diseases and Conditions—cont'd

Term	Definition
Bowen disease BŌ-ĕn	Very early form of skin cancer, which is easily curable and characterized by a red, scaly patch on the skin that has not spread beyond the epidermis; also called *squamous cell carcinoma in situ* (see Fig. 5-7). *Treatment for Bowen disease includes topical chemotherapy, curettage, cryotherapy, and surgical removal.*
cellulitis sĕl-ū-LĪ-tĭs	Diffuse (widespread), acute infection of the skin and subcutaneous tissue. *Cellulitis is characterized by a light, glossy appearance of the skin, localized heat, redness, pain, and swelling, occasionally with fever, malaise, and chills.*
chloasma klō-ĂZ-mă	Pigmentary skin discoloration usually occurring in yellowish-brown patches or spots
comedo KŎM-ē-dō	Typical small skin lesion of acne vulgaris caused by accumulation of keratin, bacteria, and dried sebum that forms when a pore gets blocked *The closed form of comedo, called a* **whitehead,** *consists of a papule from which the contents are not easily expressed.*
decubitus ulcer dē-KŪ-bĭ-tŭs ŬL-sĕr	Inflammation, sore, or skin deterioration caused by prolonged pressure from lying in one position that prevents blood flow to the tissues, usually in elderly bedridden persons; also known as *pressure ulcer* (see Fig. 5-11). *Pressure ulcers are most commonly found in skin overlying a bony projection, such as the hip, ankle, heel, shoulder, and elbow. The wounds are categorized from stage 1 to stage 4 (see Fig. 5-12).*

Figure 5-11 Decubitus ulcer. (A) Deep pressure ulcer over a bony prominence in a bedridden patient. (B) Common sites of pressure ulcers. From Goldsmith LA, Lazarus GS, Tharp MD: *Adult and Pediatric Dermatology: A Color Guide to Diagnosis and Treatment,* Philadelphia, 1997, F.A. Davis, p. 445, with permission.

Continued

Diseases and Conditions—cont'd

Term	Definition

Figure 5-12 Stages of pressure ulcer. (A) Stage 1, with shiny, reddened skin that usually appears over a bony prominence. (B) Stage 2, untreated stage 1 ulcer that becomes more serious when skin is swollen and shows a blister. (C) Stage 3, in which a crater-like ulcer goes deeper into the skin. (D) Stage 4 ulcer that goes into a muscle or bone. From Dillon PM: *Nursing Health Assessment,* ed 2, Philadelphia, 2007, F.A. Davis, p. 239, with permission.

ecchymosis
ĕk-ĭ-MŌ-sĭs

Skin discoloration consisting of a large, irregularly formed hemorrhagic area with colors changing from bluish black to greenish brown or yellow; commonly called a *bruise* (see Fig. 5-13).

Figure 5-13 Ecchymosis.

eczema
ĔK-zĕ-mă

Chronic inflammatory skin condition that is characterized by erythema, papules, vesicles, pustules, scales, crusts, and scabs and accompanied by intense itching (pruritus); also called *atopic dermatitis*

Eczema most commonly occurs during infancy and childhood, with decreasing incidence in adolescence and adulthood. Statistics support a convincing genetic component in that it tends to occur in patients with a family history of allergic conditions.

erythema
ĕr-ĭ-THĒ-mă

Redness of the skin caused by swelling of the capillaries
An example of erythema is a mild sunburn or nervous blushing.

Diseases and Conditions—cont'd

Term	Definition
eschar ĔS-kăr	Dead matter that is sloughed off from the surface of the skin, especially after a burn *Eschar material is commonly crusty or scabbed.*
impetigo ĭm-pĕ-TĪ-gō	Bacterial skin infection characterized by isolated pustules that become crusted and rupture
keloid KĒ-lōyd	Thickened scar that forms after a surgical incision or injury that is firm, raised, and often a purplish-red color (see Fig. 5-14). Figure 5-14 Keloid scar formation appears in the lower portion of the incision site after knee replacement surgery. The upper part of the scar shows normal scar formation (cicatrix).
keratosis kĕr-ă-TŌ-sĭs *kerat:* horny tissue, hard; cornea *-osis:* abnormal condition; increase (used primarily with blood cells)	Thickened area of the epidermis or any horny growth on the skin (such as a callus or wart)
lentigo lĕn-TĪ-gō	Small brown macules that are common in areas that get repeated sun exposure and usually appear in a middle-aged or older person *Lentigo are benign pigmented lesions of the skin that require no treatment unless cosmetic repair is desired; referred to as* **age spots** *or* **liver spots**.
pallor PĂL-or	Unnatural paleness or absence of color in the skin
pediculosis pĕ-dĭk-ū-LŌ-sĭs *pedicul:* lice *-osis:* abnormal condition; increase (used primarily with blood cells)	Infestation with lice (parasitic insects), transmitted by close personal contact and shared bedding, brushes, combs, and clothing
petechia pē-TĒ-kē-ă	Minute, pinpoint hemorrhage under the skin *A petechia (plural,* petechiae*) is a smaller version of an ecchymosis.*

Continued

Diseases and Conditions—cont'd

Term	Definition
pruritus proo-RĪ-tŭs	Intense itching
psoriasis sō-RĪ-ă-sĭs	Chronic skin disease characterized by itchy red patches covered by thick, dry, silvery scales and caused by excessive development of the basal layer of the epidermis (see Fig. 5-15). *Psoriasis lesions may develop anywhere on the body. The more common sites are the scalp, face, knees, elbows, and genitalia. Treatment includes topical application of various medications, keratolytics, phototherapy, and ultraviolet light therapy in an attempt to slow hyperkeratosis.* **Figure 5-15** Psoriasis. From Goldsmith LA, Lazarus GS, Tharp MD: *Adult and Pediatric Dermatology: A Color Guide to Diagnosis and Treatment,* Philadelphia, 1997, F.A. Davis, p. 258, with permission.
purpura PŬR-pŭ-ră	Any of several bleeding disorders characterized by hemorrhage into the tissues, particularly beneath the skin or mucous membranes, producing ecchymoses or petechiae *Hemorrhage into the skin shows red darkening into purple and then brownish yellow and finally disappearing in 2 to 3 weeks. Areas of discoloration do not disappear under pressure.*
scabies SKĀ-bēz	Contagious skin disease caused by the itch mite, transmitted through prolonged or close physical contact, such as living together or sexual contact; also spreads through shared clothing, bedding, or towels, though less common since the mites survive only 2 -3 days off the body *Symptoms include intense nighttime itching, a pimple-like rash, and burrow tracks on areas like the wrists, elbows, fingers, waist, and genitals. It spreads quickly in crowded places like nursing homes, daycares, and prisons.*
tinea TĬN-ē-ăh	Fungal skin infection whose name commonly indicates the body part affected; also called *ringworm* *Examples of tinea include tinea barbae (beard), tinea corporis (body), tinea pedis (athlete's foot), tinea versicolor (skin), and tinea cruris (jock itch).*

Diseases and Conditions—cont'd

Term	Definition

urticaria
ŭr-tĭ-KĂR-ē-ă

Allergic reaction of the skin characterized by the eruption of pale red, elevated patches called *wheals* or *hives* (see Fig. 5-16).

Figure 5-16 Urticaria. From Goldsmith LA, Lazarus GS, Tharp MD: *Adult and Pediatric Dermatology: A Color Guide to Diagnosis and Treatment,* Philadelphia, 1997, F.A. Davis, p. 209, with permission.

verruca
vĕr-ROO-kă

Epidermal growth caused by a virus; also known as *warts*

Verrucae may be removed by cryosurgery, electrocautery, or acids; however, they may regrow if the virus remains in the skin. Types include plantar warts, juvenile warts, and venereal warts (see Fig. 5-17).

Figure 5-17 Verruca. From Goldsmith LA, Lazarus GS, Tharp MD: *Adult and Pediatric Dermatology: A Color Guide to Diagnosis and Treatment,* Philadelphia, 1997, F.A. Davis, p. 241, with permission.

Continued

Diseases and Conditions—cont'd

Term	Definition
vitiligo vĭt-ĭl-Ī-gō	Localized loss of skin pigmentation characterized by milk-white patches (see Fig. 5-18) **Figure 5-18** Vitiligo. From Goldsmith LA, Lazarus GS, Tharp MD: *Adult and Pediatric Dermatology: A Color Guide to Diagnosis and Treatment,* Philadelphia, 1997, F.A. Davis, p. 121, with permission.

 It is time to review pathology, diseases, and conditions by completing Learning Activity 5-5.

Diagnostic, Surgical, and Therapeutic Procedures

This section introduces diagnostic, surgical, and therapeutic procedures used to treat and diagnose skin disorders. Descriptions are provided, along with pronunciations and word analyses for selected terms.

Procedure	Description
Diagnostic	
allergy skin test	Any test in which a suspected allergen or sensitizer is applied to or injected into the skin to determine the patient's sensitivity to it *The most commonly used skin tests are the intradermal, patch, and scratch tests. The intensity of the response is determined by the wheal-and-flare reaction after application of the suspected allergen. Positive and negative controls help verify normal skin reactivity (see Fig. 5-19).*

Diagnostic, Surgical, and Therapeutic Procedures—cont'd

Procedure	Description

intradermal
ĭn-tră-dĕr-măl
  intra-: in, within
  derm: skin
  -al: pertaining to
	Skin test that identifies suspected allergens by subcutaneously injecting small amounts of extracts of the suspected allergens and observing the skin for a subsequent reaction
	
	Intradermal skin tests help determine immunity to diphtheria (Schick test) and tuberculosis (Mantoux test).

patch	Skin test that identifies allergic contact dermatitis by applying a suspected allergen to a patch, which is then taped on the skin, usually the forearm, and observing the area 24 hours later for an allergic response *After patch removal, a lack of noticeable reaction indicates a negative result; skin reddening or swelling indicates a positive result and means the person is allergic to the suspected allergen.*
scratch	Skin test that identifies suspected allergens by placing a small quantity of the suspected allergen on a lightly scratched area of the skin; also called *puncture test* or *prick test* *Redness or swelling at the scratch sites within 10 minutes indicates an allergy to the substance or a positive test result. If no reaction occurs, the test result is negative.*

Figure 5-19 Allergy skin tests. (A) Patch allergy testing. (B) Scratch (prick) skin test kit for allergy testing.

Continued

Diagnostic, Surgical, and Therapeutic Procedures—cont'd

Procedure	Description
Surgical	
biopsy (Bx, bx) BĪ-ŏp-sē	Representative tissue sample removed from a body site for microscopic examination *Skin biopsies help establish or confirm a diagnosis, estimate prognosis, or follow the course of a disease. Any lesion suspected of malignancy is removed and sent to the pathology laboratory for evaluation.*
frozen section (FS)	Ultrathin slice of tissue from a frozen specimen for immediate pathological examination *FS is commonly used for rapid diagnosis of malignancy after the patient has been anesthetized to determine treatment options.*
needle	Removal of a small tissue sample for examination using a hollow needle, usually attached to a syringe
punch	Removal of a small core of tissue using a hollow punch
shave	Removal of elevated lesions using a surgical blade
Mohs MŌZ	Procedure that involves progressive removal and microscopic examination of layers of cancer-containing skin until only cancer-free tissue remains; also called *micrographic surgery.*
skin graft	Transplantation of healthy tissue to an injured site *Human, animal, or artificial skin can provide a temporary covering or permanent layer of skin over a wound or burn.*

allograft
   ĂL-ō-grăft
   allo-: other; differing from
   normal
   -graft: transplantation
	Transplantation of healthy tissue from one person to another person; also called *homograft*
	
	In an allograft, the skin donor is usually a cadaver. This type of skin graft is temporary and is used to protect the patient against infection and fluid loss. The allograft is frozen and stored in a skin bank until needed. Allografts are the most common type of tissue transplant.

autograft
   AW-tō-grăft
   auto: self, own
   -graft: transplantation
	Transplantation of healthy tissue from one site to another site in the same individual
	
	An autograft is a permanent skin graft and cannot be rejected by the body because it's from the same person with identical genetic makeup.

synthetic sĭn-THĔT-ĭk	Transplantation of artificial skin produced from collagen fibers arranged in a lattice pattern *The recipient's body does not reject synthetic skin (produced artificially), and healing skin grows into it as the graft gradually disintegrates.*

xenograft
   ZĔN-ō-grăft
   xen/o: foreign
   -graft: transplantation
	Transplantation (dermis only) from a foreign donor (usually a pig) and transferred to a human; also called *heterograft*
	
	A xenograft is a temporary graft to protect the patient against infection and fluid loss.

Diagnostic, Surgical, and Therapeutic Procedures—cont'd

Procedure	Description
Therapeutic	
chemical peel	Chemical removal of the outer layers of skin to treat acne scarring and general keratoses; also called *chemabrasion*
	Chemical peels are also commonly used for cosmetic purposes to remove fine wrinkles on the face.
cryosurgery krī-ō-SĔR-jĕr-ē	Use of subfreezing temperature (commonly liquid nitrogen) to destroy or eliminate abnormal tissue, such as tumors, warts, and unwanted, cancerous, or infected tissue
débridement dĕ-BRĒD-mĕnt	Removal of necrotized tissue from a wound by surgical excision, enzymes, or chemical agents
	Débridement is used to promote healing and prevent infection.
dermabrasion DĔRM-ă-brā-zhŭn	Rubbing (abrasion) using wire brushes or sandpaper to mechanically scrape away (abrade) the epidermis
	Dermabrasion commonly helps remove acne scars, tattoos, and scar tissue.
fulguration fŭl-gū-RĀ-shŭn	Tissue destruction by means of high-frequency electric current; also called *electrodesiccation*
	Fulguration helps remove tumors and lesions in and on the body.
laser	Uses intense focused light to remove tissue for medical or cosmetic purposes
	Laser therapy can shrink or destroy tumors, polyps, and precancerous growths. Cosmetically it is used to improve the skin's appearance or treat minor facial flaws such as fine wrinkles, age spots, or scar tissue.
photodynamic therapy (PDT)	Procedure in which cells selectively treated with an agent called a *photosensitizer* are exposed to light to produce a reaction that destroys the cells
	Various forms of photodynamic therapy are used in treatment of cancer, actinic keratosis, and macular degeneration.

Pharmacology

Various medications are available to treat skin disorders (see Table 5-3). Because of their superficial nature and location, many skin disorders respond well to topical drug therapy. Such mild, localized skin disorders as contact dermatitis, acne, poison ivy, and diaper rash can be effectively treated with topical agents available as over-the-counter products.

Widespread or particularly severe dermatological disorders may require systemic treatment. For example, poison ivy with large areas of open, weeping lesions may be difficult to treat with topical medication and may require a prescription-strength drug. In such a case, an oral steroid or antihistamine might be prescribed to relieve inflammation and severe itching.

TABLE 5-3 Drugs Used to Treat Skin Disorders

This table lists classifications of common drugs used to treat skin disorders, their therapeutic actions, and selected generic and trade names.

Classification	Therapeutic Action	Generic and Trade Names
antiacne agents	Reduce acne through multiple mechanisms *Some antiacne medications decrease bacteria in the follicles of the skin to prevent the formation of acne; others disrupt the stickiness of the follicular skin cells and decrease microcomedones (widening of the follicle, which fills with debris and bacteria to form comedones).*	**benzoyl peroxide** BĔN-zō-ĭl pĕr-ŎK-sīd *PanOxyl* **tretinoin** TRĔT-ĭ-noyn *Retin-A*
antifungals ăn-tĭ-FŬN-găls	Alter the cell wall of fungi or disrupt enzyme activity, resulting in cell death *Antifungals help treat ringworm (tinea corporis), athlete's foot (tinea pedis), and fungal infection of the nail (onychomycosis). When topical antifungals are not effective, oral or intravenous antifungal drugs may be necessary.*	**itraconazole** ĭt-ră-KŎN-ă-zōl *Sporanox (oral form only)* **terbinafine** TĔR-bĭn-ă-fēn *Lamisil* (available in both oral and topical form) **fluconazole** flū-KŎ-nă-zōl *Diflucan* (available in both intravenous and oral form)
antihistamines ăn-tĭ-HĬS-tă-mĭns	Inhibit allergic reactions of inflammation, redness, and itching caused by the release of histamine *In a case of severe itching, antihistamines may be given orally. As a group, these drugs are also known as antipruritics (pruritus means "itching").*	**diphenhydramine** dī-fĕn-HĬ-dră-mēn *Benadryl* **hydroxyzine** hī-DRŎKS-ĭzēn *Vistaril, Atarax*
antiparasitics ăn-tĭ-păr-ă-SĬT-ĭks	Kill insect parasites, such as mites and lice *Parasiticides are used to treat scabies (mites) and pediculosis (lice). The drug is applied as a cream or lotion to the body and as a shampoo to treat the scalp.*	**lindane** LĬN-dān *Kwell, Thion* **permethrin** pĕr-MĔTH-rĭn *Nix*
antiseptics ăn-tĭ-SĔP-tĭks	Topically applied agents that inhibit growth of bacteria, thus preventing infections in cuts, scratches, and surgical incisions	**ethyl or isopropyl alcohol** ĔTH-ĭl, ī-sō-PRŌ-pĭl **hydrogen peroxide** HĪ-drō-jĕn pĕ-RŎK-sīd **povidone-iodine** PŌ-vĭ-dōn Ī-ō-dīn *Betadine*

TABLE 5-3 Drugs Used to Treat Skin Disorders—cont'd

Classification	Therapeutic Action	Generic and Trade Names
corticosteroids kor-tĭ-kō-STĔR-oyds	Decrease inflammation and itching by suppressing the immune system's inflammatory response to tissue damage *Topical corticosteroids are used to treat contact dermatitis, poison ivy, insect bites, psoriasis, seborrhea, and eczema. Oral corticosteroids may be prescribed for systemic treatment of severe or widespread inflammation or itching.*	**hydrocortisone** HĪ-drō-KOR-tĭ-sōn *Cetacort, Cortaid* **triamcinolone** trī-ăm-SĬN-ō-lōn *Azmacort, Kenalog*
keratolytics kĕr-ă-tō-LĬT-ĭks	Destroy and soften the outer layer of skin so that it is sloughed off or shed *Strong keratolytics remove warts and corns and aid in penetration of antifungal drugs. Milder keratolytics promote shedding of scales and crusts in eczema, psoriasis, seborrheic dermatitis, and other conditions with dry, scaly skin. Weak keratolytics irritate inflamed skin, acting as a tonic to accelerate healing.*	**salicylic acid** săl-ĭ-SĬL-ĭkĂS-ĭd *Sebasorb, Psoriasin, and so forth* (Multiple brand names based on use) **urea** ū-RĒ-ă *Kerafoam, Keralac*
protectives prŏ-TĔK-tĭvs	Cover, cool, dry, or soothe inflamed skin *Protectives do not penetrate the skin or soften it. Rather, they allow the natural healing process to occur by forming a long-lasting film that protects the skin from air, water, and clothing.*	**lotions** *Cetaphil moisturizing lotion* **ointments** *Vaseline*
topical anesthetics ăn-ĕs-THĔT-ĭks	Block sensation of pain by numbing the skin layers and mucous membranes *These topical drugs are administered directly by means of sprays, creams, gargles, suppositories, and other preparations. They provide temporary symptomatic relief of minor burns, sunburns, rashes, and insect bites.*	**lidocaine** LĪ-dō-kān *Xylocaine* **procaine** PRŌ-kān *Novocain*

Abbreviations

This section introduces integumentary-related abbreviations and their meanings.

Abbreviation	Meaning	Abbreviation	Meaning
Bx, bx	biopsy	**IMP**	impression (synonymous with diagnosis)
BCC	basal cell carcinoma	**IV**	intravenous
CA	cancer; chronological age; cardiac arrest	**PDT**	photodynamic therapy
FS	frozen section	**TNM**	tumor-node-metastasis
ID	intradermal	**ung**	ointment
I&D	incision and drainage	**XP, XDP**	xeroderma pigmentosum

 It is time to review procedures, pharmacology, and abbreviations by completing Learning Activity 5-6.

LEARNING ACTIVITIES

The activities that follow provide a review of the integumentary system terms introduced in this chapter. Complete each activity and review your answers to evaluate your understanding of the chapter.

Visit the Medical Language Laboratory at medicallanguagelab.com. Use it to enhance your study and reinforcement of this chapter with the flash card activity. We recommend that you complete the flash card activity before starting Learning Activities 5-1 and 5-2.

Learning Activity 5-1
Medical Word Elements

Read the definition in the numbered list. Then select the elements from the table to build medical words. You may use the elements more than once.

Combining Forms		Suffixes		Prefixes	
derm/o	myc/o	-al	-oma	an-	hypo-
dermat/o	pedicul/o	-cyte	-osis	hetero-	hyper-
hidr/o	py/o	-derma	-pathy	homo-	intra-
ichthy/o	scler/o	-graft	-plasty		
kerat/o	seb/o	-ic	-rrhea		
lip/o	trich/o	-logist			
melan/o	xer/o				

1. pertaining to within the skin _____

2. cell that is black (produces pigment) _____

3. abnormal condition of lice _____

4. transplantation from different (species) _____

5. abnormal condition of excessive sweating _____

6. tumor (that is) black _____

7. pertaining to under the skin _____

8. surgical repair of the skin _____

9. cell (composed of) fat _____

10. skin (containing) pus _____

11. specialist in the study of skin disorders _____

12. skin that is dry _____

13. abnormal condition without sweat _____

14. transplantation from the same (species) _____

15. abnormal condition of dry or scaly (skin) _____

16. skin (that has) hardened _____

17. abnormal condition of a fungus _____

18. discharge or flow of sebum _____

19. disease of the hair _____

20. abnormal condition of horny tissue _____

Check your answers in Appendix A. Review any material that you did not answer correctly.

Correct Answers _____ X 5 = _____ % Score

Learning Activity 5-2
Building Medical Words

Use *adip/o* or *lip/o* (fat) to build words that mean:

1. tumor consisting of fat _____
2. hernia containing fat _____
3. resembling fat _____
4. fat cell _____

Use *dermat/o* (skin) to build words that mean:

5. inflammation of the skin _____
6. abnormal condition of a skin fungus _____

Use *onych/o* (nail) to build words that mean:

7. tumor of the nails _____
8. softening of the nails _____
9. abnormal condition of the nails _____
10. abnormal condition of the nails caused by a fungus _____
11. abnormal condition of a hidden (ingrown) nail _____
12. disease of the nails _____

Use *scler/o* (hardening; sclera) to build words that mean:

13. skin that is hardened _____
14. abnormal condition of hardening (of the skin) _____

Use *-logy* or *-logist* to build words that mean:

15. study of the skin _____
16. specialist in the study of skin (diseases) _____

Build surgical words that mean:

17. excision of fat (adipose tissue) _____
18. removal of a nail _____
19. transplantation (of skin) from one site to another site in the same individual _____
20. surgical repair (plastic surgery) of the skin _____

✓ *Check your answers in Appendix A. Review material that you did not answer correctly.*

Correct Answers _____ X 5 = _____ % Score

Learning Activity 5-3
Identifying Skin Lesions

Label the skin lesions on the lines provided, using the listed terms.

bulla   *fissure*   *nodule*   *pustule*   *ulcer*   *wheal*
excoriations   *macule*   *papule*   *tumor*   *vesicle*

Primary Lesions	**FLAT LESIONS**

Flat, discolored, circumscribed lesions of any size

Flat, pigmented, circumscribed area less than 1 cm in diameter.
Examples: Freckle, flat mole, or rash that occurs in rubella.

ELEVATED LESIONS

Solid | **Fluid-filled**

Solid, elevated lesion less than 1 cm in diameter that may be the same color as the skin or pigmented.
Examples: Nevus, wart, pimple, ringworm, psoriasis, eczema.

Elevated, circumscribed, fluid-filled lesion less than 0.5 cm in diameter.
Examples: Poison ivy, shingles, chicken pox.

Palpable, circumscribed lesion; larger and deeper than a papule (0.6 to 2 cm in diameter); extends into the dermal area.
Examples: Intradermal nevus, benign or malignant tumor.

Small, raised, circumscribed lesion that contains pus; usually less than 1 cm in diameter.
Examples: Acne, furuncle, pustular psoriasis, scabies.

Solid, elevated lesion larger than 2 cm in diameter that extends into the dermal and subcutaneous layers.
Examples: Lipoma, steatoma, dermatofibroma, hemangioma.

A vesicle or blister larger than 1 cm in diameter.
Examples: Second-degree burns, severe poison oak, poison ivy.

Elevated, firm, rounded lesion with localized skin edema (swelling) that varies in size, shape, and color; paler in the center than its surrounding edges; accompanied by itching.
Examples: Hives, insect bites, urticaria.

Secondary Lesions	**DEPRESSED LESIONS**

Depressed lesions caused by loss of skin surface

Linear scratch marks or traumatized abrasions of the epidermis.
Examples: Scratches, abrasions, chemical or thermal burns.

Small slit or cracklike sore that extends into the dermal layer; could be caused by continuous inflammation and drying.

An open sore or lesion that extends to the dermis and usually heals with scarring.
Examples: Pressure sore, basal cell carcinoma.

 Check your answers by referring to Figure 5–3 on page 100. Review material that you did not answer correctly.

Learning Activity 5-4

Matching Burn and Oncology Terms

Match each term on the left with its meaning on the right.

1. _____ metastasis
2. _____ T0
3. _____ malignant
4. _____ first-degree burn
5. _____ grading
6. _____ squamous cell carcinoma
7. _____ benign
8. _____ T1
9. _____ M0
10. _____ third-degree burns

a. develops from keratinizing epidermal cells
b. noncancerous
c. no evidence of metastasis
d. extensive damage to underlying connective tissue
e. no evidence of primary tumor
f. determines degree of abnormal cancer cells compared with normal cells
g. burn that heals without scar formation
h. cancerous; may be life-threatening
i. spread of cancer from primary site to other parts of the body
j. primary tumor size, small with minimal invasion

Check your answers in Appendix A. Review any material that you did not answer correctly.

Correct Answers _____ X 10 = _____ % Score

Learning Activity 5-5

Diseases and Conditions

Match the terms with the definitions in the numbered list.

abscess	*ecchymosis*	*pallor*	*scabies*
alopecia	*eczema*	*pediculosis*	*tinea*
Bowen disease	*erythema*	*petechiae*	*urticaria*
chloasma	*eschar*	*pruritus*	*verruca*
comedo	*impetigo*	*psoriasis*	*vitiligo*

1. acne lesion that forms when a pore becomes blocked _____
2. unnatural paleness or absence of color in the skin _____
3. chronic inflammatory skin disease that causes erythema, itching, and blistering of the skin _____
4. early form of skin cancer that is also known as *squamous cell carcinoma in situ* _____
5. chronic skin disease caused by excessive development of the basal cell layer of the epidermis _____
6. infestation with lice _____
7. skin depigmentation characterized by milk-white patches _____
8. fungal skin infection, also called *ringworm* _____
9. contagious skin disease transmitted by the itch mite _____
10. bacterial skin infection characterized by pustules that become crusted and rupture _____
11. allergic reaction of the skin, characterized by elevated red patches called *hives* _____

12. hyperpigmentation of the skin, characterized by yellowish-brown patches or spots _____

13. hemorrhagic spot or bruise on the skin _____

14. minute or small hemorrhagic spots on the skin _____

15. loss or absence of hair _____

16. localized collection of pus at the site of infection (staphylococcal) _____

17. redness of the skin caused by swelling of the capillaries _____

18. damaged tissue after a severe burn _____

19. intense itching _____

20. epidermal growth caused by a virus; also known as a *wart* _____

✓ *Check your answers in Appendix A. Review material that you did not answer correctly.*

Correct Answers _____ X 5 = _____ % Score

Learning Activity 5-6
Procedures, Pharmacology, and Abbreviations

Match the terms with the definitions in the numbered list.

antifungals	*débridement*	*intradermal test*	*patch test*
antihistamines	*dermabrasion*	*keratolytics*	*ung*
BCC	*fulguration*	*Mohs*	*xenograft*
corticosteroids	*IMP*	*parasiticides*	

1. progressive removal and microscopic examination of skin cancer until the tissue is cancer-free _____

2. tissue destruction by means of high-frequency electric current _____

3. agents that decrease inflammation and itching by suppressing the inflammatory response _____

4. removal of necrotized tissue from a wound surgically or with chemical agents _____

5. agents that kill parasitic skin infestations _____

6. agents that soften the outer layer of skin so that it sloughs off _____

7. procedure in which extracts of suspected allergens are injected subcutaneously _____

8. cancer that develops in basal cells _____

9. means ointment _____

10. transplantation taken from another species (usually a pig) to a human _____

11. topical agents to treat athlete's foot and onychomycosis _____

12. means diagnosis _____

13. inhibits allergic reactions of inflammation, redness, and itching caused by histamine release _____

14. use of wire brushes or other abrasive materials to remove scars, tattoos, or fine wrinkles _____

15. procedure in which allergens are applied topically, usually on the forearm _____

✓ *Check your answers in Appendix A. Review material that you did not answer correctly.*

Correct Answers _____ X 6.67 = _____ % Score

DOCUMENTING HEALTH-CARE ACTIVITIES

This section provides practical application activities in the form of exercises to help students develop skills in documenting patient care. First, read the medical report. Then complete the activities and exercises that follow.

Documenting Health-Care Activity 5-1
Pathology Report: Skin Lesion

General Hospital

1511 Ninth Avenue ■ ■ Sun City, USA 12345 ■ ■ (555) 802–1887

Pathology Report

Date: April 16, 20xx   Pathology: 43022
Patient: Franks, Robert   Room: 910
Physician: Dante Riox, MD

Specimen: Skin from (a) dorsum left wrist and (b) left forearm, ulnar, near elbow.

Clinical Diagnosis: Bowen disease versus basal cell carcinoma versus dermatitis.

Microscopic Description: (a) There is mild hyperkeratosis and moderate epidermal hyperplasia with full-thickness atypia of squamous keratinocytes. Squamatization of the basal cell layer exists. A lymphocytic inflammatory infiltrate is present in the papillary dermis. Solar elastosis is present. (b) Nests, strands, and columns of atypical neoplastic basaloid keratinocytes grow down from the epidermis into the underlying dermis. Fibroplasia is present. Solar elastosis is noted.

Pathological Diagnosis: (a) Bowen disease of left wrist; (b) nodular and infiltrating basal cell carcinoma of left forearm, near elbow.

Samantha Roberts, MD
Samantha Roberts, MD

sr:bg

D: 4–16-xx
T: 4–16-xx

Terminology

The terms listed in the table that follows are taken from Pathology Report: Skin Lesion. Use a medical dictionary such as *Taber's Cyclopedic Medical Dictionary*, the appendices of this book, or other resources to define each term. Then review the pronunciation for each term and practice by reading the medical record aloud.

Term	Definition
atypia ā-TĬP-ē-ă	
atypical ā-TĬP-ĭ-kăl	
basal cell layer BĀ-săl	
Bowen disease BŌ-ĕn	
dermis DĔR-mĭs	
dorsum DOR-sŭm	
epidermal hyperplasia ĕp-ĭ-DĔR-măl hī pĕr PLĀ zē ă	
fibroplasia fī-brō-PLĀ-sē-ă	
hyperkeratosis hī-pĕr-kĕr-ă- TŌ-sĭs	
infiltrate ĬN-fĭl-trāt	
keratinocytes kĕ-RĂT-ĭ-nō-sīts	
neoplastic nē-ō-PLĂS-tĭk	
papillary PĂP-ĭ-lăr-ē	

Term	Definition
pathological păth-ō-LŎJ-ĭk-ăl	
solar elastosis SŌ-lăr ĕ-lăs- TŌ-sĭs	
squamous SKWĀ-mŭs	

Visit the Medical Terminology Systems online resource center at FADavis. com to practice pronunciation and reinforce the meanings of the terms in this medical report.

Critical Thinking

Review Pathology Report: Skin Lesion to answer the questions.

1. In the specimen section, what does skin on dorsum left wrist mean?

_____

_____

_____

_____

2. What was the inflammatory infiltrate?

_____

_____

_____

_____

3. What was the pathologist's diagnosis for the left forearm?

_____

_____

_____

_____

4. Provide a brief description of Bowen disease, the pathologist's diagnosis for the left wrist.

_____

_____

_____

_____

Documenting Health-Care Activity 5-2
Patient Referral Letter: Onychomycosis

Physician Center

2422 Rodeo Drive ■ ■ **Sun City, USA 12345** ■ ■ **(555)788–2427**

May 3, 20xx

John Roberts, MD
1115 Forest Ave
Sun City, USA 12345

Dear Doctor Roberts:

Thank you for referring Alicia Gonzoles to my office. Mrs. Gonzoles presents to the office for evaluation and treatment of onychomycosis with no previous treatment. Past pertinent medical history does reveal hypertension and breast CA. Pertinent surgical history does reveal mastectomy.

Examination of patient's feet does reveal onychomycosis, 1–5 bilaterally. Vascular and neurological examinations are intact. Previous laboratory work was within normal limits except for an elevated alkaline phosphatase of 100.

Tentative diagnosis: Onychomycosis, 1–5 bilaterally

Treatment consisted of débridement of mycotic nails and bilateral feet and dispensing a prescription for Sporanox Pulse Pack to be taken for 3 months to treat the onychomycotic infection. I have also asked her to repeat her liver enzymes in approximately 4 weeks. Mrs. Gonzoles will make an appointment in 2 months for follow-up, and I will keep you informed of any changes in her progress. If you have any questions, please feel free to contact me.

Sincerely yours,

Juan Perez, MD
Juan Perez, MD

jp:az

Terminology

The terms in the table that follows are taken from Patient Referral Letter: Onychomycosis. Use a medical dictionary such as *Taber's Cyclopedic Medical Dictionary,* the appendices of this book, or other resources to define each term. Then review the pronunciation for each term and practice by reading the medical record aloud.

Term	Definition
alkaline phosphatase ĂL-kă-lĭn FŎS- fă-tās	
bilaterally bī-LĂT-ĕr-ăl-ē	
CA	
débridement dĕ-BRĒD-mĕnt	
hypertension hī-pĕr-TĔN-shŭn	
mastectomy măs-TĔK-tŏ-mē	
neurological noor-ō-LŎJ-ĭk-ăl	
onychomycosis ŏn-ĭ-kō-mī-KŌ-sĭs	
Sporanox* SPŎR-ă-nŏks	
vascular VĂS-kū-lăr	

*Refer to Table 5-3 to determine the drug classification and the generic name for Sporanox.

Visit the Medical Terminology Systems online resource center at FADavis. com to practice pronunciation and reinforce the meanings of the terms in this medical report.

Critical Thinking

Review Patient Referral Letter: Onychomycosis to answer the questions.

1. What pertinent disorders were identified in the past medical history?

   _____

   _____

   _____

2. What pertinent surgery was identified in the past surgical history?

   _____

   _____

   _____

3. Did the doctor identify any problems in the vascular system or nervous system?

   _____

   _____

   _____

4. What was the significant finding in the laboratory results?

   _____

   _____

   _____

5. What treatment did the doctor employ for the onychomycosis?

   _____

   _____

   _____

6. What did the doctor recommend regarding the abnormal laboratory finding?

   _____

   _____

   _____

Documenting Health-Care Activity 5-3
Constructing Chart Notes

To construct chart notes, replace the italicized and boldfaced terms in each of the two case studies with one of the medical terms from the list.

asymptomatic	*erythematous*	*Mohs surgery*
biopsy	*lymphadenectomy*	*oncologist*
chemotherapy	*metastasize*	*pruritic*
dermatologist		

Mr. R. is concerned about a "patch" that developed on the back of his neck. Lately, the patch has become (1) **reddened** and is (2) **itchy.** Now that the patch is crusting and bleeding, his wife advises him to see a (3) **skin specialist.** After various tests are performed, the dermatologist identifies the patch as a basal cell carcinoma. She explains that this type of cancer rarely (4) **spreads to other body sites.** The dermatologist advises that the tumor must be removed using a technique in which (5) **thin layers of cancer-containing skin are progressively removed and microscopically examined until only cancer-free tissue remains.**

1. _____
2. _____
3. _____
4. _____
5. _____

Miss M. noticed that a mole on her neck is increasing in size. Other than the increase in size, Miss M. is experiencing (6) **no other symptoms.** An appointment in the outpatient clinic is scheduled for the (7) **excision of the lesion for microscopic examination.** After evaluation of the biopsy, the pathology report indicates a diagnosis of melanoma. Miss M. is advised to see the (8) **physician who specializes in tumors.** In addition to the melanoma, the surgeon discovers metastasis of adjacent lymph glands (nodes) and (9) **removes the lymph glands (nodes).** After her discharge, Miss M. will begin (10) **treatment using chemicals** to target and destroy any remaining cancer cells.

6. _____
7. _____
8. _____
9. _____
10. _____

✓ *Check your answers in Appendix A. Review any material that you did not answer correctly.*

Correct Answers _____ X 10 = _____ % Score

CHAPTER

6

Digestive System

Chapter Outline

Objectives

Upon completion of this chapter, you will be able to:

- Locate the major organs of the digestive system and describe their structure and function.
- Describe the functional relationship between the digestive system and other body systems.
- Pronounce, spell, and build words related to the digestive system.
- Describe diseases, conditions, and procedures related to the digestive system.
- Explain pharmacology related to the treatment of digestive disorders.
- Demonstrate your knowledge of this chapter by completing the learning and documenting health-care activities.

Anatomy and Physiology

The digestive system, also called the *gastrointestinal (GI) system*, consists of a digestive tube called the *GI tract* (or *alimentary canal*) and several accessory organs whose primary function is to break down food, prepare it for absorption, and eliminate waste. The GI tract, extending from the mouth to the anus, varies in size and structure in several distinct regions.

Food passing along the GI tract is mixed with digestive enzymes and bile and broken down into nutrient molecules, which are absorbed into the bloodstream. Undigested waste materials not absorbed by the blood are then eliminated from the body through defecation. Included in the digestive system are the accessory organs of digestion: the liver, gallbladder, and pancreas. These organs combined with their associated ducts are collectively known as the *biliary system*. The process of digestion breaks down food into nutrients to nourish the body (see Fig. 6-1).

Anatomy and Physiology Key Terms

This section introduces important terms, along with their definitions and pronunciations. The key terms are highlighted in color in the Anatomy and Physiology section. Word analyses for selected terms are also provided. Pronounce the term and place a check mark in the box after you do so.

Term	Definition
bilirubin ☐ bĭl-ĭ-ROO-bĭn	Orange-yellow pigment formed during destruction of erythrocytes that is taken up by liver cells and eventually excreted in the feces *Elevated bilirubin in the blood produces yellowing of the skin (jaundice). It also indicates liver damage or disease.*
bolus ☐ BŌ-lŭs	Mass of masticated, or broken down, food ready for swallowing
exocrine ☐ ĔKS-ō-krĭn 　*exo-:* outside, outward 　*-crine:* secrete	Type of gland that secretes its products through excretory ducts to the surface of an organ or tissue or into a vessel
sphincter ☐ SFĬNGK-tĕr	Circular band of muscle fibers that constricts a passage or closes a natural opening of the body *An example of a sphincter is the lower esophageal (cardiac) sphincter, which constricts once food passes into the stomach.*
triglycerides ☐ trī-GLĬS-ĕr-īd	Most common form of fat (lipid) found in the bloodstream *Triglycerides are stored as unused calories to provide the body with energy. High blood levels increase the risk of heart disease.*

Pronunciation Help	Long Sound	ā — rate	ē — rebirth	ī — isle	ō — over	ū — unite
	Short Sound	ă — apple	ĕ — ever	ĭ — it	ŏ — not	ŭ — cut

Mouth

The process of digestion begins in the mouth (see Fig. 6-2, page 138). The mouth, also known as the (1) **oral cavity**, is a receptacle for food. It is formed by the cheeks (**bucca**), lips, teeth, tongue, and hard and soft palates. Located around the oral cavity are three pairs of salivary glands that secrete saliva. Saliva contains important digestive enzymes that help begin the chemical breakdown of food. In the mouth, food is broken down mechanically (by the teeth) and chemically (by saliva) and then formed into a **bolus**.

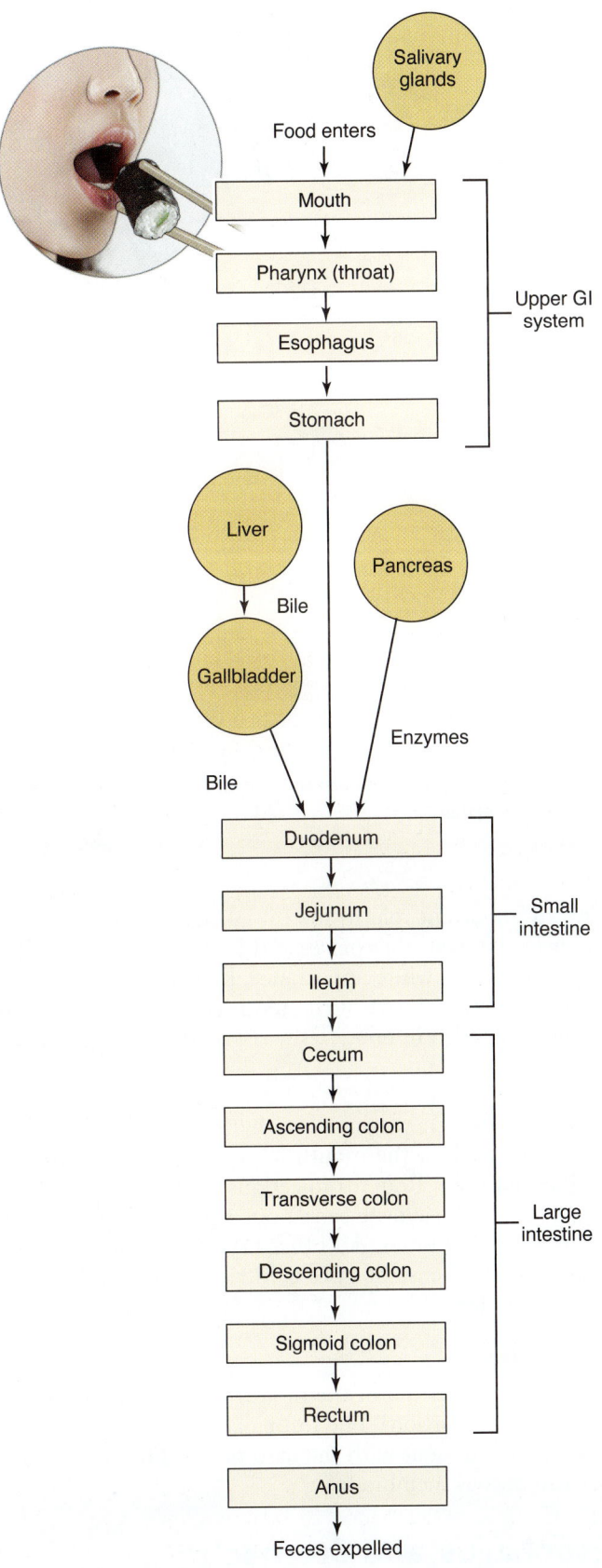

Figure 6-1 Pathway of food through the digestive system.

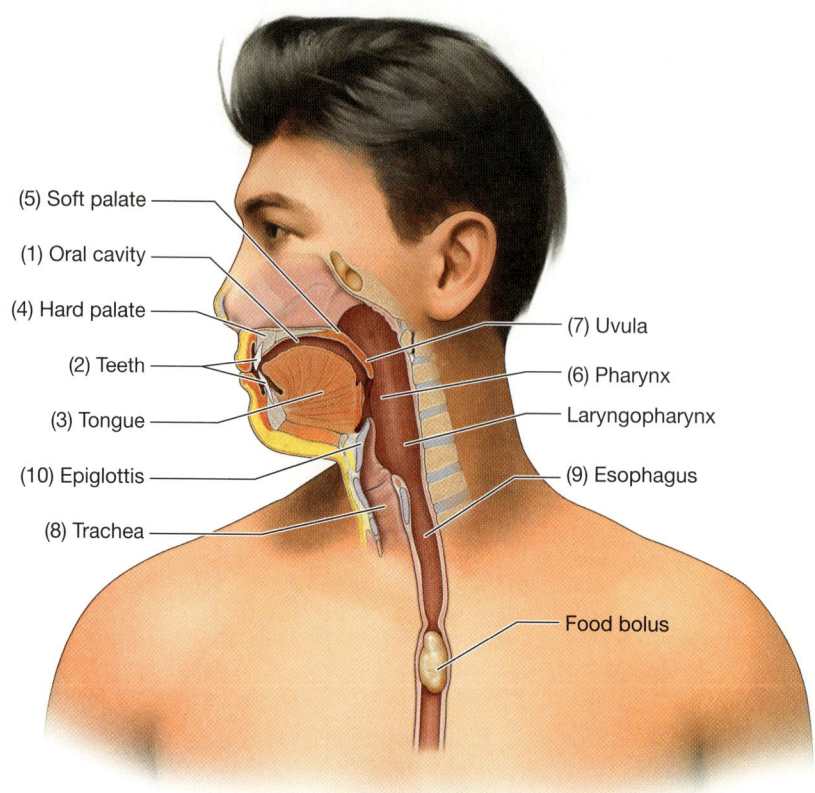

(5) Soft palate

(1) Oral cavity

(4) Hard palate

(2) Teeth

(3) Tongue

(10) Epiglottis

(8) Trachea

(7) Uvula

(6) Pharynx

Laryngopharynx

(9) Esophagus

Food bolus

Figure 6-2 Sagittal view of the head showing oral, nasal, and pharyngeal components of the digestive system.

Teeth

The (2) **teeth** play an important role in the initial stages of digestion by mechanically breaking down food (**mastication**) into smaller pieces as it is mixed with saliva. Teeth are covered by a hard enamel, giving them a smooth, white appearance. Beneath the enamel is **dentin**, the main structure of the tooth. The innermost part of the tooth is the **pulp**, which contains nerves and blood vessels. The teeth are embedded in pink, fleshy tissue known as **gums** (**gingiva**).

Tongue

The (3) **tongue** assists in the chewing process by manipulating the bolus of food during chewing and moving it to the back of the mouth for swallowing (**deglutition**). The tongue also aids in speech production and taste. Rough projections on the surface of the tongue called **papillae** contain taste buds. The four basic taste sensations registered by chemical stimulation of the taste buds are sweet, sour, salty, and bitter. All other taste perceptions are combinations of these four basic flavors. In addition, the sense of taste is intricately linked with the sense of smell, making taste perception very complex.

Hard and Soft Palates

The two structures forming the roof of the mouth are the (4) **hard palate** (anterior portion) and the (5) **soft palate** (posterior portion). The soft palate, which forms a partition between the mouth and the nasopharynx, is continuous with the hard palate. The entire oral cavity, like the rest of the GI tract, is lined with mucous membranes.

Pharynx, Esophagus, and Stomach

As the tongue pushes the bolus into the (6) **pharynx** (throat), it is guided by the soft, fleshy, V-shaped structure called the (7) **uvula**. The funnel-shaped pharynx serves as a passageway to the respiratory and GI tracts and provides a resonating chamber for speech sounds. The lowest portion of the pharynx divides into two tubes: one that leads to the lungs, called the (8) **trachea**, and one that leads to the stomach, called the (9) **esophagus**. A small flap of cartilage called the (10) **epiglottis** folds back to cover the trachea during swallowing, forcing food to enter the esophagus. At all other times, the epiglottis remains upright, allowing air to freely pass through the respiratory structures.

The **stomach**, a saclike structure located in the left upper quadrant (LUQ) of the abdominal cavity, serves as a food reservoir that continues mechanical and chemical digestion (see Fig. 6-3). The stomach extends from the (1) **esophagus** to the first part of the small intestine, the (2) **duodenum**. The terminal portion of the esophagus, the (3) **lower esophageal (cardiac) sphincter**, is composed of muscle fibers that constrict once food has passed into the stomach. It prevents the stomach contents from regurgitating back into the esophagus. The (4) **body** of the stomach, the large central portion, together with the (5) **fundus**, the upper portion, are mainly storage areas. Most digestion takes place in the funnel-shaped terminal portion, the (6) **pylorus**. The interior lining of the stomach is composed of mucous membranes and contains numerous macroscopic longitudinal folds called (7) **rugae** that gradually unfold as the stomach fills. Located within the rugae, digestive glands produce hydrochloric acid (HCl) and enzymes. Secretions from these glands coupled with the mechanical churning of the stomach turn the bolus into a semiliquid form called **chyme** that slowly leaves the stomach through the (8) **pyloric sphincter** to enter the duodenum. This **sphincter** regulates the speed and movement of chyme into the small intestine and prohibits backflow. Food is propelled through the entire GI tract by coordinated, rhythmic muscle contractions called **peristalsis**.

Small Intestine

The small intestine extends approximately 20 feet from the pyloric sphincter to the first part of the large intestine (see Fig. 6-4, page 140). It consists of three parts:

1. **duodenum**, the uppermost segment, which is approximately 10 inches long
2. **jejunum**, which is approximately 8 feet long
3. **ileum**, which is approximately 12 feet long

Digestion and nutrient absorption are completed in the small intestine with the help of additional enzymes and secretions from the (4) **pancreas** and (5) **liver**. Nutrients in chyme are

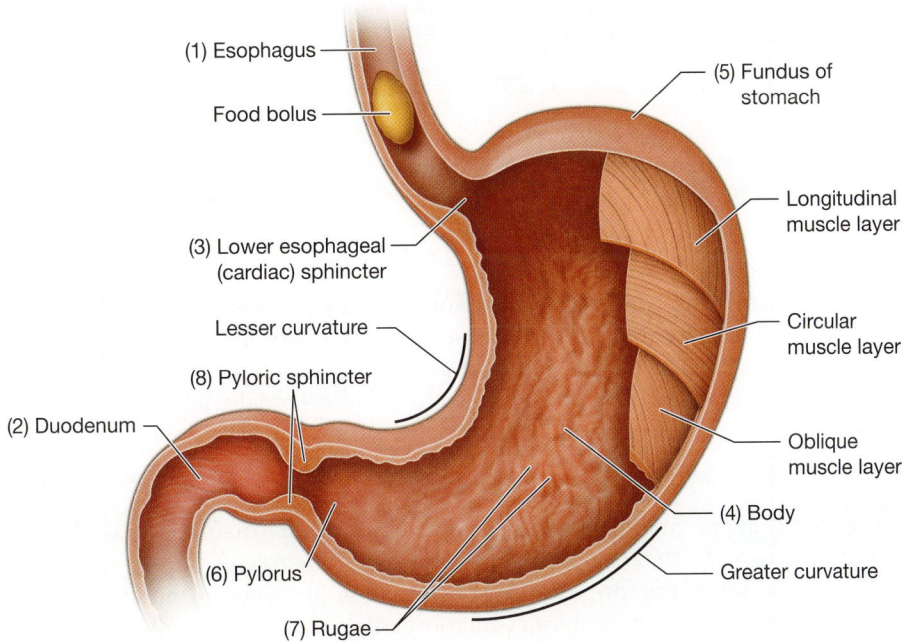

Figure 6-3 Anterior view of the stomach showing muscle layers and rugae of the mucosa.

Figure 6-4 Anterior view of the trunk and digestive organs.

absorbed through microscopic, fingerlike projections called **villi**. Nutrients enter the bloodstream and lymphatic system for distribution to the rest of the body. At the terminal end of the small intestine, a sphincter muscle called the **ileocecal valve** allows undigested or unabsorbed material from the small intestine to pass into the large intestine and eventually be excreted from the body.

Large Intestine

The large intestine is approximately 5 feet in length with a wider diameter than the small intestine, and it extends from the end of the ileum to the anus. The role of the large intestine focuses on the reabsorption of water, the formation and elimination of wastes in the form of feces (stool), and the maintenance of the gut microbiota (microorganisms like bacteria, fungi, and viruses that live in the intestines). A balanced diet rich in fiber, regular hydration, and good gut health practices are essential for the proper functioning of the large intestine. The large intestine has three main components: the cecum, colon, and rectum. The first 2 or 3 inches of the large intestine comprise the (6) **cecum**, a small pouch that hangs inferior to the ileocecal valve. Projecting downward from the cecum is the (7) **appendix**, a small, wormlike structure with no apparent function. The cecum merges as it becomes the first part of the colon. The colon is divided into ascending, transverse, descending, and sigmoid portions:

- The (8) **ascending colon** extends from the cecum to the lower border of the liver and turns left to form the (9) **hepatic flexure**.
- The (10) **transverse colon** continues across the abdomen to the left side, curving beneath the lower end of the (11) **spleen** to form the (12) **splenic flexure**.
- As the transverse colon turns downward, it becomes the (13) **descending colon**.
- The descending colon continues until it forms the (14) **sigmoid colon** and the (15) **rectum**. The rectum, the last part of the GI tract, terminates at the (16) **anus**.

Accessory Organs of Digestion

Although the liver, gallbladder, and pancreas lie outside the GI tract, they play a vital role in the proper digestion and absorption of nutrients (see Fig. 6-5).

Liver

The (1) **liver**, the largest glandular organ in the body, weighs approximately 3 to 4 pounds. It is located beneath the diaphragm in the right upper quadrant (RUQ) and the left upper quadrant (LUQ) of the abdominal cavity. The liver has a crucial role in digestion and performs many vital functions that include:

- Storing vitamins, such as B_{12}, A, D, E, and K
- Regulating glucose levels in the blood

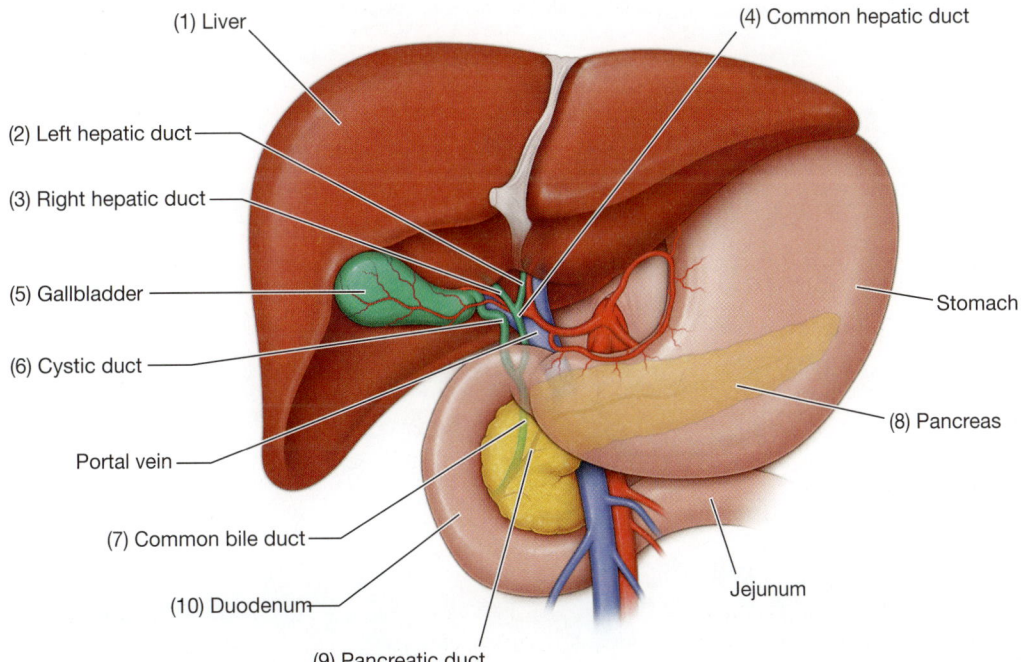

Figure 6-5 Liver, gallbladder, pancreas, and duodenum with associated ducts and blood vessels.

- Destroying or transforming toxic products into less harmful compounds
- Synthesizing proteins that circulate in the blood, such as albumin for fluid balance and pro-thrombin and fibrinogen for coagulation (blood clotting)
- Destroying old erythrocytes and releasing **bilirubin**
- Producing bile, which aids in the digestion of fat

Components of **bile** include **bilirubin, bile salts,** and cholesterol. Bilirubin is the pigment that gives bile its yellow-green color. Bile salts play the primary role of breaking down and emulsifying dietary fats, while cholesterol is carried out of the body as waste through bile.

The liver continuously produces bile that drains through two main ducts, the (2) **left hepatic duct** and the (3) **right hepatic duct,** which merge to form the (4) **common hepatic duct,** carrying bile away from the liver.

Gallbladder

The (5) **gallbladder** is a saclike structure on the inferior surface of the liver that serves as a storage reservoir for bile. After meals, when bile is needed for digestion, the gallbladder contracts, expelling bile through the (6) **cystic duct** and into the (7) **common bile duct,** toward the duodenum of the small intestine.

Pancreas

The (8) **pancreas** is an elongated, somewhat flattened organ that lies posterior and slightly inferior to the stomach. It performs endocrine and exocrine functions. As an **endocrine** gland, the pancreas secretes insulin directly into the bloodstream to maintain normal blood glucose levels. (For a comprehensive discussion of the endocrine function of the pancreas, review Chapter 13.) As an **exocrine** gland, the pancreas produces various digestive enzymes such as trypsin, which digests proteins; amylase, which digests starch; and lipase, which digests **triglycerides**. These enzymes pass into the duodenum through the (9) **pancreatic duct**. The pancreatic duct extends along the pancreas and joins with the common bile duct to enter the (10) **duodenum**.

Anatomy Review: Digestive System

To review the anatomy of the digestive system, label the illustration using the listed terms.

anus

appendix

ascending colon

cecum

descending colon

duodenum

hepatic flexure

ileum

jejunum

liver

pancreas

rectum

sigmoid colon

spleen

splenic flexure

transverse colon

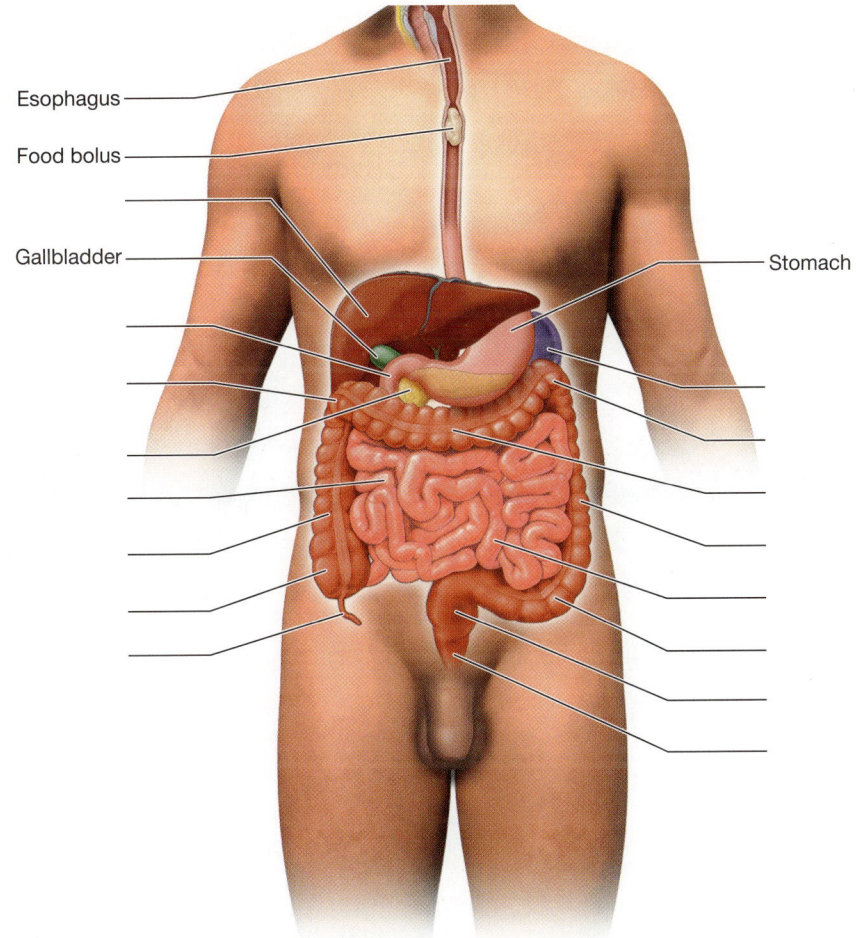

Esophagus

Food bolus

Gallbladder

Stomach

Check your answers by referring to Figure 6-4 on page 140. Review material that you did not answer correctly.

Anatomy Review: Accessory Organs of Digestion

To review the anatomy of the accessory organs of digestion, label the illustration using the listed terms.

common bile duct

cystic duct

duodenum

gallbladder

hepatic duct

left hepatic duct

liver

pancreas

pancreatic duct

right hepatic duct

Stomach

Portal vein

Jejunum

 Check your answers by referring to Figure 6–5 on page 141. Review material that you did not answer correctly.

CONNECTING BODY SYSTEMS—DIGESTIVE SYSTEM

The main function of the digestive system is to provide vital nutrients for growth, maintenance, and repair of all organs and body cells. Specific functional relationships between the digestive system and other body systems are discussed here.

Blood, Lymphatic, and Immune
- The liver regulates blood glucose levels.
- The digestive tract secretes acids and enzymes to provide a hostile environment for pathogens.
- The intestinal walls contain lymphoid nodules that help prevent the invasion of pathogens.
- The digestive system absorbs vitamin K, which is necessary for blood clotting.

Cardiovascular
- The digestive system absorbs nutrients needed by the heart.

Endocrine
- The liver eliminates hormones from the blood.
- The pancreas contains hormone-producing cells.

Female Reproductive
- The digestive system provides adequate nutrition, including fats, to make conception and normal fetal development possible.
- The digestive system provides nutrients for repair of the endometrium following menstruation.

Male Reproductive
- The digestive system provides adequate nutrients for the development of viable sperm.

Integumentary
- The digestive system supplies fats that provide insulation in the dermis and subcutaneous tissue.
- The digestive system absorbs nutrients for maintenance, growth, and repair of the skin.

Musculoskeletal
- The digestive system provides the nutrients needed for energy fuel.
- The digestive system absorbs calcium, which is needed for bone salts and muscle contraction.
- The liver removes lactic acid (resulting from muscle activity) from the blood.

Nervous
- The digestive system supplies nutrients necessary for normal neural functioning.
- The digestive system provides nutrients for the synthesis of neurotransmitters and electrolytes for the transmission of a nervous impulse.
- Approximately 90% of the neurotransmitter serotonin is found in the GI tract. There is an interplay of neurotransmitter signals from the gut to the brain and vice versa through the vagus nerve.
- The liver plays a role in maintaining the glucose levels needed for neural function.

Respiratory
- The digestive system absorbs nutrients needed by cells in the lungs and other tissues in the respiratory tract.
- The pharynx is shared by the digestive and respiratory systems. The lowest portion of the pharynx divides into two tubes: one that leads to the lungs, called the *trachea,* and one that leads to the stomach, called the *esophagus.*

Urinary
- The liver metabolizes hormones, toxins, and drugs into forms that can be excreted in the urine.

Medical Word Elements

This section introduces combining forms, suffixes, and prefixes related to the digestive system. Word analyses are also provided. From the information provided, complete the meaning of the medical words in the right-hand column. The first one is completed for you.

Element	Meaning	Word Analysis and Meaning
Combining Forms		
Mouth		
or/o	mouth	**or**/al (OR-ăl): *pertaining to the mouth* *-al:* pertaining to
stomat/o		**stomat**/itis (stŏ-mă-TĪ-tĭs): _____ *-itis:* inflammation
gloss/o	tongue	**gloss**/ectomy (glŏs-ĔK-tō-mē): _____ *-ectomy:* excision, removal
lingu/o		**lingu**/al (LĬN-gwăl): _____ *-al:* pertaining to
bucc/o	cheek	**bucc**/al (BŬK-ăl): _____ *-al:* pertaining to
cheil/o	lip	**cheil/o**/plasty (KĪ-lō-plăs-tē): _____ *-plasty:* surgical repair
labi/o		**labi**/al (LĀ-bē-ăl): _____ *-al:* pertaining to
dent/o	teeth	**dent**/ist (DĔN-tĭst): _____ *-ist:* specialist
odont/o		orth/**odont**/ist (or-thō-DŎN-tĭst): _____ *orth:* straight *-ist:* specialist *Orthodontists are dentists who specialize in correcting and preventing irregularities of abnormally aligned teeth.*
gingiv/o	gum(s)	**gingiv**/ectomy (jĭn-jĭ-VĔK-tō-mē): _____ *-ectomy:* excision, removal *Gingivectomy is a surgical treatment for periodontal disease.*
sial/o	saliva, salivary gland	**sial/o**/lith (sī-ĂL-ō-lĭth): _____ *-lith:* stone, calculus
Esophagus, Pharynx, and Stomach		
esophag/o	esophagus	**esophag/o**/scope (ē-SŎF-ă-gō-skōp): _____ *-scope:* instrument for examining

Medical Word Elements—cont'd

Element	Meaning	Word Analysis
pharyng/o	pharynx (throat)	**pharyng/o**/tonsill/itis (fă-rĭng-gō-tŏn-sĭ-LĪ-tĭs): _____ *tonsill:* tonsils *-itis:* inflammation
gastr/o	stomach	**gastr/**algia (găs-TRĂL-jē-ă): _____ *-algia:* pain *Gastralgia is also called stomachache.*
pylor/o	pylorus	**pylor/o**/spasm (pī-LOR-ō-spăzm): _____ *-spasm:* involuntary contraction, twitching *Pylorospasm occurs in the pyloric sphincter of the stomach.*
Small Intestine		
duoden/o	duodenum (first part of small intestine)	**duoden/o**/scopy (dū-ŏd-ĕ-NŎS-kō-pē): _____ *-scopy:* visual examination
enter/o	intestine (usually small intestine)	**enter/o**/pathy (ĕn-tĕr-ŎP-ă-thē): _____ *-pathy:* disease *Enteropathy typically occurs in the small intestine.*
jejun/o	jejunum (second part of small intestine)	**jejun/o**/rrhaphy (jĕ-joo-NOR-ă-fē): _____ *-rrhaphy:* suture
ile/o	ileum (third part of small intestine)	**ile/o**/stomy (ĭl-ē-ŎS-tō-mē): _____ *-stomy*:* forming an opening (mouth) *An ileostomy creates an opening on the abdominal wall to allow feces to be discharged into an external bag worn on the abdomen.*
Large Intestine		
append/o	appendix	**append/**ectomy (ăp-ĕn-DĔK-tō-mē): _____ *-ectomy:* excision, removal *An appendectomy removes a diseased appendix that is in danger of rupturing.*
appendic/o		**appendic/**itis (ă-pĕn-dĭ-SĪ-tĭs): _____ *-itis:* inflammation

*When the suffix *-stomy* is used with a combining form that denotes an organ, it refers to a surgical opening to the outside of the body.

Continued

Medical Word Elements—cont'd

Element	Meaning	Word Analysis
col/o	colon	**col/o**/stomy (kō-LŎS-tō-mē): _____ *-stomy:** forming an opening (mouth) *A colostomy creates a place for fecal matter to exit the body other than through the anus.*
colon/o		**colon/o**/scopy (kō-lŏn-ŎS-kō-pē): _____ *-scopy:* visual examination *Colonoscopy is performed with an elongated flexible endoscope called a colonoscope.*
sigmoid/o	sigmoid colon	**sigmoid/o**/tomy (sĭg-moyd-ŎT-ō-mē): _____ *-tomy:* incision
Terminal End of Large Intestine		
rect/o	rectum	**rect/o**/cele (RĔK-tŏ-sēl): _____ *-cele:* hernia, swelling *Rectocele is also known as proctocele.*
proct/o	anus, rectum	**proct/o**/logist (prŏk-TŎL-ō-jĭst): _____ *-logist:* specialist in the study of *A proctologist is a physician who specializes in treating disorders of the colon, rectum, and anus.*
an/o	anus	peri/**an**/al (pĕr-ē-Ā-năl): _____ *peri-:* around *-al:* pertaining to
Accessory Organs of Digestion		
hepat/o	liver	**hepat/o**/megaly (hĕp-ă-tō-MĔG-ă-lē): _____ *-megaly:* enlargement
pancreat/o	pancreas	**pancreat/o**/lysis (păn-krē-ă-TŎL-ĭ-sĭs): _____ *-lysis:* separation; destruction; loosening *Pancreatolysis may be related to alcohol consumption or result from inflammation, infection, or cancer.*
cholangi/o	bile vessel	**cholangi/o**/le (kō-LĂN-jē-ōl): _____ *-ole:* small, minute
chol/e**	bile, gall	**chol/e**/lith (KŌ-lē-lĭth): _____ *-lith:* calculus, stone *Gallstones are solid masses composed of bile and cholesterol that form in the gallbladder and common bile duct.*

*When the suffix *-stomy* is used with a combining form that denotes an organ, it refers to a surgical opening to the outside of the body.

**The e in *chol/e* is an exception to the rule of using the connecting vowel *o*.

Medical Word Elements—cont'd

Element	Meaning	Word Analysis
cholecyst/o	gallbladder	**cholecyst**/ectomy (kō-lē-sĭs-TĔK-tō-mē): _____ -*ectomy:* excision, removal *Cholecystectomy is performed by laparoscopic or open surgery.*
choledoch/o	bile duct	**choledoch/o**/plasty (kō-LĔD-ō-kō-plăs-tē): _____ -*plasty:* surgical repair

Suffixes

Element	Meaning	Word Analysis
-emesis	vomit	hyper/**emesis** (hī-pĕr-ĔM-ĕ-sĭs): _____ *hyper-:* excessive, above normal
-iasis	abnormal condition (produced by something specified)	chol/e/lith/**iasis** (kō-lē-lĭ-THĪ-ă-sĭs): _____ *chol/e:* bile, gall *lith:* stone, calculus *When gallstones form in the common bile duct, the condition is called choledocholithiasis.*
-megaly	enlargement	hepat/o/**megaly** (hĕp-ă-tō-MĔG-ă-lē): _____ *hepat/o:* liver *Hepatomegaly may be caused by hepatitis or infection, fatty infiltration (as in alcoholism), biliary obstruction, or malignancy.*
-orexia	appetite	an/**orexia** (ăn-ō-RĔK-sē-ă): _____ *an-:* without, not *Anorexia can result from various conditions, such as adverse effects of drugs or various physical or psychological causes.*
-pepsia	digestion	dys/**pepsia** (dĭs-PĔP-sē-ă): _____ *dys-:* bad, painful, difficult *Dyspepsia, also called indigestion, is an epigastric discomfort felt after eating.*
-phagia	swallowing, eating	aer/o/**phagia** (ĕr-ō-FĀ-jē-ă): _____ *aer/o:* air
-prandial	meal	post/**prandial** (pōst-PRĂN-dē-ăl): _____ *post-:* after, behind
-rrhea	discharge, flow	steat/o/**rrhea** (stē-ă-tō-RĒ-ă): _____ *steat/o:* fat

Continued

Medical Word Elements—cont'd

Element	Meaning	Word Analysis
Prefixes		
dia-	through, across	**dia**/rrhea (dī-ă-RĒ-ă): _____ *-rrhea:* discharge, flow *Diarrhea is a discharge or flow of fluid fecal matter through the bowel.*
peri-	around	**peri**/odont/itis (pĕr-ē-ō-dŏn-TĪ-tĭs): _____ *odont-:* tooth *-itis:* inflammation
sub-	under, below	**sub**/lingu/al (sŭb-LĬN-gwăl): _____ *lingu:* tongue *-al:* pertaining to

Visit the Medical Terminology Systems online resource center at FADavis.com for an audio exercise using the terms in this table. Other activities are also available to reinforce content.

 It is time to review medical word elements by completing Learning Activities 6-1, 6-2, and 6-3.

Disease Focus

Although some digestive disorders do not manifest symptoms (**asymptomatic**), many are associated with nausea, vomiting, bleeding, pain, and weight loss. Clinical signs, such as jaundice and edema, may indicate a hepatic disorder. Severe infection, drug toxicity, and changes in fluid and electrolyte balance can cause behavioral abnormalities. Disorders of the GI tract or any of the accessory organs (liver, gallbladder, and pancreas) may result in far-reaching metabolic or systemic problems that can eventually threaten life itself. Assessment of a suspected digestive disorder includes a thorough history and physical examination. A range of diagnostic tests can assist in identifying abnormalities of the GI tract, liver, gallbladder, and pancreas.

For diagnosis, treatment, and management of digestive disorders, the medical services of a specialist may be warranted. **Gastroenterology** is the branch of medicine concerned with digestive diseases. The physician who specializes in the diagnosis and treatment of digestive disorders is known as a **gastroenterologist**. Gastroenterologists do not perform surgeries; however, under the broad classification of surgery, they do perform such procedures as liver biopsies and endoscopic examinations.

Peptic Ulcer Disease (PUD)

An **ulcer** is a circumscribed open sore on the skin or mucous membrane of the body. Peptic ulcers are one of the most common ulcer types that occur in the digestive system. They primarily develop in the stomach and duodenum but may also occur to a lesser extent in the lower esophagus. Ulcers are named by their location in the body: *esophageal ulcer, gastric ulcer,* or *duodenal ulcer* (see Fig. 6-6).

A common cause of PUD is the erosion of the protective mucous membrane caused by infection with ***Helicobacter pylori*** (*H. pylori*) bacteria. As the mucous membrane erodes, it exposes the tissue beneath to the strong acids and digestive enzymes of the stomach, and eventually, an ulcer forms. Some individuals have more rapid gastric emptying, which—combined with hypersecretion of acid—creates a large amount of acid moving into the duodenum. As a result, peptic ulcers occur more commonly in the duodenum.

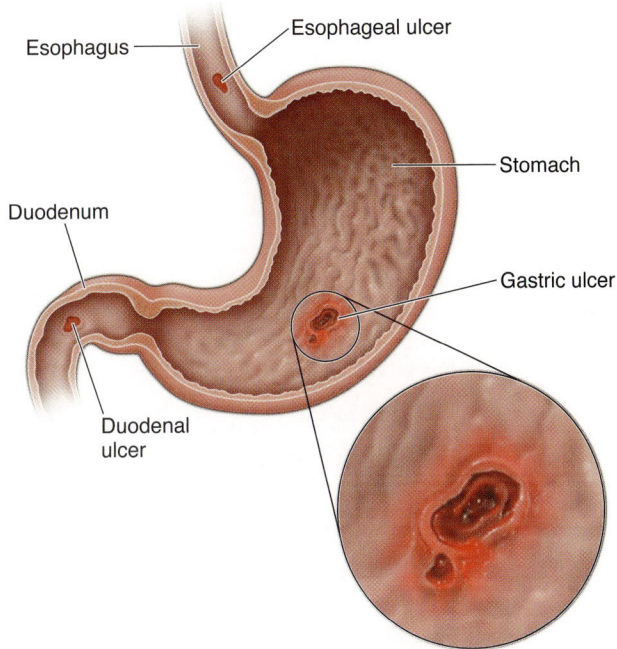

Esophageal ulcer

Esophagus

Stomach

Duodenum

Gastric ulcer

Duodenal ulcer

Figure 6-6 Peptic ulcers.

Risk factors that contribute to PUD include smoking, chewing tobacco, stress, caffeine use, and such medications as steroids, aspirin, and nonsteroidal anti-inflammatory drugs (NSAIDs). Smoking contributes to the development of peptic ulcers by enhancing the damaging effects of *H. pylori*, disrupting protective mechanisms, and reducing gastric blood flow.

Treatment of PUD includes antibiotics to destroy *H. pylori* and antacids to reduce stomach acids and allow the ulcer to heal. If left untreated, mucosal destruction produces a hole (**perforation**) in the wall lining, with resultant bleeding from the damaged area. At worst, the hole penetrates the entire wall, and the gastric contents leak into the abdominal cavity, possibly leading to inflammation of the peritoneum (**peritonitis**).

Hernia

A **hernia** is a protrusion of any organ, tissue, or structure through the wall of the cavity in which it is naturally contained (see Fig. 6-7). In general, though, the term is applied to protrusions of abdominal organs (**viscera**) through the abdominal wall.

An (1) **inguinal hernia** develops in the groin where the abdominal folds of flesh meet the thighs. In the initial stages, it may be hardly noticeable and appears as a soft lump under the skin, no larger than a marble. In the early stages, an inguinal hernia is usually reducible; that is, it can be pushed gently back into its normal place. With this type of hernia, pain may be minimal. As time passes, the pressure of the abdomen against the weak abdominal wall may increase the size of the opening and the size of the hernia lump. If the blood supply to the hernia is cut off because of pressure, a (2) **strangulated hernia** may develop, leading to necrosis with gangrene. An (3) **umbilical hernia** is a protrusion of part of the intestine at the navel. It occurs more commonly in obese women and among those who have had several pregnancies. Hernias also occur in newborn infants (**congenital**) or during early childhood. If the defect has not corrected itself by age 2, the deformity can be surgically corrected. Treatment consists of surgical repair of the hernia (**hernioplasty**) with suture of the abdominal wall (**herniorrhaphy**).

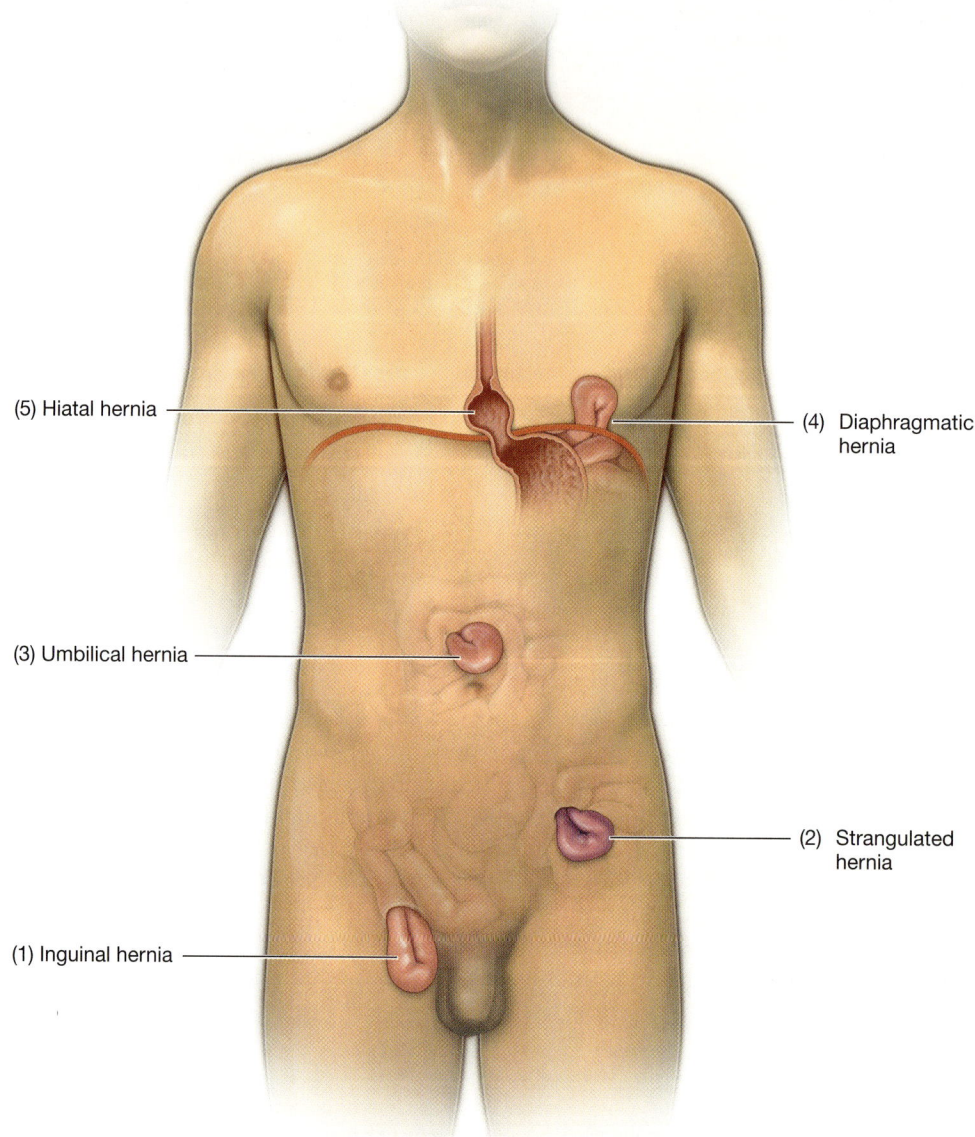

Figure 6-7 Common types and locations of hernias.

Although hernias most commonly occur in the abdominal region, they may develop in the diaphragm. Two forms of this type include (4) **diaphragmatic hernia**, a congenital disorder, and (5) **hiatal hernia**, in which the lower part of the esophagus and the top of the stomach slide through an opening **(hiatus)** in the diaphragm into the thorax. With a hiatal hernia, stomach acid backs up into the esophagus, causing heartburn, chest pain, and swallowing difficulty. Although many hiatal hernias are asymptomatic, if the disease continues for a prolonged period, it may cause **gastroesophageal reflux disease (GERD)**.

Hepatitis

Hepatitis is an inflammatory condition of the liver. The usual causes include exposure to toxic substances, especially alcohol, obstructions in the bile ducts, metabolic diseases, autoimmune diseases, and bacterial or viral infections. A growing public health concern is the increasing incidence of viral hepatitis. Even though its mortality rate is low, the disease is easily transmitted and can cause significant morbidity and prolonged loss of time from school or employment.

Although forms of hepatitis range from hepatitis A through hepatitis E, the three most common forms are hepatitis A **(HAV; infectious hepatitis)**, hepatitis B (HBV; **serum hepatitis**), and hepatitis C (HCV). The most common cause of HAV is the ingestion of contaminated food, water, or milk. HBV and HCV are usually transmitted by routes other than the mouth **(parenteral)**, such as from blood transfusions and sexual contact. Because of patient exposure, healthcare personnel are at increased risk for contracting HBV, but a vaccine that provides immunity to HBV is available. There is no vaccine available for HCV. Patients with HCV may remain asymptomatic for years, or the disease may produce only mild, flulike symptoms. Treatment for hepatitis includes antiviral drugs; however, there is no cure. As the disease progresses, scarring of the liver may become so serious that liver transplantation is the only recourse.

One of the major symptoms of many liver disorders, including hepatitis and cirrhosis, is a yellowing of the skin, mucous membranes, and sclerae of the eyes **(jaundice** or **icterus)**. This condition occurs because the liver is no longer able to remove **bilirubin**, a yellow compound formed during the destruction of erythrocytes. Jaundice may also result when the bile duct is blocked, causing bile to enter the bloodstream (see Fig. 6-8).

Figure 6-8 Jaundice. Yellow sclerae of the eye from excess bilirubin.

Diverticulosis

Diverticulosis is a condition in which small, blisterlike pockets **(diverticula)** develop in the inner lining of the large intestine and may balloon through the intestinal wall. These pockets occur most commonly in the sigmoid colon (see Fig. 6-9). They usually do not cause any problem unless they become inflamed **(diverticulitis)**. Symptoms of diverticulitis include pain, commonly in the left lower quadrant (LLQ) of the abdomen, extreme constipation **(obstipation)** or diarrhea, fever, abdominal swelling, and occasional blood in bowel movements. Treatment for mild cases of diverticulitis includes rest, antibiotics, and changes in diet. Severe cases, however, may require surgical intervention, such as excision of the affected segment of intestine.

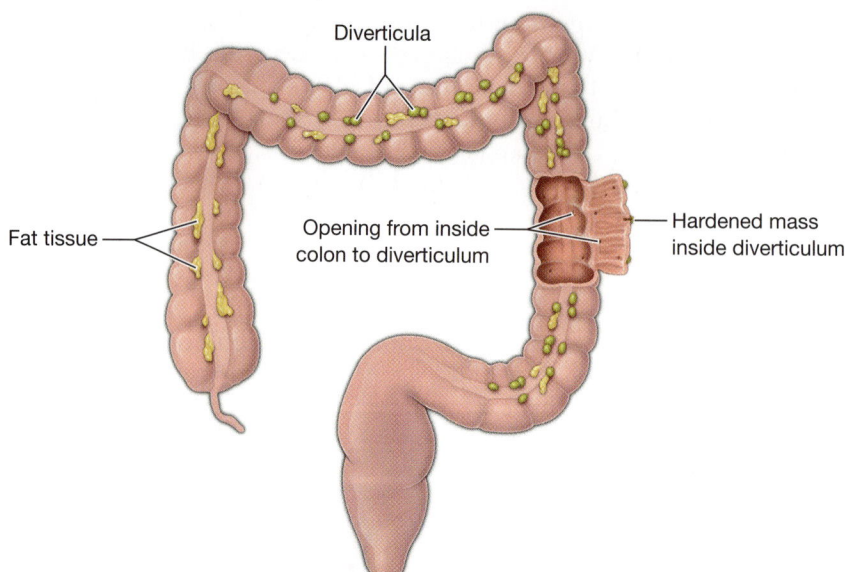

Diverticula

Fat tissue —

Opening from inside
colon to diverticulum

— Hardened mass
inside diverticulum

Figure 6-9 Diverticula of the colon.

Oncology

There are several types of GI cancers that occur in the cells, tissues, and organs of the digestive system. Like other cancers, underlying conditions, genetics, and lifestyle choices can all contribute to abnormal cell growth that ultimately causes malignancy in the digestive system. Risk factors for GI cancer, many of which are modifiable, except for increasing age and infection, include obesity, smoking, excessive alcohol consumption, and diets high in animal fats and poorly preserved food. Depending on the location of the cancer and how advanced it is, symptoms can include nausea and vomiting, abdominal pain, unintentional weight loss, changes in bowel habits, difficulty swallowing, and blood in the stool.

Although gastric (stomach) cancer is rare in the United States, it is common in many parts of the world where food preservation is problematic. It is a significant medical problem because of its high mortality rate. Men are more susceptible to stomach cancer than women. The neoplasm nearly always develops from the epithelial or mucosal lining of the stomach in the form of a cancerous glandular tumor (**gastric adenocarcinoma**). Persistent indigestion is an important warning sign of stomach cancer.

Other types of GI carcinomas include **esophageal** carcinomas, **hepatocellular** carcinomas, and **pancreatic** carcinomas. Less common GI cancers include neuroendocrine tumors (NETs), GI stromal tumors (GISTs), and anal cancer.

Colorectal cancer is the most common type of intestinal cancer in the United States. With this type of cancer, abnormal growth of cells called *polyps* arise from the epithelial lining of the colon or rectum and can occur anywhere in the large intestine. Polyps are not always cancerous and are categorized by their shape and cell pattern. Symptoms of carcinoma of the colon depend largely on the location of the malignancy and include changes in bowel habits, passage of blood and mucus in stools, rectal or abdominal pain, anemia, weight loss, varying degrees of obstruction, and perforation (see Fig. 6-10). There are several diagnostic tests and procedures used to detect and stage colorectal cancer. A procedure called a *colonoscopy* uses a thin, flexible, lighted tube with a camera (colonoscope) to directly view the entire length of the colon and rectum. Biopsies of abnormal cells can be performed through the colonoscope. Due to advances in both early detection and treatment, the prognosis of colorectal cancer is generally good when caught early. The stages of colon cancer are illustrated in Figure 6-11.

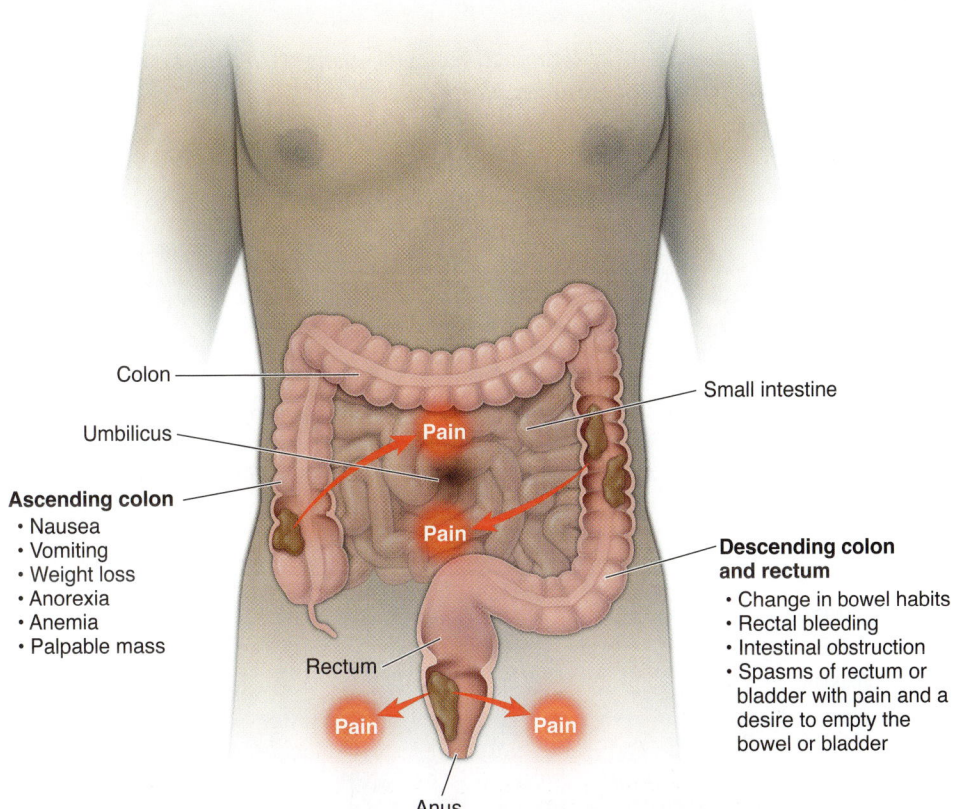

Figure 6-10 Symptoms of carcinoma of the colon, in which pain usually radiates toward the umbilicus or perianal area.

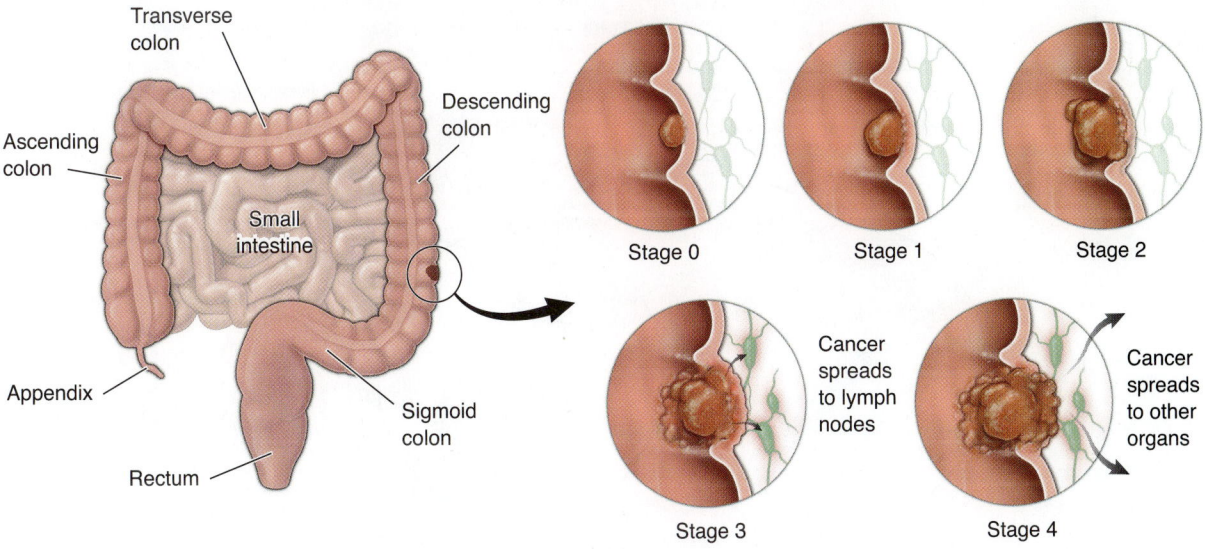

Figure 6-11 Stages of colon cancer.

Diseases and Conditions

This section introduces diseases and conditions of the digestive system, along with their meanings and pronunciations. Word analyses for selected terms are also provided.

Term	Definition
anorexia ăn-ō-RĔK-sē-ă *an-:* without, not *-orexia:* appetite	Lack or loss of appetite, resulting in the inability to eat *Anorexia should not be confused with anorexia nervosa, which is a complex psychogenic eating disorder characterized by an all-consuming desire to remain thin.*
appendicitis ă-pĕn-dĭ-SĪ-tĭs *appendic:* appendix *-itis:* inflammation	Inflammation of the appendix, usually caused by obstruction or infection *Treatment for appendicitis is open or laparoscopic appendectomy. Because of the likelihood of the appendix rupturing and causing a severe, life-threatening infection, the surgeon will remove the appendix as soon as possible (see Fig. 6-12).*

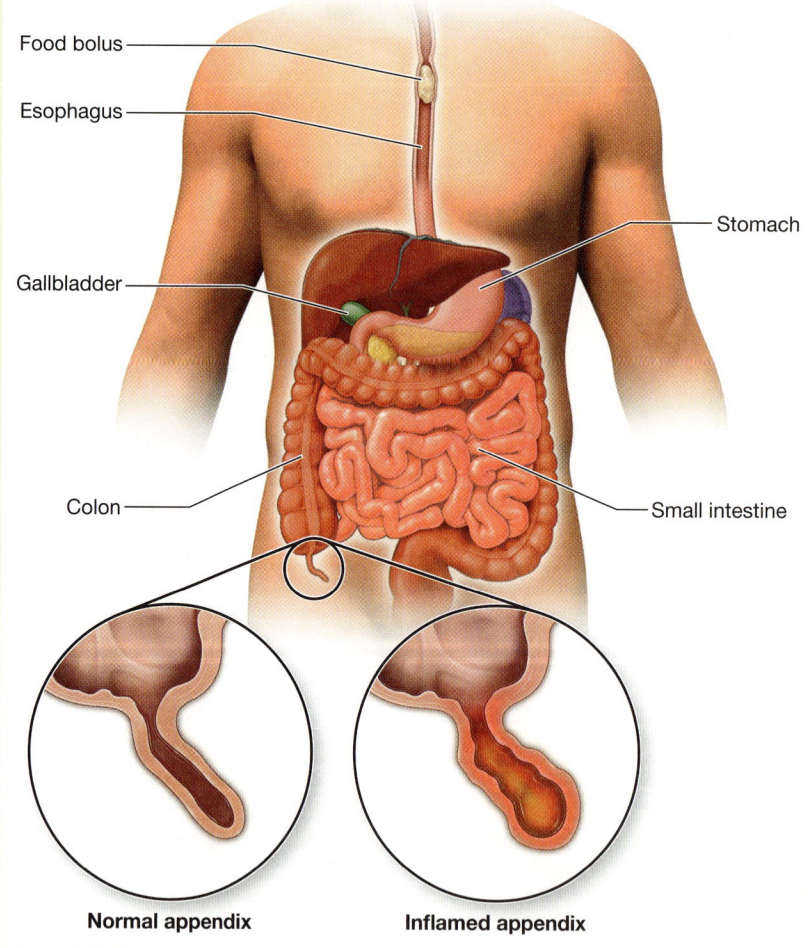

Food bolus

Esophagus

Stomach

Gallbladder

Colon

Small intestine

Normal appendix   Inflamed appendix

Figure 6-12 Appendicitis.

Diseases and Conditions—cont'd

Term	Definition
ascites ă-SĪ-tēz	Abnormal accumulation of fluid in the abdominal cavity, usually as a result of chronic liver disease, a neoplasm, or an inflammatory disorder in the abdomen *Ascites is most commonly associated with cirrhosis of the liver, especially when caused by alcoholism. Treatment includes paracentesis to remove the fluid.*
borborygmus bor-bō-RĬG-mŭs	Rumbling or gurgling noises that are audible at a distance and caused by passage of gas through the liquid contents of the intestine
cachexia kă-KĔKS-ē-ă	Physical wasting that includes loss of weight and muscle mass and is commonly associated with acquired immune deficiency syndrome (AIDS) and cancer; also called *wasting syndrome*
cholelithiasis kō-lē-lĭ-THĪ-ă-sĭs *chol/e:* bile, gall *lith:* stone, calculus *-iasis:* abnormal condition (produced by something specified)	Presence or formation of gallstones in the gallbladder *When one or more gallstones are present in the common bile duct, the condition is called choledocholithiasis. Gallstones may or may not produce symptoms (see Fig. 6-13).*

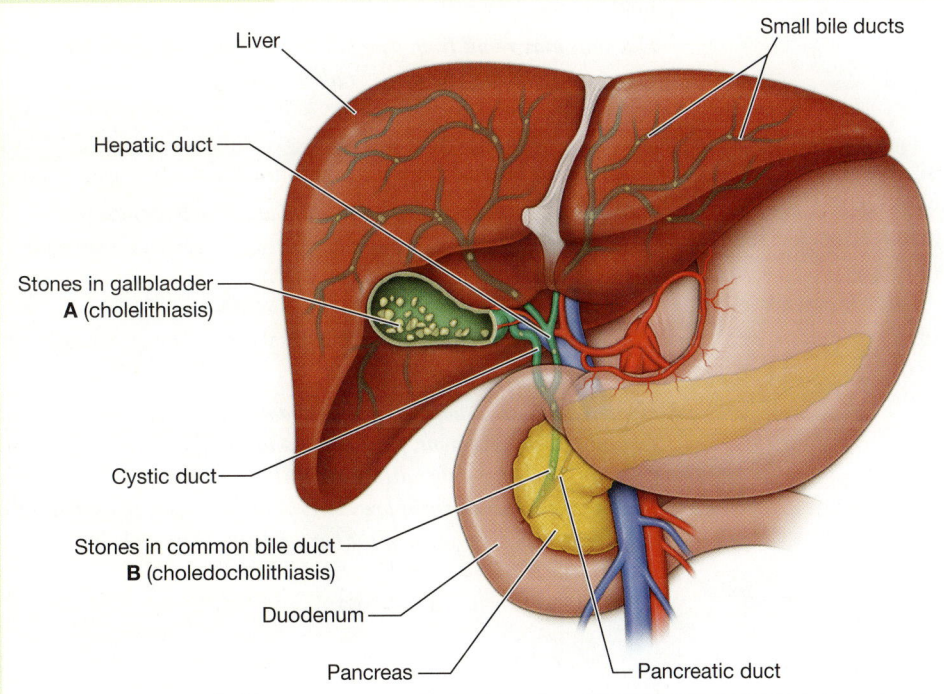

Figure 6-13 Sites of gallstones. (A) Cholelithiasis. (B) Choledocholithiasis.

Term	Definition
cirrhosis sĭr-RŌ-sĭs	Scarring and dysfunction of the liver caused by chronic liver disease *Cirrhosis is most commonly caused by chronic alcoholism. It may also be caused by toxins, infectious agents, metabolic diseases, and circulatory disorders.*

Continued

Diseases and Conditions—cont'd

Term	Definition
dysentery DĬS-ĕn-tĕr-ē	Inflammation of the intestine, especially the colon, that may be caused by ingesting water or food containing chemical irritants, bacteria, protozoa, or parasites and results in bloody diarrhea *Dysentery is common in underdeveloped countries and in times of disaster when sanitary living conditions, clean food, and safe water are not available.*
fistula FĬS-tū-lă	Abnormal passage from one organ to another or from a hollow organ to the surface *An anal fistula is located near the anus and may open into the rectum.*
flatus FLĀ-tŭs	Gas in the GI tract; expelling of air from a body orifice, especially the anus
gastroesophageal reflux disease (GERD) găs-trō-ĕ-sŏf-ă-JĒ-ăl RĒ-flŭks *gastr/o:* stomach *esophag:* esophagus *-eal:* pertaining to	Backflow of gastric contents into the esophagus as a result of a malfunction of the sphincter muscle at the inferior portion of the esophagus *GERD may occur whenever pressure in the stomach is greater than that in the esophagus and may be associated with heartburn, esophagitis, hiatal hernia, or chest pain.*
halitosis hăl-ĭ-TŌ-sĭs	Foul-smelling breath *Halitosis may result from poor oral hygiene, dental or oral infections, ingestion of certain foods, such as garlic or alcohol, use of tobacco, or a systemic disease, such as diabetes or liver disease.*
hematemesis hĕm-ăt-ĔM-ĕ-sĭs *hemat:* blood *-emesis:* vomiting	Vomiting of blood from bleeding in the stomach or esophagus *Hematemesis can be caused by an esophageal ulcer, esophageal varices (dilation of veins), or a gastric ulcer. Treatment requires correction of the underlying cause.*
hemorrhoids HĔM-ō-roydz	Swollen varicose veins in the anorectal region categorized as external or internal *Hemorrhoids are usually caused by abdominal pressure, such as from straining during bowel movement, pregnancy, and standing or sitting for long periods. Consuming a high-fiber diet and drinking plenty of water and juice play a pivotal role in hemorrhoid prevention. Treatment of an advanced condition involves surgical removal of the hemorrhoids (hemorrhoidectomy).*
inflammatory bowel disease (IBD) ĭn-FLĂM-ă-tŏr-ē BŎWL	Ulceration of the colon mucosa
Crohn disease KRŌN	Form of IBD, usually of the ileum but possibly affecting any portion of the intestinal tract; also called *regional enteritis* *Crohn disease is a chronic disease distinguished from closely related bowel disorders by its inflammatory pattern. It may cause fever, cramping, diarrhea, and weight loss.*

Diseases and Conditions—cont'd

Term	Definition
ulcerative colitis (UC) kō-LĪ-tĭs	Chronic inflammatory disease of the colon, commonly beginning in the rectum or sigmoid colon and extending upward into the entire colon *UC is characterized by profuse, watery diarrhea containing varying amounts of blood, mucus, and pus. Severe cases may require surgical creation of an opening (stoma) for bowel evacuation to a bag worn on the abdomen. UC is associated with an increased risk of colon cancer.*
intestinal obstruction ĭn-TĔS-tĭ-năl	Mechanical or functional blockage of the intestines that occurs when the contents of the intestine cannot move forward through the intestinal tract because of a partial or complete blockage of the bowel *Obstruction of the intestine causes the bowel to become vulnerable to ischemia. The intestinal mucosal barrier can suffer damage, allowing intestinal bacteria to invade the intestinal wall.*
intussusception ĭn-tĕ-sĕ-sĕp-SHĔN	Telescoping of one portion of the intestine into another, causing intestinal blockage *Intussusception is a rare but serious condition that typically occurs in the small intestine or the junction between the terminal ileum and cecum, most often in infants and young children. Barium enema is used to confirm diagnosis, and surgery is usually necessary to correct the obstruction (see Fig. 6–14A).*
volvulus VŎL-vū-lŭs	Twisting of the bowel on itself, causing obstruction *Volvulus usually requires surgery to untwist the loop of bowel (see Fig. 6–14B).*

 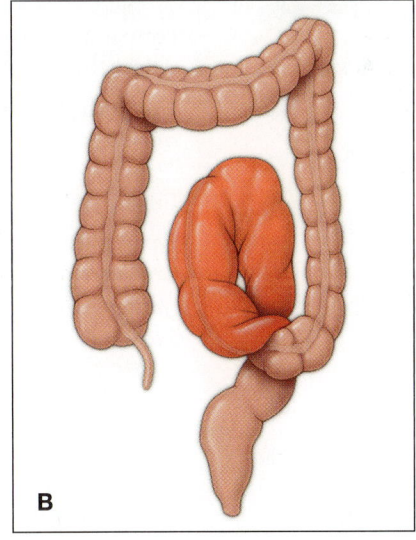

Figure 6-14 Intestinal obstruction. (A) Intussusception. (B) Volvulus. From Williams LS, Hooper PD: *Understanding medical surgical nursing,* 1999, F.A. Davis, p. 609.

Term	Definition
irritable bowel syndrome (IBS)	Symptom complex marked by abdominal pain and altered bowel function (typically constipation, diarrhea, or alternating constipation and diarrhea) for which no organic cause can be determined; also called *spastic colon* *Contributing or aggravating factors of IBS include anxiety and stress.*

Continued

Diseases and Conditions—cont'd

Term	Definition
malabsorption syndrome măl-ăb-SORP-shŭn SĬN-drōm	Symptom complex of the small intestine characterized by the impaired passage of nutrients, minerals, or fluids through intestinal villi into the blood or lymph *Malabsorption syndrome may be associated with or caused by a number of diseases, including those affecting the intestinal mucosa. It may also be caused by surgery, such as gastric resection and ileal bypass, or by antibiotic therapy.*
melena MĚL-ĕ-nă	Dark, tarlike feces that contain digested blood from bleeding in the esophagus or stomach *Treatment requires correcting the underlying cause of bleeding.*
obesity ō-BĒ-sĭ-tē	Excessive accumulation of fat that exceeds the body's skeletal and physical standards, usually an increase of 20% or more above ideal body weight or a body mass index (BMI) beginning at 30 *Obesity may be caused by excessive intake of food (exogenous) or metabolic or endocrine abnormalities (endogenous).*
morbid	Obesity in which BMI is 40 or greater than 40, and generally 100 lb or more over ideal body weight *Morbid obesity is a disease with serious psychological, social, and medical ramifications and one that threatens necessary body functions such as respiration.*
obstipation ŏb-stĭ-PĀ-shŭn	Severe constipation, which may be caused by an intestinal obstruction
oral leukoplakia OR-ăl loo-kō-PLĀ-kē-ă *leuk/o:* white *-plakia:* plaque	Formation of white spots or patches on the mucous membrane of the tongue, lips, or cheek caused primarily by irritation *Oral leukoplakia is a precancerous condition, usually associated with pipe or cigarette smoking or ill-fitting dentures.*
pancreatitis păn-krē-ă-TĪ-tĭs *pancreat:* pancreas *-itis:* inflammation	Inflammation of the pancreas *Pancreatitis occurs when digestive enzymes attack pancreatic tissue, causing damage to the gland. The most common causes of pancreatitis are alcoholism, gallstone obstruction, drug toxicity, and infection of the pancreas caused by bacteria or viruses.*

Diseases and Conditions—cont'd

Term	Definition
pyloric stenosis pī-LOR-ĭk stĕ-NŌ-sĭs *pylor:* pylorus *-ic:* pertaining to *sten:* narrowing, stricture *-osis:* abnormal condition; increase (used primarily with blood cells)	An uncommon condition appearing within 3 to 5 weeks after birth resulting in a stricture or narrowing of the pyloric sphincter (circular muscle of the pylorus) at the outlet of the stomach, causing an obstruction that blocks the flow of food into the small intestine *Surgery, called a pyloromyotomy, where a portion of the muscle fibers of the pyloric sphincter are cut to allow food to enter the small intestine, corrects the defect (see Fig. 6-15).*

Stomach

Pylorus

Small intestine

Junction of stomach and duodenum

Narrowed (stenosed) pyloric sphincter

Figure 6-15 Pyloric stenosis.

regurgitation rē-gŭr-jĭ-TĀ-shŭn	A backward flow, as in the return of solids or fluids to the mouth from the stomach

 It is time to review pathology, diseases, and conditions by completing Learning Activity 6–4.

Diagnostic, Surgical, and Therapeutic Procedures

This section introduces diagnostic, surgical, and therapeutic procedures used to diagnose and treat digestive system disorders. Descriptions are provided, along with pronunciations and word analyses for selected terms.

Procedure	Description
Diagnostic	
Endoscopic	
endoscopy ĕn-DŎS-kō-pē *endo-:* in, within *-scopy:* visual examination	Visual examination of the interior of organs and cavities with a specialized lighted instrument called an *endoscope* *The organ, cavity, or canal being examined dictates the name of the endoscopic procedure. A camera and video recorder are commonly used during the procedure to provide a permanent record.*
capsule	Endoscopy using a tiny, wireless camera the size of a vitamin pill that is swallowed and travels through the digestive tract taking thousands of photos that are transmitted to a recorder worn on a belt around the waist *Capsule endoscopy allows the small intestine to be reached more easily than traditional endoscopy to diagnose gastrointestinal bleeding, cancer, polyps, and inflammatory bowel disease such as Crohn disease (see Fig. 6-16).*

Large intestine

Small intestine

Endoscopic capsule
in small intestine

Figure 6-16 Capsule endoscopy.

upper GI	Endoscopy of the esophagus (esophagoscopy), stomach (gastroscopy), and duodenum (duodenoscopy) *Endoscopy of the upper GI tract is performed to identify tumors, esophagitis, gastroesophageal varices, peptic ulcers, and the source of upper GI bleeding. It is also used to confirm the presence and extent of varices in the lower esophagus and stomach in patients with liver disease.*

Diagnostic, Surgical, and Therapeutic Procedures—cont'd

Procedure	Description
lower GI	Endoscopy of the colon (colonoscopy), sigmoid colon (sigmoidoscopy), and rectum and anal canal (proctoscopy).

Endoscopy of the lower GI tract is used to identify pathological conditions in the colon (see Fig. 6-17). It may also be used to perform a polypectomy, a simple procedure used to remove polyps that are discovered in the colon and then examined microscopically to detect abnormal or cancerous cells. Larger size colon polyps have a high risk of developing into colorectal cancer (see Fig. 6-18).

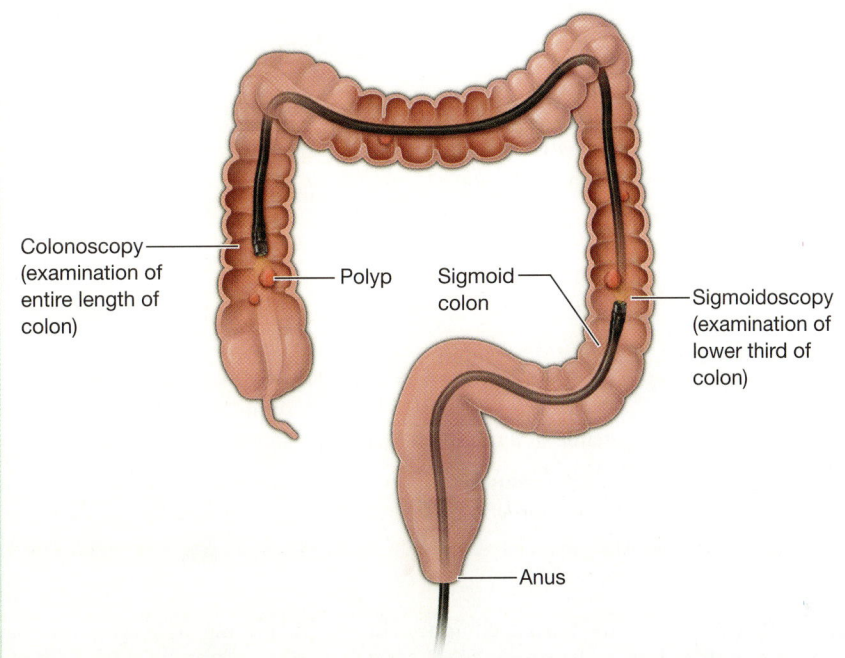

Colonoscopy (examination of entire length of colon)

Polyp

Sigmoid colon

Sigmoidoscopy (examination of lower third of colon)

Anus

Figure 6-17 Colonoscopy and sigmoidoscopy.

Figure 6-18 Polypectomy.

Continued

Diagnostic, Surgical, and Therapeutic Procedures—cont'd

Procedure	Description
Laboratory	
hepatitis panel hĕp-ă-TĪ-tĭs *hepat:* liver *-itis:* inflammation	Panel of blood tests that identifies the specific virus—HAV, HBV, or HCV—that is causing hepatitis by testing serum using antibodies to each of these antigens
liver function tests (LFTs)	Group of blood tests that evaluate liver injury, liver function, and conditions commonly associated with the biliary tract *LFTs evaluate liver enzymes, bilirubin, and proteins produced by the liver.*
serum bilirubin SĒ-rŭm bĭl-ĭ-ROO-bĭn	Measurement of the level of bilirubin in the blood *Elevated serum bilirubin indicates excessive destruction of erythrocytes, liver disease, or biliary tract obstruction.*
stool culture	Test to identify microorganisms or parasites present in feces that are causing a GI infection *Feces are examined microscopically after being placed in a growth medium.*
stool guaiac GWĪ-ăk	Test that applies a substance called *guaiac* to a stool sample to detect the presence of occult (hidden) blood in the feces; also called *Hemoccult* (trade name of a modified guaiac test) *A stool guaiac test helps detect colon cancer and bleeding associated with digestive disorders.*
Imaging	
computed tomography (CT) kŏm-PŪ-tĕd tō-MŎG-ră-fē *tom/o:* to cut *-graphy:* process of recording	Imaging technique achieved by rotating an x-ray emitter around the area to be scanned and measuring the intensity of transmitted rays from different angles *In CT scanning, a computer generates a detailed cross-sectional image that appears as a slice (see Fig. 4-7D). In the digestive system, CT scans aid in visualizing the gallbladder, bowel, liver, bile ducts, and pancreas. They also aid in the diagnosis of tumors, cysts, inflammation, abscesses, perforation, bleeding, and obstruction.*

Diagnostic, Surgical, and Therapeutic Procedures—cont'd

Procedure	Description
lower gastrointestinal series găs-trō-ĭn-tĕs-tĭn-ăl	Radiographic images of the rectum and colon following administration of barium into the rectum; also called *lower GI series* or *barium enema (BE)* *Barium is retained in the lower GI tract during fluoroscopic and radiographic studies. It helps diagnose obstructions, tumors, and other abnormalities of the colon (see Fig. 6-19).*

Figure 6-19 Barium enema done poorly (A) and correctly (B).

Procedure	Description
oral cholecystography (OCG) kō-lē-sĭs-TŎG-ră-fē *chol/e:* bile, gall *cyst/o:* bladder *-graphy:* process of recording	Radiographic images taken of the gallbladder after administration of a contrast material containing iodine, usually in the form of a tablet *OCG evaluates gallbladder function and identifies the presence of disease or gallstones.*
magnetic resonance imaging (MRI) RĔZ-ō-năns ĬM-ăj-ĭng	Technique that uses radio waves and a strong magnetic field, rather than an x-ray beam, to produce highly detailed, multiplanar, cross-sectional views of soft tissues *Abdominal MRI provides detailed imaging of the abdomen and pelvis with the advantages of detailed soft tissue contrast and noninvasiveness to diagnose a spectrum of GI disease processes.*
magnetic resonance cholangiopancreatography (MRCP) kō-lăn-jē-ō-păn-krē-ă-TŎG-ră-fē *cholangi/o:* bile vessel *pancreat/o:* pancreas *-graphy:* process of recording	Special MRI technique that produces detailed images of the hepatobiliary and pancreatic systems, including the liver, gallbladder, bile ducts, pancreas, and pancreatic duct *MRCP requires no contrast medium. It can help determine whether gallstones are lodged in any of the ducts surrounding the gallbladder. It may also detect tumors, inflammation, infection, or pancreatitis.*

Continued

Diagnostic, Surgical, and Therapeutic Procedures—cont'd

Procedure	Description
ultrasonography (US) ŭl-tră-sŏn-ŎG-ră-fē *ultra-:* excess, beyond *son/o:* sound *-graphy:* process of recording	Test in which high-frequency sound waves (ultrasound) are directed at soft tissue and reflected as "echoes" to produce an image on a monitor of an internal body structure; also called *ultrasound, sonography,* and *echo* *US is a noninvasive procedure that does not require a contrast medium. It helps detect diseases and abnormalities in the digestive organs, such as the gallbladder, liver, and pancreas. It also helps locate abdominal masses outside the digestive organs.*
abdominal ăb-DŎM-ĭ-năl *abdomin:* abdomen *-al:* pertaining to	Ultrasound visualization of the abdominal aorta, liver, gallbladder, bile ducts, pancreas, kidneys, ureters, and bladder *An abdominal US helps diagnose and locate cysts, tumors, and malformations, document the progression of various diseases, and guide the insertion of instruments during surgical procedures.*
endoscopic ĕn-dō-SKŎP-ĭk *endo:* in; within *scop:* to view *-ic:* pertaining to	Combination of endoscopy and ultrasound that examines and obtains images of the digestive tract and the surrounding tissues and organs *In endoscopic US, a long, flexible tube (endoscope) inserted via the mouth or rectum emits high-frequency sound waves (ultrasound) that produce images of the organs and structures.*
upper gastrointestinal series (UGIS) gĂS-trō-ĭn-tĕs-tĭn-ăl	Radiographic images of the esophagus, stomach, and small intestine following oral administration of barium; also called *barium swallow* *UGIS is most commonly used with patients who are experiencing difficulty swallowing. It also helps identify ulcers, tumors, or an obstruction in the esophagus, stomach, or small intestine.*
Surgical	
anastomosis ă-năs-tō-MŌ-sĭs	Surgical joining of two ducts, vessels, or bowel segments to allow flow from one to another
ileorectal ĭl-ē-ō-RĔK-tăl *ile/o:* ileum *rect:* rectum *-al:* pertaining to	Surgical connection of the ileum and rectum after total colectomy, as is sometimes performed in the treatment of UC
intestinal ĭn-TĔS-tĭ-năl	Surgical connection of two portions of the intestines
appendectomy ăp-ĕn-DĔK-tō-mē *append:* appendix *-ectomy:* excision, removal	Excision of a diseased appendix using an open or laparoscopic procedure *Appendectomy usually occurs within 24 to 48 hours of symptom onset. Delay in treatment may result in rupture of the appendix, causing peritonitis as fecal matter enters the peritoneal cavity.*

Diagnostic, Surgical, and Therapeutic Procedures—cont'd

Procedure	Description
laparoscopic lăp-ă-rō-SKŎP-ĭk	Minimally invasive appendectomy using three to four small incisions into the abdominal wall, typically less than an inch in length, to insert trocars that serve as entry points for the surgical instruments and a camera. The surgeon views the enlarged image of the surgical site projected on a screen while performing surgery. *Laparoscopic surgery reduces recovery time with less postoperative pain and risk of infection, and the patient often returns home the same day (see Fig. 6-20).* **Figure 6-20** Laparoscopic appendectomy with trocars (access devices used to insert laparoscopic instruments).
open	Excision of a diseased appendix through a 2- to 3-inch incision in the right lower quadrant of the abdomen
bariatric surgery băr-ē-Ă-trĭk	Group of surgical procedures designed to promote weight loss and lower the risk of medical problems associated with obesity through restriction or malabsorption of food.

A   Normal stomach   B   Adjustable gastric band (AGB)   C   Roux-en-Y gastric bypass (RYGB)   D   Vertical sleeve gastrectomy (VSG)

Figure 6-21 Bariatric surgery. (A) Normal stomach. (B) Adjustable gastric band (AGB). (C) Roux-en-Y gastric bypass (RYGB). (D) Vertical sleeve gastrectomy (VSG).

Continued

Diagnostic, Surgical, and Therapeutic Procedures—cont'd

Procedure	Description
adjustable gastric band (AGB) GĂS-trĭk	Bariatric surgery that involves the placement of a band (**Lap-Band**) around the upper portion of the stomach that creates a small pouch, thereby restricting the amount of food that can be consumed; also called *Lap-Band* and *gastric band*. *This is one of the least invasive bariatric surgeries and is reversible, but it does not lead to significant weight loss compared with Roux-en-Y gastric bypass (RYGB) or vertical sleeve gastrectomy (VSG), described in the following sections (see Fig. 6-21B).*
Roux-en-Y gastric bypass (RYGB) rū-ĕn-WĪ GĂS-trĭk	Bariatric surgery that involves stapling the stomach to decrease its size and then directly connecting it to the jejunum so food will bypass much of the stomach and duodenum, thereby reducing absorption of calories and fats; also called *gastric bypass with gastroenterostomy*. *RYGB can be performed laparoscopically or as an open procedure (laparotomy), depending on the health of the patient (see Fig. 6-21C).*
sleeve gastrectomy, vertical sleeve gastrectomy (VSG) găs-TRĔK-tō-mē	Bariatric surgery that involves removing a large portion of the stomach, leaving a smaller, sleeve-shaped pouch that greatly reduces the stomach's capacity, thereby restricting the amount of food a person can eat; also reduces the production of the hunger-producing hormone **ghrelin**. *Sleeve gastrectomy is less complex than RYGB and does not affect the absorption of nutrients in the intestines. VSG is the most commonly performed bariatric surgery due to its effectiveness and lower complication rates compared with other types of weight loss surgeries (see Fig. 6-21D).*
colostomy kō-LOS-tō-mē *col/o:* colon *-stomy:* forming an opening (mouth)	Surgical procedure in which a surgeon forms an opening (stoma) by drawing the healthy end of the colon through an incision in the anterior abdominal wall and suturing it into place *A colostomy diverts fecal flow to a colostomy bag and provides a new path for waste material to leave the body (see Fig. 6-22).*

Diagnostic, Surgical, and Therapeutic Procedures—cont'd

Procedure	Description

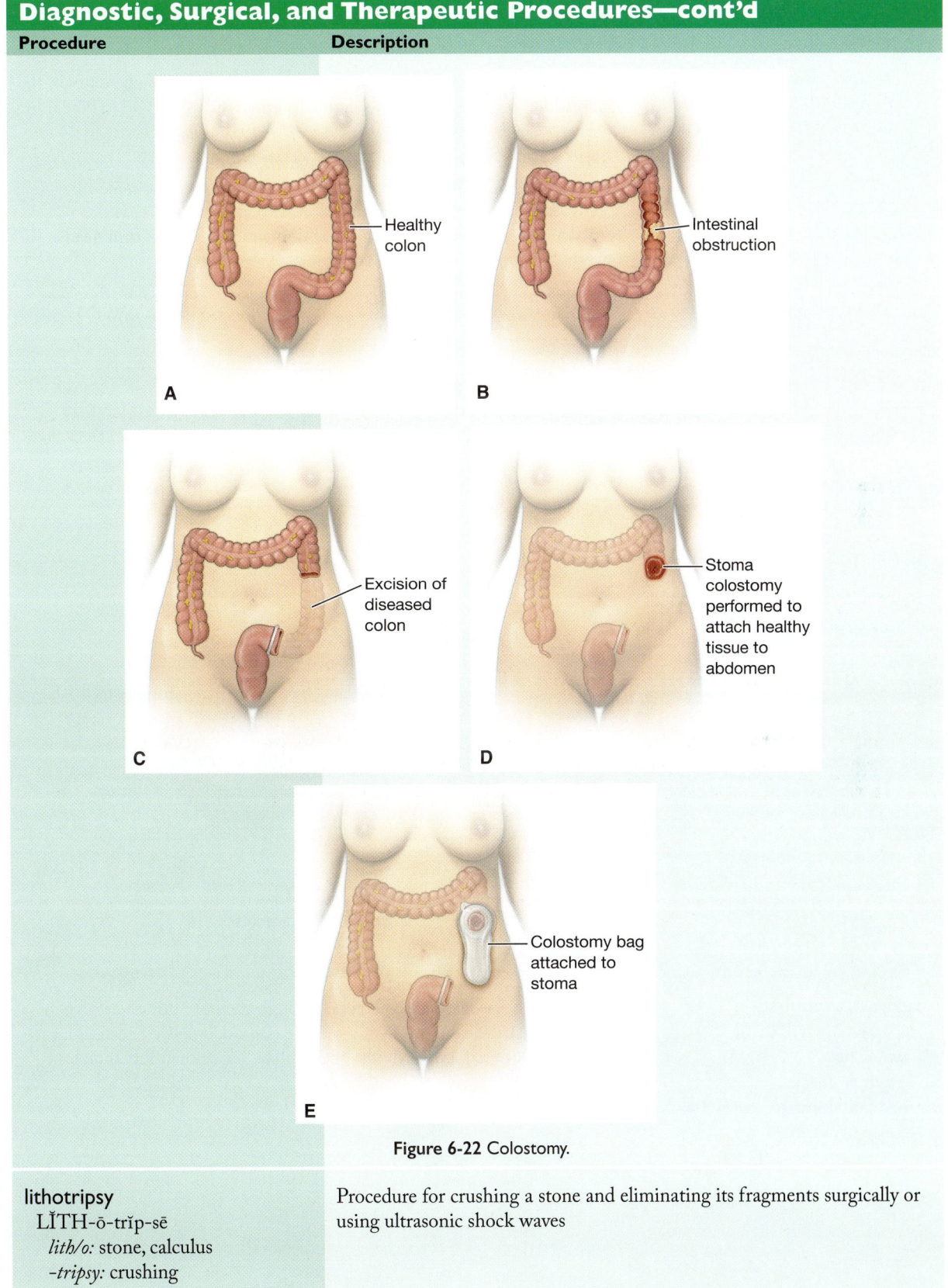

A — Healthy colon

B — Intestinal obstruction

C — Excision of diseased colon

D — Stoma colostomy performed to attach healthy tissue to abdomen

E — Colostomy bag attached to stoma

Figure 6-22 Colostomy.

lithotripsy
LĬTH-ō-trĭp-sē
   lith/o: stone, calculus
   -tripsy: crushing

Procedure for crushing a stone and eliminating its fragments surgically or using ultrasonic shock waves

Continued

Diagnostic, Surgical, and Therapeutic Procedures—cont'd

Procedure	Description
extracorporeal shock- wave lithotripsy (ESWL) ĕks-tră-kor-POR-ē-ăl SHŎK-wăv	Use of shock waves as a noninvasive method to help break up stones in the gallbladder or biliary ducts to clear obstruction and allow bile to flow more freely *ESWL can be used as long as the gallbladder is functioning normally and the stones are small. ESWL is used more commonly to treat kidney stones.*
paracentesis păr-ă-sĕn-TĒ-sĭs *para-:* near, beside, beyond *-centesis:* surgical puncture	Procedure to remove fluid from the abdomen using a long, thin needle inserted through the belly; also called *abdominocentesis* *The fluid is sent to a laboratory for analysis to find the cause of the fluid accumulation. Paracentesis may also relieve abdominal pressure or pain in patients with cancer, cirrhosis, or ascites (see Fig. 6–23).* Liver — Stomach — Ascites — Rectum — Ascites fluid **Figure 6-23** Paracentesis.

Therapeutic

nasogastric intubation nā-zō-GĂS-trĭk ĭn-tū-BĀ-shŭn *nas/o:* nose *gastr:* stomach *-ic:* pertaining to	Insertion of a nasogastric (NG) tube through the nose into the stomach to relieve gastric distention by removing gas, food, or gastric secretions; to instill medication, food, or fluids; or to obtain a specimen for laboratory analysis

Pharmacology

Various pharmaceutical agents are available to counteract abnormal conditions that occur in the GI tract. Antacids counteract or decrease excessive stomach acid, the cause of heartburn, gastric discomfort, and gastric reflux. Antidiarrheals and antiemetics help preserve water and electrolytes, which are essential for body hydration and homeostasis. Medications that increase or decrease peristalsis help regulate the speed at which food passes through the GI tract. These drugs include agents that relieve "cramping" (**antispasmodics**) and those that help in the movement of material through a sluggish bowel (**laxatives**; see Table 6-1).

TABLE 6-1 Drugs Used To Treat Digestive Disorders

This table lists common drug classifications used to treat digestive disorders, their therapeutic actions, and selected generic and trade names.

Classification	Therapeutic Action	Generic and Trade Names
antacids ănt-ĂS-ĭds	Counteract or neutralize acidity, usually in the stomach *Antacids treat and prevent heartburn and acid reflux.*	**calcium carbonate** KĂL-sē-ŭm KĂR-bŏn-āt *Rolaids, Tums* **aluminum hydroxide and magnesium hydroxide** ă-LŪ-mĭ-nŭm hī-DRŎKS-īd, măg-NĒ-zē-ŭm hī-DRŎKS-īd *Maalox, Mylanta*
antidiarrheals an-tĭ-dī-ă-RĒ-ăls	Control loose stools and relieve diarrhea by absorbing excess water in the bowel or slowing peristalsis in the intestinal tract	**loperamide** lō-PĔR-ă-mīd *Imodium* **kaolin/pectin** KĀ-ō-lĭn, PĔK-tĭn *Donnagel-MB, Kapectolin*
antiemetics ăn-tĭ-ē-MĔT-ĭks	Control nausea and vomiting by blocking nerve impulses to the vomiting center of the brain *Some antiemetics act by hastening movement of food through the digestive tract.*	**prochlorperazine** prō-klor-PĔR-ă-zēn *Compazine, Compro* **ondansetron** ŏn-DĂN-sĕ-trŏn *Zofran*
antispasmodics ăn-tē-spăz-MŎD-ĭks	Decrease GI spasms by slowing peristalsis and motility throughout the GI tract *Antispasmodics help treat IBS, spastic colon, and diverticulitis.*	**glycopyrrolate** glī-kō-PĬR-rō-lāt *Robinul* **dicyclomine** dī-SĪ-klō-mēn *Bentyl*
histamine-2 (H₂) blockers	Inhibit secretion of stomach acid from the gastric cells by blocking the H_2 receptor *H_2 blockers treat acid reflux and gastric or duodenal ulcers.*	**ranitidine** ră-NĬ-tĭ-dēn *Zantac* **famotidine** fă-MŌ-tĭ-dēn *Pepcid*

(continued)

TABLE 6-1 Drugs Used To Treat Digestive Disorders—cont'd

Classification	Therapeutic Action	Generic and Trade Names
laxatives LĂK-să-tĭvs	Treat constipation by increasing peristaltic activity in the large intestine or absorbing water into the bowel to induce defecation	**senna, sennosides** SĔN-ă, SĔN-ō-sīdz *Senokot, Senolax* **psyllium** SĬL-ē-ŭm *Metamucil, Natural Fiber Supplement*
proton pump inhibitors	Inhibit the acid-producing pump in the gastric cells *Proton pump inhibitors treat gastric and duodenal ulcers and acid reflux. These drugs are more potent acid inhibitors than the H_2 blockers.*	**omeprazole** ō-MĔP-ră-zōl *Prilosec* **esomeprazole** ĕs-ō-MĔP-ră-zōl *Nexium*

Abbreviations

This section introduces digestive-related abbreviations and their meanings.

Abbreviation	Meaning	Abbreviation	Meaning
AIDS	acquired immune deficiency syndrome	GI	gastrointestinal
BE	barium enema	GISTs	gastrointestinal stromal tumors
BM	bowel movement	HAV	hepatitis A virus
BMI	body mass index	HBV	hepatitis B virus
CT	computed tomography	HCV	hepatitis C virus
EGD	esophagogastroduodenoscopy	IBD	inflammatory bowel disease
ESWL	extracorporeal shock-wave lithotripsy	IBS	irritable bowel syndrome
EUS	endoscopic ultrasonography (x-ray studies)	LFT	liver function test
GBS	gallbladder series	LUQ	left upper quadrant
GER	gastroesophageal reflux	MRCP	magnetic resonance cholangiopancreatography
GERD	gastroesophageal reflux disease	NETs	neuroendocrine tumors

Abbreviation	Meaning	Abbreviation	Meaning
NG	nasogastric	RYGB	Roux-en-Y gastric bypass
NSAID	nonsteroidal anti-inflammatory drugs	SBO	small bowel obstruction
OCG	oral cholecystography	UC	ulcerative colitis
PE	physical examination; pulmonary embolism; pressure-equalizing (tube)	UGIS	upper gastrointestinal series
PUD	peptic ulcer disease	US	ultrasound; ultrasonography
R/O	rule out	VSG	vertical sleeve gastrectomy
RUQ	right upper quadrant		

It is time to review procedures, pharmacology, and abbreviations by completing Learning Activity 6–5.

LEARNING ACTIVITIES

The activities that follow provide a review of the digestive system terms introduced in this chapter. Complete each activity and review your answers to evaluate your understanding of the chapter.

Medical Language Lab
Turning terminology into language

Visit the Medical Language Laboratory at medicallanguagelab.com. Use it to enhance your study and reinforcement of this chapter with the flash card activity. We recommend that you complete the flash card activity before starting Learning Activities 6-1 and 6-2.

Learning Activity 6-1
Medical Word Elements

Use the listed elements to build medical words. You may use the elements more than once.

Combining Forms		Suffixes		Prefixes
an/o	hepat/o	-al	-phagia	an-
colon/o	jejun/o	-emesis	-plasty	dys-
dent/o	pharyng/o	-ic	-rrhaphy	hypo-
esophag/o	sial/o	-itis	-scope	peri-
gastr/o	stomat/o	-lith	-scopy	
gingiv/o		-pathy		
hemat/o		-pepsia		

1. surgical reshaping (repair) of the gum(s) _____

2. visual examination of the colon _____

3. inflammation of the liver _____

4. pertaining to under or below the stomach _____

5. bad, painful, or difficult digestion _____

6. calculus in a salivary gland or duct _____

7. disease of the mouth _____

8. pertaining to around the anus _____

9. suture of the jejunum (second part of the small intestine) _____

10. inflammation of the pharynx _____

11. instrument to examine the esophagus _____

12. without an appetite _____

13. vomiting blood _____

14. pertaining to the teeth _____

15. bad, painful, or difficult swallowing or eating _____

Check your answers in Appendix A. Review any material that you did not answer correctly.

Correct Answers _____ X 6.67 = _____ % Score

Learning Activity 6-2
Building Medical Words

Use *esophag/o* (esophagus) to build words that mean

1. pain in the esophagus _____
2. spasm of the esophagus _____
3. stricture or narrowing of the esophagus _____

Use *gastr/o* (stomach) to build words that mean

4. surgical repair of the stomach _____
5. pain in the stomach _____
6. disease of the stomach _____

Use *duoden/o* (duodenum), *jejun/o* (jejunum), or *ile/o* (ileum) to build words that mean

7. excision of all or part of the jejunum _____
8. relating to the duodenum _____
9. forming an opening (mouth) in the ileum _____
10. pertaining to the jejunum and ileum _____

Use *enter/o* (usually small intestine) to build words that mean

11. inflammation of the small intestine _____
12. disease of the small intestine _____
13. inflammation of the small intestine and colon _____

Use *col/o* (colon) to build words that mean

14. inflammation of the colon _____
15. pertaining to the colon and rectum _____
16. prolapse or downward displacement of the colon _____
17. disease of the colon _____

Use *proct/o* (anus, rectum) or *rect/o* (rectum) to build words that mean

18. narrowing or constriction of the rectum _____
19. herniation of the rectum _____
20. paralysis of the anus (anal muscles) _____

Use *chol/e* (bile, gall) to build words that mean

21. excision of the gallbladder _____
22. abnormal condition of a gallstone _____

Use *hepat/o* (liver) or *pancreat/o* (pancreas) to build words that mean

23. tumor of the liver _____
24. enlargement of the liver _____
25. inflammation of the pancreas _____

✓ *Check your answers in Appendix A. Review material that you did not answer correctly.*

Correct Answers _____ X 4 = _____ % Score

Learning Activity 6-3
Building Surgical Words

Build a surgical word that means

1. excision of gums (tissue) _____
2. partial or complete excision of the tongue _____
3. repair of the esophagus _____
4. removal of part or all of the stomach _____
5. forming an opening between the stomach and jejunum _____
6. excision of (part of) the esophagus _____
7. forming an opening between the stomach, small intestine, and colon _____
8. surgical repair of the small intestine _____
9. fixation of the small intestine (to the abdominal wall) _____
10. suture of the bile duct _____
11. surgical puncture of the abdomen _____
12. crushing of a gallstone _____
13. surgical repair of a hernia _____
14. excision of a hemorrhoid _____
15. instrument to cut the intestine _____
16. forming an opening into the colon _____
17. fixation of a movable liver (to the abdominal wall) _____
18. surgical repair of the anus or rectum _____
19. removal of the gallbladder _____
20. surgical repair of a bile duct _____

✓ *Check your answers in Appendix A. Review material that you did not answer correctly.*

Correct Answers _____ X 5 = _____ % Score

Learning Activity 6-4
Diseases and Conditions

Match the terms with the definitions in the numbered list.

anorexia	*Crohn disease*	*hemorrhoids*	*obstipation*
ascites	*dysphagia*	*hiatal hernia*	*steatorrhea*
borborygmus	*fistula*	*intussusception*	*volvulus*
cachexia	*flatus*	*leukoplakia*	
cirrhosis	*halitosis*	*melena*	

1. obstruction caused by a twisting of the bowel _____
2. difficulty swallowing or inability to swallow _____
3. varicose veins in the rectal area _____
4. foul-smelling breath _____
5. loss of appetite _____
6. dark, tarry stools caused by presence of blood in the GI tract _____
7. yellowing of the skin caused by liver disease _____
8. state of ill health, malnutrition, and wasting _____
9. intractable constipation _____
10. gurgling audible noises caused by passing of gas through the liquid contents of the stomach _____
11. abnormal accumulation of fluid in the abdominal cavity _____
12. form of inflammatory bowel disease, usually of the ileum _____
13. passage of fat in large amounts in the feces _____
14. formation of white patches on the mucous membrane of the cheek _____
15. gas in the gastrointestinal tract _____
16. bad-smelling breath _____
17. abnormal passage from one organ to another or from a hollow organ to the surface _____
18. severe constipation _____
19. telescoping of the intestines _____
20. protrusion of the upper part of the stomach through the diaphragm _____

Check your answers in Appendix A. Review any material that you did not answer correctly.

Correct Answers _____ X 5 = _____ % Score

Learning Activity 6-5

Procedures, Pharmacology, and Abbreviations

Match the terms with the definitions in the numbered list.

anastomosis	*gastroscopy*	*liver function tests*	*PUD*
antacids	*GERD*	*lower GI series*	*stool culture*
antiemetics	*IBS*	*MRCP*	*stool guaiac*
antispasmodics	*intubation*	*paracentesis*	*upper GI series*
endoscopy	*laxatives*	*proctosigmoidoscopy*	*VSG*

1. procedure to visualize biliary and pancreatic ducts by using magnetic resonance imaging _____

2. bariatric surgery that involves removing a large portion of the stomach, leaving a smaller, sleeve-shaped pouch _____

3. disorder that affects the colon and causes constipation and diarrhea; also called *spastic colon* _____

4. agents that alleviate muscle spasms _____

5. removal of fluid from the abdomen using a long, thin needle _____

6. administration of a barium enema while a series of radiographs is taken of the colon _____

7. visual examination of the stomach _____

8. agents that control nausea and vomiting _____

9. insertion of a tube into any hollow organ _____

10. surgical formation of a passage or opening between two hollow viscera or vessels _____

11. detects presence of blood in the feces; also called *Hemoccult* _____

12. visual examination of a cavity or canal using a specialized lighted instrument _____

13. used to treat constipation _____

14. neutralize excess acid in the stomach and help to relieve gastritis and ulcer pain _____

15. test to identify microorganisms present in feces _____

16. measures the levels of certain enzymes, bilirubin, and various proteins _____

17. causes heartburn from backflow of gastric contents into the esophagus _____

18. erosion of the mucous membrane layer of the esophagus, stomach, or duodenum caused by *Helicobacter pylori* (*H. pylori*) bacteria _____

19. endoscopic procedure for visualization of the rectosigmoid colon _____

20. radiographic imaging of the esophagus, duodenum, and stomach after ingestion of barium _____

✓ *Check your answers in Appendix A. Review material that you did not answer correctly.*

Correct Answers _____ X 5 = _____ % Score

DOCUMENTING HEALTH-CARE ACTIVITIES

This section provides practical application activities in the form of exercises to help students develop skills in documenting patient care. First, read the medical report. Then complete the activities and exercises that follow.

Documenting Health-Care Activity 6-1
Chart Note: GI Evaluation

Damian, Mary Age: 52

April 10, 20xx

Chief Complaint: Right-sided abdominal pain

History of Present Illness: Patient reports intermittent waves of abdominal pain that have become continuous, deep, and right sided over the last week. She reports abdominal bloating, nausea, and diarrhea. It does not cause any vomiting, does not trigger any urge to defecate, and is not alleviated by passage of flatus. She reports that she had a cholecystectomy about 2 years ago after experiencing episodic intermittent, sharp epigastric pain and was found to have cholecystitis with cholelithiasis.

Past Medical History: Significant for tonsillectomy, appendectomy, and cholecystectomy.

Physical Examination: No hepatomegaly or splenomegaly. The rectal examination confirmed normal sphincter tone and heme-negative stool. Abnormal, high-pitched bowel sounds upon auscultation of the abdomen.

Impression: Abdominal pain. R/O partial small bowel obstruction secondary to adhesions.

Plan: Schedule abdominopelvic CT scan with contrast for possible SBO.

Joseph Bogata, MD
Joseph Bogata, MD

bcg

Terminology

The terms listed in the table that follows are taken from "Chart Note: GI Evaluation." Use a medical dictionary such as *Taber's Cyclopedic Medical Dictionary,* the appendices of this book, or other resources to define each term. Then review the pronunciation for each term and practice by reading the medical record aloud.

Term	Definition
appendectomy ăp-ĕn-DĔK-tō-mē	
cholecystectomy kō-lē-sĭs-TĔK- tō-mē	
cholecystitis kō-lē-sĭs-TĪ-tĭs	
cholelithiasis kō-lē-lĭ-THĪ-ă-sĭs	
defecate DĔF-ĕ-kāt	
flatus FLĀ-tŭs	
heme-negative stool hēm-NĔG-ă-tĭv	
hepatomegaly hĕp-ă-tō-MĔG-ă-lē	
intermittent ĭn-tĕr-MĬT-ĕnt	
nausea NAW-sē-ă	
PE	
PMH	
SBO	
R/O	
splenomegaly splē-nō-MĔG-ă-lē	
tonsillectomy tōn-sĭl-ĔK-tō-mē	

 Visit the Medical Terminology Systems online resource center at FADavis. com to practice pronunciation and reinforce the meanings of the terms in this medical report.

Critical Thinking

Review *Chart Note: GI Evaluation* to answer the questions.

1. Referring to Figure 6-4, describe the location of the gallbladder in relation to the liver.

_____

_____

_____

_____

2. Why did the patient undergo the cholecystectomy?

_____

_____

_____

_____

3. What were the patient's prior surgeries?

_____

_____

_____

_____

4. How does the patient's most recent episode of pain differ from the initial pain she described?

_____

_____

_____

_____

5. What finding in the physical examination is a possible symptom of an SBO?

_____

_____

_____

_____

Operative Report: Esophagogastroduodenoscopy with Biopsy

OPERATIVE REPORT

Date:	May 14, 20xx	Physician:	Dante Riox, MD
Patient:	Franks, Roberta	Room:	703

Preoperative Diagnosis: Hematemesis of unknown etiology.

Postoperative Diagnosis: Diffuse gastritis and duodenitis.

Procedure: Esophagogastroduodenoscopy with biopsy.

Specimen: Biopsies from gastric antrum and duodenal bulb.

Estimated Blood Loss: No significant blood loss observed.

Complications: None.

Time Under Sedation: 20 minutes.

Procedure and Findings: After obtaining informed consent regarding the procedure, the patient was taken to the GI laboratory, where she was placed on the examining table in the left lateral recumbent position. She was given nasal oxygen at 3 liters per minute and monitored with a pulse oximeter throughout the procedure. Through a previously inserted intravenous line, the patient was sedated with a total of 50 mg of Demerol plus 4 mg of Midazolam throughout the procedure. The Fujinon computed tomography scan videoendoscope was then readily introduced, and the following organs were evaluated:

Esophagus: There was evidence of prior esophageal varices, but the esophageal mucosa otherwise appeared normal throughout.

Stomach: There was diffuse erythema with old blood seen within the stomach. No ulcerations, erosions, or fresh bleeding was seen. A representative biopsy was obtained from the gastric antrum and submitted to the pathology laboratory.

Duodenum: Punctate erythema was noted in the duodenal bulb. There was some friability. No ulcerations, erosions, or active bleeding was seen. A bulbar biopsy was obtained. The second portion of the duodenum appeared normal. The patient tolerated the procedure well. Patient was transferred to the recovery room in stable condition.

Dante Riox, MD
Dante Riox, MD

dr:bg

D: 5-14-20xx; T: 5-14-20xx

Terminology

The terms listed in the table that follows are taken from *Operative Report: Esophagogastro-duodenoscopy with Biopsy*. Use a medical dictionary such as *Taber's Cyclopedic Medical Dictionary*, the appendices of this book, or other resources to define each term. Then review the pronunciation for each term and practice by reading the medical record aloud.

Term	Definition
Demerol DĔM-ĕr-ŏl	
duodenal bulb dū-ō-DĒ-năl bŭlb	
duodenitis dū-ŏd-ĕ-NĪ-tĭs	
erythema ĕr-ĭ-THĒ-mă	
esophageal varices ĕ-sŏf-ă-JĒ-ăl VĂR-ĭ-sēz	
esophagogastro-duodenoscopy ĕ-sŏf-ă-gō-găs-trō-doo-ō-dĕn-ŎS-kō-pē	
etiology ē-tē-ŎL-ō-jē	
friability frī-ă-BĬL-ĭ-tē	
gastric antrum GĂS-trĭk ĂN-trŭm	
gastritis găs-TRĪ-tĭs	
hematemesis hĕm-ăt-ĔM-ĕ-sĭs	
lateral recumbent LĂT-ĕr-ăl rē-KŬM-bĕnt	
Midazolam mĭ-dā-zōl-ăm	
oximeter ŏk-SĬM-ĕ-tĕr	

Continued

Term	Definition
punctate erythema PŬNK-tāt ĕr-ĭ-THĒ-mă	
tomography tō-MŎG-ră-fē	
videoendoscope vĭd-ē-ō-ĔND- ō-skōp	

Visit the Medical Terminology Systems online resource center at FADavis.
com to practice pronunciation and reinforce the meanings of the terms in this
medical report.

Critical Thinking

Review the medical report Operative Report: Esophagogastroduodenoscopy with Biopsy to answer the questions.

1. What caused the hematemesis?

_____

_____

_____

2. What procedures were carried out to determine the cause of bleeding?

_____

_____

_____

3. How much blood did the patient lose during the procedure?

_____

_____

_____

4. Were any ulcerations or erosions found during the exploratory procedure that might account for the bleeding?

_____

_____

_____

5. What type of sedation was used during the procedure?

_____

_____

_____

6. What did the doctors find when they examined the stomach and duodenum?

_____

_____

_____

Documenting Health-Care Activity 6-3

Constructing Chart Notes

To construct chart notes, replace the italicized and boldfaced terms in each of the two case studies with one of the listed medical terms.

anorexia	*gastric reflux*	*jaundice*
antacids	*hepatomegaly*	*nausea*
dyspepsia	*hiatal hernia*	*sclerae*
dysphagia		

During her annual checkup, Mrs. L. complains that she has (1) ***difficulty swallowing.*** Also, she is awakened at night with a feeling of (2) ***difficult or painful digestion.*** She further complains of (3) ***regurgitation of stomach acid*** and has been taking Tums and Rolaids. She feels that the (4) ***medications*** to neutralize the backflow of acid from her stomach have not been effective. After a thorough examination along with some radiographic procedures, the doctor suspects her symptoms are caused by a (5) ***part of her stomach herniating through the opening of the diaphragm.***

1. _____
2. _____
3. _____
4. _____
5. _____

Mr. K recently returned from Haiti where he worked with other volunteers from his church. Their purpose was to help homeless families rebuild their communities. Lately, he complains of (6) ***no appetite*** and feeling feverish. He also complains of (7) ***unpleasant queasy sensations of discomfort in the region of his stomach.*** Today, he presents to the clinic, and his doctor notes that the (8) ***whites of his eyes*** are now (9) ***yellow in color.*** After further examination and a series of blood tests, the doctor suspects that Mr. K suffers from an (10) ***enlarged liver*** and should undergo further testing for hepatitis A.

6. _____
7. _____
8. _____
9. _____
10. _____

✓ *Check your answers in Appendix A. Review any material that you did not answer correctly.*

Correct Answers _____ X 10 = _____ % Score

Respiratory System

Chapter Outline

Objectives

Upon completion of this chapter, you will be able to:

- Locate and describe the structures of the respiratory system.
- Describe the functional relationship between the respiratory system and other body systems.
- Pronounce, spell, and build words related to the respiratory system.
- Describe diseases, conditions, and procedures related to the respiratory system.
- Explain pharmacology related to the treatment of respiratory disorders.
- Demonstrate your knowledge of this chapter by completing the learning and documenting health-care activities.

Anatomy and Physiology

The respiratory system is responsible for the exchange of **oxygen (O_2)** and **carbon dioxide (CO_2)**. O_2 is essential for life. It is carried to all cells of the body in exchange for CO_2, a waste product. The lungs and airways transport O_2 enriched air from the atmosphere to the lungs and carry waste CO_2 from the lungs to the atmosphere by a process called **breathing (ventilation)**. Breathing helps regulate the **pH** (acidity/alkalinity) of the blood, thereby helping maintain a stable internal environment of the body **(homeostasis)**.

Anatomy and Physiology Key Terms

This section introduces important respiratory system terms and their definitions. The key terms are highlighted in color in the Anatomy and Physiology section. Word analyses for selected terms are also provided. Pronounce the term and place a check mark in the box after you do so.

Term	Definition
carbon dioxide (CO_2) ☐ KĂR-bŏn dī-ŎK-sīd	Tasteless, colorless, odorless gas produced by body cells during metabolism *The blood carries CO_2 to the lungs, which then exhale it.*
cartilage ☐ KĂR-tĭ-lĭj	Tough, elastic connective tissue that is more rigid than ligaments but less dense than bone *The tip of the nose and the outer ear are composed of cartilage.*
cilia ☐ SĬL-ē-ă	Minute, hairlike structures that extend from the surface of a cell *Cilia in the trachea move particles upward to the pharynx, a mechanism called the cilia escalator. Habitual smoking destroys the cilia escalator.*
diffuse ☐ dĭ-FŪZ	To move or spread out a substance at random, rather than by chemical reaction or application of external forces
oxygen (O_2) ☐ ŎK-sĭ-jĕn	Tasteless, odorless, colorless gas essential for human respiration
pH ☐	Symbol that indicates the degree of acidity or alkalinity of a substance *Increasing acidity is expressed as a number less than 7; increasing alkalinity is expressed as a number greater than 7; 7 indicates a neutral substance.*

serous membrane ☐
SĒR-ūs MĔM-brăn
  ser: serum
  -ous: pertaining to
	Thin layer of tissue that covers internal body cavities and secretes a fluid that keeps the membrane moist; also called *serosa*

Pronunciation Help	Long Sound	ā — rate	ē — rebirth	ī — isle	ō — over	ū — unite
	Short Sound	ă — alone	ĕ — ever	ĭ — it	ŏ — not	ŭ — cut

Upper Respiratory Tract

The breathing process begins with inhalation (see Fig. 7-1). Air is drawn into the (1) **nasal cavity**, a chamber lined with **mucous membranes** and tiny hairs called *cilia*. Here, air is filtered, heated, and moistened to prepare it for its journey to the lungs. The nasal cavity is divided into a right and left side by a vertical partition of **cartilage** called the **nasal septum**.

Figure 7-1 Anterior view of the upper and lower respiratory tracts.

Olfactory neurons are receptors for the sense of smell. They are covered with a layer of mucus and located deep in the nasal cavity, embedded among the epithelial cells lining the nasal tract. Because they are located higher in the nasal passage than air normally travels during breathing, a person must sniff or inhale deeply to identify weak odors. Air passes from the nasal cavity to the throat **(pharynx)**, a muscular tube that serves as a passageway for food and air. The pharynx consists of three sections: the (2) **nasopharynx**, posterior to the nose; the (3) **oropharynx**, posterior to the mouth; and the (4) **laryngopharynx**, superior to the larynx.

Within the nasopharynx is a collection of lymphoid tissue known as (5) **adenoids** (pharyngeal tonsils). The (6) **palatine tonsils**, more commonly known as **tonsils,** are located in the oropharynx. They protect the opening to the respiratory tract from microscopic organisms that may attempt entry by this route. The (7) **larynx** (voice box) contains the structures that make vocal sounds possible. A leaf-shaped structure on top of the larynx, the (8) **epiglottis**, seals off the air passage to the lungs during swallowing. This function ensures that food or liquids do not obstruct the flow of air to the lungs. The larynx is a short passage that joins the pharynx with the (9) **trachea** (windpipe). The trachea is composed of smooth muscle embedded with C-shaped rings of cartilage, which provide rigidity to keep the air passage open.

Lower Respiratory Tract

The trachea divides into two branches called (10) **bronchi** (singular, **bronchus**). One branch leads to the (11) **right lung** and the other to the (12) **left lung**. The inner walls of the trachea and bronchi are composed of **mucous membrane (mucosa)** embedded with cilia. This membrane traps incoming particles, and the cilia move the entrapped material upward into the pharynx, where it is expelled by coughing, sneezing, or swallowing. Like the trachea, bronchi contain C-shaped rings of cartilage.

Each bronchus divides into smaller and smaller branches, eventually forming (13) **bronchioles**. At the end of the bronchioles are tiny air sacs called (14) **alveoli** (singular, **alveolus**). An alveolus resembles a small balloon because it expands and contracts with inflow and outflow of air. The (15) **pulmonary capillaries** lie next to the thin tissue membranes of the alveoli. CO_2 **diffuses** from the blood within the pulmonary capillaries and enters the alveolar spaces, and O_2 from the alveoli diffuses into the blood. After the exchange of gases, freshly oxygenated blood returns to the heart. O_2 is now ready for delivery to all body tissues.

The lungs are divided into lobes: three lobes in the right lung and two lobes in the left lung. The space between the right and left lungs is called the (16) **mediastinum**. It contains the heart, aorta, esophagus, and bronchi. A **serous membrane**, the pleura, covers the lobes of the lungs and folds over to line the walls of the thoracic cavity. The membrane lying closest to the lung is the (17) **visceral pleura**; the membrane that lines the thoracic cavity is the (18) **parietal pleura**. The space between these two membranes is the (19) **pleural cavity**. It contains a small amount of lubricating fluid, which permits the visceral pleura to glide smoothly over the parietal pleura during breathing.

Ventilation depends on a pressure differential between the atmosphere and chest cavity. A large muscular partition, the (20) **diaphragm**, lies between the chest and abdominal cavities. The diaphragm assists in changing the volume of the thoracic cavity to produce the needed pressure differential for ventilation. When the diaphragm contracts, it partially descends into the abdominal cavity, thus decreasing the pressure within the chest and drawing air into the lungs **(inspiration)**. When the diaphragm relaxes, it slowly reenters the thoracic cavity, thus increasing the pressure within the chest. As pressure increases, air leaves the lungs **(expiration)**. The intercostal muscles assist the diaphragm in changing the volume of the thoracic cavity by elevating and lowering the rib cage (see Fig. 7-2).

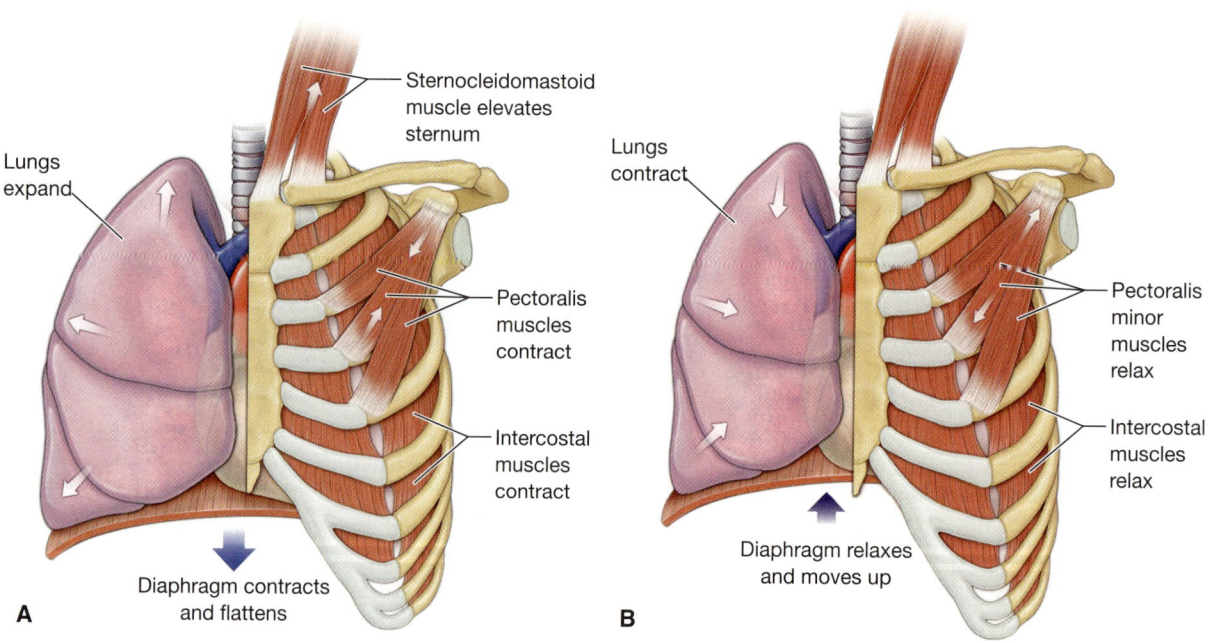

Figure 7-2 Breathing muscles. (A) Inspiration. (B) Expiration.

Pulmonary Respiration

Pulmonary respiration is the process by which O_2 is taken from air and carried to body cells for their use, and the waste products generated by these cells, CO_2, are carried to the lungs and returned to the environment (see Fig. 7-3). Respiration includes four stages:

I. **Pulmonary ventilation (breathing)**: nervous stimulation of the diaphragm and inter-costal muscles and changes in blood O_2 and CO_2 levels trigger an involuntary action that moves air into (inspiration) and out of the lungs (expiration).
II. **External respiration**: the exchange of O_2 and CO_2 between the alveoli and the blood in the pulmonary capillaries.
III. **Transport of gases**: the movement of O_2 to body cells and CO_2 to the lungs by means of the cardiovascular system.
IV. **Internal respiration**: the exchange of O_2 and CO_2 between body cells and the blood in systemic capillaries.

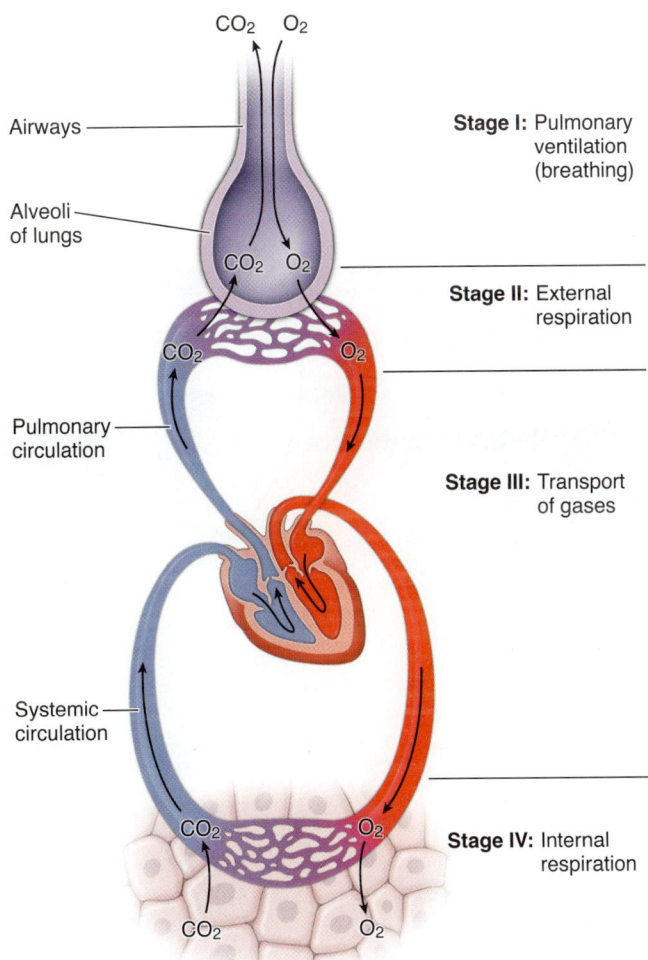

Figure 7-3 Pulmonary respiration.

Anatomy Review: Respiratory System

To review the anatomy of the respiratory system, label the illustration using the listed terms.

adenoids	*epiglottis*	*nasal cavity*	*pleural cavity*
alveoli	*laryngopharynx*	*nasopharynx*	*pulmonary capillaries*
bronchi	*larynx*	*oropharynx*	*right lung*
bronchiole	*left lung*	*palatine tonsils*	*trachea*
diaphragm	*mediastinum*	*parietal pleura*	*visceral pleura*

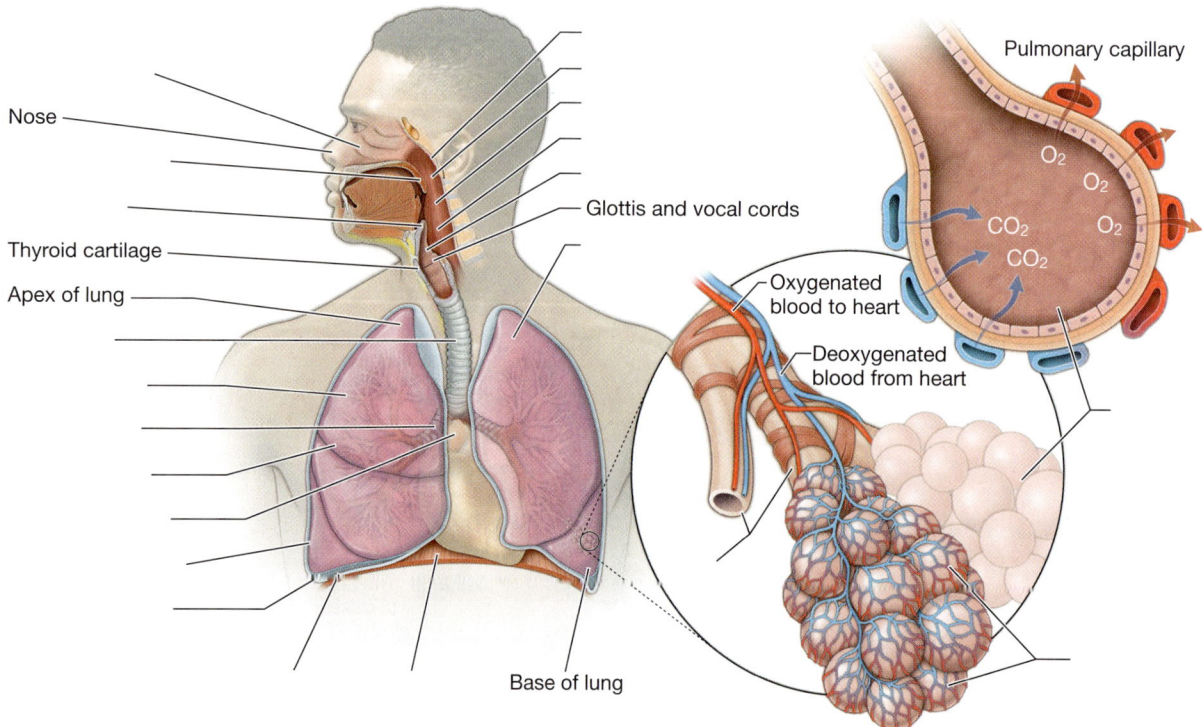

Nose

Thyroid cartilage

Apex of lung

Glottis and vocal cords

Base of lung

Pulmonary capillary

O_2 O_2

CO_2 O_2

CO_2

Oxygenated blood to heart

Deoxygenated blood from heart

 Check your answers by referring to Figure 7–1 on page 189. Review material that you did not answer correctly.

CONNECTING BODY SYSTEMS—RESPIRATORY SYSTEM

The main function of the respiratory system is to provide O_2 to the entire body and expel CO_2 from the body. Specific functional relationships between the respiratory system and other body systems are summarized here.

Blood, Lymphatic, and Immune
- The tonsils, adenoids, and other immune structures in the respiratory tract protect against pathogens that attempt entry through respiratory passageways.

Cardiovascular
- The respiratory system provides O_2 and removes CO_2 from cardiac tissue.

Digestive
- The respiratory system provides O_2 needed for digestive functions.
- The respiratory system removes CO_2 produced by the organs of digestion.
- The respiratory and digestive systems share the pharynx, an anatomic structure of digestion.

Endocrine
- The respiratory system helps maintain a stable pH required for proper functioning of the endocrine glands.

Female Reproductive
- Respiratory rate increases in response to sexual activity.
- Fetal respiration occurs during pregnancy.

Integumentary
- The respiratory system furnishes O_2 and disposes of CO_2 to maintain healthy skin.

Male Reproductive
- Respiratory rate increases in response to sexual activity.
- The respiratory system helps maintain pH for gonadal hormone function.
- O_2 is supplied to reproductive structures to maintain viable sperm.

Musculoskeletal
- The respiratory system provides O_2 for muscle contraction.
- The respiratory system eliminates CO_2 produced by muscles.
- The respiratory system provides O_2 for bone development.

Nervous
- The respiratory system provides O_2 for brain, spinal cord, and sensory organ functions.
- The respiratory system helps maintain a stable pH for neural function.

Urinary
- The respiratory system supplies O_2 and removes CO_2 to maintain proper functioning of urinary structures.
- The respiratory system assists the urinary structures in regulating pH by removing CO_2.

Medical Word Elements

This section introduces combining forms, suffixes, and prefixes related to the respiratory system. Word analyses are also provided. From the information provided, complete the meaning of the medical words in the right-hand column. The first one is completed for you.

Element	Meaning	Word Analysis
Combining Forms		
Upper Respiratory Tract		
nas/o	nose	**nas**/al (NĀ-zl): *pertaining to the nose* -*al:* pertaining to
rhin/o		**rhin/o**/plasty (RĬ-nō-plăs-tē): _____ -*plasty:* surgical repair *Rhinoplasty is performed to correct birth defects or for cosmetic purposes.*
sept/o	septum	**sept/o**/plasty (SĔP-tō-plăs-tē): _____ -*plasty:* surgical repair *Septoplasty is commonly performed to correct a deviated septum.*
sinus/o	sinus, cavity	**sinus/o**/tomy (sī-nŭs-ŎT-ō-mē): _____ -*tomy:* incision *Sinusotomy is performed to improve breathing or for drainage in unresponsive sinusitis.*
pharyng/o	pharynx (throat)	**pharyng/o**/scope (făr-ĬN-gō-skōp): _____ *scope:* instrument for examining
adenoid/o	adenoids	**adenoid**/ectomy (ăd-ĕ-noyd-ĔK-tō-mē): _____ -*ectomy:* excision, removal
tonsill/o	tonsils	peri/**tonsill**/ar (pĕr-ĭ-TŎN-sĭ-lăr): _____ *peri-:* around -*ar:* pertaining to
epiglott/o	epiglottis	**epiglott**/itis (ĕp-ĭ-glŏt-Ī-tĭs): _____ -*itis:* inflammation *Because the epiglottis seals the opening to the lungs, inflammation can lead to severe airway obstruction and death. Epiglottitis is treated as a medical emergency.*
laryng/o	larynx (voice box)	**laryng/o**/plegia (lă-rĭn-gō-PLĒ-jē-ă): _____ -*plegia:* paralysis
trache/o	trachea (windpipe)	**trache/o**/plasty (TRĀ-kē-ō-plăs-tē): _____ -*plasty:* surgical repair *Tracheoplasty is performed to correct a narrow or stenotic trachea.*

Medical Word Elements—cont'd

Element	Meaning	Word Analysis
Lower Respiratory Tract		
bronchi/o	bronchus (plural, bronchi)	**bronchi**/ectasis (brŏng-kē-ĔK-tă-sĭs): _____ *-ectasis:* dilation, expansion *Bronchiectasis is associated with various lung conditions and is commonly accompanied by chronic infection.*
bronch/o		**bronch/o**/scope (BRŎNG-kō-skōp): _____ *-scope:* instrument for examining *A bronchoscope is a flexible tube that is passed through the nose or mouth to enable inspection of the lungs and collection of tissue biopsies and secretions for analysis.*
bronchiol/o	bronchiole	**bronchiol**/itis (brŏng-kē-ō-LĪ-tĭs): _____ *-itis:* inflammation
alveol/o	alveolus; air sac	**alveol**/ar (ăl-VĒ-ō-lăr): _____ *-ar:* pertaining to
pleur/o	pleura	**pleur/o**/scopy (ploo-RŎS-kō-pē): _____ *-scopy:* visual examination *Pleuroscopy involves insertion of a specialized endoscope through a small incision in the chest to allow an inspection of the pleural space, obtain lung tissue for analysis, inject medications, and perform other diagnostic or therapeutic procedures.*
pneum/o	air; lung	**pneum/o**/lith (NŪ-mō-lĭth): _____ *-lith:* stone, calculus
pneumon/o		**pneumon**/ia (nū-MŌ-nē-ă): _____ *-ia:* condition
pulmon/o	lung	**pulmon/o**/logist (pŭl-mŏ-NŎL-ŏ-jĭst): _____ *-logist:* specialist in the study of
Other		
anthrac/o	coal, coal dust	**anthrac**/osis (ăn-thră-KŌ-sĭs): _____ *-osis:* abnormal condition; increase (used primarily with blood cells) *Anthracosis (black lung disease) is a chronic occupational disease found in coal miners and those associated with the coal industry.*
atel/o	incomplete; imperfect	**atel**/ectasis (ăt-ĕ-LĔK-tă-sĭs): _____ *-ectasis:* dilation, expansion *Atelectasis (airless or collapsed lung) is usually caused by a blocked airway, trauma to the chest cavity, or infection.*

Continued

Medical Word Elements—cont'd

Element	Meaning	Word Analysis
coni/o	dust	pneum/o/**coni**/osis (nū-mō-kō-nē-Ō-sĭs): _____ *pneum/o:* air; lung *-osis:* abnormal condition; increase (used primarily with blood cells) *Pneumoconiosis is caused by mineral dusts of occupational or environmental origin and includes silicosis, asbestosis, and anthracosis.*
cyan/o	blue	**cyan**/osis (sī-ă-NŌ-sĭs): _____ *-osis:* abnormal condition; increase (used primarily with blood cells) *Cyanosis results from poor circulation or inadequate oxygenation of the blood.*
lob/o	lobe	**lob**/ectomy (lō-BĔK-tō-mē): _____ *-ectomy:* excision *Lobectomies are performed when a malignancy is confined to a single lobe of any lobed organ, such as the lungs, liver, and thyroid gland.*
orth/o	straight	**orth/o**/pnea (or-THŎP-nē-ă): _____ *-pnea:* breathing *Discomfort in breathing that is relieved by sitting or standing in an erect position.*
ox/o	oxygen (O_2)	hyp/**ox**/emia (hī-pŏks-Ē-mē-ă): _____ *hyp-:* under, below, deficient *-emia:* blood condition *Hypoxemia is an abnormal decrease of oxygen in arterial blood.*
pector/o	chest	**pector**/algia (pĕk-tō-RĂL-jē-ă): _____ *-algia:* pain *Pectoralgia is also called thoracalgia or thoracodynia.*
steth/o		**steth/o**/scope (STĔTH-ō-skōp): _____ *-scope:* instrument for examining *A stethoscope enables evaluation of sounds in the chest and the abdomen, an assessment technique known as auscultation.*
thorac/o		**thorac/o**/pathy (thō-răk-ŎP-ă-thē): _____ *-pathy:* disease
phren/o	diaphragm; mind	**phren/o**/spasm (FRĔN-ō-spăzm): _____ *-spasm:* involuntary contraction, twitching
spir/o	breathe	**spir/o**/meter (spī-RŎM-ĕt-ĕr): _____ *-meter:* instrument for measuring *A spirometer evaluates the movement of air into and out of the lungs (ventilation).*

Medical Word Elements—cont'd

Element	Meaning	Word Analysis

Suffixes

Element	Meaning	Word Analysis
-capnia	carbon dioxide (CO_2)	hyper/**capnia** (hī-pĕr-KĂP-nē-ă): _____ *hyper-:* excessive, above normal
-osmia	smell	an/**osmia** (ăn-ŎZ-mē-ă): _____ *an-:* without, not *Anosmia is a loss, usually partial, of the sense of smell. It mostly occurs as a temporary condition resulting from an upper respiratory infection (URI) or a condition that causes intranasal swelling.*
-phonia	voice	dys/**phonia** (dĭs-FŌ-nē-ă): _____ *dys-:* bad, painful, difficult *Dysphonia usually signifies dysfunction in the muscles needed to produce sound.*
-pnea	breathing	a/**pnea** (ĂP-nē-ă): _____ *a-:* without, not
-ptysis	spitting	hem/o/**ptysis** (hē-MŎP-tĭ-sĭs): _____ *hem/o:* blood *Hemoptysis is usually a sign of a serious condition of the lungs.*
-thorax	chest	hem/o/**thorax** (hē-mō-THŌ-răks): _____ *hem/o:* blood *Hemothorax is a type of pleural effusion containing blood, commonly associated with severe trauma to the chest.*

Prefixes

Element	Meaning	Word Analysis
brady-	slow	**brady**/pnea (brăd-ĭp-NĒ-ă): _____ *-pnea:* breathing
dys-	bad, painful, difficult	**dys**/pnea (DĬSP-nē-ă): _____ *-pnea:* breathing
eu-	good, normal	**eu**/pnea (ŪP-nē-ă): _____ *-pnea:* breathing
tachy-	rapid	**tachy**/pnea (tăk-ĭp-NĒ-ă): _____ *-pnea:* breathing

 Visit the Medical Terminology Systems online resource center at FADavis. com for an audio exercise of the terms in this table. Other activities are also available to reinforce content.

 It is time to review medical word elements by completing Learning Activities 7–1 on page 220 and 7–2 on page 221.

Disease Focus

Common signs and symptoms of many respiratory disorders include cough (dry or productive), chest pain (**thoracodynia**), altered breathing patterns, shortness of breath (SOB), cyanosis, fever, and exercise intolerance. Many disorders of the respiratory system, including bronchitis and emphysema, begin as an acute problem but become chronic over time. Chronic respiratory diseases are not curable, and their damaging effects are often irreversible. However, there are various forms of treatment that help to open the air passageway to improve SOB and the quality of life for those living with these conditions.

For diagnosis, treatment, and management of respiratory disorders, the medical services of a specialist may be warranted. **Pulmonology** is the medical specialty concerned with disorders of the respiratory system. The physician who treats these disorders is called a **pulmonologist**.

Chronic Obstructive Pulmonary Disease

Chronic obstructive pulmonary disease (COPD) is a progressive and chronic respiratory disorder characterized by airflow limitation and long-term respiratory symptoms with increased difficulty in breathing (**dyspnea**). COPD is insidious and is commonly first diagnosed after the patient has already lost some lung capacity. It is possible to have early stages of COPD without knowing it (see Table 7-1). The three major disorders of COPD are asthma, chronic bronchitis, and emphysema (see Fig. 7-4).

Asthma

Asthma produces spasms in the bronchial passages (**bronchospasms**) that may be sudden and violent (**paroxysmal**), causing dyspnea. Asthma is caused by exposure to allergens or irritants. Other causes include stress, cold, and exercise. During recovery, coughing episodes produce large amounts of mucus (**productive cough**). Over time, the epithelium of the bronchial passages thickens, breathing becomes more difficult, and flare-ups (**exacerbations**) occur more frequently. Treatment includes agents that loosen and break down mucus (**mucolytics**) and medications that expand the bronchi (**bronchodilators**) by relaxing their smooth muscles. Most cases of asthma can be treated effectively. However, when treatment does not reverse bronchospasm, a life-threatening condition called **status asthmaticus** can occur, requiring hospitalization.

TABLE 7-1 Stages of COPD

This table lists the levels of severity of COPD and describes their characteristics.

Severity Level	Description
At risk, mild	• Minor difficulty with airflow
	• Possible presence of chronic cough with sputum production
	• Patient possibly unaware of disease
Moderate	• Apparent limitation in airflow
	• Possible shortness of breath
	• Patient possibly seeking medical intervention at this level
Severe	• Inadequate airflow
	• Increase in shortness of breath with activity
	• Patient experiencing diminished quality of life
Very severe	• Severe airflow limitations
	• Significant impairment in quality of life
	• Possible life-threatening exacerbations
	• Possible development of complications, such as respiratory or heart failure

Excess mucus production

Enlarged alveoli

Inflamed airway

Distended bronchiole

Extra mucus

Constricted smooth muscle

A Chronic bronchitis   **B** Emphysema   **C** Asthma

Figure 7-4 Chronic obstructive pulmonary disease (COPD). (A) Chronic bronchitis with inflamed airways and excessive mucus. (B) Emphysema with distended bronchioles and alveoli. (C) Asthma with narrowed bronchial tubes and swollen mucous membranes.

Chronic Bronchitis

Chronic bronchitis is an inflammation of the bronchi caused mainly by smoking and air pollution. However, other agents, such as viruses and bacteria, may also cause the disorder. Bronchitis is characterized by swelling of the mucosa and a heavy, productive cough accompanied by chest pain. Patients commonly seek medical help when they suffer exercise intolerance, wheezing, and SOB. Bronchodilators and medications that aid in the removal of mucus (**expectorants**) help widen air passages. Steroids are prescribed if the disease progresses or becomes chronic.

Emphysema

Emphysema is characterized by decreased elasticity of the alveoli. The alveoli expand (**dilate**) but are unable to contract to their original size, making it difficult to exhale. The air that remains trapped in the chest results in a characteristic "barrel-chested" appearance. Emphysema commonly occurs with another respiratory disorder, such as asthma, tuberculosis, or chronic bronchitis, and in long-term heavy smokers. Most emphysema sufferers find it easier to breathe when sitting upright or standing erect (**orthopnea**). As the disease progresses, relief—even in the orthopneic position—is not possible. Treatment for emphysema is similar to that for chronic bronchitis.

Pneumonia

Pneumonia is an inflammatory condition affecting the lungs, primarily the microscopic air sacs (**alveoli**). As inflammatory fluids collect in the alveoli, lung tissue loses its spongy texture and becomes swollen and engorged (**consolidation**), and oxygen exchange becomes difficult. Causes of pneumonia include bacterial and viral infections, but fungi, chemicals, and even inhaled substances such as food, vomitus, or liquids (**aspiration pneumonias**) can also cause pneumonia.

Lobar pneumonia is generally of bacterial origin and affects a large portion or an entire lobe of a lung. Typically, this disease occurs in young, healthy adults and thus is considered a primary pneumonia. Antibiotic therapy is effective in the treatment of this disease.

Bronchopneumonia is caused by a wider variety of organisms and is centered in the bronchi and surrounding alveoli. It tends to occur in infants, the elderly, and those suffering from other illnesses, including cancer, heart failure, and immune disorders. Because of this association, it is considered a secondary pneumonia.

Pneumocystis pneumonia (PCP) is a type of pneumonia closely associated with AIDS. Recent evidence suggests that it is caused by an organism that resides in or on most people (**normal flora**) but causes no harm as long as the individual remains healthy. When the immune system begins to fail, this organism becomes infectious (**opportunistic**).

Thoracodynia, dyspnea, hemoptysis, and coughing up sputum containing white blood cells (**mucopurulent sputum**) are common signs and symptoms of pneumonia.

Auscultation, percussion, chest x-ray (CXR), and blood tests help diagnose pneumonia. For elderly patients, especially those who are hospitalized with other health issues, a pleural fluid culture and computed tomography (CT) scan aid in determining a diagnosis.

Acute Respiratory Distress Syndrome

Acute respiratory distress syndrome (ARDS) is a condition in which the lungs no longer function effectively, threatening the life of the patient. It usually occurs as a result of very serious lung conditions, such as trauma, severe pneumonia, and other major infections that affect the entire body (**systemic infections**) or blood (**sepsis**). In ARDS, the alveoli fill with fluid (**edema**) caused by inflammation and then collapse, making oxygen exchange impossible. Mechanical ventilation is commonly required to save the life of the patient.

Neonatal respiratory distress syndrome (NRDS) is a form of respiratory distress syndrome seen in preterm infants or infants born to diabetic mothers. It is caused by insufficient **surfactant**, a phospholipid substance that helps keep alveoli open. With insufficient surfactant, the alveoli collapse, and breathing becomes labored. Clinical signs may include blueness (**cyanosis**) of the extremities. Flaring of the nostrils (**nares**), rapid breathing (**tachypnea**), and a characteristic grunt audible during exhalation are signs of this disorder. Radiography shows a membrane that has a ground-glass appearance (**hyaline membrane**), bilateral decrease in lung volume, and fluid in the alveoli (**alveolar consolidation**). Although severe cases of hyaline membrane disease (HMD) result in death, some forms of therapy are effective.

Oncology

Lung Cancer

Lung cancer, malignant tumors growing in the bronchi and lungs, is the leading cause of cancer death in the United States and worldwide. Most lung cancers are associated with cigarette smoking but can also occur in nonsmokers. Signs and symptoms of lung cancer may not appear until after the cancer has spread to other parts of the body (**metastasized**), making it more difficult to treat, resulting in a poor outcome (**prognosis**). The extent (**stage**) and the type of cancer are important factors that affect the treatment and prognosis. There are two main types of lung cancer: non-small cell lung cancer and small cell lung cancer.

Non-small cell lung cancer (NSLC) comprises most lung cancers and includes three subtypes, based on the lung cell origin. *Adenocarcinomas* begin in the cells that line the alveoli and make substances such as mucus. *Squamous cell carcinoma* forms in the thin, flat cells lining the inside of the lungs. *Large cell carcinoma* may begin in several types of large cells located throughout the lungs.

Small cell lung cancer (SCLC), also known as *oat cell cancer,* is characterized by small, round cells resembling oat grain. They tend to grow rapidly and metastasize faster than NSLC.

Treatments for lung cancer include surgical removal of tumors, radiation, chemotherapy, targeted therapy, and immunotherapy. Often, a combination of these is used.

Screening high-risk individuals has the potential to dramatically improve lung cancer survival rates by finding the disease at an earlier stage when it is more likely to be treatable. The **spiral or helical CT scan** provides a detailed image of lung tissue and has shown to be superior to CXRs in detecting new growths.

Diseases and Conditions

This section introduces diseases and conditions of the respiratory system, along with their definitions and pronunciations. Word analyses for selected terms are also provided.

Term	Definition
abnormal breath sounds	Abnormal breath sounds heard during respiration with the use of a stethoscope (**auscultation**), commonly leading to a diagnosis of a respiratory or cardiac condition; also called *adventitious breath sounds*
crackle KRĂK-ĕl	Intermittent sounds caused by exudates, spasms, hyperplasia, or when air enters moisture-filled alveoli; also called *rale*
rhonchus RŎNG-kŭs	Continuous sound heard during inspiration and expiration caused by secretions in the larger airways and commonly resembling snoring
stridor STRĪ-dor	High-pitched, harsh sound caused by a spasm or swelling of the larynx or an obstruction in the upper airway *The presence of stridor may be life-threatening and requires immediate intervention.*
wheeze HWĒZ	Whistling or sighing that results from narrowing of the lumen of the respiratory passageway *Wheezing is a sign of asthma, croup, hay fever, obstructive emphysema, and other obstructive respiratory conditions.*
acidosis ăs-ĭ-DŌ-sĭs *acid:* acid *-osis:* abnormal condition; increase (used primarily with blood cells)	Excessive acidity of body fluids *Respiratory acidosis is commonly associated with pulmonary insufficiency and the subsequent retention of carbon dioxide.*
apnea ĂP-nē-ă *a-:* without, not *-pnea:* breathing	Disorder in which breathing stops repeatedly during sleep, resulting in blood deoxygenation, causing the patient to awaken, gasping for air; also called *sleep apnea* *Apneic episodes may be as seldom as once per hour or as often as once every 5 minutes.*
central (CSA)	A form of sleep apnea that occurs when the brain fails to stimulate breathing muscles, causing brief pauses in breathing *Cheyne-Stokes, a type of periodic respiration related to CSA, is commonly associated with heart failure.*
obstructive (OSA)	Most common form of sleep apnea caused by an upper airway blockage that prevents an adequate flow of air to the lungs *Causes of OSA include enlarged tonsils or adenoids or decreased muscle tone of the soft palate that causes it to collapse over the airway, blocking air passages and leading to reduction or absence of breathing during sleep. Symptoms include frequent waking, snoring, gasping, or choking (see Fig. 7-5).*
mixed	Type of sleep apnea that occurs when CSA and OSA occur simultaneously

Continued

Diseases and Conditions—cont'd

Term	Definition

A   Normal airway   **B**   Sleep apnea

Figure 7-5 Obstructive sleep apnea (OSA). (A) Airway is open and throat muscles that support the back of the roof of the mouth (soft palate), tongue, and sides of the throat are positioned to create an open airway for breathing. (B) OSA occurs when the airway narrows or closes due to the muscles in the back of the throat relaxing, causing a blocked airway with resulting snoring, gasping, or choking. The brain senses the apnea and awakens the person from sleep so the airway can reopen.

Term	Definition

atelectasis
ăt-ĕ-LĔK-tă-sĭs
  atel: incomplete, imperfect
  -ectasis: dilation, expansion
	Collapsed or airless state of the lung, which may be acute or chronic and affects all or part of a lung
	
	Atelectasis is a potential complication of some surgical procedures, especially those of the chest, because of shallow breathing to avoid pain from the surgical incision.

coronavirus kŭh RŌ nŭh vī rŭs	Group of viruses that can cause illnesses such as the common cold and severe acute respiratory syndrome (SARS) that are highly contagious and mainly spread through respiratory droplets produced when an infected person breathes, talks, sneezes, or coughs
coronavirus disease 2019 (COVID-19)	Pandemic of new coronavirus that originated in China in 2019; common symptoms include loss of taste and smell, fever, cough, tiredness, and difficulty breathing, with some experiencing worsened SOB and pneumonia after a week of onset (see Fig. 7-6). *Those who are older, have existing chronic medical conditions, or immunosuppression are at an increased risk of severity. New vaccinations offer protection from several of the most recent strains of the virus.*

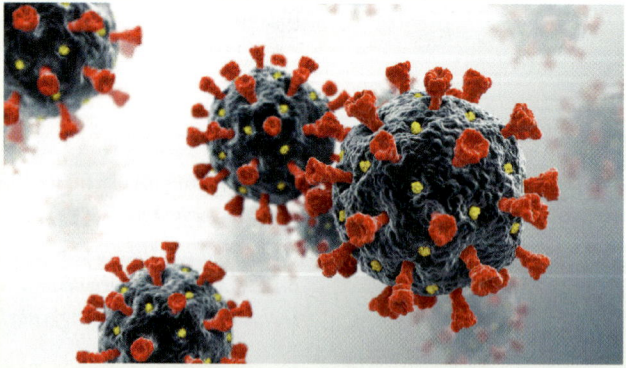

Figure 7-6 COVID-19 cells close-up under a microscope.

Diseases and Conditions—cont'd

Term	Definition
coryza kŏ-RĪ-ză	Acute inflammation of the membranes of the nose; also called *rhinitis* *Causes of coryza include bacteria, viruses, irritants, and allergens.*
croup CROOP	Common childhood condition involving inflammation of the larynx, trachea, and bronchial passages and sometimes involving the lungs *Signs and symptoms of croup include a resonant, barking cough with suffocative, difficult breathing; laryngeal spasms; and, sometimes, the narrowing of the top of the air passages.*
cystic fibrosis (CF) SĬS-tĭk fī-BRŌ-sĭs *cyst:* bladder *-ic:* pertaining to *fibr:* fiber, fibrous tissue *-osis:* abnormal condition; increase (used primarily with blood cells)	Life-threatening genetic disease that causes mucus to become unusually thick and sticky, plugging tubes and ducts, especially in the lungs and pancreas *There are different types of CF with varying levels of severity. Currently, there is no cure for CF. Treatment consists of supportive measures that help the patient lead a normal life to the extent possible and that prevent pulmonary infection.*
deviated nasal septum DĒ-vē-āt-ĕd NĀ-zl SĔP-tŭm *nas:* nose *-al:* pertaining to	Displacement of the cartilage dividing the nostrils that causes reduced airflow and sometimes causes nosebleed
epiglottitis ĕp-ĭ-glŏt-Ī-tĭs *epiglott:* epiglottis *-itis:* inflammation	Severe, life-threatening infection of the epiglottis and supraglottic structures that occurs most commonly in children between ages 2 and 12 years *Signs and symptoms of epiglottitis include fever, dysphagia, inspiratory stridor, and severe respiratory distress. Intubation or tracheostomy may be required to open the obstructed airway.*
epistaxis ĕp-ĭ-STĂK-sĭs	Nasal hemorrhage; also called *nosebleed*
hypoxemia hī-pŏks-Ē-mē-ă *hyp-:* under, below, deficient *ox:* oxygen *-emia:* blood condition	O_2 deficiency in arterial blood, which is usually a sign of respiratory impairment and commonly causes hypoxia
hypoxia hī-PŎKS-ē-ă *hyp-:* under, below, deficient *-oxia:* oxygen	O_2 deficiency in the body or a region of the body that commonly causes cyanosis

Continued

Diseases and Conditions—cont'd

Term	Definition
influenza ĭn-floo-ĔN-ză	Acute, contagious viral disorder of the respiratory tract, characterized by weakness, fever, chills, and muscle pain, especially in the back, arms, and legs; also called *flu* *Flu viruses are constantly changing, with new strains appearing regularly. Guidelines recommend vaccination each flu season because flu can cause serious complications, including pneumonia, bronchitis, sinusitis, and asthma flare-up.*
pertussis pĕr-TŬS-ĭs	Acute, infectious disease characterized by a cough that has a characteristic "whoop" sound; also called *whooping cough* *Immunization of infants as part of the diphtheria-pertussis-tetanus (DPT) vaccination is effective in preventing pertussis.*
pleural effusion PLOO-răl ĕ-FŪ-zhŭn *pleur:* pleura *-al:* pertaining to	Abnormal accumulation of fluid in the pleural cavity that impairs breathing by limiting the expansion of the lungs *Pleural effusions are described as exudates when the effusion is high in protein and immune cells or as transudates when the fluid resembles serum and does not contain inflammatory cells.*
empyema ĕm-pī-Ē-mă	Exudative effusion characterized by collection of pus in the pleural cavity, commonly as a result of bacterial pneumonia that spreads from the lungs; also called *pyothorax*
pneumothorax nū-mō-THŌ-răks *pneum/o:* air, lung *-thorax:* chest	Presence of air in the pleural cavity, commonly caused by a blunt or penetrating chest injury or as the result of a thoracic surgery *Pneumothorax commonly causes a partial or complete collapse of a lung (atelectasis)(see Fig. 7-7).*

Diseases and Conditions—cont'd

Term	Definition

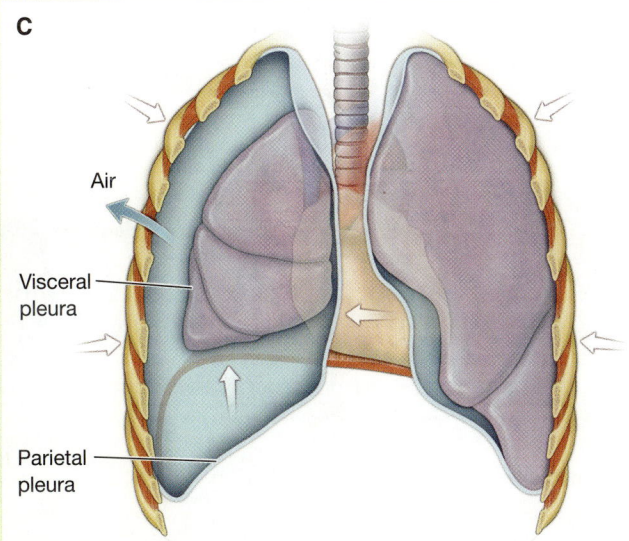

Figure 7-7 Pneumothorax. (A) Normal lungs. (B) Open pneumothorax during inspiration. (C) Open pneumothorax during expiration.

Term	Definition
pleurisy PLOO-rĭs-ē *pleur:* pleura *-isy:* state of, condition	Inflammation of the pleural membrane characterized by a stabbing pain that is intensified by coughing or deep breathing; also called *pleuritis*
pulmonary edema PŬL-mō-nĕ-rē ĕ-DĒ-mă *pulmon:* lung *-ary:* pertaining to	Accumulation of extravascular fluid in lung tissues and alveoli, most commonly caused by heart failure *Excessive fluid in the lungs induces coughing and dyspnea.*

Continued

Diseases and Conditions—cont'd

Term	Definition

pulmonary embolism (PE)
PŬL-mō-nĕ-rē ĔM-bō-lĭzm
pulmon: lung
-ary: pertaining to
embol: plug
-ism: condition

Blockage in an artery of the lungs caused by a mass of undissolved matter (such as a blood clot, tissue, air bubbles, or bacteria) that has traveled to the lungs from another part of the body.

PE is commonly caused by a deep vein thrombosis (DVT) that travels from the leg to the lungs (see Fig. 7-8).

The embolus lodges in the pulmonary arteries and blocks blood flow and oxygen exchange

Embolus travels through the heart and into the lungs

Embolus forms in a deep vein of the leg and travels to the heart

Figure 7-8 Pulmonary embolism.

sudden infant death syndrome (SIDS)

Completely unexpected and unexplained death of an apparently normal, healthy infant, usually less than age 12 months; also called *crib death*

The rate of SIDS has decreased more than 30% since parents have been instructed to place babies on their backs for sleeping, rather than on their stomachs.

Diseases and Conditions—cont'd

Term	Definition
tuberculosis (TB) tū-bĕr-kū-LŌ-sĭs *tubercul:* little swelling *-osis:* abnormal condition; increase (used primarily with blood cells)	Potentially fatal contagious disease spread through respiratory droplets, affecting any organ of the body but primarily the lungs and causing chest pain, hemoptysis, weight loss, fatigue, and night sweats *Many strains of TB are resistant to treatment. Therefore, patients with TB require administration of multiple antibiotics taken for several months to eradicate the organism.*

 It is time to review diseases and conditions by completing Learning Activity 7–3 on p. 222.

Diagnostic, Surgical, and Therapeutic Procedures

This section introduces diagnostic, surgical, and therapeutic procedures used to diagnose and treat respiratory disorders. Descriptions are provided, along with pronunciations and word analyses for selected terms.

Procedure	Description
Diagnostic	
Clinical	
Mantoux test măn-TŪ	TB screening test in which an injection of tuberculin purified protein derivative (PPD) is placed just beneath the surface of the skin to identify a previous exposure to TB *A positive test result is indicated by a lump that is hardened, red, and swollen at the injection site after 2 days. A positive test is followed up with a CXR to confirm whether or not the patient has active TB.*
oximetry ŏk-SĬM-ĕ-trē *ox/i:* oxygen *-metry:* act of measuring	Noninvasive method of monitoring the percentage of hemoglobin (Hb) saturated with O_2; also called *pulse oximetry* *In pulse oximetry, a small cliplike device is attached to the patient's finger or earlobe that measures the O_2 level of the blood; normal reading is 95% to 100%.*
polysomnography pŏl-ē-sŏm-NOG-ră-fē *poly:* many, much *somn/o:* sleep *-graphy:* process of recording	Test of sleep cycles and stages using electroencephalograms (EEGs), which are continuous recordings of brain waves, as well as electrical activity of muscles, eye movement, respiratory rate, blood pressure, blood O_2 saturation, heart rhythm, and sometimes direct observation of the person during sleep using a video camera (see Fig. 7-9).

Continued

Diagnostic, Surgical, and Therapeutic Procedures—cont'd

Procedure	Description

Figure 7-9 Polysomnography. (A) Patient in the hospital undergoing polysomnography, also known as a sleep study, to diagnose sleep disorders. (B) The technician checks the transmitted recordings on the monitor in an adjacent room to make sure everything is working properly.

pulmonary function tests (PFTs)
PŬL-mō-nĕ-rē
pulmon: lung
-*ary:* pertaining to

Noninvasive tests to assess the capacity of the lungs during inhalation and exhalation that measure the lung volume, capacity, rates of flow, and gas exchange (see Fig. 7-10)

PFTs help evaluate patients with SOB to diagnose respiratory disease, evaluate effectiveness of current treatment, and monitor disease progression. PFTs are commonly performed by respiratory therapists.

spirometry
spī-RŎM-ĕ-trē
spir/o: breathe
-*metry:* act of measuring

PFT that measures the volume and rate of air movement in and out of the lungs using a device called a *spirometer*

Spirometry is often one of the first tests performed to assess lung health. Spirometry results are compared with reference values based on sex, age, height, and other factors to determine the presence of lung impairment. It is also used to assess lung function before surgery.

Figure 7-10 Pulmonary function testing. The respiratory therapist instructs the patient to forcefully exhale into the tube attached to the recording device, with a tight seal with the lips to prevent air leakage. The nose clip ensures that air only flows out of the mouth so the volume of air into the lungs can be measured accurately.

Diagnostic, Surgical, and Therapeutic Procedures—cont'd

Procedure	Description

Endoscopy

bronchoscopy
brŏng-KŎS-kō-pē
bronch/o: bronchus
-scopy: visual examination

Visual examination of the bronchi using an endoscope (flexible fiberoptic or rigid) inserted through the mouth and trachea for direct viewing of structures or for projection on a monitor (see Fig. 7-11)

Attachments on the bronchoscope can help suction mucus, remove foreign bodies, collect sputum, or perform biopsy.

Figure 7-11 Bronchoscopy with direct visualization of bronchus displayed on the bedside monitor. From Ray AS, Holden VK, Sachdeva A, Nasim F: Equipment and procedural setup for interventional pulmonology procedures in the intensive care unit, *J Thorac Dis* 13(8):5331–5342, 2021. https://doi:10.21037/jtd-20-3595.

laryngoscopy
lăr-ĭn-GŎS-kō-pē
laryng/o: larynx (voice box)
-scopy: visual examination

Visual examination of the larynx to detect tumors, foreign bodies, nerve or structural injury, or other abnormalities

mediastinoscopy
mē-dē-ăs-tĭ-NŎS-kō-pē
mediastin/o: mediastinum
-scopy: visual examination

Visual examination of the mediastinal structures, including the heart, trachea, esophagus, bronchus, thymus, and lymph nodes

The mediastinoscope is inserted through a small incision made above the sternum. The attached camera projects images on a monitor. The surgeon may make additional incisions to remove nodes or perform other diagnostic or therapeutic procedures. The mediastinoscope is especially useful to locate problems related to lung cancer.

Laboratory

arterial blood gas (ABG)
ăr-TĒ-rē-ăl
arteri/o: artery
-al: pertaining to

Test that measures dissolved O_2 and CO_2 in arterial blood

ABG analysis evaluates acid-base state and how well O_2 is being carried to body tissues.

Continued

Diagnostic, Surgical, and Therapeutic Procedures—cont'd

Procedure	Description
COVID-19 tests	Laboratory tests performed to detect the presence of antibodies or the presence of the COVID-19 virus
antibody	Blood test to detect the presence of antibodies to determine past infection with the virus that causes COVID-19 *It can take 2 to 3 weeks to develop enough antibodies for detection and is important that testing not be done too soon*
nose swab	Long swab is used to take a sample from the upper nasal cavity that is then sent to a laboratory for testing (see Fig. 7-12).

Figure 7-12 Doctor in protective workwear taking nose swab test from middle-aged man wearing a face mask during the COVID-19 pandemic outbreak.

Procedure	Description
sputum culture SPŪ-tŭm	Microbial test used to identify disease-causing organisms of the lower respiratory tract, especially those that cause pneumonias
sweat test	Measurement of the amount of salt (sodium chloride) in sweat *A sweat test is used almost exclusively in children to confirm CF and is commonly considered the gold standard in diagnosis.*
throat culture	Test used to identify pathogens, especially group A streptococci *Untreated streptococcal infections may lead to serious secondary complications, including kidney and heart disease.*
Imaging	
CXR	Radiographic test that aids in identifying lung conditions such as pneumonia, lung cancer, COPD, and pneumothorax *When CXR results are inconclusive, other imaging tests are performed.*

Diagnostic, Surgical, and Therapeutic Procedures—cont'd

Procedure	Description
computed tomography (CT) kŏm-PŪ-tĕd tō-MŎG-ră-fē *tom/o:* to cut *-graphy:* process of recording	Imaging technique that rotates an x-ray emitter around the area to be evaluated and measures the intensity of transmitted rays from different angles *In a CT scan, the computer generates a detailed cross-sectional image that appears as a slice. It may detect tumor masses, bone displacement, and fluid accumulation. This technique may be used with or without a contrast medium.*
helical computed tomography (HCT) HĔL-ĭ-căl kŏm-PŪ-tĕd tō-MŎG-ră-fē *tom/o:* to cut *-graphy:* process of recording	CT scan that works by continuously rotating the x-ray source and detector around the patient while the patient is simultaneously moved through the scanner, providing a more comprehensive view of anatomical structures and abnormalities and an image that is clearer, more accurate, and completed more quickly than a traditional CT; also called *spiral CT scan* *HCT is employed in various screening programs to detect early signs of diseases like lung cancer or cardiovascular conditions. Its ability to capture detailed images of the body aids in identifying small abnormalities at an earlier stage that lead to earlier treatment and better outcomes.*
computed tomography pulmonary angiography (CTPA) kŏm-PŪ-tĕd tō-MŎG-ră-fē PŬL-mō-nĕr-ē ăn-jē-ŎG-ră-fē *tom/o:* to cut *-graphy:* process of recording *pulmon:* lung *-ary:* pertaining to *angi/o:* vessel (usually blood or lymph) *-graphy:* process of recording	Minimally invasive imaging that combines CT scanning and angiography to produce images of the pulmonary arteries *CTPA is highly sensitive and specific for the presence of PE.*
ventilation-perfusion (V-Q) scan	Nuclear test scan that evaluates airflow (ventilation) and blood flow (perfusion) in the lungs for evidence of a blood clot in the lungs; also called *V-Q lung scan*
Surgical	
pleurectomy ploor-ĔK-tō-mē *pleur:* pleura *-ectomy:* excision, removal	Excision of part of the pleura, usually the parietal pleura *Pleurectomy helps reduce pain caused by a tumor mass or prevent the recurrence of pleural effusion but is generally ineffective in the treatment of malignancy of the pleura.*

Continued

Diagnostic, Surgical, and Therapeutic Procedures—cont'd

Procedure	Description
pneumonectomy nū-mŏn-ĔK-tō-mē *pneumon:* air; lung *-ectomy:* excision, removal	Excision of a lung or a portion of the lung, commonly for treatment of cancer (see Fig. 7-13). Figure 7-13 Types of pneumonectomy.
septoplasty sĕp-tō-PLĂS-tē *sept/o:* septum *-plasty:* surgical repair	Surgical repair of a deviated nasal septum that is usually performed when the septum is encroaching on the breathing passages or nasal structures *Common complications of a deviated septum include interference with breathing and a predisposition to sinus infections.*
thoracentesis thō-ră-sĕn-TĒ-sĭs	Surgical puncture and drainage of the pleural cavity; also called *pleurocentesis* or *thoracocentesis* *Thoracentesis as a diagnostic procedure helps determine the nature and cause of an effusion; as a therapeutic procedure, it relieves the discomfort caused by the effusion (see Fig. 7-14).*

Diagnostic, Surgical, and Therapeutic Procedures—cont'd

Procedure	Description

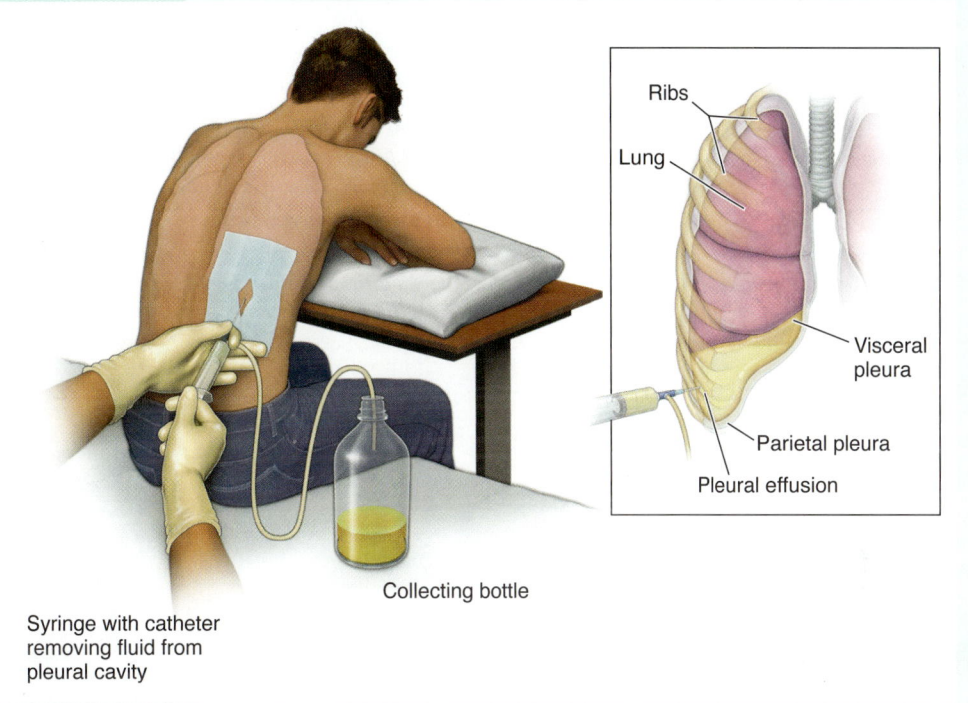

Syringe with catheter removing fluid from pleural cavity

Collecting bottle

Ribs
Lung
Visceral pleura
Parietal pleura
Pleural effusion

Figure 7-14 Thoracentesis.

tracheostomy
trā-kē-ŎS-tō-mē
trache/o: trachea
-stomy: forming an opening (mouth)

Surgical procedure in which an opening is made in the neck and into the trachea into which a breathing tube may be inserted (see Fig. 7-15).

A

Epiglottis
Trachea
Thyroid gland
Tracheostomy tube
Expanding balloon

B

Figure 7-15 Tracheostomy. (A) Lateral view with tracheostomy tube in place. (B) Frontal view.

Continued

Diagnostic, Surgical, and Therapeutic Procedures—cont'd

Procedure	Description
Therapeutic	

aerosol therapy
ĂR-ō-sŏl THĔR-ă-pē

Lung treatment using various techniques to deliver medication in mist form directly to the lungs or air passageways

Techniques include nebulizer mist treatments (NMTs), metered-dose inhalers (MDIs), and dry powder inhalers (DPIs). Nebulizers change liquid medications into droplets to be inhaled through a mouthpiece (see Fig. 7-16). MDIs deliver a specific amount when activated. Children and the elderly can use a spacer to synchronize inhalation with medication release (see Fig. 7-17). DPIs are activated by a quick inhalation by the user.

Figure 7-16 Nebulizer.

Metered-dose inhaler

Spacer

Metered-dose inhaler without spacer

Figure 7-17 Metered-dose inhaler.

Diagnostic, Surgical, and Therapeutic Procedures—cont'd

Procedure	Description
antral lavage ĂN-trăl lă-VĂZH	Washing or irrigating of the paranasal sinuses to remove mucopurulent material in an immunosuppressed patient or one with known sinusitis that has failed to respond to medical management
continuous positive airway pressure (CPAP)	Medical device used to treat sleep apnea that delivers a continuous stream of air at a set pressure level to keep the airway open during sleep and ensure a consistent flow of oxygen to the lungs (see Fig. 7-18). Figure 7-18 Continuous positive airway pressure (CPAP) with a nasal mask connected to a pump, where pressure level is set, to keep the airway open during sleep and prevent periods of apnea, snoring, and choking.
endotracheal intubation ĕn-dŏ-TRĀ-kē-ăl ĭn-tū-BĀ-shŭn *endo-:* in, within *trache:* trachea *-al:* pertaining to	Procedure in which a plastic tube is inserted into the trachea to maintain an open airway *Endotracheal intubation is commonly performed before surgery when the patient is first placed under sedation or in emergency situations to facilitate ventilation if necessary (see Fig. 7-19).* Figure 7-19 Endotracheal intubation.

Continued

Diagnostic, Surgical, and Therapeutic Procedures—cont'd

Procedure	Description
postural drainage PŎS-tū-răl	Method of positioning a patient so that gravity aids in the drainage of secretions from the bronchi and lobes of the lungs to make breathing easier
supplemental oxygen therapy	Provides additional O_2 to patients whose blood levels are below normal to help increase the O_2 in the bloodstream and improve delivery throughout the tissues and organs of the body; several types of methods are available and depend on the specific medical condition of the patient
nasal cannula	Delivers O_2 directly into the nose through small prongs inserted into each nostril that are attached by a loose tube attached to an oxygen source (see Fig. 7-20A)
oxygen masks	Delivers higher concentration of O_2 through a mask that covers the mouth and nose (see Fig. 7-20B)

Figure 7-20 Supplemental oxygen therapy. (A) Nasal cannula. (B) Oxygen mask.

Diagnostic, Surgical, and Therapeutic Procedures—cont'd

Procedure	Description
hyperbaric chamber	Delivers pure O_2 at a higher than normal atmospheric pressure in a sealed chamber that allows the bloodstream to absorb more O_2 *Hyperbaric O_2 therapy (HBOT) is used to promote wound healing and fight infection, for carbon monoxide poisoning, and to treat decompression sickness (DCS), which occurs when nitrogen dissolved in the body under high pressure forms bubbles, "the bends," after rapid ascent from deep depths of underwater diving (see Fig. 7-21)*

Figure 7-21 Patient receiving oxygen therapy in a hyperbaric chamber.

Pharmacology

Several classes of drugs are prescribed to treat pulmonary disorders. These include antibiotics, which are used to treat respiratory infections, and bronchodilators, which are especially effective in treating COPD and exercise-induced asthma (see Table 7-2). Steroidal and nonsteroidal anti-inflammatory drugs are important in the control and management of many pulmonary disorders.

TABLE 7-2 Drugs Used to Treat Respiratory Disorders

This table lists common drug classifications used to treat respiratory disorders, their therapeutic actions, and selected generic and trade names.

Classification	Therapeutic Action	Generic and Trade Names
antibiotics ăn-tĭ-bī-ĂW-tĭks	Destroy or inhibit the growth of bacteria by disrupting their membranes or one or more of their metabolic processes	**azithromycin** ā-ZĬTH-rō-mī-sĭn *Zithromax* **amoxicillin** ă-MŎX-ĭ-cĭl-ĭn **clavulanate** clă-vū-LĂN-āt *Augmentin*

(continued)

TABLE 7-2 Drugs Used to Treat Respiratory Disorders—cont'd

Classification	Therapeutic Action	Generic and Trade Names
antihistamines ăn-tĭ-HĬS-tă-mēnz	Block histamines from binding with histamine receptor sites in tissues *Histamines cause sneezing, runny nose, itchiness, and rashes. Antihistamines are commonly combined with decongestants, antitussives, or analgesics for cold and flu symptom relief.*	**fexofenadine** fĕk-sō-FĔN-ă-dēn *Allegra* **loratadine** lor-ĂH-tă-dēn *Claritin*
antituberculars ăn-tĭ-too-BĔR-kū-lărs	Used to treat tuberculosis, an infectious disease caused by *mycobacterium tuberculosis*; infection mainly affects the lungs but can also affect other organs *Several antituberculars are used in combination for effective treatment.*	**rifampin** rĭ-FĂM-pĭn *Rifadin, Rimactane* **isoniazid** ī-sĭ-NĪ- ă-zĭd *Niazid*
antitussives ăn-tĭ-T ŬS-ĭvz	Relieve or suppress coughing by blocking the cough reflex in the medulla of the brain *Antitussives alleviate nonproductive dry coughs and should not be used with productive coughs.*	**hydrocodone*** hī-drō-KŌ-dōn **dextromethorphan** dĕk-strō-mĕth-OR-făn *Delsym*
bronchodilators brŏng-kō-DĪ-lā-torz	Stimulate bronchial muscles to relax, thereby expanding air passages, resulting in increased airflow *Bronchodilators help treat chronic symptoms and prevent acute attacks in respiratory diseases, such as asthma and COPD, and may be delivered by an inhaler, orally, or intravenously. Because bronchodilators are commonly used in conjunction with corticosteroids, combination products are available.*	**albuterol** ăl-BŪ-tĕr-ŏl *Proventil, Ventolin* **salmeterol** săl-MĔT-ĕr-ŏl *Serevent* **budesonide/formoterol** bū-DĔS-ō-nīd for-MŌ-tĕr-ŏl *Symbicort*
corticosteroids kor-tĭ-kō-STĔR-oyds	Act on the immune system by blocking production of substances that trigger allergic and inflammatory actions *Corticosteroids are available as nasal sprays, in metered-dose inhalers (inhaled steroids), and in oral forms (pills or syrups) to treat chronic lung conditions, such as asthma and COPD.*	**beclomethasone** bĕ-klō-MĔTH-ă-sōn *Qvar (metered-dose inhaler)* **mometasone** mō-MĔT-ă-sōn *Nasonex (nasal spray)*
decongestants dē-kŏn-JĔST-ănts	Constrict blood vessels of nasal passages and limit blood flow, which causes swollen tissues to shrink so that air can pass more freely through the passageways *Decongestants are commonly prescribed for allergies and colds and are usually combined with antihistamines in cold remedies. They can be administered orally or topically as nasal sprays and nasal drops.*	**oxymetazoline** ŏks-ē-mĕt-ĂZ-ō-lēn *Afrin (available for nasal instillation only)* **pseudoephedrine** soo-dō-ĕ-FĔD-rĭn *Sudafed (oral product)*
expectorants ĕk-SPĔK-tō-rănts	Liquefy respiratory secretions so that they are more easily dislodged during coughing episodes *Expectorants are prescribed for productive coughs.*	**guaifenesin** gwī-FĔN-ĕ-sĭn *Robitussin, Mucinex*

*Available only in generic form

Abbreviations

This section introduces respiratory-related abbreviations and their meanings.

Abbreviation	Meaning	Abbreviation	Meaning
ABG	arterial blood gas(es)	**HMD**	hyaline membrane disease
AIDS	acquired immunodeficiency syndrome	**MDI**	metered-dose inhaler
ARDS	acute respiratory distress syndrome	**NMT**	nebulized mist treatment
CF	cystic fibrosis	**NRDS**	neonatal respiratory distress syndrome
CO$_2$	carbon dioxide	**NSCLC**	nonsmall cell lung cancer
COPD	chronic obstructive pulmonary disease	**O$_2$**	oxygen
COVID-19	coronavirus disease 2019	**OSA**	obstructive sleep apnea
CPAP	continuous positive airway pressure	**PCO$_2$**	partial pressure of carbon dioxide
CT	computed tomography	**PCP**	*Pneumocystis* pneumonia; primary care physician
CTPA	computed tomography pulmonary angiography	**PE**	physical examination; pulmonary embolism; pressure-equalizing (tube)
CXR	chest x-ray, chest radiograph	**PFT**	pulmonary function test
DCS	decompression sickness	**pH**	degree of acidity or alkalinity
DPI	dry powder inhaler	**PO$_2$**	partial pressure of oxygen
DPT	diphtheria, pertussis, tetanus	**PPD**	purified protein derivative
DVT	deep vein thrombosis	**SCLC**	small cell lung cancer
EEG	electroencephalogram	**SIDS**	sudden infant death syndrome
Hb, Hgb	hemoglobin	**SOB**	shortness of breath
HBOT	hyperbaric oxygen therapy	**TB**	tuberculosis
HCT	helical computed tomography	**URI**	upper respiratory infection

It is time to review procedures, pharmacology, and abbreviations by completing Learning Activity 7-4.

LEARNING ACTIVITIES

The activities that follow provide a review of the respiratory system terms introduced in this chapter. Complete each activity and review your answers to evaluate your understanding of the chapter.

Medical Language Lab
Turning terminology into language

Visit the Medical Language Laboratory at medicallanguagelab.com. Use it to enhance your study and reinforcement of this chapter with the flash card activity. We recommend that you complete the flash card activity before starting Learning Activities 7-1 and 7-2.

Learning Activity 7-1
Medical Word Elements

Use the listed elements to build medical words. You may use these elements more than once.

Combining Forms

bronch/o	pneumon/o
bronchi/o	sept/o
cyan/o	sinus/o
ox/o	steth/o
pleur/o	tonsill/o

Suffixes

-capnia	-osmia
-centesis	-phonia
-ectasis	-plasty
-ectomy	-pnea
-ia	-scope
-osis	-tomy

Prefixes

an-
brady-
dys-
eu-
hyper-
hyp-

1. surgical puncture of the pleura _____

2. instrument for examining the bronchus _____

3. excision of the tonsils _____

4. slow breathing _____

5. difficult voice _____

6. abnormal condition of blue(ness) _____

7. condition of decrease of oxygen _____

8. absence of the sense of smell _____

9. surgical repair of the septum _____

10. incision of the sinus _____

11. excessive carbon dioxide _____

12. good, normal breathing _____

13. expansion of a bronchi _____

14. instrument to examine the sounds in the chest _____

15. condition of the lungs _____

✓ *Check your answers in Appendix A. Review any material that you did not answer correctly.*

Correct Answers _____ X 6.67 = _____ % Score

Learning Activity 7-2
Building Medical Words

Use *rhin/o* (nose) to build words that mean:

1. discharge from the nose _____
2. inflammation of (mucous membranes of) the nose _____

Use *laryng/o* (larynx [voice box]) to build words that mean:

3. visual examination of the larynx _____
4. inflammation of the larynx _____
5. stricture or narrowing of the larynx _____

Use *bronch/o* or *bronchi/o* (bronchus) to build words that mean:

6. dilation or expansion of the bronchus _____
7. pertaining to origin in the bronchi _____
8. involuntary contraction of the bronchus _____

Use *pneumon/o* or *pneum/o* (air; lung) to build words that mean:

9. air in the chest (pleural space) _____
10. abnormal condition of dust in the lung _____

Use *pulmon/o* (lung) to build words that mean:

11. specialist in lung (diseases) _____
12. pertaining to the bronchi and lung _____

Use *-pnea* (breathing) to build words that mean:

13. difficult breathing _____
14. slow breathing _____
15. rapid breathing _____
16. absence of breathing _____

Build surgical words that mean:

17. surgical procedure to create an opening (through the neck) into the trachea _____
18. surgical puncture of the chest _____
19. removal of a lobe (in the lung) _____
20. repair of a deviated septum _____

Check your answers in Appendix A. Review material that you did not answer correctly.

Correct Answers _____ X 5 = _____ % Score

Learning Activity 7-3
Diseases and Conditions

Match the terms with the definitions in the numbered list.

atelectasis	*cystic fibrosis*	*hemoptysis*	*pleurisy*
consolidation	*deviated septum*	*hypoxemia*	*pulmonary edema*
COPD	*emphysema*	*hypoxia*	*pulmonary embolism*
Coryza	*empyema*	*OSA*	*rhonchus*
COVID-19	*epistaxis*	*pertussis*	*tuberculosis*

1. collapsed or airless lung _____

2. pus in the pleural cavity _____

3. abnormal breath sound commonly resembling snoring _____

4. deficiency of oxygen (in the tissues) _____

5. recent virus in 2019 causing a public health emergency of international concern that is highly contagious and mainly spreads through respiratory droplets _____

6. group of respiratory disorders characterized by asthma, chronic bronchitis, and emphysema _____

7. deficiency of oxygen in atrial blood _____

8. genetic disease causing mucus to become unusually thick and sticky _____

9. acute, contagious viral disorder of the respiratory tract _____

10. disease characterized by a decrease in alveolar elasticity _____

11. spitting of blood _____

12. nosebleed; nasal hemorrhage _____

13. excessive fluid in the lungs that induces cough and dyspnea _____

14. sudden blockage of a pulmonary artery caused by a blood clot that has traveled from another part of the body _____

15. displacement of the cartilage dividing the nostrils _____

16. acute inflammation of the membranes of the nose; also called *rhinitis* _____

17. sleep apnea caused by an upper airway blockage that prevents an adequate flow of air to the lungs _____

18. inflammation of the pleural membrane _____

19. loss of sponginess of lungs due to engorgement _____

20. whooping cough _____

Check your answers in Appendix A. Review material that you did not answer correctly.

Correct Answers _____ X 5 = _____ % Score

Learning Activity 7-4

Procedures, Pharmacology, and Abbreviations

Match the terms with the definitions in the numbered list.

ABGs	CPAP	Mantoux test	septoplasty
aerosol therapy	CXR	oximetry	sputum culture
antihistamine	decongestant	pneumonectomy	sweat test
antitussive	expectorant	polysomnography	thoracentesis
antral lavage	HBOT	pulmonary function test	throat culture

1. microbial test used to identify disease-causing organisms of the lower respiratory tract _____

2. test of sleep cycles and stages _____

3. imaging procedure to evaluate the lungs _____

4. washing or irrigating sinuses _____

5. relieves sneezing, runny nose, itchiness, and rashes _____

6. relieves or suppresses coughing _____

7. used primarily in children to confirm cystic fibrosis _____

8. noninvasive test used to monitor the percentage of hemoglobin saturated with oxygen _____

9. surgical puncture and drainage of the pleural cavity _____

10. inhalation of medication directly into the respiratory system via a nebulizer _____

11. decreases mucous membrane swelling by constricting blood vessels _____

12. intradermal test to determine tuberculin sensitivity _____

13. laboratory tests to assess gases and pH of arterial blood _____

14. reduces the viscosity of sputum to facilitate productive coughing _____

15. used to identify pathogens, especially group A streptococci _____

16. multiple tests used to determine the ability of lungs and capillary membranes to exchange oxygen _____

17. promotes wound healing and fights infection by delivering pure oxygen at a higher than normal atmospheric pressure in a sealed chamber _____

18. procedure to correct a deviated nasal septum _____

19. excision of the entire lung _____

20. medical device used to treat sleep apnea _____

✓ *Check your answers in Appendix A. Review any material that you did not answer correctly.*

Correct Answers _____ X 5 = _____ % Score

DOCUMENTING HEALTH-CARE ACTIVITIES

This section provides practical application activities in the form of exercises to help develop skills in documenting patient care. First, read the medical report. Then complete the activities and exercises that follow.

Documenting Health-Care Activity 7-1
SOAP Note: Respiratory Evaluation

Emergency Department Record

Date: February 1, 20xx   Time Registered: 1345 hours
Patient: Flowers, Richard   Physician: Samara Batichara, MD
Chief Complaint: SOB

S: This 49-year-old married, Caucasian male presents with chief complaint of shortness of breath over the past few days. He denies having a fever, cough, or sputum production. Patient was a heavy smoker and states that he quit smoking for a short time but now smokes 3–4 cigarettes a day. He has a history of difficult breathing, hypertension, COPD, and peripheral vascular disease. The patient underwent triple bypass surgery in 19xx.

O: T: 98.9 F. BP: 180/90. Pulse: 80 and regular. R: 20 and shallow. Physical examination indicates scattered bilateral wheezes and rhonchi heard anteriorly and posteriorly. Compared with a portable chest film taken 22 months earlier, the current study most likely indicates interstitial vascular congestion. Some superimposed inflammatory change cannot be excluded. There may also be some pleural reactive change.

A: 1. Acute exacerbation of chronic obstructive pulmonary disease.
    2. Heart failure.
    3. Hypertension.
    4. Peripheral vascular disease.

P: Admit to hospital. Continue the following medication: Vytorin 10/20 mg daily; Toprol-XL 50 mg daily; Azmacort 2 puffs three times a day; Proventil 2 puffs every 6 hours.

Samara Batichara, MD
Samara Batichara, MD

SB:icc

D: 2/1/20xx; T: 2/1/20xx

Terminology

The terms listed in the table that follows are taken from *SOAP Note: Respiratory Evaluation*. Use a medical dictionary such as *Taber's Cyclopedic Medical Dictionary*, the appendices of this book, or other resources to define each term. Then review the pronunciation for each term and practice by reading the medical record aloud.

Term	Definition
anteriorly ăn-TĒR-ē-or-lē	
bilateral bī-LĂT-ĕr-ăl	
COPD	
exacerbation ĕks-ăs-ĕr-BĀ-shŭn	
heart failure	
Hx	
hypertension hī-pĕr-TĔN-shŭn	
interstitial ĭn-tĕr-STĬSH-ăl	
peripheral vascular disease pĕr-ĬF-ĕr-ăl VĂS-kū-lăr	
pleural PLOO-răl	
posteriorly pŏs-TĒR-ē-or-lē	
rhonchi RŎNG-kī	
SOB	
wheezes HWĒZ-ĕz	

Visit the Medical Terminology Systems online resource center at FADavis.com to practice pronunciation and reinforce the meanings of the terms in this medical report.

Critical Thinking

Review *SOAP Note: Respiratory Evaluation* to answer the questions.

1. What symptom caused the patient to seek medical help?

2. What was the patient's previous history?

3. What were the abnormal findings of the physical examination?

4. What changes were noted from the previous film?

5. What are the present assessments?

6. What new diagnosis was made that did not appear in the previous medical history?

SOAP Note: Chronic Interstitial Lung Disease

O'Malley, Robert   09/01/20xx

S: Patient is an 84-year-old male with chief complaint of dyspnea with activity and pedal edema. He carries the dx cardiomyopathy, renal insufficiency, COPD, and pulmonary fibrosis. He also has peripheral neuropathy, which has improved with amitriptyline therapy.

O: BP: 140/70. Pulse: 76. Neck is supple without thyromegaly or adenopathy. Mild kyphosis without scoliosis is present. Auscultation of the chest reveals basilar crackles without wheezing or rhonchi. Cardiac examination shows trace edema without clubbing or murmur. Abdomen is soft and nontender. ABGs on room air demonstrate a PO_2 of 55, PCO_2 of 45, and pH of 7.42.

A: Chronic interstitial lung disease, likely a combination of pulmonary fibrosis and heart failure. We do believe he would benefit from further diuresis, which was implemented by Dr. Lu. Should there continue to be concerns about his volume status or lack of response to Lasix therapy, then he might benefit from right heart catheterization.

P: Supplemental oxygen to be continued. We plan no change in his pulmonary medication at this time and will see him in return visit in 4 months. He has been told to contact us should he worsen in the interim.

Samara Batichara, MD
Samara Batichara, MD

SB:icc

Terminology

The terms listed in the table that follows are taken from *SOAP Note: Chronic Interstitial Lung Disease.* Use a medical dictionary such as *Taber's Cyclopedic Medical Dictionary,* the appendices of this book, or other resources to define each term. Then review the pronunciations for each term and practice by reading the medical record aloud.

Term	Definition
adenopathy ăd-ĕ-NŎP-ă-thē	
amitriptyline ă-mĭ-TRĬP-tĭ-lēn	
basilar crackles BĂS-ĭ-lăr KRĂK-ĕlz	
cardiomyopathy kăr-dē-ō-mī-ŎP-ă-thē	
diuresis dī-ū-RĒ-sĭs	
fibrosis fī-BRŌ-sĭs	
interstitial ĭn-tĕr-STĬSH-ăl	
kyphosis kī-FŌ-sĭs	
Lasix LĀ-sĭks	
neuropathy nū-RŎP-ă-thē	
pedal edema PĔD-ăl ĕ-DĒ-mă	
pulmonary fibrosis PŬL-mō-nĕ-rē fī-BRŌ-sĭs	
renal insufficiency RĒ-năl ĭn-sŭ-FĬSH-ĕn-sē	
scoliosis skō-lē-Ō-sĭs	

Visit the Medical Terminology Systems online resource center at FADavis. com to practice pronunciation and reinforce the meanings of the terms in this medical report.

Critical Thinking

Review *SOAP Note: Chronic Interstitial Lung Disease* to answer the following questions.

1. When did the patient notice dyspnea?

2. Other than the respiratory system, what other body systems are identified in the history of present illness?

3. What were the findings regarding the neck?

4. What abnormal lung sounds were heard upon auscultation?

5. What appears to be the likely cause of the chronic interstitial lung disease?

6. What did the cardiac examination reveal?

Constructing Chart Notes

To construct chart notes, replace the italicized and boldfaced terms in each of the two case studies with one of the listed medical terms.

antitussive	dyspnea	septoplasty
cephalodynia	myalgia	sinusitis
coryza	pharyngitis	T&A
deviated nasal septum		

Billy P., a 2-year-old boy, was referred to the ENT clinic by his pediatrician. His mother states that when he is sleeping, Billy experiences (1) *difficult breathing*, starts gasping for air, and then wakes up crying. This is especially true when he has a (2) *head cold*. The examination of his nasal passages shows a (3) *septum displaced to one side*, causing impaired airflow through the nostrils. His tonsils and adenoids are also enlarged, making breathing even more difficult. The physician schedules a (4) *surgical repair of the septum* and (5) *removal of the tonsils and adenoids.*

1. _____
2. _____
3. _____
4. _____
5. _____

Betty L. presents to the student health services on campus. She complains of (6) *muscle pain* and (7) *headache*. Betty states that she was up the entire night with a dry, hacking cough. Upon examination, the physician confirms that Betty has the flu and states that her headache was probably a result of (8) *inflamed sinuses*. He further notes an (9) *inflammation of the throat* without evidence of strep infection. Betty is advised to drink clear fluids and take Tylenol, as needed, to reduce fever and general discomfort. The physician also prescribes Hycodan, a (10) *medication to control coughing*.

6. _____
7. _____
8. _____
9. _____
10. _____

✓ *Check your answers in Appendix A. Review any material that you did not answer correctly.*

Correct Answers _____ X 10 = _____ % Score

Cardiovascular System

Chapter Outline

Objectives

Upon completion of this chapter, you will be able to:

- Locate and describe the structures of the cardiovascular system.
- Describe the functional relationship between the cardiovascular system and other body systems.
- Pronounce, spell, and build words related to the cardiovascular system.
- Describe diseases, conditions, and procedures related to the cardiovascular system.
- Explain pharmacology related to the treatment of cardiovascular disorders.
- Demonstrate your knowledge of this chapter by completing the learning and documenting health-care activities.

Anatomy and Physiology

The cardiovascular (CV) system is composed of the heart and blood vessels. The heart is a hollow, muscular organ lying in the mediastinum, the center of the thoracic cavity between the lungs. The pumping action of the heart propels blood that contains oxygen (O_2), nutrients, and other vital products from the heart to body cells through a vast network of blood vessels called **arteries**. Arteries branch into smaller vessels until they become microscopic vessels called **capillaries**. At the capillary level, an exchange of products occurs between body cells and blood. Capillaries merge to form larger blood vessels called **venules**, which then combine to form **veins**, the vessels that return blood to the heart to begin the cycle again. Millions of body cells rely on the CV system for their survival. When it fails, life at the cellular level is not possible and, ultimately, death occurs.

Anatomy and Physiology Key Terms

This section introduces important terms, along with their definitions and pronunciations. The key terms are highlighted in color in the Anatomy and Physiology section. Word analyses for selected terms are also provided. Pronounce the term and place a check mark in the box after you do so.

Term	Definition
leaflets ☐	Flat, leaf-shaped structures that comprise the valves of the heart and prevent the backflow of blood
lumen ☐ LŪ-mĕn	Tubular space or channel within an organ or structure of the body; space within an artery, vein, intestine, or tube
regurgitation ☐ rē-gŭr-jĭ-TĀ-shŭn	Backflow or ejecting of contents through an opening
sphincters ☐ SFĬNGK-tĕr	Circular muscles found in a tubular structure or hollow organ that constrict or dilate to regulate passage of substances through its opening
vasoconstriction ☐ văs-ō-kŏn-STRĬK-shŭn	Narrowing of the lumen of a blood vessel that limits blood flow, usually as a result of diseases, medications, or physiological processes
vasodilation ☐ văs-ō-dī-LĀ-shŭn	Widening or relaxation of the lumen of a blood vessel associated with an increased blood flow that occurs in response to various physiological factors or medications
viscosity ☐ vĭs-KŎS-ĭ-tē	Thickness or a measure of how resistant a liquid is to flowing *A solution that has a high viscosity is relatively thick and flows slowly.*

Pronunciation Help	Long Sound	ā — rate	ē — rebirth	ī — isle	ō — over	ū — unite
	Short Sound	ă — apple	ĕ — ever	ĭ — it	ŏ — not	ŭ — cut

Vascular System

Three major types of vessels—(1) **artery**, (2) **capillary**, and (3) **vein**—carry blood throughout the body (see Fig. 8-1). Each type of vessel differs in structure, depending on its function.

Arteries

Arteries carry blood from the heart to all cells of the body. Because the pumping action of the heart propels blood through the arteries, the walls of the arteries must be strong and flexible enough to withstand the surge of blood that results from each contraction.

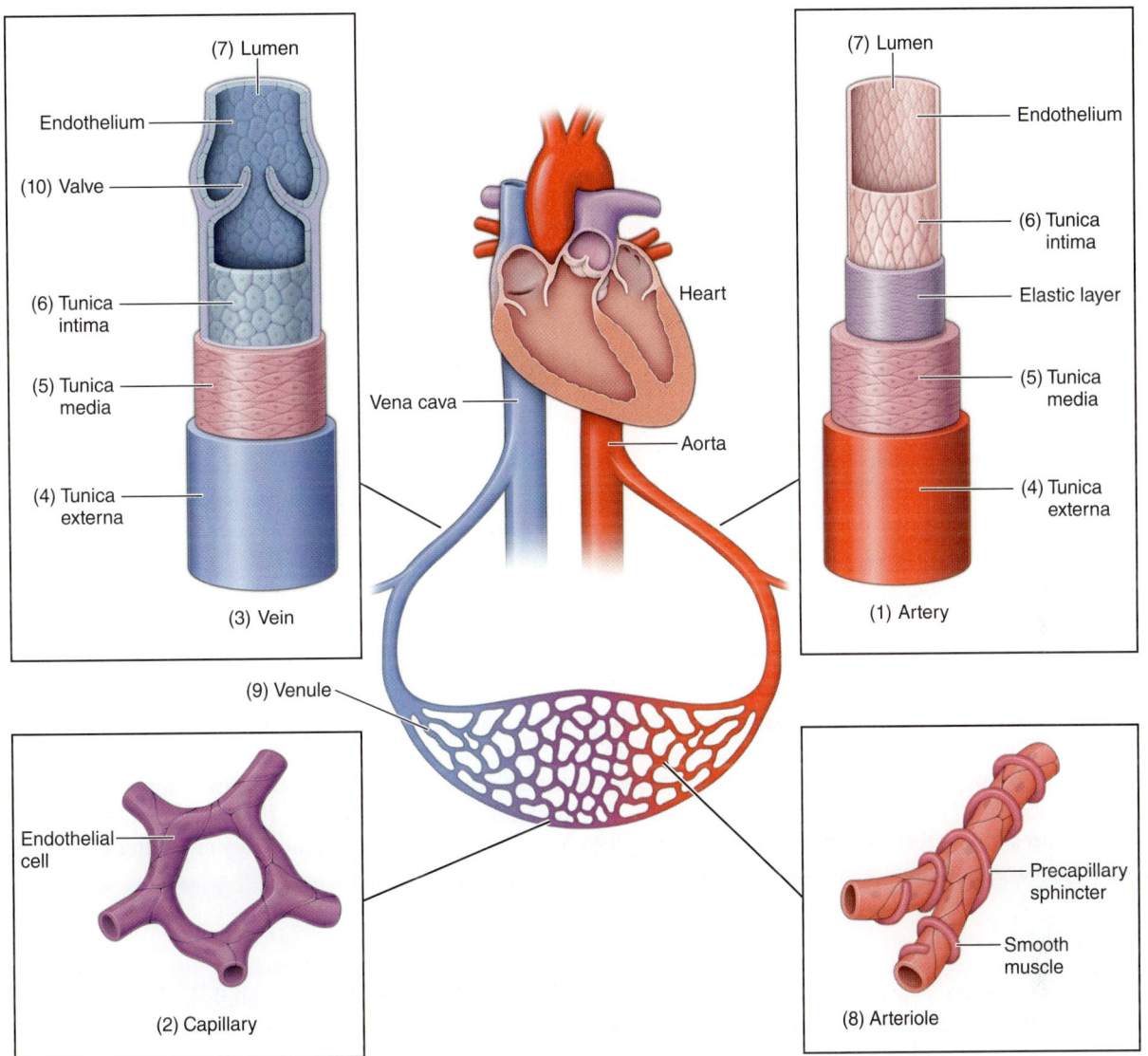

Figure 8-1 Vascular structures.

The walls of large arteries have three layers to provide toughness and elasticity. The (4) **tunica externa** is the outer coat, composed of connective tissue that provides strength and flexibility. The (5) **tunica media** is the middle layer, composed of smooth muscle. Depending on the needs of the body, this muscle can alter the size of the (7) **lumen** of the vessel. When it contracts, the tunica media causes **vasoconstriction**, resulting in decreased blood flow. When it relaxes, it causes **vasodilation**, resulting in increased blood flow. The (6) **tunica intima** is the thin, inner lining of the lumen of the vessel, composed of endothelial cells that provide a smooth surface on the inside of the vessel.

The surge of blood felt in the arteries when blood is pumped from the heart is referred to as a **pulse**. Because of the pressure against arterial walls associated with the pumping action of the heart, a cut or severed artery may lead to profuse bleeding.

Arterial blood (except for that found in the pulmonary artery) contains a high concentration of **oxygen** (O_2) and appears bright red in color. Oxygenated blood travels to smaller arteries called (8) **arterioles,** and finally to the smallest vessels, the capillaries.

Capillaries

Capillaries are microscopic vessels that join the arterial system with the venous system. These are the smallest, most numerous blood vessels in the body. Because capillary walls are composed of only a single layer of endothelial cells, they are very thin, enabling the exchange of water, respiratory gases, macromolecules, metabolites, and wastes between the blood and the cells adjacent to the capillary bed. The vast number of capillaries branching from arterioles causes blood to flow very slowly, providing sufficient time for exchange of essential substances.

Blood flow through the capillary networks is slow and intermittent, rather than steady, and is regulated by the precapillary **sphincters**. When tissues require more blood, these sphincters open; when less blood is required, they close. Once the exchange of products is complete, blood enters the venous system for its return to the heart.

Veins

Veins return deoxygenated blood from the body's tissues back to the heart. They are formed from smaller vessels called (9) **venules** that develop from the union of capillaries. Compared to arteries, veins have thinner walls and lower pressure, so they use other methods to return blood to the heart, including the following:

- skeletal muscle contraction
- gravity
- respiratory activity
- one way valves

The (10) **valves** are small structures within veins that prevent the backflow of blood. As blood moves toward the heart, these valves open, allowing blood to flow through. Once the blood has passed, the valves close to prevent backflow. This valve mechanism is especially important in the lower extremities where it assists in overcoming the challenge of gravity and helps maintain efficient blood circulation back to the heart. Large veins, especially in the abdomen, contain smooth muscle that provides peristalsis and helps propel blood toward the heart.

Blood carried in veins (except for the blood in the pulmonary veins) contains a low concentration of O_2 and a correspondingly high concentration of carbon dioxide (CO_2). This blood takes on a characteristic purple color and is said to be deoxygenated. It continuously circulates from the heart to the lungs so that CO_2 can be exchanged for O_2.

Heart

The **heart** is a muscular pump that propels blood to the entire body through a closed vascular network. It allows a dual circulatory system: pulmonary circulation provided by the right side of the heart and systemic circulation provided by the left side of the heart. **Pulmonary circulation** is the pathway where the right side of the heart pumps deoxygenated blood from the body to the lungs for oxygenation and release of carbon dioxide, then returns oxygenated blood to the left side of the heart to be pumped to the rest of the body through systemic circulation. **Systemic circulation** delivers the oxygen rich blood from the left side of the heart to body tissues and organs, and returns deoxygenated blood back to the right side of the heart. Both systemic and pulmonary circulatory activities occur simultaneously (see Fig. 8-2).

Pericardial Membranes and Heart Wall

The heart is enclosed in a protective two-layer sac called the **pericardium**. The outermost layer, the **fibrous pericardium**, functions as structural support. The inner layer, the **serous pericardium**, is further subdivided into the parietal layer and visceral layer (also known as the epicardium). Between these two layers is a small fluid-filled space called the **pericardial cavity** that contains pericardial fluid. This fluid allows the heart to beat and move smoothly within the pericardial sac by reducing friction between the heart and surrounding structures (see Fig. 8-3).

The heart wall is composed of three distinct layers. The **epicardium** covers the heart surface, making it the outermost layer of the heart wall. The **myocardium** is the middle and thickest layer, composed of muscle tissue, responsible for the contractions that pump blood throughout the body. The innermost layer, the **endocardium**, is a serous membrane that lines the four chambers of the heart and its valves and is continuous with the endothelium of the arteries and veins (see Fig. 8-3).

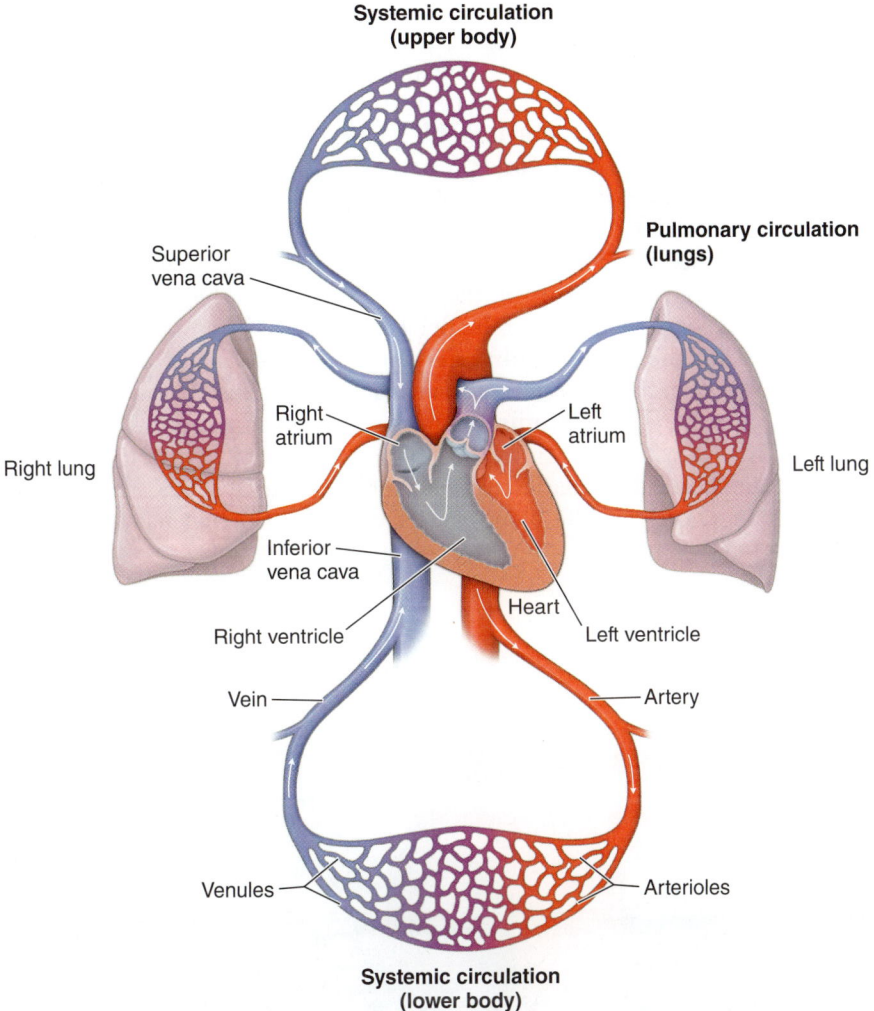

Figure 8-2 Systemic and pulmonary circulation.

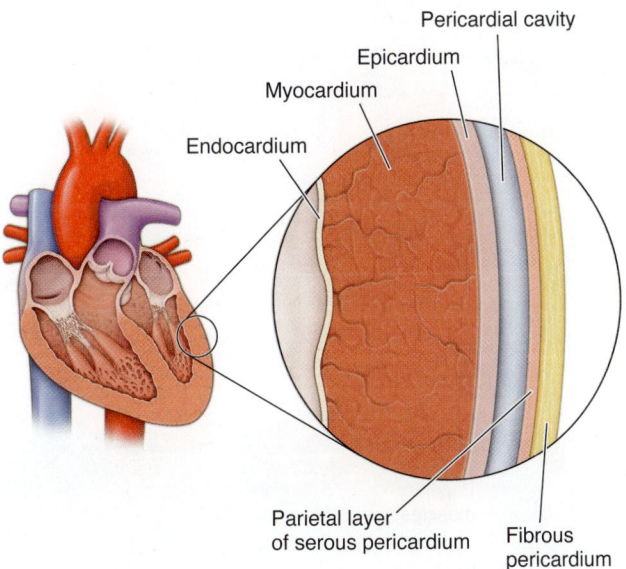

Figure 8-3 Pericardial membrane and heart wall

Cardiac Circulation

The heart is divided into four chambers (see Fig. 8-4, see below). The two upper chambers, the (1) **right atrium (RA)** and (2) **left atrium (LA)**, collect blood. The two lower chambers, the (3) **right ventricle (RV)** and (4) **left ventricle (LV)**, pump blood from the heart. The RV pumps deoxygenated blood to the lungs (**pulmonary circulation**) for oxygenation, and the LV pumps oxygenated blood to the entire body (**systemic circulation**).

Deoxygenated blood from the body returns to the RA by way of two large veins: the (5) **superior vena cava**, which collects and carries blood from the upper body, and the (6) **inferior vena cava**, which collects and carries blood from the lower body. From the RA, blood passes through the (7) **tricuspid valve**, consisting of three **leaflets**, to the RV. When the heart contracts, blood leaves the RV by way of the (8) **left pulmonary artery** and (9) **right pulmonary artery** and travels to the lungs. During contraction of the ventricle, the tricuspid valve closes to prevent a backflow of blood to the RA. The (10) **pulmonic valve** (or **pulmonary semilunar valve**) prevents **regurgitation** of blood into the RV from the pulmonary artery. In the lungs, the pulmonary artery branches into millions of capillaries, each lying close to an alveolus. Here, in the process of pulmonary gas exchange, CO_2 in the blood is exchanged for O_2 that has been drawn into the lungs during inhalation.

Figure 8-4 Internal structures of the heart, with red arrows designating oxygen-rich blood flow and blue arrows designating oxygen-poor blood flow.

Through the convergence of smaller vessels within the lungs, four pulmonary veins are formed, two (11) **right pulmonary veins** and two (12) **left pulmonary veins**. These vessels carry oxygenated blood back to the heart via the LA. Blood then passes to the LV through the (13) **mitral (bicuspid) valve**, a structure consisting of two leaflets. Upon contraction of the ventricles, the oxygenated blood leaves the heart through the largest artery of the body, the (14) **aorta**. The aorta contains the (15) **aortic semilunar valve (aortic valve)**, which permits blood to flow in only one direction—from the LV to the aorta. The aorta branches into many smaller arteries that carry blood to all parts of the body, contributing to systemic circulation.

Coronary Arteries

It is important to understand that the myocardium cannot use the blood that passes through the chambers of the heart as a source of O_2 and nutrients. Instead, an arterial system composed of the coronary arteries branches from the aorta and provides the myocardium with its own blood supply (see Fig. 8-5). The artery vascularizing the right side of the heart is the (1) **right coronary artery**. The artery vascularizing the left side of the heart is the (2) **left coronary artery**. The left coronary artery divides into two branches, the (3) **left anterior descending artery** and the

Figure 8-5 Anterior view of the heart showing coronary arteries.

(4) **circumflex artery**. If blood flow in the coronary arteries is diminished, it can lead to reduced O_2 supply to the heart muscle, potentially causing chest pain, or in severe cases a heart attack. Damage to the heart muscle may result, and when severe damage occurs, part of the heart muscle may die (**ischemia**).

Conduction System of the Heart

Within the heart, specialized cardiac tissue known as **conduction tissue** has the sole function of initiating and spreading contraction impulses (see Fig. 8-6). This tissue consists of four masses of highly specialized cells that possess characteristics of both nervous and cardiac tissue:

• sinoatrial (SA) node
• atrioventricular (AV) node
• bundle of His (AV bundle)
• Purkinje fibers

The (1) **sinoatrial (SA) node** is located in the upper portion of the RA and possesses its own intrinsic rhythm. Without being stimulated by external nerves, it can initiate and propagate each heartbeat, thereby setting the basic pace for the cardiac rate. For this reason, the SA node

Figure 8-6 Conduction system.

is commonly known as the **pacemaker** of the heart. The cardiac rate may be altered by impulses from the **autonomic nervous system**. Such an arrangement allows outside influences to accelerate or decelerate heart rate. For example, the heart beats more quickly during physical exertion and more slowly during rest. Each electrical impulse discharged by the SA node is transmitted to the (2) **atrioventricular (AV) node**, causing the atria to contract. The AV node is located at the base of the RA. From this point, a tract of conduction fibers called the (3) **bundle of His (or AV bundle)**, composed of a right and left branch, relays the impulse to the (4) **Purkinje fibers**, which extend up the ventricle walls. The Purkinje fibers transmit the impulse to the RVs and LVs, causing them to contract. Blood is now forced from the heart through the pulmonary artery and aorta. The sequence of the four structures responsible for conduction of a contraction impulse is as follows:

SA node → AV node → bundle of His → Purkinje fibers

Impulse transmission through the conduction system generates weak electrical impulses on the surface of the body. These impulses can be recorded on graph paper by an instrument called an **electrocardiograph** (ECG, EKG). The needle deflection of the ECG produces waves or peaks designated by the letters P, Q, R, S, and T, each representing different phases of the cardiac cycle (see Fig. 8-6) as follows:

- The **P wave** is the depolarization (contraction) of the atria.
- The **QRS complex** is the depolarization (contraction) of the ventricles.
- The **ST segment** is the interval between ventricular depolarization and repolarization (recovery).
- The **T wave** is the repolarization (recovery) of the ventricles.

Blood Pressure

Blood pressure (BP) is the force exerted by blood against the arterial walls during two phases of a heartbeat: the contraction phase **(systole)** when the blood is forced out of the heart and the relaxation phase **(diastole)** when the ventricles are filling with blood. A **sphygmomanometer** measures blood pressure in millimeters of mercury (mm Hg), which you record as two figures separated by a diagonal line. When recording a blood pressure reading, list systolic pressure first, followed by diastolic pressure. For example, a blood pressure reading of *120/80 mm Hg* means a systolic pressure of 120 with a diastolic pressure of 80. Guidelines for blood pressure are listed in Figure 8-7.

Several factors influence blood pressure:

- resistance of blood flow in blood vessels
- pumping action of the heart
- **viscosity** of blood
- elasticity of arteries
- quantity of blood in the vascular system

BLOOD PRESSURE	Systolic Mm Hg (Top Number)		Diastolic Mm Hg (Bottom Number)
Normal	<120	and	<80
Elevated	120–129	and	<80
High Blood Pressure Stage 1 hypertension	130–139	and	80–90
High Blood Pressure Stage 2 hypertension	>140	or	>90
Hypertensive Crisis Seek medical attention	>180	and/or	>120

Figure 8-7 Blood pressure guidelines.

Anatomy Review: Cardiovascular System

To review the anatomy of the heart, label the illustration using the listed terms.

aorta

aortic semilunar valve

inferior vena cava

left atrium

left pulmonary artery

left pulmonary veins

left ventricle

mitral (bicuspid) valve

pulmonic valve

right atrium

right pulmonary artery

right pulmonary veins

right ventricle

superior vena cava

tricuspid valve

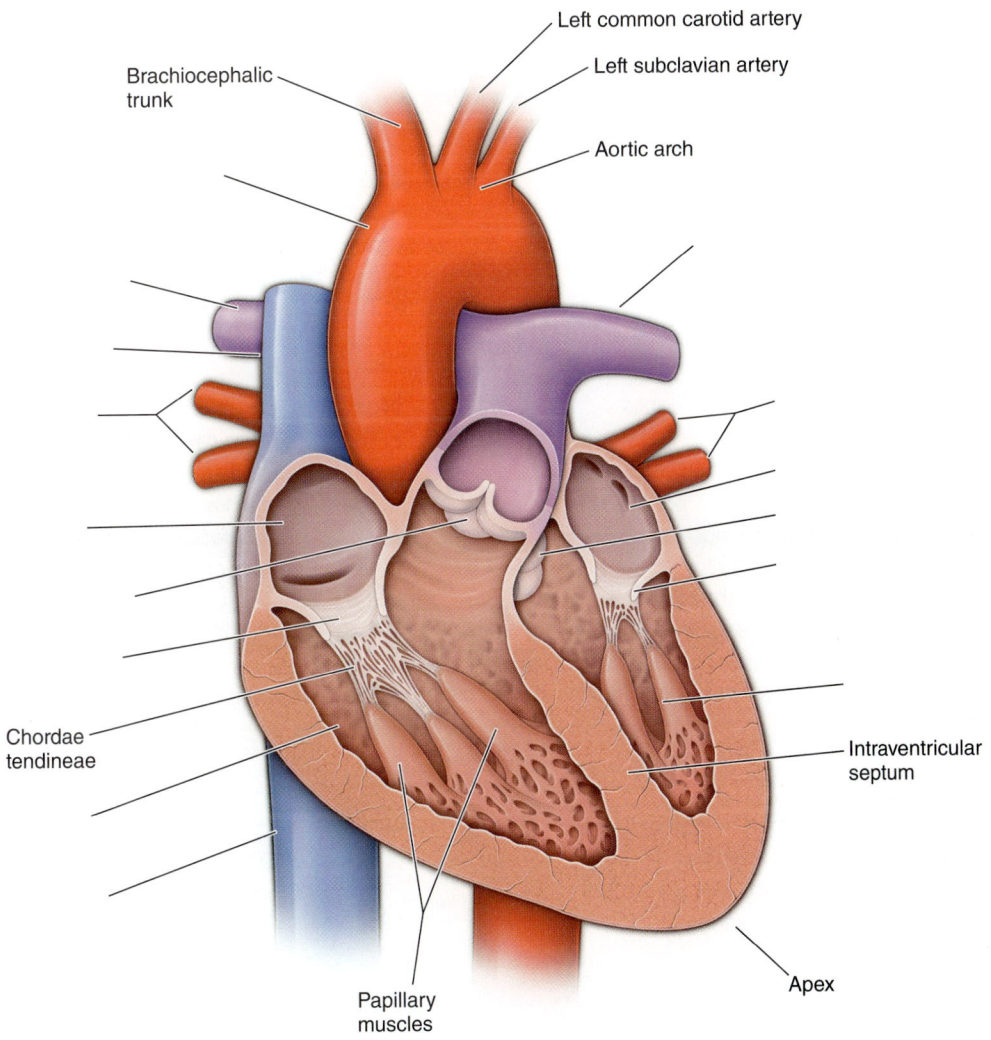

Left common carotid artery

Left subclavian artery

Brachiocephalic trunk

Aortic arch

Chordae tendineae

Intraventricular septum

Apex

Papillary muscles

 Check your answers by referring to Figure 8–4 on page 236. Review material that you did not answer correctly.

CONNECTING BODY SYSTEMS—CARDIOVASCULAR SYSTEM

The main function of the cardiovascular (CV) system is to provide a network of vessels through which blood is pumped by the heart to all body cells. Specific functional relationships between the CV system and other body systems are discussed here.

Blood, Lymphatic, and Immune
- The CV system transports the products of the immune system, such as antibodies, immune cells, and nutrients, throughout the body.
- Inflammation can affect blood vessels and contribute to CV conditions.

Digestive
- The CV system delivers hormones that affect the glandular activity of the digestive tract.
- The vessels of the CV system in the walls of the small intestine absorb nutrients.

Endocrine
- The CV system delivers O_2 and nutrients to the endocrine glands.
- The CV system transports hormones from glands to target organs.

Female Reproductive
- The CV system transports hormones that regulate the menstrual cycle.
- The CV system influences the normal function of reproductive organs.
- During pregnancy, the vessels of the CV system in the placenta exchange nutrients and waste products.

Integumentary
- The blood vessels of the CV system in the skin regulate body temperature.
- The CV system transports clotting factors to the skin to control bleeding.

Male Reproductive
- The CV system transports reproductive hormones.
- The CV system influences the normal function of sex organs, especially erectile tissue.

Musculoskeletal
- The CV system removes heat and waste products generated by muscle contraction.
- The CV system delivers oxygen for energy to sustain muscle contraction.
- The CV system delivers calcium and nutrients and removes metabolic waste from skeletal structures.
- The CV system delivers hormones that regulate skeletal growth.

Nervous
- The CV system carries electrolytes for transmission of electrical impulses.
- The CV system and nervous system communicate closely to regulate heart rate and blood pressure.

Respiratory
- The CV system transports O_2 and CO_2 between lungs and tissues.

Urinary
- The CV system delivers O_2 and nutrients to organs in the urinary system.
- Blood pressure maintains kidney function.

Medical Word Elements

This section introduces combining forms, suffixes, and prefixes related to the cardiovascular system. Word analyses are also provided. From the information provided, complete the meaning of the medical words in the right-hand column. The first one is completed for you.

Element	Meaning	Word Analysis
Combining Forms		
aneurysm/o	aneurysm (widened blood vessel)	**aneurysm/o**/rrhaphy (ăn-ū-rĭz-MOR-ă-fē): *suture of an aneurysm* *-rrhaphy:* suture
angi/o	vessel (usually blood or lymph)	**angi/o**/plasty (ĂN-jē-ō-plăs-tē): _____ *-plasty:* surgical repair *Angioplasty is a procedure that reopens narrowed blood vessels and restores blood flow using a balloon-tipped catheter.*
vascul/o		**vascul**/itis (văs-kū-LĪ-tĭs): _____ *-itis:* inflammation
aort/o	aorta	**aort/o**/stenosis (ā-or-tō-stě-NŌ-sĭs): _____ *-stenosis:* narrowing, stricture
arteri/o	artery	**arteri/o**/rrhexis (ăr-tē-rē-ō-RĔK-sĭs): _____ *-rrhexis:* rupture
arteriol/o	arteriole	**arteriol**/itis (ăr-tēr-ē-ō-LĪ-tĭs): _____ *-itis:* inflammation
atri/o	atrium	**atri/o**/megaly (ā-trē-ō-MĔG-ă-lē): _____ *-megaly:* enlargement
ather/o	fatty plaque	**ather**/oma (ăth-ĕr-Ō-mă): _____ *-oma:* tumor *Atheromas are formed when fatty plaque builds up on the inner lining of arterial walls.*
cardi/o	heart	**cardi/o**/megaly (kăr-dē-ō-MĔG-ă-lē): _____ *-megaly:* enlargement
coron/o		**coron**/ary (KOR-ō-nă-rē): _____ *-ary:* pertaining to *Coronary artery disease (CAD) is the most common type of heart disease and the leading cause of death in the United States in men and women.*
electr/o	electricity	**electr/o**/cardi/o/gram (ē-lĕk-trō-KĂR-dē-ō-grăm): _____ *cardi/o:* heart *-gram:* record, recording *An electrocardiogram helps detect many heart problems including heart attacks, arrhythmias, and heart failure.*

Continued

Medical Word Elements—cont'd

Element	Meaning	Word Analysis
embol/o	embolus (plug)	**embol**/ectomy (ĕm-bō-LĔK-tō-mē): _____ *-ectomy:* excision, removal *An embolectomy is performed in emergency situations to open blood vessels and reestablish blood flow.*
hemangi/o	blood vessel	**hemangi**/oma (hē-măn-jē-Ō-mă): _____ *-oma:* tumor *Hemangiomas, also called* **strawberry marks** *and found mostly in neonates, are benign tumors of cells that line blood vessels and usually disappear over time.*

my/o	muscle	**my/o**/cardi/al (mī-ō-KĂR-dē-ăl): _____
		   cardi: heart
		   -al: pertaining to

phleb/o	vein	**phleb**/ectasis (flĕ-BĔK-tă-sĭs): _____ *-ectasis:* dilation, expansion
ven/o		**ven/o**/stasis (vē-nō-STĀ-sĭs): _____ *-stasis:* standing still *Venostasis, also called* **phlebostasis,** *is an abnormally slow blood flow in the veins and is a major risk factor for clot formation.*

scler/o	hardening; sclera (white of eye)	**arteri/o**/scler/osis (ăr-tē-rē-ō-sklĕ-RŌ-sĭs): _____
		   arteri/o: artery
		   -osis: abnormal condition; increase (used primarily with blood cells)
		
		The most common cause of arteriosclerosis is the presence of an atheroma in the vessel. Other causes include smoking, diabetes, high blood pressure, obesity, and familial tendency.

sept/o	septum	**sept/o**/stomy (sĕp-TŎS-tō-mē): _____ *-stomy:* forming an opening (mouth) *Septostomy is a temporary procedure performed to increase systemic oxygenation in infants with congenital heart defects until corrective surgery can be performed.*
sphygm/o	pulse	**sphygm**/oid (SFĬG-moyd): _____ *-oid:* resembling
sten/o	narrowing, stricture	**sten/o**/tic (stĕ-NŎT-ĭk): _____ *-tic:* pertaining to
thromb/o	blood clot	**thromb/o**/lysis (thrŏm-BŎL-ĭ-sĭs): _____ *-lysis:* separation; destruction; loosening *In thrombolysis, enzymes that destroy blood clots are infused into the occluded vessel.*

Medical Word Elements—cont'd

Element	Meaning	Word Analysis
valv/o	valve	**valv/o**/tomy (văl-VŎT-ō-mē): _____ *-tomy:* incision *Valvotomy commonly involves use of a balloon catheter passed through a blood vessel in the groin to gain access to a stenosed valve of the heart.*
valvul/o		**valvul/o**/plasty (VĂL-vū-lō-plăs-tē): _____ *-plasty:* surgical repair
ventricul/o	ventricle (of the heart or brain)	**ventricul**/ar (vĕn-TRĬK-ū-lăr): _____ *-ar:* pertaining to
Suffixes		
-cardia	heart condition	tachy/**cardia** (tăk-ē-KĂR-dē-ă): _____ *tachy-:* rapid
-stenosis	narrowing, stricture	aort/o/**stenosis** (ā-or-tō-stĕ-NŌ-sĭs): _____ *aort/o:* aorta
Prefixes		
brady-	slow	**brady**/cardia (brăd-ē-KĂR-dē-ă): _____ *-cardia:* heart condition

endo-	in, within	**endo**/vascul/ar (ĕn-dō-VĂS-kū-lăr): _____
		  vascul: vessel (usually blood or lymph)
		  -ar: pertaining to
		
		Endovascular procedures are those that occur within the lumen of a vessel.

extra-	outside	**extra**/vascul/ar (ĕks-tră-VĂS-kū-lăr): _____
		  vascul: vessel (usually blood or lymph)
		  -ar: pertaining to

peri-	around	**peri**/cardi/al (pĕr-ĭ-KĂR-dē-ăl): _____
		  cardi: heart
		  -al: pertaining to
		
		Pericardial refers to the membrane that surrounds the heart, the pericardium.

trans-	across	**trans**/sept/al (trăns-SĔP-tăl): _____
		  sept: septum
		  -al: pertaining to

Visit the Medical Terminology Systems online resource center at FADavis.com for an audio exercise of the terms in this table. Other activities are also available to reinforce content.

It is time to review medical word elements by completing Learning Activities 8–1 and 8–2.

Disease Focus

Many cardiac disorders, especially coronary artery disease, and valvular disorders are associated with a genetic predisposition. Some of the most serious cardiovascular diseases have few signs and symptoms, but when they occur, they may include chest pain (**angina**), breathing difficulties, cardiac irregularities, and loss of consciousness.

For diagnosis, treatment, and management of cardiovascular disorders, the medical services of a **cardiologist** may be warranted. **Cardiology** is the medical specialty concerned with disorders of the cardiovascular system.

Arteriosclerosis and Atherosclerosis

Arteriosclerosis is a general term referring to the thickening and hardening of the arteries that can restrict the flow of blood to tissues and organs. **Atherosclerosis** is a specific type of arteriosclerosis characterized by the buildup of a plaquelike substance composed of cholesterol, lipids, calcium, and cellular debris (**atheroma**) on the interior arterial wall. Over time, the atheroma hardens (**atherosclerosis**) and increases in size, causing the lumen of the artery to narrow. In some instances, blood hemorrhages into the plaque and forms a clot (**thrombus**) that may break loose, travel through the vascular system (now an **embolus**), and lodge in a more distal area of the artery. Arterial emboli that completely block circulation cause localized tissue death (**infarction**) in the surrounding area. A partial blocking of circulation causes inadequate blood supply to a part of the body (**ischemia**), leading to reduced O_2 and nutrient delivery to tissues (see Fig. 8-8).

Arteries usually affected by arteriosclerosis include the coronary, carotid, cerebral, and femoral arteries and the aorta. Both arteriosclerosis and atherosclerosis can cause similar signs and symptoms, but atherosclerosis specifically involves the buildup of plaque in the arteries as the underlying etiology. Signs and symptoms vary depending on the artery involved. For example, if the carotid and cerebral arteries are involved, weakness or paralysis on one side of the body (**hemiplegia**), blurred vision, and confusion can result. However, if there is arteriosclerosis in the femoral arteries, muscle pain (**myalgia**) and numbness or tingling in the calves, thighs, and feet can occur.

Major risk factors for developing arteriosclerosis include an elevated level of fatty substances in the blood (**hyperlipidemia**), age, family history, smoking, stress, hypertension, diabetes, and lack

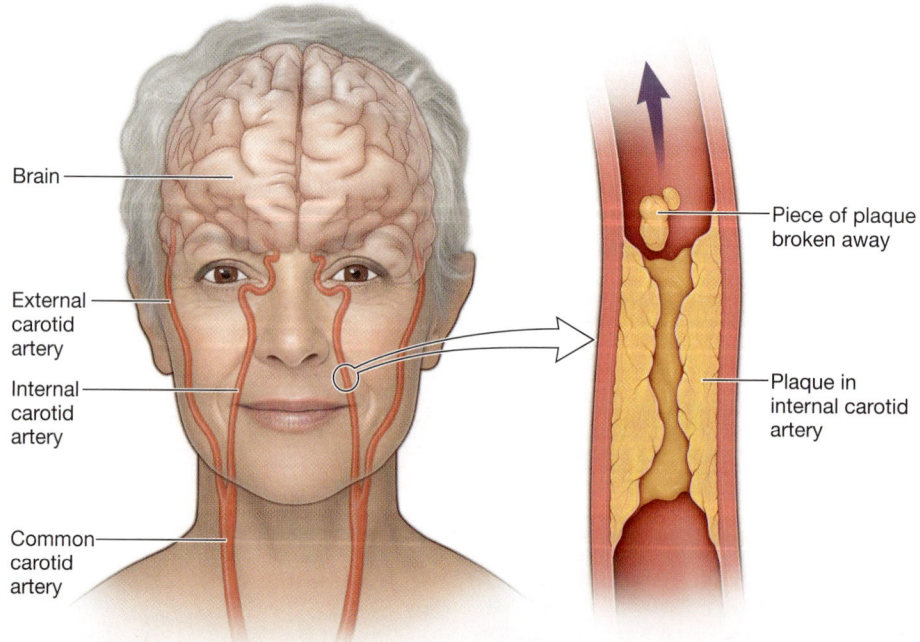

Figure 8-8 Atherosclerosis of the internal carotid artery.

of physical activity. Treatment varies depending on the location and symptoms. Drugs that slow down or reverse fat buildup (**statins**) in arteries, those that control blood pressure (**antihypertensives**), and those that reduce thrombus formation (**anticoagulants**) are helpful. Surgical treatments include repairing the affected vessels (**angioplasty**) and surgical removal of fatty deposits from the inside of the artery (**endarterectomy**). Physicians commonly use endarterectomy to treat carotid artery disease, **peripheral artery disease (PAD)**, and diseases of the renal artery and aortic arch (see Fig. 8-9).

Coronary Artery Disease (CAD)

For the heart to function effectively, the myocardium must receive an adequate and uninterrupted supply of blood from the coronary arteries. **Coronary artery disease (CAD)** is a CV condition characterized by the buildup of atherosclerotic plaques in the coronary arteries that can narrow or block the arteries, reducing blood flow to the heart muscle. Some key contributors to CAD include hypertension, diabetes, hyperlipidemia, smoking, stress, lack of physical activity, obesity, age, and gender. Insufficient blood supply (**ischemia**) to the myocardium can lead to chest pain (**angina**). Ischemia can be temporary and reversible if blood flow is restored in time. However, when ischemia is prolonged, tissue death occurs in the heart muscle, resulting in a **myocardial infarction (MI)** (see Fig. 8-10).

As the heart muscle undergoes necrotic changes, it releases several highly specific substances, including enzymes, proteins, and hormones. Rapid elevation in the levels of these substances indicates myocardial damage, and diagnostically will help differentiate MI from pericarditis, **abdominal aortic aneurysm (AAA)**, and acute **pulmonary embolism (PE)**.

Endocarditis

Endocarditis is an inflammation of the inner lining of the heart and its valves. It is usually caused by bacteria (**infective endocarditis**) that have entered the bloodstream from infections in remote regions of the body (gut, skin, mouth) and have lodged on damaged endocardial tissue or abnormal valves. Once established in the heart, bacteria and other cellular material form clumps (**vegetations**) on the valves, especially the mitral valve. This results in the narrowing of the valve (**mitral valve stenosis**) that impedes blood flow to the ventricle, or a prevention of the valve from closing properly (**mitral valve insufficiency**), commonly causing a backflow of blood into the atrium (**regurgitation**; see Fig. 8-11). Although medications may prove helpful, if heart failure develops as a result of damaged heart valves, surgery to correct the damaged valves (**valvuloplasty**) may be the only treatment option. Whenever possible, the original valve is repaired. When the damage is extensive, a mechanical device or one made of human or animal tissue (**bioprosthetic**) may be used.

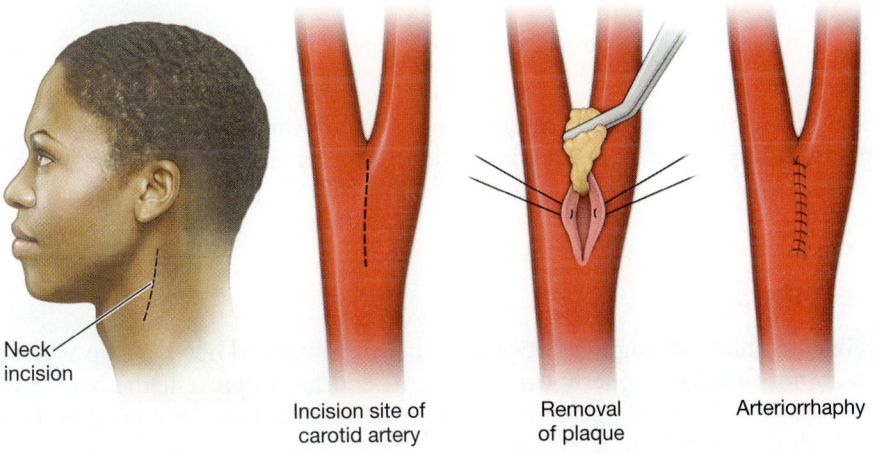

Neck incision

Incision site of carotid artery

Removal of plaque

Arteriorrhaphy

Figure 8-9 Endarterectomy of the common carotid artery.

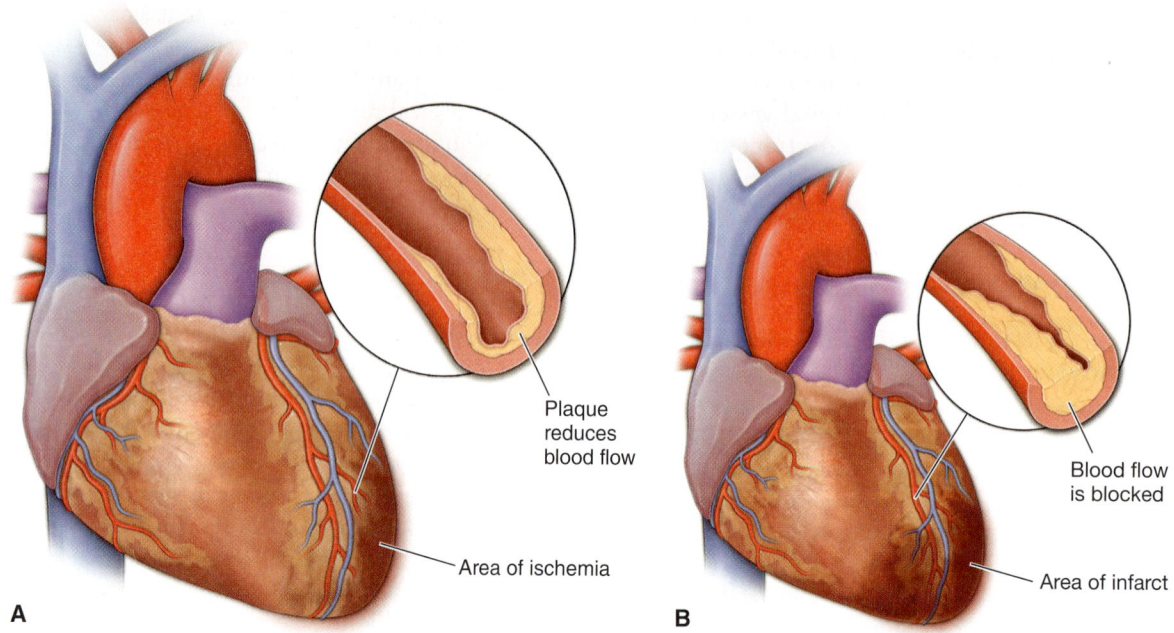

Figure 8-10 Coronary artery occlusions. (A) Partial occlusion showing area of ischemia. (B) Complete occlusion showing myocardial infarction.

Figure 8-11 Valvular defects. (A) Mitral stenosis. (B) Mitral insufficiency.

Congenital valvular defects, scarlet fever, rheumatic fever, mitral valve prolapse, and prosthetic valves are predisposing factors for developing endocarditis. Patients susceptible to endocarditis are given antibiotic treatment to protect against infection before invasive procedures **(prophylactic treatment)**.

Varicose Veins

Varicose veins are enlarged, engorged, twisted, superficial veins. They develop when the valves of the veins do not function properly **(incompetent)** and fail to prevent the backflow of blood. Varicose veins may develop in almost any part of the body, including the esophagus **(varices)** and rectum **(hemorrhoids),** but occur most commonly in the greater and lesser saphenous veins of the lower legs (see Fig. 8-12). Varicose veins of the legs are not typically painful but may be unsightly

A   Normal vein with   Varicose vein with   **B**
         competent valves   incompetent valves

Figure 8-12 Healthy and unhealthy veins and valves. (A) Valve function in competent and incompetent valves. (B) Varicose veins.

in appearance. Treatment of mild cases of varicose veins includes use of elastic stockings and rest periods, during which the legs are elevated.

However, if pain, open lesions, or inflammation of the vein (**phlebitis**) develops, treatment may be required. Destroying the tissue within the vein (**endovenous ablation**) is an effective and minimally invasive technique in treating varicose veins. Common endovenous options include treatments that employ lasers, heat (**radiofrequency ablation**), extreme cold (**cryoablation**), or chemicals (**sclerotherapy**). The goal of this procedure is to close off or seal a damaged or enlarged vein from the inside, allowing blood to be rerouted through healthier veins. Endovascular methods of treatment are replacing the more invasive, complicated ligation and stripping, which is more painful and requires a longer convalescent time.

Oncology

Malignant tumors that originate in the heart (primary tumors) are very rare and are called primary **cardiac sarcomas**. When cardiac sarcomas do occur, they develop in the soft tissues, including muscle tissue, and are classified based on the specific type of cell they resemble. Although still rare, an **angiosarcoma** is the most frequently diagnosed type of cardiac sarcoma that tends to arise in the right atrium. A tumor in this particular location causes obstruction of blood circulation, leading to symptoms of fluid in the lungs (**pulmonary edema**) and swelling (**edema**) of the lower extremities and abdomen.

Most cancers of the heart are secondary or metastatic tumors, where the cancer cells originate from the primary tumor site in another area of the body and spread to the heart (**metastasize**) through the bloodstream. The most common primary sites of metastasis to the heart include the lungs, breast, and skin.

The treatment of malignant cardiac tumors is challenging due to their rarity, aggressive nature, and limited treatment options. Treatment approaches vary depending on factors such as the type of tumor, its size, location, extent of spread, and the patient's overall health and preferences.

Diseases and Conditions

This section introduces diseases and conditions of the cardiovascular system, along with their meanings and pronunciations. Word analyses for selected terms are also provided.

Term	Definition
aneurysm ĂN-ū-rĭzm	Localized abnormal dilation of a vessel, usually an artery (see Fig. 8-13). *An aneurysm can lead to serious complications, with rupture being the most dangerous, causing internal bleeding, stroke, shock, or sudden death. It may also form clots that travel and damage vital organs.*

A

B

C

Figure 8-13 Types of aneurysm. (A) Fusiform, with dilation of the entire circumference of the artery. (B) Saccular, with dilation of one side of the artery. (C) Dissecting, in which a tear in the inner layer causes a cavity to form between the layers of the artery that fills with blood and expands with each heartbeat.

Diseases and Conditions—cont'd

Term	Definition
angina ĂN-jĭ-nă *angin:* choking pain *-a:* noun ending	Chest pain or discomfort, caused by obstructions or spasms of the coronary arteries that decrease blood flow to the myocardium; also called *angina pectoris* *Anginal pain typically radiates down the left arm or into the shoulder, neck, jaw, or back (see Fig. 8-14).*

Typical distribution
of referred pain

Figure 8-14 Common locations of anginal pain, which may vary in combination and intensity.

Term	Definition
arrhythmia ă-RĬTH-mē-ă	Irregularity in the rate or rhythm of the heart; also called *dysrhythmia*

bradycardia
   brăd-ē-KĂR-dē-ă
     brady-: slow
     -cardia: heart condition
	Abnormally slow heart rate, usually fewer than 60 beats per minute (bpm) in a resting adult

fibrillation fĭ-brĭl-Ā-shŭn	Abnormally rapid, uncoordinated quivering of the myocardium that can affect the atria or the ventricles

tachycardia
   tăk-ē-KĂR-dē-ă
     tachy-: rapid
     -cardia: heart condition
	Abnormally fast but regular rhythm, with the heart possibly beating up to 200 bpm
	
	Patients with tachycardia may experience palpitations.

bruit BRWĒ	Soft, blowing sound heard over a blood vessel on auscultation often associated with turbulent blood flow; it can indicate an underlying vascular issue, such as an obstruction or narrowing in the blood vessel

Continued

Diseases and Conditions—cont'd

Term	Definition
cardiomyopathy kăr-dē-ō-mī-ŎP-ă-thē *cardi/o:* heart *my/o:* muscle *–pathy:* disease	Group of diseases that affect the heart muscle and diminish cardiac function; can lead to heart failure, arrhythmias, or other complications *There are various types of cardiomyopathy, including dilated, hypertrophic, and restrictive, each with distinct characteristics and causes. Causes of cardiomyopathy include viral or bacterial infections, metabolic disorders, alcohol or substance abuse, and general systemic disease.*
coarctation kō-ărk-TĀ-shŭn	Narrowing of a vessel, especially the aorta *Coarctation of the aorta is a congenital heart defect that typically requires medical intervention, such as surgery or catheter-based procedures, to correct the narrowing and restore proper blood flow.*
embolism ĔM-bō-lĭzm *embol:* embolus (plug) *–ism:* condition	Intravascular mass that dislodges from one part of the body and causes a blockage in another area, commonly leading to life-threatening situations *The deadliest form of embolism is a pulmonary embolism, which blocks blood flow to the lungs, causing chest pain, hypoxemia, tachycardia, and even sudden death. When treated, mortality rate drops considerably.*
heart block	Interference with the normal transmission of electrical impulses from the SA node to the Purkinje fibers *Heart block is usually specified by the location of the block and the type.*
first-degree	Atrioventricular (AV) block in which the atrial electrical impulses are delayed by a fraction of a second before being conducted to the ventricles *First-degree AV block is recognized on ECG by a prolonged PR interval. There is no specific treatment for first-degree AV block, but the condition is monitored because it may precede higher degrees of block.*
second-degree	AV block in which occasional electrical impulses from the SA node fail to be conducted to the ventricles *Because of the dropped beats in second-degree AV block, the QRS complexes are dropped periodically, usually every second, third, or fourth beat.*
third-degree	AV block in which the electrical impulses from the atria fail to reach the ventricles; also called *complete heart block (CHB)* *Treatment for second- or third-degree heart block consists of atropine (drug used to increase heart rate) or pacemaker insertion.*
heart failure (HF)	Inability of the heart to pump sufficient blood to meet the metabolic needs of the body *Common causes of HF include CAD, hypertension, diabetes, and obesity.*
congestive	Congestive heart failure (CHF) is a specific type of HF that occurs when blood returning to the heart backs up, causing fluid to accumulate in the lungs (pulmonary edema) and other parts of the body such as the liver, abdomen, and lower extremities

Diseases and Conditions—cont'd

Term	Definition
hyperlipidemia hī-pĕr-lĭp-ĭ-DĒ-mē-ă *hyper-:* excessive, above normal *lipid:* fat *-emia:* blood condition	Excessive amounts of lipids (cholesterol, phospholipids, and triglycerides) in the blood *Hyperlipidemia is associated with an increased risk of atherosclerosis.*
hypertension (HTN) hī-pĕr-TĔN-shŭn *hyper-:* excessive, above normal *-tension:* to stretch	Elevated blood pressure levels persistently exceeding the normal range; measured in millimeters of mercury (mm Hg; see Fig. 8-7)
hypotension hī-pō-TĔN-shŭn *hypo-:* under, below, deficient *-tension:* to stretch	A medical condition characterized by persistently low blood pressure, generally less than 90/60 mm Hg
mitral valve prolapse (MVP) MĪ-trăl, PRŌ-lăps	Structural defect in which the mitral (bicuspid) valve leaflets prolapse into the LA during ventricular contraction (systole), resulting in incomplete closure and backflow of blood *Common signs and symptoms of MVP include a characteristic murmur heard on auscultation and palpitations of the heart.*
murmur	Abnormal heart sound heard with a stethoscope caused by turbulent blood flow through the heart *Heart murmurs may be a sign of a defective heart valve or disease or may be a mild form not associated with disease. Murmurs are described by their volume, sound, and when they occur in the cardiac cycle.*
palpitation păl-pĭ-TĀ-shŭn	Sensation of an irregular heartbeat, commonly described as pounding, racing, skipping a beat, or flutter
peripheral artery disease (PAD) pĕr-ĬF-ĕr-ăl ĂR-tĕr-ē	Common circulatory disorder characterized by a reduced flow of blood to the extremities, especially the legs, resulting in muscle cramping and pain, and commonly the result of atherosclerosis *If PAD is caused by plaque, it may signal disease in the arteries of vital organs, including the heart (heart attack) and brain (stroke).*
phlebitis flĕ-BĪ-tĭs *phleb:* vein *-itis:* inflammation	Inflammation of a deep or superficial vein of the arms or legs (more commonly the legs)
thrombophlebitis thrŏm-bō-flĕ-BĪ-tĭs	Inflammation of a vein with the formation of a blood clot.

Continued

Diseases and Conditions—cont'd

Term	Definition
rheumatic heart disease (RHD) roo-MĂT-ĭk	Serious pathological condition resulting from rheumatic fever, a condition that can occur as a result of untreated or inadequately treated streptococcal throat infections *Chronic RHD remains the leading cause of mitral valve stenosis and valve replacement in adults.*
syncope SĬN-kō-pē	Partial or complete loss of consciousness usually caused by a decreased supply of blood to the brain; also called *fainting*
thrombosis thrŏm-BŌ-sĭs *thromb:* blood clot *-osis:* abnormal condition; increase (used primarily with blood cells)	Abnormal condition in which a blood clot develops in a vessel and obstructs it at the site of its formation
deep vein thrombosis (DVT) thrŏm-BŌ-sĭs *thromb:* blood clot *-osis:* abnormal condition; increase (used primarily with blood cells)	Blood clot that forms in the deep veins of the body, especially those in the legs or thighs; also called *deep venous thrombosis* (see Fig. 8-15) *In DVT, blood clots may break away from the vein wall and travel in the body, especially to the lungs.*

Blood flow to heart and lungs

Muscle

Superficial vein

Skin

Thrombosis in deep vein

Swelling and inflammation below blockage

Figure 8-15 Deep vein thrombosis (DVT).

It is time to review pathology, diseases, and conditions by completing Learning Activity 8-3.

Diagnostic, Surgical, and Therapeutic Procedures

This section introduces diagnostic, surgical, and therapeutic procedures used to diagnose and treat cardiovascular disorders. Descriptions are provided, along with pronunciations and word analyses for selected terms.

Procedure	Description
Diagnostic	
Clinical	

electrocardiography (ECG)
ē-lĕk-trō-kăr-dē-ŎG-ră-fē
electr/o: electricity
cardi/o: heart
-graphy: process of recording

Test that records the electrical activity of the heart using small metal electrodes applied to the chest, arms, and legs

ECG helps diagnose abnormal heart rhythms and myocardial damage (see Fig. 8-16).

Figure 8-16 Screening electrocardiograph.

Holter monitor test
HŌL-tĕr

Procedure that uses a small, portable system to record and store the electrical activity of the heart over a 24- to 48-hour period; also called *event monitor test* (see Fig. 8-17)

Holter monitoring is particularly useful in diagnosing a cardiac arrhythmia that would be missed during an ECG of only a few minutes' duration. The patient also maintains a record of any symptoms experienced during this time frame to aid in identifying and capturing potential cardiac events.

stress test

ECG taken under controlled exercise stress conditions, typically involving a stationary bicycle or treadmill; a pharmacological (chemical) stress test is used when the patient is unable to perform exercise where medications are administered to simulate the effects of exercise by increasing the heart rate

A stress test may show abnormal ECG tracings that do not appear during an ECG taken when the patient is resting. Nuclear imaging or echocardiography may also be performed to assess blood flow and heart function.

Continued

Diagnostic, Surgical, and Therapeutic Procedures—cont'd

Procedure	Description

Figure 8-17 Patient wearing a Holter monitor.

Laboratory

Procedure	Description
cardiac enzymes KĂR-dē-ăk ĔN-zīmz *cardi:* heart *-ac:* pertaining to	Measures the presence and amount of specific enzymes released into the bloodstream by the heart when it is damaged or under stress *Cardiac enzymes include creatine kinase MB (CK-MB), also known as creatine phosphokinase (CPK), and lactate dehydrogenase (LDH). Levels of CK-MB and LDH begin to rise within hours following an MI. The higher the levels the more severe the MI.*
lipid panel LĬP-ĭd	Series of blood tests that measure levels of various fats: total cholesterol, high-density lipoprotein (HDL), low-density lipoprotein (LDL), and triglycerides (TG); used to help assess risk of CV disease
partial thromboplastin time (PTT) thrŏm-bō-PLĂS-tĭn	Blood test to measure the time it takes for a clot to form that is used to monitor coagulation therapy and to detect deficiencies of certain clotting factors *PTT is often ordered with prothrombin time (PT), a blood test that measures other clotting factors that aren't part of the PTT.*
troponin I and troponin T trō-PŎH-nĭn	Measures the level of two proteins released into the bloodstream by damaged cardiac muscle cells and is a highly sensitive and specific indicator of recent MI *Elevated levels of troponin can be detected within a few hours of MI and remain elevated for several days. Troponin levels are performed in conjunction with cardiac enzymes and are used to diagnose MI.*

Diagnostic, Surgical, and Therapeutic Procedures—cont'd

Procedure	Description

Imaging

angiography
ăn-jē-ŎG-ră-fē

angi/o: vessel (usually blood or lymph)
-graphy: process of recording

Procedure that records a radiographic image of the inside of a blood vessel (angiogram) after injection of a contrast medium

Angiography of an artery is called arteriography. Angiography of a vein is called venography.

    aortography
    ā-or-TŎG-ră-fē

    aort/o: aorta
    -graphy: process of recording

Angiography of the aorta and its branches after injection of a contrast medium

Aortography helps diagnose aortic insufficiency.

    coronary angiography
    KOR-ō-nă-rē

    coron: heart
    -ary: pertaining to

Specialized type of angiography that helps diagnose stenosis or obstruction of the arteries that supply blood to the heart muscle

Doppler ultrasound (US)
DŎP-lĕr

Ultrasonography used to assess the direction and speed of blood flow through blood vessels by reflecting sound waves off red blood cells; also called *ultrasonography using sound pitch*

Various Doppler techniques help diagnose blood clots, valvular disorders, arterial occlusions, and aneurysms.

    carotid artery US
    kă-RŎT-ĭd ĂR-tĕr-ē

US procedure that determines blood flow problems caused by blood clots, plaque, or tears on the walls of the carotid arteries (see Fig. 8-18)

Figure 8-18 Carotid artery ultrasound.

    echocardiography (ECHO)
    ĕk-ō-kăr-dē-ŎG-ră-fē

    echo-: repeated sound
    cardi/o: heart
    -graphy: process of recording

US test that produces moving images of blood passing through the heart, valves, and chambers, and assesses cardiac output

ECHO involves placement of a transducer on the chest to direct ultrahigh frequency sound waves toward cardiac structures. Reflected echoes are displayed on a monitor (see Fig. 8-19).

Continued

Diagnostic, Surgical, and Therapeutic Procedures—cont'd

Procedure	Description

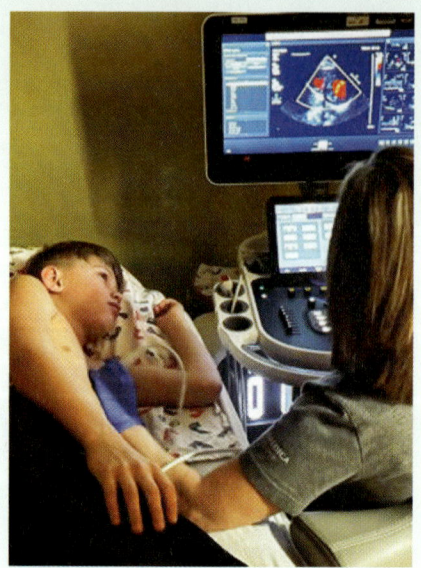

Figure 8-19 Echocardiography (ECHO).

Procedure	Description
myocardial perfusion imaging (MPI) mī-ō-KĂR-dē-ăl pĕr-FŪ-zhŭn *my/o:* muscle *cardi:* heart *-al:* pertaining to	Noninvasive imaging test using a radioactive tracer in conjunction with a stress test to show how well blood flows through (perfuses) the heart muscle at rest and during exercise; also called *nuclear stress test* *Typically, MPI involves intravenous administration of such radioactive substances as Cardiolite and thallium during the test. A gamma camera identifies areas of reduced blood flow that show up as "cold spots," an indication of myocardial damage.*
single-photon emission computed tomography (SPECT) tō-MŎG-ră-fē *tom/o:* to cut *-graphy:* process of recording	Myocardial perfusion test that involves injection of a radioactive tracer into the blood while a gamma camera moves in a circle around the patient to create individual images as "slices" of the heart (tomography) *SPECT shows how well blood is flowing to the heart and how efficiently the heart is pumping with the patient at rest or during exercise.*
cardiac magnetic resonance imaging (MRI) KĂR-dē-ăk *cardi:* heart *-ac:* pertaining to	Specialized MRI procedure that provides images of the heart chambers, valves, major vessels, and pericardium *Cardiac MRI helps evaluate the effects of coronary heart disease, plan treatment strategies, and monitor the progression of disorders over time.*
magnetic resonance angiography (MRA) măg-NĔT-ĭk RĔZ-ĕn-ăns ăn-jē-ŎG-ră-fē *angi/o:* vessel (usually blood or lymph) *-graphy:* process of recording	Type of MRI that provides highly detailed images of blood vessels *Unlike angiography, MRA detects blood flow, the condition of blood vessel walls, and blockages without using a contrast medium.*

Diagnostic, Surgical, and Therapeutic Procedures—cont'd

Procedure	Description
multiple-gated acquisition (MUGA) scan	Nuclear procedure that uses radioactive tracers and a gamma camera to detect how effectively the heart walls move as they contract and then calculates the ejection fraction rate (amount of blood the ventricle can pump out in one contraction) *The ejection fraction is the most accurate predictor of overall heart function.*

Other

cardiac catheterization (CC) KĂR-dē-ăk kăth-ĕ-tĕr-ĭ-ZĀ-shŭn *cardi:* heart *-ac:* pertaining to	Passage of a catheter into the heart through a vein or artery to provide a comprehensive evaluation of the heart and in certain cases to perform minimally invasive interventions; also called a *cardiac cath* *CC gathers information about the heart, including blood supply through the coronary arteries and blood flow and pressure through the heart's chambers and enables blood sample collection and x-rays of the heart (see Fig. 8–20).*

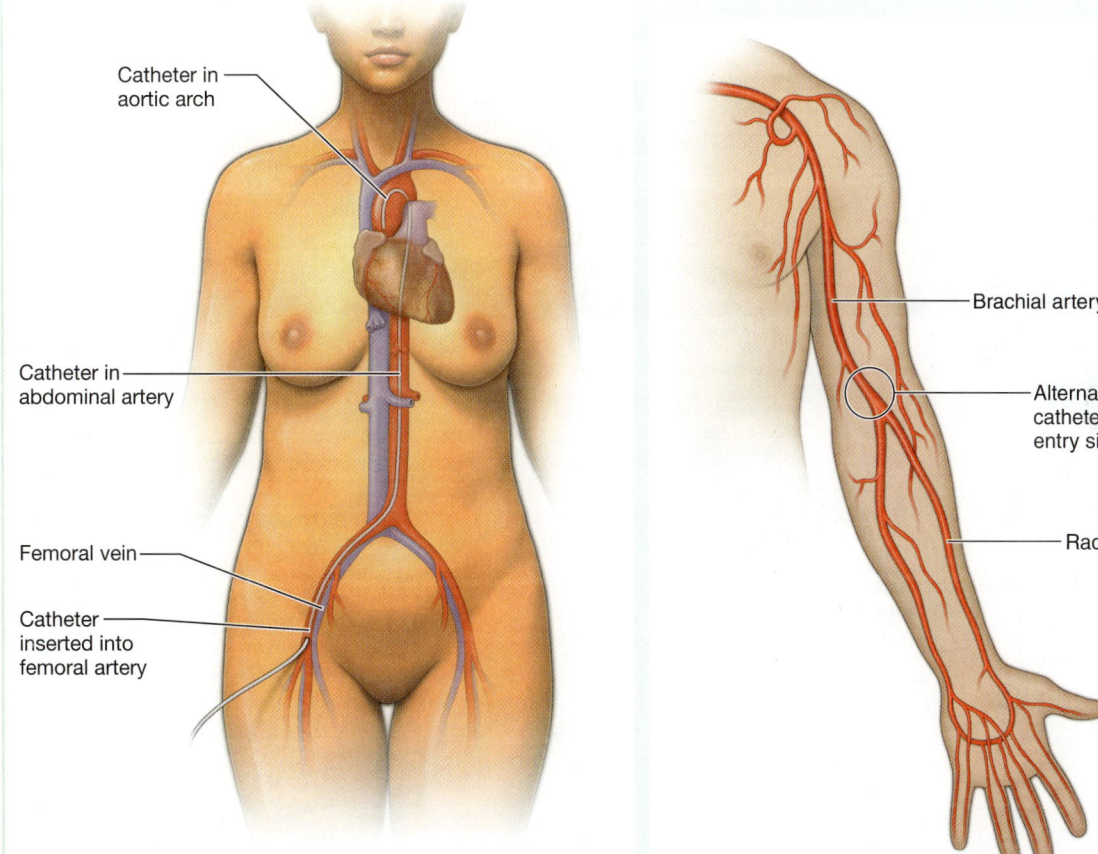

Figure 8-20 Cardiac catheterization.

electrophysiology study (EPS) ē-lĕk-trō-fĭz-ē-ŎL-ō-jē *electr/o:* electricity *physi/o:* physical *-logy:* study of	A specialized catheterization test that involves insertion of electrode catheters into the heart to examine and map the conduction system, enabling the safe replication of abnormal heart rhythms, allowing for a thorough study of their effect on the patient's heart *The information derived from EPS helps determine the best medication, treatment, or device to control or correct the abnormal rhythm.*

Continued

Diagnostic, Surgical, and Therapeutic Procedures—cont'd

Procedure	Description
Surgical	

angioplasty
ĂN-jē-ō-plăs-tē
angi/o: vessel (usually blood or lymph)
-plasty: surgical repair

Endovascular procedure that reopens narrowed or blocked arteries to restore forward blood flow

Angioplasty is most commonly performed on coronary, carotid, renal, or peripheral arteries occluded by atherosclerosis.

percutaneous transluminal coronary angioplasty (PTCA)
pĕr-kū-TĂ-nē-ŭs
trăns-LŪ-mĭ-năl
KOR-ō-nă-rē
ĂN-jē-ō-plăs-tē
per–: through
cutane: skin
-ous: pertaining to

Angioplasty of the coronary arteries that involves insertion of a balloon catheter through the right femoral artery to the site of the stenosis to enlarge the lumen of the artery and restore blood flow

After the balloon opens the lumen, the practitioner deflates and removes it. This procedure is commonly performed in conjunction with stent placement, a device that remains in the artery after the procedure is complete (see Fig. 8-21).

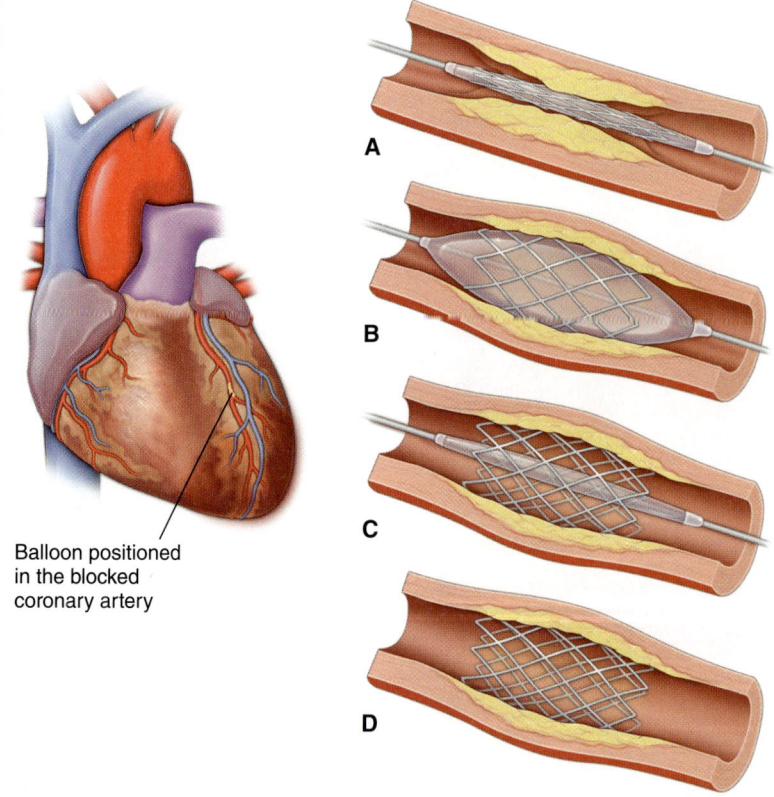

Balloon positioned in the blocked coronary artery

A

B

C

D

Figure 8-21 Percutaneous transluminal coronary angioplasty (PTCA) with stent placement. (A) Catheter is threaded through the sheath into the artery and navigated to the coronary artery with a small deflated balloon to the site of plaque blockage. (B) Balloon is inflated when positioned at the site of stenosis. (C) Deflation and removal of the balloon after enlargement of the artery. (D) Stent remaining in the artery to hold it open after the procedure is complete.

Diagnostic, Surgical, and Therapeutic Procedures—cont'd

Procedure	Description
cardiac ablation KĂR-dē-ăk ăb-LĀ-shŭn *cardi:* heart *-ac:* pertaining to	Minimally invasive procedure performed through a catheter that is inserted into the heart to deliver radiofrequency (heat) or cryoablation (extreme cold) to destroy targeted tissue producing irregular electrical signals and causing arrhythmias *Cardiac ablation causes scarring of heart tissue that results in blocking the abnormal pathways of the arrythmia to restore a normal heart rhythm.*
coronary artery bypass graft (CABG) KOR-ō-nă-rē ĂR-tĕr-ē *coron:* heart *-ary:* pertaining to	Placement of a healthy vessel graft from another part of the body to bypass the blocked or narrowed area of a coronary artery and restore blood supply to the heart muscle (see Fig. 8-22) *The two most common vessels for coronary grafts are the internal mammary arteries and the saphenous veins of the leg.* **Figure 8-22** Coronary artery bypass graft (CABG).
implantable cardioverter defibrillator (ICD) KĂR-dē-ō-vĕr-tĕr dē-FĬB-rĭ-lă-tor	Small, battery-powered device placed under the skin into the chest of a patient who is at high risk for developing an arrhythmia, such as ventricular tachycardia, ventricular fibrillation, or cardiac arrest; also called *automatic implantable cardioverter-defibrillator (AICD)* *The ICD monitors and restores the heart to a normal rhythm by delivering an electrical shock to the heart (see Fig. 8-23).*

Continued

Diagnostic, Surgical, and Therapeutic Procedures—cont'd

Procedure	Description

Electrodes in heart

Electrodes inserted into cephalic vein leading to heart

AICD implanted under the skin

Right atrium

Right ventricle

Lead delivering electrical shock

Electrical charge

Figure 8-23 Implantable cardioverter defibrillator.

Procedure	Description
open heart surgery	Surgical procedure in which the sternum is cut in half vertically to open the chest and expose the heart, its valves, or the arteries *During the operation, a heart–lung machine takes over circulation and oxygen exchange to allow surgery on the resting (nonbeating) heart. Types of open heart surgery include CABG, valve replacement, and heart transplant.*
pacemaker insertion PĀS-māk-ĕr	Implantation of a battery-powered device under the skin in the chest, usually near the collar bone, to help regulate and stabilize the heart rate and rhythm *The pacemaker uses a wire positioned in the heart to coordinate the heartbeat with an electrical pulse.*

Diagnostic, Surgical, and Therapeutic Procedures—cont'd

Procedure	Description

Therapeutic

cardioversion
KĂR-dē-ō-vĕr-zhŭn
cardi/o: heart
-version: turning

Defibrillation technique using low-energy shocks to reset an abnormal heart rhythm, such as atrial fibrillation or atrial flutter, back to its normal pattern

Cardioversion helps treat arrhythmias that antiarrhythmic drugs cannot treat. This procedure is not typically performed in an emergency situation but as a scheduled outpatient procedure (see Fig. 8-24).

Atrial fibrillation before cardioversion

Normal ECG after cardioversion

Figure 8-24 Cardioversion procedure.

defibrillation
dē-fĭb-rĭ-LĀ-shŭn

Lifesaving emergency treatment to restart the heart in cardiorespiratory arrest by delivering high-voltage electrical current through the heart

An automated external defibrillator (AED) analyzes heart rhythm and delivers an electrical shock to stimulate a heart in cardiac arrest. These devices are designed for use by laypersons and are located at airports, sports stadiums, health fitness centers, and other areas where large numbers of people congregate, as well as in ambulances.

Pharmacology

A healthy, functional cardiovascular system ensures adequate blood circulation and efficient delivery of oxygen and nutrients to all parts of the body. When any part of the cardiovascular system malfunctions or becomes diseased, drug therapy plays an integral role in establishing and maintaining perfusion and homeostasis.

Medications treat a variety of cardiovascular conditions, including angina pectoris, myocardial infarction, heart failure (HF), arrhythmias, hypertension, hyperlipidemia, and vascular disorders (see Table 8-1). Many cardiovascular drugs treat multiple problems simultaneously.

TABLE 8-1 Drugs Used to Treat Cardiovascular Disorders

This table lists common drug classifications used to treat CV disorders, their therapeutic actions, and selected generic and trade names.

Classification	Therapeutic Action	Generic and Trade Names
angiotensin-converting enzyme (ACE) inhibitors ăn-jē-ō-TĔN-sĭn ĔN-zīm ĭn-HĬB-ĭ-tōrs	Lower blood pressure by inhibiting the conversion of angiotensin I (an inactive enzyme) to angiotensin II (a potent vasoconstrictor) *ACE inhibitors treat hypertension alone or with other agents and aid in the management of HF.*	**benazepril** bĕn-ā-ză-prĭl *Lotensin* **lisinopril** lĭ-SĬN-ō-prĭl *Prinivil, Zestril*
angiotensin II receptor blockers (ARBs)	Lower blood pressure by blocking the angiotensin II enzyme from causing vasoconstriction	**losartan** lō-SĂR-tăn *Cozaar* **valsartan** văl-SĂR-tăn *Diovan*
antiarrhythmics ăn-tē-ă-RĬTH-mĭks	Prevent, alleviate, or correct cardiac arrhythmias (dysrhythmias) by stabilizing the electrical conduction of the heart *Antiarrhythmics help treat atrial and ventricular arrhythmias. There are several classes of antiarrhythmic drugs, each targeting specific mechanisms of the electrical system of the heart.*	**amiodarone** ă-mē-Ō-dă-rōn *Cordarone* **adenosine** ă-DĔN-ŭh-sēn *Adenocard, Adenoscan*
anticoagulants ăn-t ĭ-kō-ĂG-ū-lăntz	Inhibit the body's natural coagulation response to prevent the formation of clots in blood vessels *Clots can embolize, or travel, to vital organs and cause heart attacks or strokes.*	**warfarin** WĂR-fa-rĭn *Coumadin* **enoxaparin** ĕn-ŎX-ĕ-pār-ĭn *Lovenox* **heparin** *Heparin*
beta blockers BĀ-tă	Block the effect of adrenaline, primarily targeting beta-adrenergic receptors, which slows nerve pulses through the heart, causing a decrease in heart rate *Beta blockers are prescribed for hypertension, angina, and arrhythmias (dysrhythmias).*	**atenolol** ă-TĔN-ō-lŏl *Tenormin* **metoprolol** mĕ-TŌ-prō-lŏl *Lopressor, Toprol-XL*
calcium channel blockers KĂL-sē-ŭm	Block movement of calcium (required for blood vessel contraction) into myocardial cells and arterial walls, causing heart rate and blood pressure to decrease *Calcium channel blockers help treat angina pectoris, hypertension, arrhythmias, and HF.*	**amlodipine** ăm-LŌ-dĭ-pēn *Norvasc* **diltiazem** dĭl-TĪ-ă-zĕm *Cardizem CD* **nifedipine** nī-FĔD-ĭ-pēn *Adalat CC, Procardia*

TABLE 8-1 Drugs Used to Treat Cardiovascular Disorders—cont'd

Classification	Therapeutic Action	Generic and Trade Names
diuretics dī-ū-RĔT-ĭks	Act on kidneys to increase excretion of water and sodium *Diuretics reduce fluid buildup in the body, including fluid in the lungs, a common symptom of HF. Diuretics also help treat hypertension.*	**furosemide** fū-RŌ-sĕ-mīd *Lasix* **hydrochlorothiazide** hī-drō-klō-rō-THĪ-a-zīd *HydroDIURIL*
nitrates NĪ-trāts	Dilate blood vessels of the heart, causing an increase in the amount of O$_2$ delivered to the myocardium and widen blood vessels of the body, allowing more blood flow to the heart *Nitrate administration can be sublingual as a spray or tablet, oral as a tablet, transdermal as a patch, topical as an ointment, or intravenous in an emergency setting.*	**nitroglycerin** nī-trō-GLĬS-ĕr-ĭn *Nitrolingual, Nitrogard, Nitrostat* **isosorbide mononitrate** ī-sō-SŌR-bīd mŏn-ō-NĪ-trāt *Imdur*
statins STĂ-tĭnz	Lower cholesterol in the blood and reduce its production in the liver by blocking the enzyme that produces it *A combination of Vytorin, a statin drug, with a cholesterol absorption inhibitor not only lowers cholesterol in the blood and reduces its production in the liver but also decreases absorption of dietary cholesterol from the intestine.*	**atorvastatin** ăh-tor-vă-STĂ-tĭn *Lipitor* **simvastatin** SĬM-vă-stă-tĭn *Zocor* **simvastatin and ezetimibe** SĬM-vă-stă-tĭn, ĕ-ZĔ-tĭ-mīb *Vytorin*

Abbreviations

This section introduces cardiovascular–related abbreviations and their meanings.

Abbreviation	Meaning	Abbreviation	Meaning
AAA	abdominal aortic aneurysm	**BPM, bpm**	beats per minute
ACE	angiotensin-converting enzyme (inhibitor)	**CA**	cancer; cardiac arrest; chronological age
AED	automated external defibrillator	**CABG**	coronary artery bypass graft
AICD	automatic implantable cardioverter-defibrillator	**CAD**	coronary artery disease
ARB	angiotensin receptor blocker	**CC**	cardiac catheterization, chief complaint
AV	atrioventricular; arteriovenous	**CHB**	complete heart block
BP	blood pressure	**CHF**	congestive heart failure

Continued

Abbreviation	Meaning	Abbreviation	Meaning
CK	creatine kinase (cardiac enzyme); conductive keratoplasty	mm Hg	millimeters of mercury
CK-MB	creatine kinase MB	MPI	myocardial perfusion imaging
CO_2	carbon dioxide	MRA	magnetic resonance angiogram, magnetic resonance angiography
CPK	creatine phosphokinase	MRI	magnetic resonance imaging
CV	cardiovascular	MUGA scan	multiple-gated acquisition scan
DVT	deep vein thrombosis, deep venous thrombosis	O_2	oxygen
ECG, EKG	electrocardiogram, electrocardiography	PAD	peripheral artery disease
ECHO	echocardiogram, echocardiography; echoencephalogram, echoencephalography	PT	prothrombin time
EPS	electrophysiology studies	PTCA	percutaneous transluminal coronary angioplasty
HDL	high-density lipoprotein	PTT	partial thromboplastin time
HTN	hypertension	RA	right atrium
ICD	implantable cardioverter-defibrillator	RHD	rheumatic heart disease
LA	left atrium	RV	right ventricle; residual volume
LDH	lactate dehydrogenase	SA	sinoatrial
LDL	low-density lipoprotein	SPECT	single photon emission computed tomography
LV	left ventricle	TG	triglycerides
MI	myocardial infarction	US	ultrasound

It is time to review procedures, pharmacology, and abbreviations by completing Learning Activity 8–4.

LEARNING ACTIVITIES

The activities that follow provide a review of the cardiovascular system terms introduced in this chapter. Complete each activity and review your answers to evaluate your understanding of the chapter.

Medical Language Lab
Turning terminology into language

Visit the Medical Language Laboratory at medicallanguagelab.com. Use it to enhance your study and reinforcement of this chapter with the flash card activity. We recommend that you complete the flash card activity before starting Learning Activities 8-1 and 8-2.

Learning Activity 8-1
Medical Word Elements

Use the listed elements to build medical words. You may use the elements more than once.

Combining Forms		Suffixes		Prefixes
aneurysm/o	scler/o	-ar	-lysis	a-
aort/o	sept/o	-al	-megaly	brady-
arteri/o	sten/o	-cardia	-oma	peri-
ather/o	thromb/o	-ectasis	-osis	trans-
cardi/o	valvul/o	-ectomy	-plasty	
phleb/o	ventricul/o	-gram	-therapy	
rrhythm/o		-ia		

1. slow heart (rate) _____

2. tumor composed of fatty plaque _____

3. condition of narrowing _____

4. pertaining to a ventricle _____

5. pertaining to across (or through) the septum _____

6. dilation or expansion of a vein _____

7. record of the aorta _____

8. surgical repair of a valve _____

9. abnormal condition of hardening _____

10. treatment that hardens (a varicose vein) _____

11. destruction of a blood clot _____

12. condition (of the heart) without a rhythm _____

13. pertaining to around an artery_____

14. enlargement of the heart _____

15. excision of an aneurysm _____

Check your answers in Appendix A. Review any material that you did not answer correctly.

Correct Answers _____ X 6.67 = _____ % Score

Learning Activity 8-2
Building Medical Words

Use *ather/o* (fatty plaque) to build words that mean:

1. tumor of fatty plaque _____
2. abnormal condition of fatty plaque hardening _____

Use *phleb/o* (vein) to build words that mean:

3. inflammation of a vein (wall) _____
4. abnormal condition of a blood clot in a vein _____

Use *ven/o* (vein) to build words that mean:

5. a small vein _____
6. spasm of a vein _____

Use *cardi/o* (heart) to build words that mean:

7. specialist in the study of the heart _____
8. rupture of the heart _____
9. disease of the heart muscle _____
10. enlargement of the heart _____

Use *angi/o* (vessel) to build words that mean:

11. surgical repair of a vessel _____
12. tumor of a vessel _____

Use *thromb/o* (blood clot) to build words that mean:

13. beginning or formation of a blood clot _____
14. abnormal condition of a blood clot _____

Use *aort/o* (heart) to build words that mean:

15. abnormal condition of narrowing or stricture of the aorta _____
16. process of recording the aorta _____

Build surgical words that mean:

17. puncture of the heart _____
18. suture of an artery _____
19. removal of an embolus _____
20. separation, destruction, or loosening of a blood clot _____

✓ *Check your answers in Appendix A. Review material that you did not answer correctly.*

Correct Answers _____ X 5 = _____ % Score

Learning Activity 8-3
Diseases and Conditions

Match the terms with the definitions in the numbered list.

aneurysm	*bruit*	*fibrillation*	*ischemia*
angina	*CHF*	*heart block*	*palpitation*
arrhythmia	*coarctation*	*hyperlipidemia*	*regurgitation*
arteriosclerosis	*diaphoresis*	*hypertension*	*syncope*
bradycardia	*embolism*	*infarction*	*tachycardia*

1. area of tissue that undergoes necrosis _____

2. pain, usually in the chest, that is associated with lack of oxygen to the myocardium _____

3. failure of a valve to close completely _____

4. abnormally rapid heart rate _____

5. loss of consciousness usually caused by a decreased supply of blood to the brain _____

6. soft, blowing sound heard on auscultation _____

7. heart failure that occurs when blood returning to the heart backs up into the lungs or other parts of the body causing congestion _____

8. sensation of an irregular heartbeat _____

9. abnormally rapid, uncoordinated quivering of the myocardium _____

10. localized abnormal dilation of a vessel _____

11. condition in which a mass (usually a blood clot) blocks a blood vessel _____

12. inability of the heart to maintain a normal rhythm _____

13. backflow of blood due to valve failure _____

14. profuse sweating _____

15. hardening of the wall of an artery _____

16. persistent elevated blood pressure _____

17. excessive amounts of lipids in the blood _____

18. narrowing of a vessel, especially the aorta _____

19. high cholesterol _____

20. interference with normal conduction of electrical impulses in the heart _____

Check your answers in Appendix A. Review any material that you did not answer correctly.

Correct Answers _____ X 5 = _____ % Score

Learning Activity 8-4
Procedures, Pharmacology, and Abbreviations

Match the terms with the definitions in the numbered list.

anticoagulants	Doppler	ICD	sclerotherapy
CABG	ECG	LDL	statins
cardioversion	ECHO	nitrates	stent placement
defibrillation	endarterectomy	PTCA	stress test
diuretics	Holter monitor test	PTT	troponin

1. 24-hour ECG tracing taken with a small, portable recording system _____
2. ultrasound test used to visualize internal cardiac structures _____
3. blood test to measure the time it takes for a blood clot to form _____
4. agents used to treat angina _____
5. drugs that have lipid-lowering properties _____
6. agents that increase urine output _____
7. measures protein released into the bloodstream by damaged heart muscle _____
8. ultrasound procedure that assesses blood flow direction and speed through blood vessels _____
9. ECG taken under controlled exercise conditions _____
10. lifesaving emergency treatment to restart the heart _____
11. defibrillation technique that restores the normal heart rhythm _____
12. graphically records the electrical activity of the heart _____
13. device inserted in the chest that corrects potential fatal arrhythmias _____
14. insertion of a device that holds open tubular structures _____
15. prevent the formation of clots in blood vessels _____
16. treatment of a varicose vein using a chemical irritant _____
17. surgery that creates a bypass around a blocked segment of a coronary artery _____
18. removal of occluding material from the interior of an artery _____
19. abbreviation for a type of coronary angioplasty _____
20. measures the level of low density fat in the bloodstream _____

Check your answers in Appendix A. Review any material that you did not answer correctly.

Correct Answers _____ X 5 = _____ % Score

DOCUMENTING HEALTH-CARE ACTIVITIES

This section provides practical application activities in the form of exercises to help students develop skills in documenting patient care. First, read the medical report. Then complete the activities and exercises that follow.

Documenting Health-Care Activity 8-1
Chart Note: Acute Myocardial Infarction

Gately, Mary   March 15, 20xx

Chief Complaint: Severe substernal pain with radiation to the back.

History of Present Illness: This 68-year-old woman has had a history of sudden onset of chest pain. Similarly, approximately 2 hours before hospitalization, she had severe substernal pain with radiation to the back. ECG and cardiac enzyme tests showed evidence of abnormalities. She was given streptokinase and treated with heparin at 800 units per hour.

Past History: Patient has a history of an inferior MI in 19xx. She was seen in 20xx, but she was stable at that time and underwent a treadmill stress test. Test results showed no ischemia and she had no chest pain.

Impression: Acute lateral anterior myocardial infarction and a previously healed inferior myocardial infarction.

Plan: Patient admitted for acute anterior myocardial infarction. She will be evaluated with a partial thromboplastin time and cardiac enzymes in the morning. At this time the patient is stable, is in the CCU, and will be given appropriate follow-up and supportive care.

Juan Perez, MD
Juan Perez, MD

D: 03–15–20xx
T: 03–15–20xx

bg

Terminology

The terms listed in the table that follows are taken from *Chart Note: Acute Myocardial Infarction*. Use a medical dictionary such as *Taber's Cyclopedic Medical Dictionary*, the appendices of this book, or other resources to define each term. Then review the pronunciation for each term and practice by reading the medical record aloud.

Term	Definition
acute	
cardiac enzymes KĂR-dē-ăk ĔN-zīmz	
ECG	
heparin HĔP-ă-rĭn	
infarction ĭn-FĂRK-shŭn	
ischemia ĭs-KĒ-mē-ă	
lateral LĂT-ĕr-ăl	
MI	
myocardial mī-ō-KĂR-dē-ăl	
partial thrombo- plastin time thrŏm-bō-PLĂS-tĭn	
streptokinase strĕp-tō-KĪ-nās	
substernal sŭb-STĔR-năl	

Visit the Medical Terminology Systems online resource center at FADavis. com to practice pronunciation and reinforce the meanings of the terms in this medical report.

Critical Thinking

Review *Chart Note: Acute Myocardial Infarction* to answer the questions.

1. How long had the patient experienced chest pain before she was seen at the hospital?

_____

_____

_____

2. Did the patient have a previous history of chest pain?

_____

_____

_____

3. Initially, what medications were administered to stabilize the patient?

_____

_____

_____

4. What two laboratory tests will be used to evaluate the patient?

_____

_____

_____

5. During the current admission, what part of the heart was damaged?

_____

_____

_____

6. Was the location of damage to the heart for this admission the same as that for the initial MI?

_____

_____

_____

SOAP Note: Deep Venous Thrombosis

Progress Note

Franks, Robert   May 14, 20XX

CC: The patient is a 62-year-old man referred for an opinion regarding deep venous thrombosis (DVT) of the right leg.

Subjective: Patient reports a history of a stress fracture of the right foot 5 months ago, resulting in placement of a cast for 3 months. He had some problems with swelling of the right leg. A subsequent right leg ultrasound demonstrated evidence of acute thrombosis of the right popliteal veins and a thrombus in one of the tibial veins in the calf. The patient was then placed on anticoagulation, first with Lovenox and eventually warfarin. Initial swelling in the leg has improved but he still complains of some discomfort, decrease in mobility, and difficulty weightbearing on the right foot.

Objective: On physical examination, the patient appears his stated age. He is awake and alert. Blood pressure is 132/78. Pulse is 74 and regular. Lungs are clear to auscultation. Heart tones are regular. Abdominal examination reveals a soft, nontender abdomen. His aortic pulsation feels normal. Femoral, popliteal, and pedal pulses are palpable bilaterally. There is some very mild swelling in the right ankle and foot, but no swelling in the calf. He has no venous varicosities.

Assessment: Right popliteal and calf vein DVT, most likely due to immobilization of the right leg due to a foot fracture and casting. Based on his physical examination, he does not have a significant venous outflow obstruction because there is minimal to no swelling at this point.

Plan: Continue anticoagulation with warfarin for a period of three to six months. We would recommend a popliteal ultrasound at three months to look for vein recanalization. Following the period of anticoagulation, a knee-high support stocking is recommended. We will plan to see the patient back on a p.r.n. basis. The patient verbalizes understanding of the plan and is in agreement with the stated recommendations.

Dante Riox, MD
Dante Riox, MD

dr:bg

D: 5–14–20xx; T: 5–14–20xx

Terminology

The terms listed in the table that follows are taken from "SOAP Note: Deep Venous Thrombosis." Use a medical dictionary such as *Taber's Cyclopedic Medical Dictionary*, the appendices of this book, or other resources to define each term. Then review the pronunciation for each term and practice by reading the medical record aloud.

Term	Definition
anticoagulation ăn-tĭ-kō-ĂG-ū-lā-shŭn	
auscultation aws-kŭl-TĀ-shŭn	
deep venous thrombosis VĒ-nŭs thrŏm-BŌ-sĭs	
DVT	
Lovenox LŎ-vēn-ŏx	
palpable PĂL-pă-b'l	
popliteal pŏp-LĬT-ē-ăl	
p.r.n.	
recanalization rē-CĂN-ă-lĭz-ā-shŭn	
varicosities văr-ĭ-KŎS-ĭ-tēz	
venous VĒ-nŭs	
warfarin WĂR-fă-rĭn	

Visit the Medical Terminology Systems online resource center at FADavis. com to practice pronunciation and reinforce the meanings of the terms in this medical report.

Critical Thinking

Review *SOAP Note: Deep Venous Thrombosis* to answer the questions.

1. What were the findings on the ultrasound of the right leg?

2. How was the DVT initially treated?

3. What is causing the continued weightbearing difficulty on the right foot?

4. What is the risk factor for DVT in this patient?

5. What are the recommendations for follow-up?

Constructing Chart Notes

To construct chart notes, replace the italicized and boldfaced terms in each of the two case studies with one of the listed medical terms.

angina pectoris	*edema*	*myocardial infarction*
angioplasty	*hypertension*	*palpitations*
catheter	*ischemia*	*stent*
diaphoresis		

Mr. J. presented to the emergency room with complaints of (1) **chest pains,** (2) **profuse sweating,** and (3) **an awareness of his heart skipping beats.** He takes medication for (4) **persistent high blood pressure.** He also takes diuretics to promote urine excretion and to control fluid retention that is causing (5) **puffiness** in his ankles and legs.

1. _____
2. _____
3. _____
4. _____
5. _____

Mrs. R has a family history of coronary artery disease. Her 60-year-old uncle died of a (6) **heart attack** 2 years ago. Last year, her father was diagnosed with an occlusion of the coronary artery. He was also diagnosed with (7) **decreased blood flow** of the coronary vessels. He was admitted to the hospital for a (8) **surgical repair of the vessel.** During this surgery, the surgeon threaded a (9) **tube** with a deflated balloon into the blocked vessel and used it to press the fatty plaque against the arterial walls. The surgeon then inserted an (10) **expandable mesh tube** to keep the artery open after surgery.

6. _____
7. _____
8. _____
9. _____
10. _____

Check your answers in Appendix A. Review any material that you did not answer correctly.

Correct Answers _____ X 10 = _____ % Score

Blood, Lymphatic, and Immune Systems

Objectives

Upon completion of this chapter, you will be able to:

- Identify and describe the components of blood.
- Locate and identify the structures associated with the lymphatic system.
- Explain the various types of immune processes.
- Describe the mechanisms of protection provided through innate immunity.
- List the cells associated with the acquired immune response and describe their function.
- Describe the functional relationships among the blood, lymphatic, and immune systems and other body systems.
- Pronounce, spell, and build words related to the blood, lymphatic, and immune systems.
- Describe diseases, conditions, and procedures related to the blood, lymphatic, and immune systems.
- Explain pharmacology related to the treatment of blood, lymphatic, and immune disorders.
- Demonstrate your knowledge of this chapter by completing the learning and documenting health-care activities.

Anatomy and Physiology

The **blood, lymphatic,** and **immune systems** have separate but interrelated functions in maintaining a healthy environment within the body **(homeostasis).**

Blood is responsible for transporting oxygen (O_2) and carbon dioxide (CO_2) and provides cells that defend against disease. It also protects the body from loss of blood by the action of clotting.

The lymphatic system helps maintain fluid balance and is responsible for cellular communication by delivering nutrients, hormones, and other needed products to body cells while removing their waste products as it drains tissue fluid back to the vascular system. It also provides the cells of the immune system needed to defend the body against disease.

The immune system defends the body against harmful invaders. In its most simple form, it uses barriers that exclude unwanted substances from entering the body. In its most complex form, it uses cells of the lymphatic system to undertake the intricate processes that identify and destroy pathogens and protect the body against future encounters with previously encountered infectious agents.

Anatomy and Physiology Key Terms

This section introduces important blood, lymphatic, and immune system terms and their definitions. The key terms are highlighted in color in the Anatomy and Physiology section. Word analyses for selected terms are also provided. Pronounce the term, and place a check mark in the box after you do so.

Term	Definition
antibody ☐ ĂN-tĭ-bŏd-ē	Proteins produced by B lymphocytes in response to the presence of foreign substances called *antigens;* also known as *immunoglobulins* *Antibodies are highly specific and recognize and bind to specific antigens to destroy or neutralize their harmful effects on the body.*
antigen ☐ ĂN-tĭ-jĕn	Foreign substances, recognized as harmful to the body, that induce an immune response with the production of antibodies *Antigens include bacteria, viruses, fungi, cancerous cells, and any substance considered toxic to the body.*
bile pigments ☐ BĪL	Substances derived from the breakdown of hemoglobin and excreted by the liver *Bilirubin and biliverdin are the main pigments in bile.*
bilirubin ☐ bĭl-ĭ-RŪ-bĭn	A yellow pigment produced during the normal breakdown of red blood cells (RBCs) and excreted in bile *Jaundice occurs when there is an accumulation of bilirubin and causes yellowing of the skin and sclera (white of the eye) of the eyes.*
biliverdin ☐ bĭl-ĭ-vĕr-dĭn	A green pigment excreted in bile; the oxidized form of bilirubin
cytokine ☐ SĪ-tō-kīn	Small, nonstructural proteins that play a key role in signaling other cells to regulate the inflammatory and immune responses *Dysregulation of cytokine response can lead to autoimmune disorders, inflammatory conditions, certain cancers, and other diseases.*
dendritic cell ☐ dĕn-DRĬT-ĭk *dendr:* tree *-itic:* pertaining to	Specialized antigen presenting cells found in tissues throughout the body that initiate and regulate specific immune responses

Anatomy and Physiology Key Terms—cont'd

Term	Definition
immunocompetent ĭm-ū-nō-KŎM-pĕ-tĕnt	Possessing the ability to develop an immune response
natural killer (NK) cells	Specialized lymphocytes that destroy cells that display signs of infection, stress, or abnormality by releasing chemicals that disrupt their cell membranes, ultimately inducing cellular death *NK cells are components of the innate immune system and do not require prior sensitization to engage in cell destruction.*

Pronunciation Help	Long Sound	ā — rate	ē — rebirth	ī — isle	ō — over	ū — unite
	Short Sound	ă — apple	ĕ — ever	ĭ — it	ŏ — not	ŭ — cut

Blood

Blood is connective tissue composed of a liquid medium called **plasma** in which solid components are suspended. The solid components of blood include the following:

- red blood cells (**erythrocytes**)
- white blood cells (**leukocytes**)
- platelets (**thrombocytes**; see Fig. 9-1)

The body produces millions of blood cells every second to replace those that are destroyed or worn out. In adults, blood cells form in the bone marrow of the skull, ribs, sternum, vertebrae, pelvis, and ends of the long bones of the arms and legs. The stem cells in the bone marrow give rise to embryonic (**blastic**) forms of all blood cell types. In the embryonic stages, monocytes and lymphocytes migrate to the lymphatic system for maturation and specialization. All other embryonic cells remain in the bone marrow to complete their development. Once blood cells mature, they enter the circulatory system. The development of blood cells into their mature forms is called *hematopoiesis* or *hemopoiesis* (see Fig. 9-2).

Plasma (55% of total volume)

Formed elements (45% of total volume)

Thrombocytes (platelets)

Erythrocytes

Monocyte

Lymphocyte

Neutrophil

Eosinophil

Basophil

Leukocytes

Figure 9-1 Blood composition.

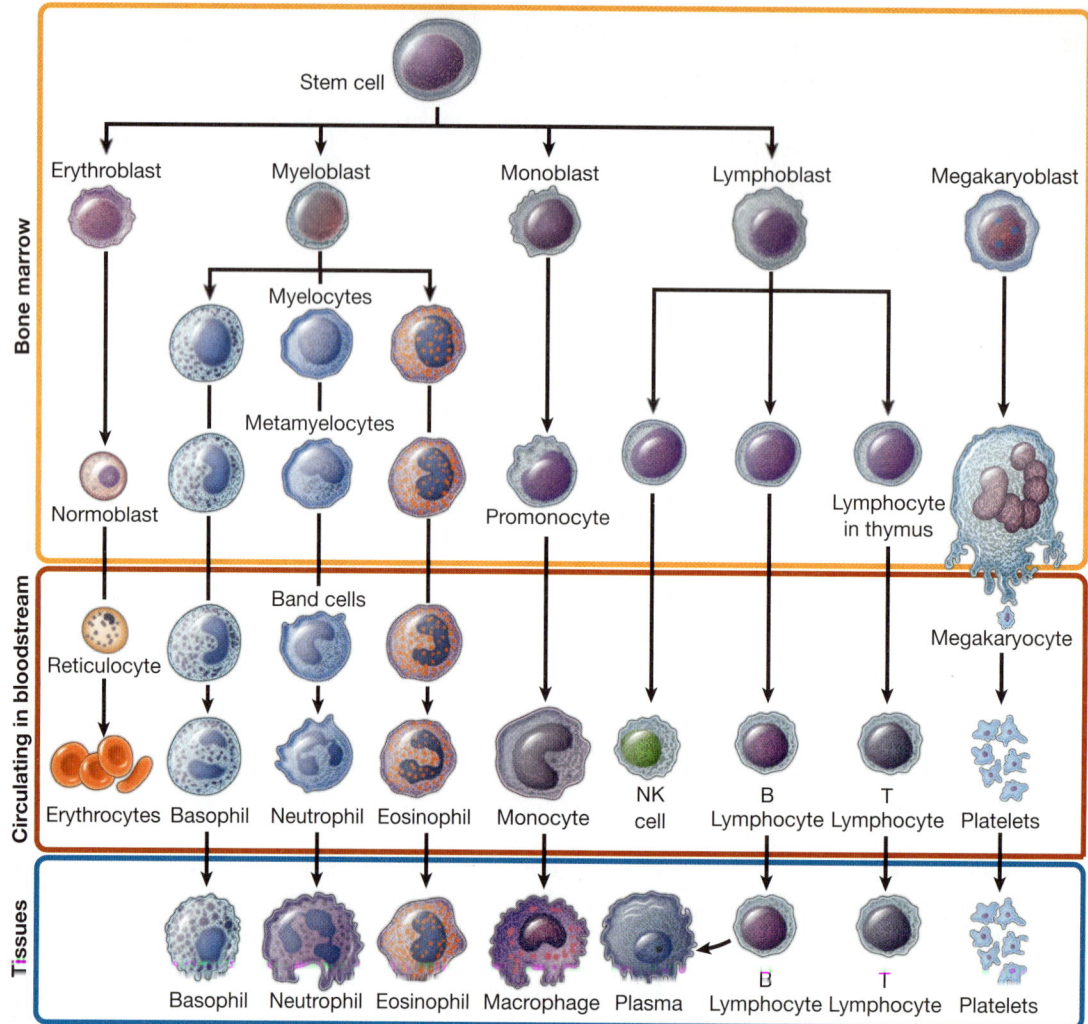

Figure 9-2 Hematopoiesis.

Red Blood Cells

Red blood cells (RBCs), or **erythrocytes,** transport O_2 and CO_2. They are the most numerous of the circulating blood cells. During RBC development **(erythropoiesis),** they decrease in size and, just before reaching maturity, extrude their nuclei. They also develop a specialized iron-containing compound called **hemoglobin (Hb, Hgb)** that gives them their red color. Hemoglobin carries O_2 to body tissues and exchanges it for CO_2. When mature, RBCs are shaped like biconcave disks of approximately the same size and hemoglobin concentration.

RBCs live about 120 days and then rupture, releasing hemoglobin and cell fragments. Hemoglobin breaks down into an iron compound called **hemosiderin** and several **bile pigments.** Most hemosiderin returns to the bone marrow for reuse in a different form to manufacture new blood cells. The two main bile pigments, **bilirubin** and **biliverdin,** are eventually excreted by the liver.

White Blood Cells

White blood cells (WBCs), or **leukocytes,** protect the body against invasion by pathogens and foreign substances, remove debris from injured tissue, and aid in the healing process. Leukocytes are crucial to the body's defense against disease because of their ability to ingest and destroy bacteria and other foreign particles through **phagocytosis** (see Fig. 9-3). Unlike RBCs that remain in the bloodstream, WBCs migrate through endothelial walls of capillaries and venules **(diapedesis)** and enter tissue spaces as part of the inflammatory response (see Fig. 9-4).

Figure 9-3 Phagocytosis.

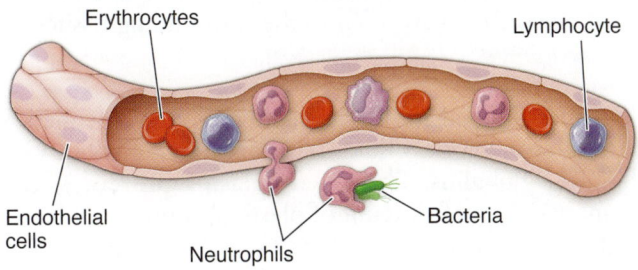

Figure 9-4 Diapedesis.

The two major types of leukocytes are classified according to the presence of granules in their cytoplasm (**granulocytes**) or absence of granules in their cytoplasm (**agranulocytes**) when observed microscopically. The granulocytic leukocytes are further classified as **neutrophils**, **eosinophils**, and **basophils** according to the staining reaction of their cytoplasmic granules during the preparation of blood smears for microscopic examination. The nuclei of mature granulocytes are so deeply lobed, especially in neutrophils, that these cells appear to have multiple nuclei, providing an alternative naming classification as **polymorphonuclear leukocytes (PMNLs, polys)**. This nuclear characteristic is not typical of agranulocytes, **lymphocytes**, and **monocytes**. Therefore, agranulocytes are more commonly called **mononuclear lymphocytes (MNLs)**. Because each type of leukocyte performs a different function, it is important for diagnostic purposes to identify their type and know whether their quantity falls within the normal range of bloodwork values. Table 9-1 summarizes important information regarding the five major types of leukocytes.

TABLE 9-1 White Blood Cells

This table lists the five types of leukocytes, their identifying morphology, and their function.

Cell Type	Nucleus	Cytoplasm	Function
Granulocytes			
Neutrophil	Polymorphonuclear	Lilac granules	• First cell to arrive at a site of injury • Provides nonspecific protection by phagocytosis • Dies as a result of phagocytosis
Eosinophil	Polymorphonuclear	Red granules	• Combats multicellular parasites (worm infestations) • Controls mechanisms associated with allergies
Basophil	Polymorphonuclear	Purple granules	• Initiates inflammation
Agranulocytes			
Lymphocytes	Mononuclear	Agranular	• Provides acquired (specific) immunity
Monocytes	Mononuclear	Agranular	• Performs mildly phagocytic function • Becomes a macrophage when it enters tissues and functions in immunity

Platelets

Platelets (**thrombocytes**) are the smallest formed elements found in blood. They are not true cells but merely cell fragments. Platelets initiate blood clotting or **coagulation** when they encounter vessel walls that have been injured or traumatized. Initially, platelets become sticky and aggregate at the injury site to form a barrier to control blood loss. Clotting factors in platelets and injured tissue release **thromboplastin,** a substance that initiates clot formation. In the final step of coagulation, **fibrinogen** (a soluble blood protein) becomes insoluble and forms fibrin strands that act as a net, entrapping blood cells. This jellylike mass of blood cells and fibrin (**thrombus, blood clot**) impedes the flow of blood (**hemostasis**) into the surrounding tissues.

Plasma

Plasma is the liquid portion of blood in which blood cells are suspended. Without blood cells, plasma appears as a thin, almost colorless fluid. It is composed of about 92% water and contains such products as albumins, globulins, fibrinogen (**plasma proteins**), clotting factors, gases, nutrients, salts, and hormones. A small amount of plasma continuously leaks from capillaries and delivers these products to surrounding cells and exchanges them for waste material produced by body cells. This exchange makes cellular communication possible throughout the body. **Blood serum** is a product of blood plasma formed when fibrinogen and clotting factors are removed from blood plasma (see Fig. 9-1).

Blood Types

Human blood is divided into four types, A, B, AB, and O, based on the presence or absence of specific **antigens** on the surface of RBCs. In each of these four blood types, the erythrocyte carries the antigen that gives the name of the blood type. The plasma contains the opposite **antibody;** for example, type A blood contains A antigen on the surface of the RBC, and the plasma contains B **antibody** (see Fig. 9-5).

Blood types are medically important in transfusions, transplants, and maternal-fetal incompatibilities. In addition to antigens of the four blood types, there are numerous other antigens that may be present on RBCs, but most of these are not of medical concern.

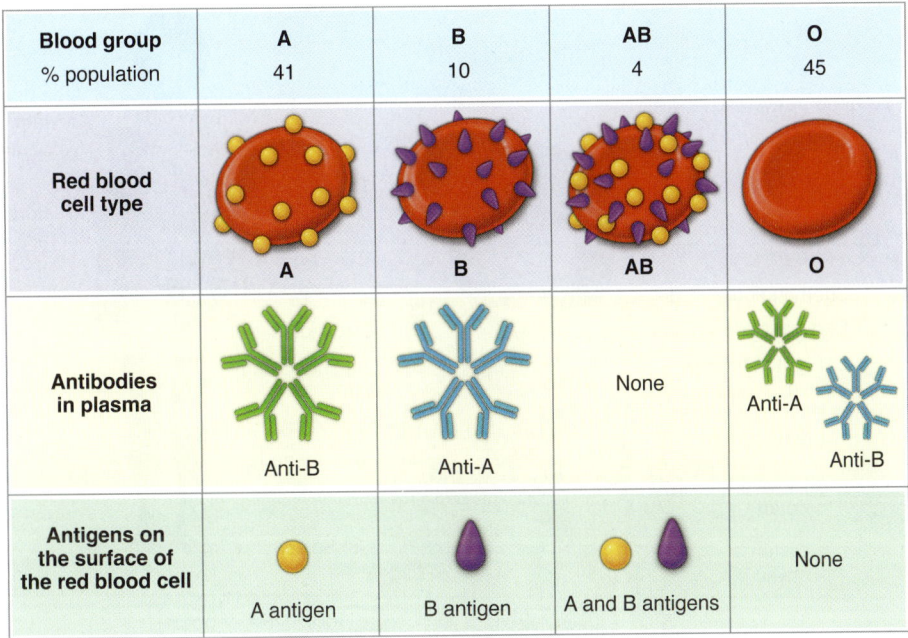

Blood group % population	A 41	B 10	AB 4	O 45
Red blood cell type	A	B	AB	O
Antibodies in plasma	Anti-B	Anti-A	None	Anti-A Anti-B
Antigens on the surface of the red blood cell	A antigen	B antigen	A and B antigens	None

Figure 9-5 ABO blood types.

Lymphatic System

The lymphatic system consists of a fluid called **lymph** that contains lymphocytes and monocytes, a network of transporting vessels called **lymph vessels,** and a multiplicity of other structures, including nodes, the spleen, the thymus, and the tonsils. Functions of the lymphatic system include the following:

- maintaining fluid balance of the body by draining interstitial fluid from tissue spaces and returning it to the blood
- transporting lipids away from the digestive organs for use by body tissues
- filtering and removing unwanted or infectious products in lymph nodes

Lymph vessels are thin-walled vessels that carry lymph throughout the body and begin as closed-ended capillaries in tissue spaces (see Fig. 9-6). As whole blood circulates, a small amount of plasma seeps from (1) **blood capillaries** and enters surrounding tissue. This fluid, now called **interstitial** or **tissue fluid,** carries needed products to tissue cells while removing their wastes. As interstitial fluid moves through tissues, it collects cellular debris, bacteria, and particulate matter. Upon completing these functions, interstitial fluid returns to the surrounding venules to become plasma or enters closed-ended microscopic vessels called (2) **lymph capillaries** to become lymph. Lymph passes into increasingly larger vessels on its return trip to the bloodstream. Before it reaches its final destination, it first enters (3) **lymph nodes** through afferent vessels. In the node, macrophages phagocytize bacteria and other harmful material, and T cells and B cells exert their protective influence. When a local infection exists, the number of bacteria entering a node is so great and the destruction by T cells and B cells so powerful that the node commonly enlarges and becomes tender. Once filtered, lymph exits the node by way of efferent vessels to continue its return to the circulatory system.

Lymph vessels from the right chest and arm join the (4) **right lymphatic duct.** This duct drains into the (5) **right subclavian vein,** a major vessel in the cardiovascular system. Lymph from all other areas of the body enters the (6) **thoracic duct** and drains into the (7) **left subclavian vein.** Lymph is redeposited into the circulating blood and becomes plasma. This cycle continually repeats itself.

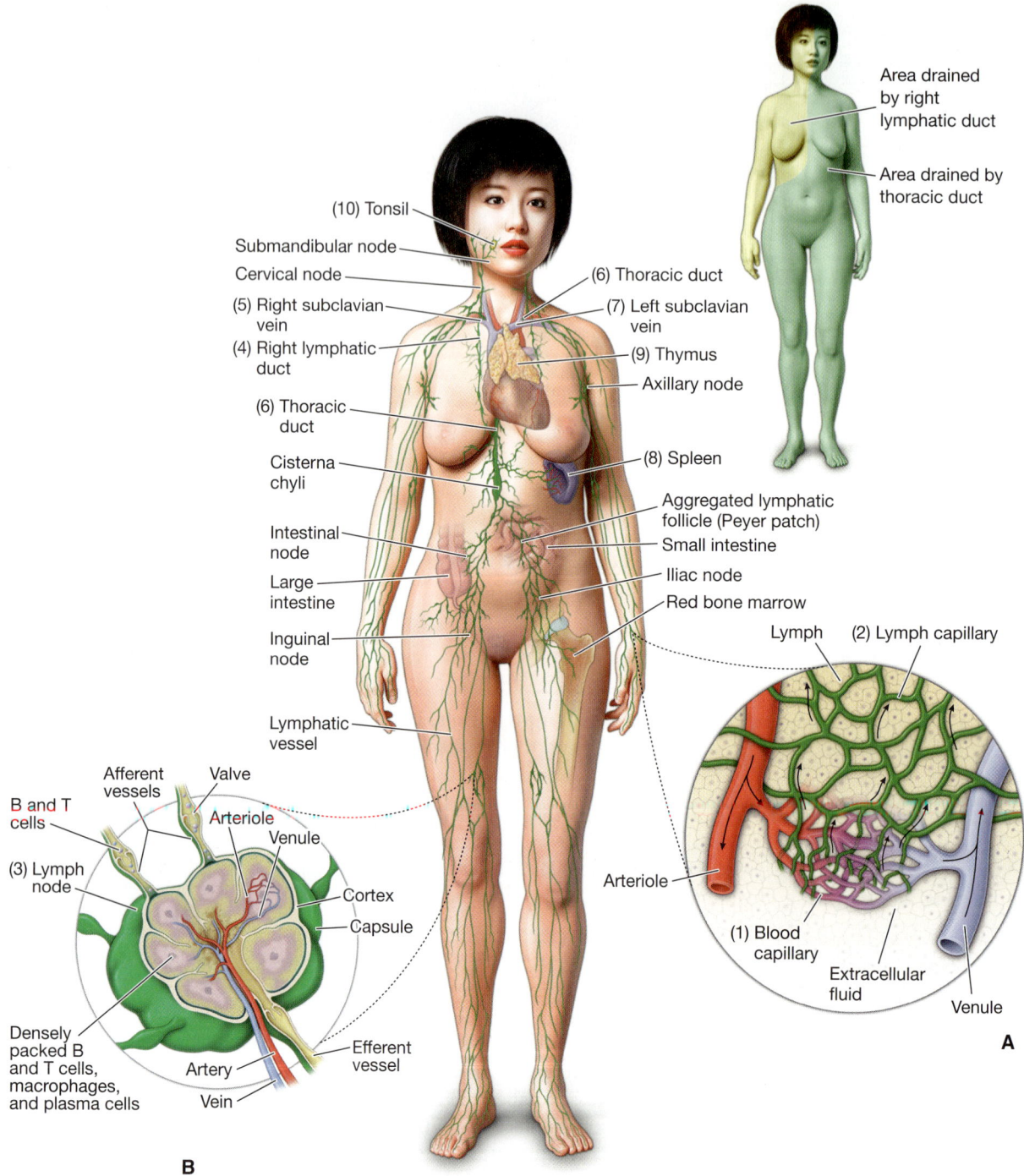

Area drained by right lymphatic duct

Area drained by thoracic duct

(10) Tonsil
Submandibular node
Cervical node
(5) Right subclavian vein
(4) Right lymphatic duct
(6) Thoracic duct
Cisterna chyli
Intestinal node
Large intestine
Inguinal node
Lymphatic vessel

(6) Thoracic duct
(7) Left subclavian vein
(9) Thymus
Axillary node
(8) Spleen
Aggregated lymphatic follicle (Peyer patch)
Small intestine
Iliac node
Red bone marrow

Lymph   (2) Lymph capillary

Arteriole

(1) Blood capillary
Extracellular fluid
Venule

A

Afferent vessels   Valve
B and T cells
Arteriole
Venule
(3) Lymph node
Cortex
Capsule
Densely packed B and T cells, macrophages, and plasma cells
Artery
Vein
Efferent vessel

B

Figure 9-6 Lymphatic system. (A) Lymph capillary. (B) Lymph node.

The (8) **spleen** resembles a lymph node because it acts as a filter by removing cellular debris, bacteria, parasites, and other infectious agents. However, the spleen also destroys old RBCs and serves as a repository for healthy blood cells. The (9) **thymus** is located in the upper part of the chest (**mediastinum**). It partially controls the immune system by transforming certain lymphocytes into T cells to function in the immune system. The (10) **tonsils** are masses of lymphatic tissue located in the pharynx. They act as filters to protect the upper respiratory structures from invasion by pathogens.

Immune System

The function of the immune system is to protect the body against harmful invaders such as bacteria, viruses, fungi, and parasites, as well as abnormal cells such as cancer cells. The immune system's key role is to initiate the immune response. This is a complex and highly orchestrated effort between the blood and lymphatic system to identify, neutralize, and destroy potentially harmful invaders while protecting the body's own tissues. The immune response provides the body with numerous defenses called *immunity* that work together to protect against harmful invaders and disease.

There are two major types of immunity that protect the body against disease-causing organisms (**pathogens**). The first type, called **innate immunity,** includes barriers designed to keep the pathogen from entering the body. The second type, called **acquired (adaptive) immunity,** identifies and destroys pathogens once they enter the body (see Fig. 9-7).

Innate Immunity

Innate immunity begins functioning at birth or immediately afterward. Because it is present at the very beginning of life, it is called the **innate immune system.** It provides protective barriers to the entry of pathogens into the body and stops their spread should they successfully overcome the barriers. This system does not differentiate the various types of pathogens and defends the body with an immediate response. Therefore, the innate immune system is also considered **nonspecific** (see Fig. 9-8). The innate immune system provides two types of barriers:

- **first-line barriers,** including the skin, mucous membranes, tears, saliva, and gastric secretions, keep pathogens from entering the body
- **second-line barriers,** including phagocytic cells, **natural killer cells**, and inflammation, stop the spread of pathogens once they have entered the body

Acquired Immunity

Acquired or **adaptive immunity** develops after birth in an **immunocompetent** individual and is a lifelong monitoring system (see Fig. 9-9). During each encounter with an antigen, the acquired immune system produces unique cells and processes that destroy the particular antigen. The method of destroying the antigen is "custom made" for each specific antigenic encounter. The response of acquired immunity is **specific** and of a delayed onset and performed by monocytes and lymphocytes.

Figure 9-7 Types of immunity.

Figure 9-8 Innate immunity.

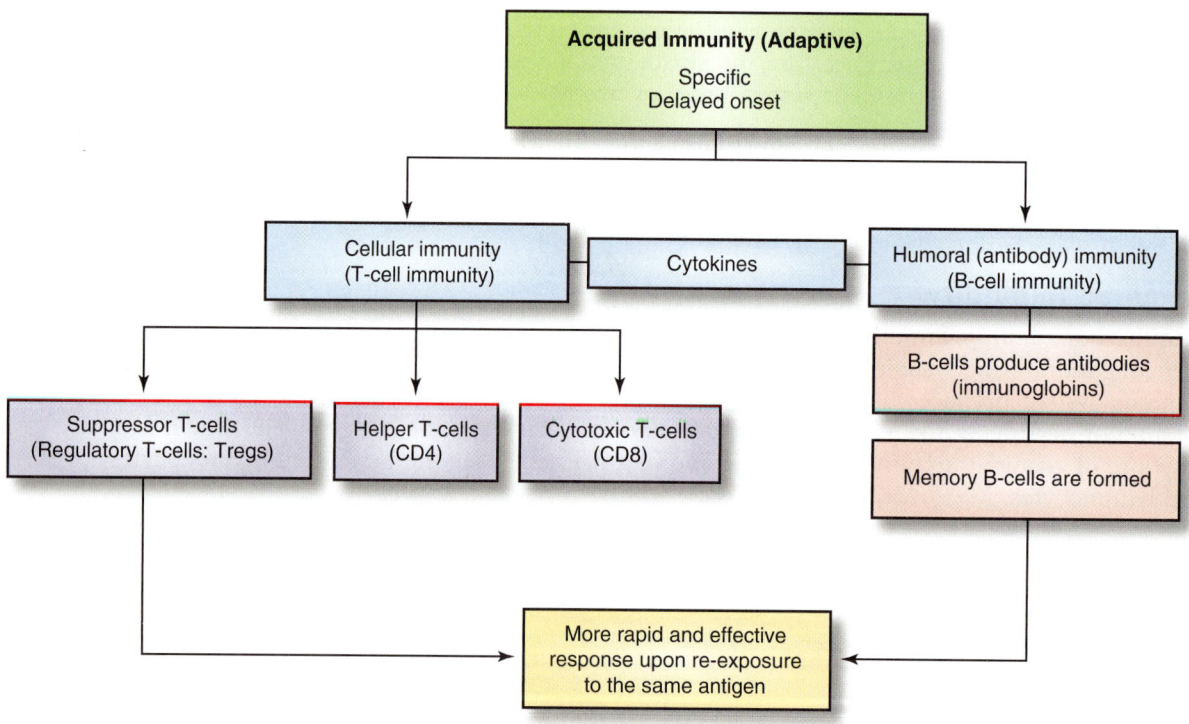

Figure 9-9 Acquired immunity.

Monocytes

Monocytes play a crucial role in the immune response between the innate and acquired immune system. Monocytes leave the bloodstream and enter tissues where they undergo differentiation into phagocytic **macrophages.** In this form, the macrophage ingests pathogens and other harmful substances, processing them while maintaining their distinctive antigenic properties. Subsequently, these preserved properties are exhibited on the macrophage surface and signal the acquired immune system to the presence of a pathogen. The macrophage is now considered an **antigen-presenting cell (APC). Dendritic cells** also have the ability to act as APCs. The dendritic cells migrate to lymph nodes, where they present the antigen to T cells, to initiate the acquired immune response. Upon this encounter, the acquired immune system begins the systematic destruction of the antigen.

Lymphocytes

Two types of lymphocytes, B cells (**B lymphocytes**) and T cells (**T lymphocytes**), are the active cells of the acquired immune response. When B cells respond as the principal defense, **humoral** or **antibody immunity** results. When T cells respond as the main defense system, **cellular immunity results**. Although each of these defenses is identified singly, there is a great deal of interaction between them. **Cytokines**, hormonelike chemicals, serve as messengers facilitating communication between these two defense systems (see Fig. 9-9). They control the magnitude and duration of responses while enabling intracellular communication among their diverse cell types. Table 9-2 provides information on the cells associated with the acquired immune system.

TABLE 9-2 Lymphocytes and Immune Response

This table provides the functions of the major lymphocytes of the immune system.

Lymphocyte	Function
B cells	• Function in humoral immunity
	• Originate and mature in bone marrow
	• Protect against extracellular antigens
	• Respond to stimulation by a compatible T cell and begin producing plasma cells
plasma cells	• Create highly specific antibodies that bind to their corresponding antigens forming unique molecules called *antigen–antibody complexes* that lead to the destruction of the antigen by the immune system
memory B cells	• Retreat to lymphatic system and remain prepared to repeat the same procedure upon a subsequent encounter with the same antigen
NK (natural killer) cells	• Provide rapid and nonspecific defense against infected or abnormal cells
	• Recognize infected cells before they are coated with antibodies
	• Release chemicals to destroy infected cells
	• Important in surveillance and elimination of cancer cells and destruction of tumor cells
T cells	• Function in cellular immunity
	• Originate in bone marrow and mature in lymphatic system
	• Protect against intracellular pathogens and cancer cells
cytotoxic T (CD8) cells	• Determine and attack the specific weakness of the cell and destroy it
helper T (CD4) cells	• Provide essential assistance to maintain B-cell activity
	• Produce cytokines that activate, direct, and regulate most of the other components of the immune system
	• Require a threshold number to avoid a shutdown of the entire immune system
suppressor T cells	• Monitor and terminate humoral and cellular response when infection resolves
	• Prevent immune overactivity to protect against autoimmune disease
memory T cells	• Migrate to lymphatic system and remain prepared for a second encounter should the same antigen reappear

The memory component is unique to the acquired immune response. Memory B and memory T cells are able to recognize previous antigens and are able to respond with a more rapid and effective attack. This long-lasting immunity is referred to as **active immunity**. Active immunity can be acquired through natural exposure to an infectious agent, such as a person getting infected with a flu virus, or through vaccination, such as the injection of the flu vaccine.

Anatomy Review: Lymphatic System

To review the anatomy of the lymphatic system, label the illustration that follows using the listed terms.

blood capillary   *right lymphatic duct*   *thoracic duct*

left subclavian vein   *right subclavian vein*   *thymus*

lymph capillary   *spleen*   *tonsil*

lymph node

Area drained by right lymphatic duct

Area drained by thoracic duct

Submandibular node

Cervical node

Axillary node

Cisterna chyli

Aggregated lymphatic follicle (Peyer patch)

Intestinal node

Small intestine

Large intestine

Iliac node

Red bone marrow

Inguinal node

Lymph

Lymphatic vessel

Afferent vessels

Valve

B and T cells

Arteriole

Venule

Cortex

Capsule

Arteriole

Densely packed B and T cells, macrophages, and plasma cells

Artery

Efferent vessel

Extracellular fluid

Venule

Vein

A

B

Check your answers by referring to Figure 9-6 on page 286. Review material that you did not answer correctly.

CONNECTING BODY SYSTEMS—BLOOD, LYMPHATIC, AND IMMUNE SYSTEMS

The main functions of the blood, lymphatic, and immune systems are to provide a way to transport and exchange products throughout the body and protect and repair cells that are damaged by disease or trauma. Specific functional relationships between the blood, lymphatic, and immune systems and other body systems are summarized here.

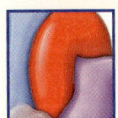

Cardiovascular
- Blood delivers oxygen needed for contraction of the heart.
- The lymphatic system returns interstitial fluid to the vascular system to maintain blood volume.
- The immune system protects against infections.

Digestive
- Blood transports products of digestion to nourish body cells.
- The immune system provides surveillance mechanisms to detect and destroy cancer cells in the digestive tract.
- As an innate component of the immune system, the acidic environment of the stomach helps control pathogens in the digestive tract.
- Specialized lymphoid nodules located in the lining of the small intestine, known as *Peyer patches*, contain immune cells to detect and respond to pathogens from ingested food to protect the body from infections and maintain intestinal homeostasis.

Endocrine
- The blood and lymphatic systems transport hormones to target organs.
- The immune system protects against infection in endocrine glands.

Female Reproductive
- The blood, lymphatic, and immune systems transport nourishing and defensive products across the placental barrier for the developing fetus.
- The immune system provides specific defense against pathogens that enter the body through the reproductive tract.
- The immune system supplies antibodies for breast milk that protect the baby until its immune system is established.

Integumentary
- The skin is the body's first line of defense against pathogenic invaders.
- Blood provides leukocytes, especially neutrophils, to the integumentary system when breaches or injury occurs in the skin.
- The lymphatic system supplies antibodies to the dermis for defense against pathogens.
- Blood in the skin, the largest organ of the body, helps maintain temperature homeostasis.

Male Reproductive
- The immune system provides surveillance against cancer cells.
- Blood delivers hormones and other essential products for male fertility.
- Lymph maintains fluid balance in the male organs of reproduction.

Musculoskeletal
- Blood removes lactic acid that accumulates in muscles during strenuous exercise.
- Blood transports calcium to bones for strength and healing.
- The lymphatic system maintains interstitial fluid balance in muscle tissue.
- The immune system aids in the repair of muscle tissue following trauma.

Nervous
- The immune system responds to nervous stimuli to identify injury or infection sites and initiate tissue defense and repair.
- Plasma and lymph provide the media in which nervous stimuli cross from one neuron to another.
- The lymphatic system removes excess interstitial fluid from tissues surrounding nerves.

Continued

CONNECTING BODY SYSTEMS—BLOOD, LYMPHATIC, AND IMMUNE SYSTEMS—cont'd

Respiratory
- RBCs transport respiratory gases to and from the lungs.
- The tonsils harbor immune cells to combat pathogens that enter through the nose and mouth.

Urinary
- Blood transports waste products, especially urea, to the kidneys for removal via the production of urine.
- Blood in peritubular capillaries reabsorbs essential products that have been filtered by the nephron.

Medical Word Elements

This section introduces combining forms, suffixes, and prefixes related to the blood, lymphatic, and immune systems. Word analyses are also provided. From the information provided, complete the meaning of the medical words in the right-hand column. The first one is completed for you.

Element	Meaning	Word Analysis
Combining Forms		
aden/o	gland	**aden/o**/pathy (ăd-ĕ-NŎP-ă-thē): *disease of a gland* *-pathy:* disease
agglutin/o	clumping, gluing	**agglutin**/ation (ă-gloo-tĭ-NĀ-shŭn): _____ *-ation:* process (of)
blast/o	embryonic cell	erythr/o/**blast**/osis (ĕ-rĭth-rō-blăs-TŌ-sĭs): _____ *erythr/o:* red *-osis:* abnormal condition; increase (used primarily with blood cells) *Erythroblasts are normally found only in bone marrow and develop into mature erythrocytes during hematopoiesis.*
chrom/o	color	hypo/**chrom**/ic (hī-pō-KRŌM-ĭk): _____ *hypo-:* under, below, deficient *-ic:* pertaining to *Hypochromic cells are erythrocytes that appear lighter in color than normal because of a deficiency of hemoglobin, a compound that gives erythrocytes their red color.*
erythr/o	red	**erythr/o**/cyte (ĕ-RĬTH-rō-sīt): _____ *-cyte:* cell *An erythrocyte is an RBC.*
granul/o	granule	**granul/o**/cyte (GRĂN-ū-lō-sīt): _____ *-cyte:* cell

Medical Word Elements—cont'd

Element	Meaning	Word Analysis
hem/o	blood	**hem/o**/phobia (hē-mō-FŌ-bē-ă): _____ *–phobia:* fear
hemat/o		*People who suffer from hemophobia commonly faint at the sight of blood.* **hemat**/oma (hē-mă-TŌ-mă): _____ *–oma:* tumor *A hematoma is a mass of extravasated, usually clotted blood, caused by a break or leak in a blood vessel. It may be found in any organ, tissue, or space within the body.*
immun/o	immune, immunity, safe	**immun/o**/logy (ĭm-ū-NŎL-ō-jē): _____ *–logy:* study of *Immunology includes the study of autoimmune diseases, hypersensitivities, and immune deficiencies.*
leuk/o	white	**leuk**/emia (loo-KĒ-mē-ă): _____ *–emia:* blood condition *Leukemia causes a profoundly elevated WBC count and a very low RBC count.*
lymph/o	lymph	**lymph**/oid (LĬM-foyd): _____ *–oid:* resembling
lymphaden/o	lymph gland (node)	**lymphaden/o**/pathy (lĭm-făd-ĕ-NŎP-ă-thē): _____ *–pathy:* disease *Lymphadenopathy is characterized by changes in the size, consistency, or number of lymph nodes.*
lymphangi/o	lymph vessel	**lymphangi**/oma (lĭm-făn-jē-Ō-mă): _____ *–oma:* tumor
morph/o	form, shape, structure	**morph/o**/logy (mor-FŎL-ō-jē): _____ *–logy:* study of

myel/o	bone marrow; spinal cord	**myel/o**/gen/ic (mī-ĕ-lō-JĔN-ĭk): _____
		  gen: forming, producing, origin
		  –ic: pertaining to
		Acute myelogenic leukemia (AML) is a common form of leukemia; also called acute myelogenous leukemia.

nucle/o	nucleus	mono/**nucle**/ar (m ŏn-ō-NŪ-klē-ăr): _____
		  mono–: one
		  –ar: pertaining to
		Mononuclear WBCs, the monocytes and lymphocytes, are also called **agranulocytes.**

phag/o	swallowing, eating	**phag/o**/cyte (FĂG-ō-sīt): _____ *–cyte:* cell *The neutrophil is an important phagocytic leukocyte of the innate immune system.*

Continued

Medical Word Elements—cont'd

Element	Meaning	Word Analysis
poikil/o	varied, irregular	**poikil/o**/cyte (POY-kĭl-ō-sīt): _____ *-cyte:* cell *A poikilocyte is an irregularly shaped RBC, such as a sickle cell.*
ser/o	serum	**ser/o**/logy (sē-RŎL-ō-jē): _____ *-logy:* study of *Serology includes the study of antigens and antibodies in serum and sources other than serum, including plasma, saliva, and urine.*
sider/o	iron	**sider/o**/penia (sĭd-ĕr-ō-PĒ-nē-ă): _____ *-penia:* decrease, deficiency *Common causes of sideropenia include inadequate iron uptake and hemorrhage.*
splen/o	spleen	**splen/o**/megaly (splē-nō-MĔG-ă-lē): _____ *-megaly:* enlargement *Serious forms of infectious mononucleosis commonly cause enlargement of the spleen and liver.*
thromb/o	blood clot	**thromb**/osis (thrŏm-BŌ-sĭs): _____ *-osis:* abnormal condition; increase (used primarily with blood cells)
thym/o	thymus gland	**thym/o**/pathy (thī-MŎP-ă-thē): _____ *-pathy:* disease
Suffixes		

-blast	embryonic cell	hem/o/cyt/o/**blast** (hē-mō-SĪ-tō-blăst): _____
		   hem/o: blood
		   cyt/o: cell
		
		A hemocytoblast is a bone marrow cell capable of giving rise to all types of blood cells.

-globin	protein	hem/o/**globin** (HĒ-mō-glō-bĭn): _____ *hem/o:* blood *Hemoglobin is an iron-containing protein found in RBCs that transports O_2 and gives blood its red color.*
-penia	decrease, deficiency	monocyt/o/**penia** (mŏn-ō-sī-tō-PĒ-nē-ă): _____ *monocyt/o:* monocyte *Some of the causes of monocytopenia include acute infections, leukemia, and reactions to certain drugs.*
-phil	attraction for	neutr/o/**phil** (NŪ-trō-fĭl): _____ *neutr/o:* neutral, neither *Neutrophils are the most numerous type of leukocyte. They provide phagocytic protection for the body.*

Medical Word Elements—cont'd

Element	Meaning	Word Analysis
-phylaxis	protection	ana/**phylaxis** (ăn-ă-fĭ-LĂK-sĭs): _____ *ana-:* against; up; back *Anaphylaxis is an exaggerated, life-threatening hypersensitivity reaction to a previously encountered antigen. It is treated as a medical emergency.*
-poiesis	formation, production	hem/o/**poiesis** (hē-mō-poy-Ē-sĭs): _____ *hem/o:* blood
-stasis	standing still	hem/o/**stasis** (hē-mō-STĀ-sĭs): _____ *hem/o:* blood *Hemostasis is the control or arrest of bleeding, commonly using chemical agents.*

Prefixes

aniso-	unequal, dissimilar	**aniso**/cyt/osis (ăn-ī-sō-sō-TŌ-sĭs): _____
		   cyt: cell
		   -osis: abnormal condition; increase (used primarily with blood cells)
		
		Normally, RBCs do not vary in size. When abnormally large RBCs (macrocytes) or abnormally small RBCs (microcytes) are present, the condition is called anisocytosis.

 Visit the Medical Terminology Systems online resource center at FADavis.com for an audio exercise of the terms in this table. Other activities are also available to reinforce content.

 It is time to review medical word elements by completing Learning Activities 9–1 and 9–2.

Disease Focus

Anemias, leukemias, and coagulation disorders typically share common signs and symptoms that include paleness, weakness, shortness of breath, and heart palpitations. Lymphatic disorders are commonly associated with edema and lymphadenopathy. Immune disorders include abnormally heightened immune responses (**hypersensitivities**), depressed responses (**immunodeficiencies** or **immune deficiencies**), and responses where the immune system fails to recognize its own tissue (**autoimmunity**).

For diagnosis, treatment, and management of diseases that affect blood and blood-forming organs, the medical services of a specialist may be warranted. **Hematology** is the branch of medicine that studies blood cells, blood-clotting mechanisms, bone marrow, and lymph nodes. The physician who specializes in this branch of medicine is called a **hematologist**. **Allergy and immunology** is the branch of medicine involving disorders of the immune system, including asthma and anaphylaxis, adverse reactions to drugs, autoimmune diseases, organ transplantations, and malignancies of the immune system. Physicians who specialize in this combined branch of medicine are called **allergists** and **immunologists**.

Anemias

Anemia (**erythropenia, erythrocytopenia**) is a deficiency in the number of erythrocytes or in the amount of hemoglobin within the RBCs (**hypochromia**). It is considered a condition, not a disease, and often functions as a symptom indicating an underlying problem.

An important hereditary anemia that primarily affects individuals of African ancestry is **sickle cell anemia.** This anemia results from a defective hemoglobin molecule **(hemoglobinopathy)** that causes RBCs to assume bizarre shapes, commonly resembling a crescent, or sickle, when oxygen levels are low. Sickle cells are fragile and easily break apart **(hemolyze).** They have difficulty passing through the small capillaries (see Fig. 9-10). Tissue distal to the blockage undergoes ischemia, resulting in severe pain called a **sickle cell crisis** that can last from several hours to several days. Sickle cell anemia affects only those who have inherited the trait from both parents. If the trait is inherited from only one parent, the offspring will be a carrier but will not have the disorder. Treatment focuses on managing symptoms and preventing complications. Folic acid is commonly recommended because it is essential for the production of new RBCs. Some medications are also proving to be helpful in controlling the disease. Table 9-3 provides information on common anemias.

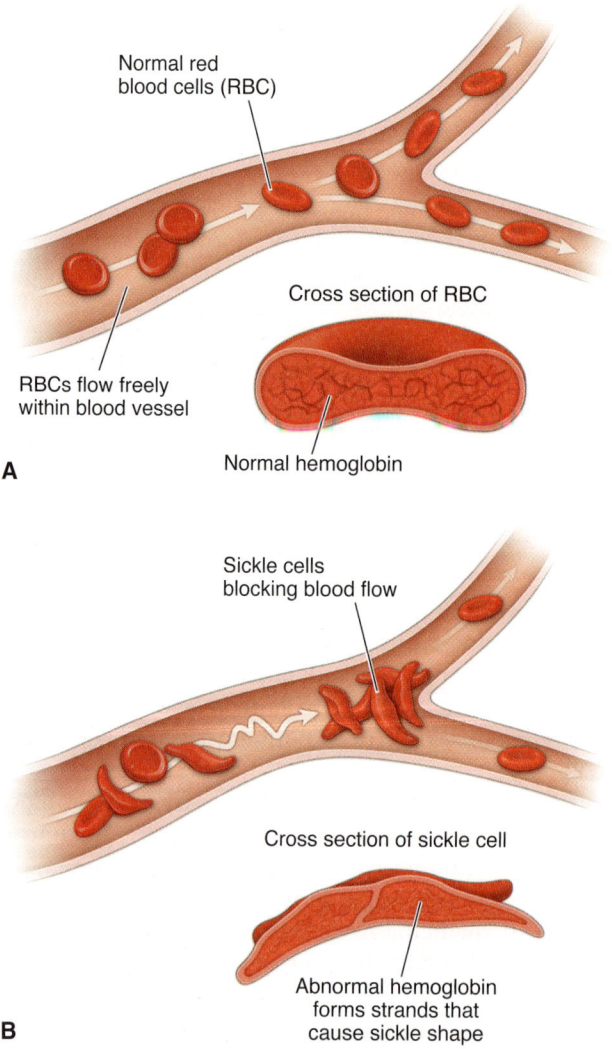

Normal red blood cells (RBC)

Cross section of RBC

RBCs flow freely within blood vessel

Normal hemoglobin

A

Sickle cells blocking blood flow

Cross section of sickle cell

Abnormal hemoglobin forms strands that cause sickle shape

B

Figure 9-10 Sickle cell anemia. (A) Normal red blood cells (RBCs) passing easily through capillaries. (B) Sickle cells becoming trapped and obstructing normal blood flow.

TABLE 9-3 Common Anemias

This table lists various types of anemia, along with descriptions and causes.

Type of Anemia	Description	Causes
Aplastic (hypoplastic)	Serious form of anemia associated with bone marrow failure, resulting in erythropenia, leukopenia, and thrombocytopenia	Commonly caused by some autoimmune disorders, chemotherapy, radiation therapy, and exposure to certain cytotoxic agents
Folic acid deficiency anemia	Inability to produce sufficient RBCs because of the lack of folic acid, a B vitamin essential for erythropoiesis	Caused by insufficient folic acid intake resulting from poor diet, impaired absorption, prolonged drug therapy, or increased requirements (pregnancy or rapid growth as seen in children)
Hemolytic	Destruction of RBCs, commonly resulting in jaundice	Associated with some inherited immune and blood (sickle cell anemia) disorders, medications, and incompatible transfusions
Iron-deficiency anemia	Lack of sufficient iron in RBCs	Caused by a greater demand for stored iron than can be supplied, usually as a result of inadequate dietary iron intake or malabsorption of iron
Pernicious anemia (PA)	Chronic, progressive anemia found mostly in people older than age 50 resulting from a lack of sufficient vitamin B_{12} needed for blood cell development	Caused by lack of intrinsic factor in the stomach, which is essential for absorption of vitamin B_{12}
Sickle cell anemia	Inherited anemia that causes RBCs to become crescent- or sickle-shaped when O_2 levels are low	Caused by a defect in the gene responsible for hemoglobin synthesis

Allergy

An **allergy** occurs when the immune system reacts to normally harmless substances called **allergens** as if they were dangerous invaders. This exaggerated immune response leads to the release of chemicals that cause allergy symptoms. An allergy requires an initial exposure (**sensitization**) to an allergen (**antigen**). Subsequent exposures to the allergen trigger the release of **histamines** and **leukotrienes** that cause a broad range of inflammatory changes, including hives (**urticaria**), eczema, allergic rhinitis, asthma, and, in the extreme, **anaphylaxis,** a life-threatening condition (see Fig. 9-11). Anaphylaxis requires immediate medical treatment. A person with previous anaphylaxis is prescribed epinephrine delivered by an EpiPen that is to be in close proximity at all times for emergency use to reverse the symptoms (see Fig. 9-12).

Sensitivity tests for allergies, involving the introduction of an allergen suspension into the skin, help identify the specific allergens causing a reaction. If the patient has an allergy to the suspected allergen, the area becomes red, swollen, and hardened (**indurated**).

Allergy shots (**immunotherapy, biotherapy**) can help with an allergy response to pollens, pet dander, molds, dust mites, and venom (bee stings) but not to foods. Immunotherapy involves repeated injections of the allergen, beginning with a highly diluted solution and increasing the concentration over a period of weeks or months. When administered as an injection, the body treats the allergen like a vaccine and begins to produce antibodies against the allergen. The newly formed antibodies desensitize the patient and reduce the reaction of the patient to the offending allergen. Allergy shots have been very successful in reducing or even eliminating the symptoms associated with the allergy.

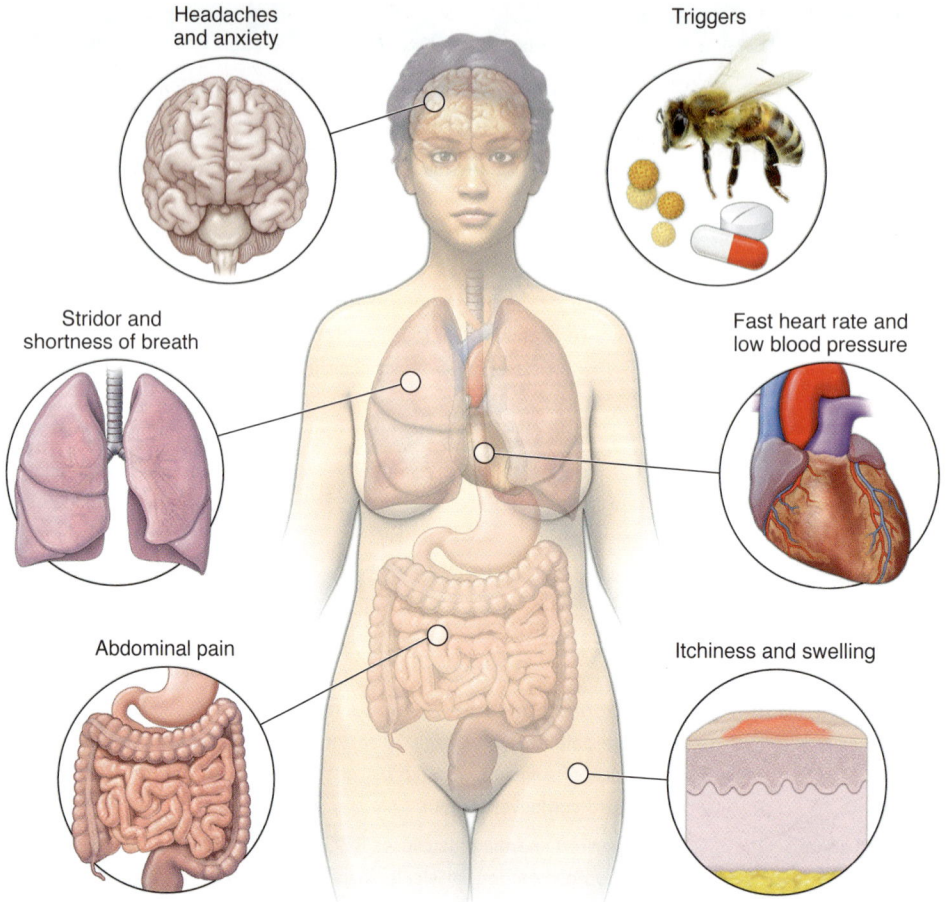

Figure 9-11 Anaphylaxis is a severe and potentially life-threatening reaction that can occur rapidly after exposure to an allergen such as a bee sting, pollen, or medication. The immune response affects multiple organ systems in the body as illustrated and requires immediate medical treatment.

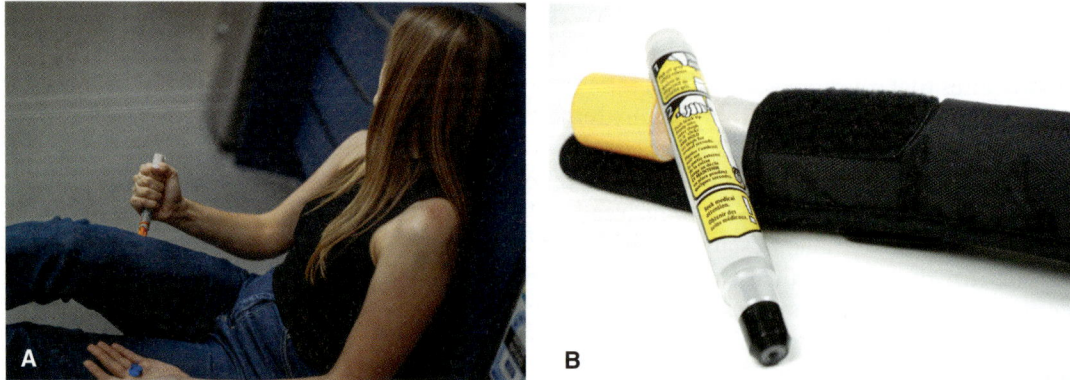

Figure 9-12 (A) A young woman delivers epinephrine with an EpiPen by a jab into the thigh and listens for a click that signals epinephrine is being delivered. The EpiPen remains in place for three seconds to complete the injection. EpiPen injections can deliver epinephrine through clothing. (B) EpiPens prescribed by a physician should be in close reach at all times by those who have had a previous anaphylactic reaction.

Autoimmune Disease

When the immune system fails to accurately differentiate foreign antigens from the body's own antigens found on cells and tissues (**autoantigens**) and begins its destructive behavior to the detriment of the individual, the disorder is considered an **autoimmune disease.** In this abnormal response, the immune system produces **autoantibodies** directed at one or more of the individual's cells or tissues until they are destroyed. Types of autoimmune disorders range from those that affect only a single organ to those that affect many organs and systems (**multisystemic**). Autoimmune diseases include rheumatoid arthritis (RA), systemic lupus erythematosus (SLE), multiple sclerosis (MS), myasthenia gravis, Addison disease, Crohn disease, and Graves disease. Most autoimmune diseases have periods of flare-ups (**exacerbations**) and latencies (**remissions**).

Treatment goals include reducing symptoms and controlling the autoimmune process while maintaining the body's ability to fight disease. Autoimmune diseases are usually chronic, requiring lifelong care and monitoring, even when the person may look or feel well. Currently, few autoimmune diseases can be cured; however, with treatment, those afflicted can live relatively normal lives.

Oncology

The major types of blood cancers include multiple myelomas that affect a single type of bone marrow cell, lymphomas that arise in the lymphatic system, and leukemias that affect blood and bone marrow.

Leukemia

Leukemia is an oncological disorder that affects the blood and bone marrow and is characterized by an overgrowth (proliferation) of blood cells. It is the most common cancer in children, adolescents, and young adults. With this condition, the body replaces healthy blood and bone marrow cells with immature, nonfunctional cells, leading to anemias, infections, and bleeding disorders. The various types of leukemia are generally identified by the type of leukocyte population affected as either granulocytic (myelogenous) or lymphocytic. They are further classified by the rate of progression as chronic or acute.

In the acute form, the disease has a sudden onset and blood cells are highly embryonic (blastic) with few mature forms. Severe anemia, infections, and bleeding disorders appear early in the disease. This form of leukemia is life-threatening.

In the chronic form, signs and symptoms are slow to develop because there are usually enough mature cells to carry on the functions of the various cell types. As the chronic form progresses, signs and symptoms develop.

Although the causes of leukemia are unknown, research has implicated viruses, environmental conditions, high-dose radiation, and genetic factors. Bone marrow aspiration and bone marrow biopsy help diagnose leukemia. Treatment includes chemotherapy, radiation, bone marrow transplant, or a combination of these modalities. Recent advances in treatment, such as monoclonal antibody therapy, cancer vaccines, and donor lymphocyte infusions, are becoming more prevalent in treatment. Leukemias are fatal if left untreated.

Diseases and Conditions

This section introduces diseases and conditions of the blood, lymphatic, and immune systems, along with their meanings and pronunciations. Word analyses for selected terms are also provided.

Term	Definition
acquired immunodeficiency syndrome (AIDS) ĭm-ūn dě-FĬSH-ěn-sē SĬN-drōm	Infectious disease causes the human immunodeficiency virus (HIV) that destroys the CD4 (helper T) cells of the immune system to such an extent that the patient falls victim to infections that usually do not affect healthy individuals (opportunistic infections) *Early stages of HIV infection (HIV disease) may remain asymptomatic for many years, especially when the patient receives medical care. Untreated, the disease ultimately develops into full-blown AIDS, a potentially fatal disease.*
coagulation disorders kō-ăg-ū-LĀ-shŭn	Any disruption or impairment in the ability to form blood clots or control bleeding *Causes include deficiency in coagulating factors, certain plasma proteins, or platelet production.*
disseminated intravascular coagulation (DIC) ĭn-tră-VĂS-kū-lăr kō-ăg-ū-LĀ-shŭn *intra-:* in, within *vascul:* vessel (usually blood or lymph) *-ar:* pertaining to	A life-threatening condition characterized by widespread blood clotting (**hypercoagulation**) blocking small blood vessels, cutting off O$_2$ supply *DIC leads to simultaneous thrombosis and hemorrhage and organ damage throughout the body. It is most often the result of a complication of an underlying medical condition such as sepsis, cancer, trauma, severe immune reactions, or certain types of infection (see Fig. 9-13).* **Figure 9-13** Extensive hemorrhage into the skin in disseminated intravascular coagulation (DIC), with an area outlined in pen to assess whether the hemorrhage is spreading. From Harmening DM: *Clinical hematology and fundamentals of hemostasis,* ed 3, Philadelphia, 1997, F.A. Davis, p. 520, with permission.

Diseases and Conditions—cont'd

Term	Definition
hemophilia hē-mō-FĬL-ē-ă *hem/o:* blood *philia:* attraction for	Congenital hereditary disorder characterized by a deficiency in clotting factor VIII (hemophilia A) or clotting factor IX (hemophilia B), resulting in prolonged bleeding; also called *bleeder's disease* *Mild symptoms include nosebleeds and hematomas. Severe symptoms include bleeding into the joints (hemarthrosis) and sudden shock; death is possible. The main treatment for hemophilia involves replacing the missing blood clotting factors, typically through infusions. Medications may also be prescribed to stimulate the release of clotting factors.*
thrombocytopenia thrŏm-bō-sī-tō-PĒ-nē-ă *thromb/o:* blood clot *cyt/o:* cell *-penia:* decrease, deficiency	Abnormal decrease in platelets caused by low production or increased destruction in the blood vessels, spleen, or liver *A common sign of thrombocytopenia is the development of pinpoint hemorrhages (petechiae) that appear primarily on the lower leg (see Fig. 9–14).* **Figure 9-14** Petechiae on the skin from thrombocytopenia. From Goldsmith L, Tharp MD: *Adult and pediatric dermatology: a color guide to diagnosis and treatment,* Philadelphia, 1997, F.A. Davis, p. 61, with permission.
graft rejection GRĂFT	Process in which a recipient's immune system identifies the transplanted graft as "foreign" and attacks or destroys it *Rejection can be lessened by a close tissue match between donor and recipient or administration of medications that depress the immune system.*
graft-versus-host disease (GVHD) GRĂFT	Complication that occurs following a stem cell or bone marrow transplant in which the transplant produces antibodies against the recipient's organs, commonly severely enough to cause death
hemoglobinopathy hē-mō-glō-bĭ-NŎP-ă-thē *hem/o:* blood *globin/o:* protein *-pathy:* disease	Group of inherited blood disorders affecting the hemoglobin molecule *Hemoglobinopathies include sickle cell anemia, thalassemia, and hemolytic anemia.*

Continued

Diseases and Conditions—cont'd

Term	Definition
infectious mononucleosis ĭn-FĔK-shŭs mŏn-ō-nū-klē-Ō-sĭs *mono-:* one *nucle:* nucleus *-osis:* abnormal condition; increase (used primarily with blood cells)	Acute infectious disease caused by the Epstein-Barr virus (EBV) that primarily affects young adults and children and causes fatigue, malaise, sore throat, and lymphadenopathy of the neck or armpits; also called *mono* and *kissing disease* *Rest and adequate fluid intake are important to recovery. Infectious mononucleosis usually resolves spontaneously and without complications. Recovery usually ensures lasting immunity.*
Kaposi sarcoma (KS) KĂP-ō-sē săr-KŌ-mă *sarc:* flesh, connective tissue *-oma:* tumor	Cancer caused by the human herpes virus 8 (HHV-8) that mainly affects the skin and mucous membranes but may also cause extensive visceral organ involvement; also called *malignant neoplasm of soft tissue* *Although several forms of KS are clinically identified, AIDS-related KS is the most common and most aggressive form (see Fig. 9-15).* **Figure 9-15** Kaposi sarcoma in an individual infected with AIDS virus. From Radu O, Pantanowitz L: Kaposi sarcoma, *Arch Pathol Lab Med* 137(2):289–294, 2013. https://doi.org/10.5858/arpa.2012-0101-RS.

Diseases and Conditions—cont'd

Term	Definition
lymphedema lĭmf-ĕ-DĒ-mă *lymph:* lymph *-edema:* swelling	Swelling, primarily in a single arm or leg, resulting from an accumulation of lymph within tissues caused by obstruction or disease in the lymph vessels *The most common causes of lymphedema are surgery, radiation therapy, and infection of the lymph vessels (see Fig. 9–16).*

Figure 9-16 Lymphedema of the leg.

Term	Definition
lymphoma lĭm-FŌ-mă *lymph:* lymph *-oma:* tumor	Any malignancy involving lymphocytes (B cells, T cells, or both) that commonly affects lymph nodes and other lymphatic tissue
Hodgkin (HL) HŎJ-kĭn	Malignancy of B cells that occurs in lymph nodes of the neck or chest and may spread to nearby lymph nodes and the spleen and sometimes to the bone marrow; also called *classical Hodgkin lymphoma, Hodgkin disease* *HL is characterized by the presence of Reed-Sternberg cells. Symptoms include a painless swelling of cervical nodes, fever, chills, and itchy skin. Treatment includes radiation therapy, chemotherapy, or bone marrow transplant.*
non-Hodgkin Lymphoma (NHL)	Any malignancy of B cells, T cells, or NK cells that does not involve Reed-Sternberg cells *More than 60 subtypes of NHL have been identified. Prognosis depends on the type, stage, grade of the disease, and age and general health of the patient.*
multiple myeloma (MM) mī-ĕ-LŌ-mă *myel:* bone marrow; spinal cord *-oma:* tumor	Malignancy of the bone marrow that affects plasma cells, leading to proliferation of abnormal antibodies, destruction of healthy bone marrow cells, and weakening of bone tissue *Serious consequences of the disease include low blood counts, bone and kidney disorders, and infections.*

Continued

Diseases and Conditions—cont'd

Term	Definition
sepsis SĔP-sĭs	Presence of bacteria or their toxins in the blood; also called *septicemia* or *blood poisoning* *Usual causes of sepsis are peritonitis, urinary tract infections, meningitis, cellulitis, and bacterial pneumonias.*
systemic lupus erythematosus (SLE) sĭs-TĔM-ĭk LŪ-pŭs ĕr-ĭ-thē-mă-TŌ-sŭs	Widespread chronic autoimmune inflammatory disease that affects the collagen in the skin, internal organs, and joints; also called *discoid lupus* if symptoms are limited to the skin *A typical "butterfly rash" appears over the nose and cheeks in about 50% of people afflicted with SLE; this tends to get worse in direct sunlight (see Fig. 9–17).*

Figure 9-17 Red papules and plaques of systemic lupus erythematosus (SLE) in a butterfly pattern on the face. From Goldsmith L, Tharp MD: *Adult and pediatric dermatology: a color guide to diagnosis and treatment,* Philadelphia, 1997, F.A. Davis, p. 230, with permission.

Term	Definition
thrombocythemia thrŏm-bō-sī-THĒ-mē-ă	Overproduction of platelets, leading to thrombosis or bleeding disorders as a result of platelet malformations

 It is time to review pathology, diseases, and conditions by completing Learning Activity 9–3.

Diagnostic, Surgical, and Therapeutic Procedures

This section introduces diagnostic, surgical, and therapeutic procedures used to treat and diagnose blood, lymphatic, and immune system disorders. Descriptions are provided, along with pronunciations and word analyses for selected terms.

Procedure	Description
Diagnostic	
Laboratory	
antinuclear antibody (ANA) ăn-tĭ-NŪ-klē-ăr ĂN-tĭ-bŏd-ē *anti-:* against *nucle:* nucleus *-ar:* pertaining to	Test that identifies the antibodies that attack the nucleus of the individual's own body cells (autoantibodies) *The presence of ANAs indicates the potential for autoimmunity and directs the physician to explore possible autoimmune diseases.*
blood culture	Test to determine the presence of pathogens in the bloodstream
complete blood count (CBC)	Series of tests that includes hemoglobin, hematocrit, RBC and WBC counts, platelet count, and differential (diff) count *CBC is a broad screening test for anemias, coagulation disorders, and infections.*
monospot	Nonspecific, rapid serological test for the presence of the heterophile antibody, which develops several days after infection by Epstein-Barr virus, the organism that causes infectious mononucleosis
partial thromboplastin time (PTT) thrŏm-bō-PLĂS-tĭn	Screening test for deficiencies in clotting factors by measuring the length of time it takes blood to clot; also called *activated partial thromboplastin time (APTT)* *PTT is a valuable tool in preoperative screening for bleeding tendencies.*
prothrombin time (PT) prō-THRŎM-bĭn	Test used to detect and diagnose bleeding disorders or excessive clotting disorders; also called *pro time* *PT is commonly used to monitor blood thinning medications, diagnose liver problems, and assess the blood's ability to clot before undertaking surgical procedures.*
Imaging	
bone marrow magnetic resonance imaging (MRI)	Highly sensitive imaging procedure that detects lesions and changes in bone tissue and bone marrow, especially in diagnosing multiple myeloma
lymphangiography lĭm-făn-jē-ŎG-ră-fē *lymph:* lymph *angi/o:* vessel *-graphy:* process of recording	Visualization of lymph channels and lymph nodes using a contrast medium to determine blockages or other pathologies of the lymphatic system *Because lymph nodes filter and trap cancer cells, this test is commonly used to determine lymph flow in areas that contain malignancy.*

Continued

Diagnostic, Surgical, and Therapeutic Procedures—cont'd

Procedure	Description
lymphoscintigraphy lĭm-fō-sĭn-TĬG-ră-fē	Introduction of a radioactive tracer into the lymph channels to determine lymph flow, identify obstructions, and locate the sentinel node *Lymphoscintigraphy is also used to biopsy the sentinel node, assess the stage of cancer, and determine a plan of treatment.*
Surgical	
bone marrow aspiration BŌN MĂR-ō ăs-pĭ-RĀ-shŭn	Removal of bone marrow (usually from the pelvis) for microscopic examination using a thin aspirating needle (see Fig. 9-18) *Bone marrow aspiration aids in identifying blood disorders (leukemias or anemias), infections, and fevers of unknown origin.*

Biopsy needle

Skin

Bone

Bone marrow

Iliac crest

Pelvic

Figure 9-18 Bone marrow aspiration.

bone marrow transplant (BMT) BŌN MĂR-ō TRĂNS-plănt	Infusion of healthy bone marrow stem cells after destroying the diseased bone marrow by chemotherapy, radiation therapy, or both and commonly used to treat leukemia, aplastic anemia, and certain cancers; also called *stem cell transplant* *In an autologous transplant, the donor and recipient are the same individual. In a homologous transplant, the donor and recipient are different individuals.*
lymphadenectomy lĭm-făd-ĕ-NĔK-tō-mē *lymph:* lymph *aden:* gland *-ectomy:* excision	Removal of lymph nodes, especially in surgical procedures undertaken to remove malignant tissue, in an effort to control the spread of cancer *A limited or modified lymphadenectomy removes only some of the lymph nodes in the area around a tumor; a total, or radical, lymphadenectomy removes all of the lymph nodes in the area.*

Diagnostic, Surgical, and Therapeutic Procedures—cont'd

Procedure	Description
sentinel node excision SĔNT-ĭ-nĕl NŌD	Removal of the first node (sentinel node) that receives drainage from cancer-containing areas and the one most likely to contain malignant cells *If the sentinel node does not contain malignant cells, there may be no need to remove regional lymph nodes during cancer surgery (see Fig. 9-19).*

Figure 9-19 Sentinel node.

Therapeutic

Procedure	Description
immunotherapy ĭm-ū-nō-THĔR-ă-pē *immun/o:* immune, immunity, safe *-therapy:* treatment	Any form of treatment that alters, enhances, stimulates, or restores the body's own natural immune mechanisms to treat diseases; also called *biological therapy*
immunoglobulin (IG) therapy ĭm-ū-nō-GLŎB-ū-lĭn THĔR-ă-pē	Treatment using antibody mixtures, administered via intravenous, subcutaneous, or intramuscular routes *IG therapy is commonly used to treat immunodeficiencies and autoimmune diseases.*
plasmapheresis plăz-mă-fĕr-Ē-sĭs	Removal, treatment, and return of blood plasma from the body for the purpose of removing harmful antibodies; also known as *apheresis* *Autoimmune diseases treated using plasmapheresis include myasthenia gravis, Guillain-Barre syndrome, multiple sclerosis, and muscular dystrophy.*
transfusion trăns-FŪ-zhŭn	Infusion of blood or blood products from one person (donor) to another (recipient) *Transfusion is usually performed as a lifesaving maneuver when there is serious blood loss or for the treatment of severe anemias.*

Continued

Diagnostic, Surgical, and Therapeutic Procedures—cont'd

Procedure	Description
vaccination văk-sĭ-NĀ-shŭn	Administration of a vaccine, typically containing a weakened (**attenuated**) or inactivated form of the disease-causing microorganism, to stimulate the immune system and provide protection against a specific infectious disease *Vaccinations have been effective in preventing the spread of many infectious diseases and reducing the morbidity and mortality associated with them, for example, polio and diphtheria. It is a major intervention for controlling and eradicating certain diseases and protecting individuals and communities from illness.*

Pharmacology

Various pharmaceutical agents are available to treat blood, lymphatic, and immune system disorders. These drugs act directly on individual components of each system. For example, anticoagulants help prevent clot formation but are ineffective in destroying formed clots. Instead, thrombolytics help dissolve clots that obstruct coronary, cerebral, or pulmonary arteries. Conversely, hemostatics help prevent or control hemorrhage. In addition, chemotherapy and radiation are common treatments for diseases of the blood and immune systems. For example, antineoplastics prevent cellular replication to halt the spread of cancer in the body; antiretrovirals prevent viral replication within cells and have been effective in slowing the progression of HIV and AIDS (see Table 9-4).

TABLE 9-4 Drugs Used to Treat Blood, Lymphatic, and Immune Disorders

This table lists common drug classifications used to treat blood, lymphatic, and immune disorders, along with their therapeutic actions and selected generic and trade names.

Classification	Therapeutic Action	Generic and Trade Names
anticoagulants an-tĭ-kō-ĂG-ū-lănts	Prevent blood clot formation by inactivating one or more clotting factors or inhibiting their synthesis *Anticoagulants prevent deep vein thrombosis (DVT) and postoperative clot formation and decrease the risk of stroke.*	**heparin** HĔP-ă-rĭn *heparin sodium* **warfarin** WĂR-făr-ĭn *Coumadin* **dabigatran** dă-BĬG-ă-trăn *Pradaxa*
antifibrinolytics ăn-tĭ-fī-brĭ-nō-LĬT-ĭks	Neutralize fibrinolytic chemicals in the mucous membranes of the mouth, nose, and urinary tract to prevent the breakdown of blood clots *Antifibrinolytics are used to treat serious bleeding following certain surgeries and dental procedures, especially in patients with hemophilia.*	**aminocaproic acid** a-mē-nō-kă-PR Ō-ĭk ĂS-ĭd *Amicar*

TABLE 9-4 Drugs Used to Treat Blood, Lymphatic, and Immune Disorders—cont'd

Classification	Therapeutic Action	Generic and Trade Names
antimicrobials ăn-tĭ-mī-KR Ō-bē-ălz	Destroy bacteria, fungi, and protozoa, depending on the particular drug, generally by interfering with the functions of the cell membrane or the reproductive cycle *Patients with HIV are commonly treated prophylactically with antimicrobials to prevent the development of Pneumocystis pneumonia (PCP).*	**trimethoprim, sulfamethoxazole** trĭ-MĔTH-ō-prĭm, sŭl-fă-mĕth- ŎK-să-zōl *Bactrim, Septra* **metronidazole** mĕ-trō-NĬ-dă-zōl *Flagyl*
antiretrovirals ăn-tĭ-rĕ-trō-VĪ-rălz	Prevent replication of viruses within host cells *Antiretrovirals are used in the treatment of HIV infection and AIDS. Resistance to these agents is common, so they are generally given in combination to avoid this problem.*	**nelfinavir** nĕl-FĬN-ă-vēr *Viracept* **lamivudine/zidovudine** lă-MĬV-ū-dēn, zī-D Ō-vū-dēn *Combivir*
immunosuppressants ĭm-ū-nō-sū-PRĔSS-ănts	Decrease inflammation by suppressing the body's natural immune response *Immunosuppressants are used to treat autoimmune disorders that cause inflammation, such as rheumatoid arthritis; they are also used in transplant patients to prevent graft rejection.*	**prednisone** PRĔD-n ĭ-zōn **cyclosporine** SĪ-klō-spor-ēn *Neoral* **mycophenolate mofetil** mī-cō-FĔN-ō-lāt MŎF-ĕ-tĭl *CellCept*
thrombolytics thrŏm-bō-LĬT-ĭks	Dissolve blood clots by destroying their fibrin strands *Thrombolytics are used to break apart, or lyse, thrombi, especially those that obstruct coronary, pulmonary, and cerebral arteries.*	**alteplase** ĂL-tĕ-plās *Activase, t-PA* **streptokinase** strĕp-tō-KĪ-nās *Streptase*

Abbreviations

This section introduces blood, lymphatic, and immune system abbreviations and their meanings.

Abbreviation	Meaning	Abbreviation	Meaning
A, B, AB, O	blood types in ABO blood group	**Ig**	immunoglobulin
AB, Ab, ab	antibody, abortion	**KS**	Kaposi sarcoma
AIDS	acquired immunodeficiency syndrome	**MM**	multiple myeloma
AML	acute myelogenic leukemia	**MNL**	mononuclear leukocyte
ANA	antinuclear antibody	**MRI**	magnetic resonance imaging
APC	antigen-presenting cell	**MS**	multiple sclerosis
APTT	activated partial thromboplastin time	**NHL**	non-Hodgkin lymphoma
BMT	bone marrow transplant	**NK cell**	natural killer cell
CBC	complete blood count	**O₂**	oxygen
CO₂	carbon dioxide	**PA**	pernicious anemia
DIC	disseminated intravascular coagulation	**PCP**	*Pneumocystis* pneumonia; primary care physician
diff	differential count (white blood cells)	**PMNL, poly**	polymorphonuclear leukocyte
DVT	deep vein thrombosis	**PT**	prothrombin time, physical therapy
EBV	Epstein-Barr virus	**PTT**	partial thromboplastin time
GVHD	graft-versus-host disease	**RA**	right atrium; rheumatoid arthritis
Hb, Hgb	hemoglobin	**RBC, rbc**	red blood cell
HIV	human immunodeficiency virus	**SLE**	systemic lupus erythematosus
HL	Hodgkin lymphoma	**WBC, wbc**	white blood cell

It is time to review procedures, pharmacology, and abbreviations by completing Learning Activity 9–4.

LEARNING ACTIVITIES

The activities that follow provide a review of the blood, lymphatic, and immune system terms introduced in this chapter. Complete each activity and review your answers to evaluate your understanding of the chapter.

Visit the Medical Language Laboratory at medicallanguagelab.com. Use it to enhance your study and reinforcement of this chapter with the flash card activity. We recommend that you complete the flash card activity before starting Learning Activities 9-1 and 9-2.

Learning Activity 9-1
Medical Word Elements

Use the listed elements to build medical words. You may use elements more than once.

Combining Forms		Suffixes		Prefixes
aden/o	lymphangi/o	-ar	-oma	a-
chrom/o	morph/o	-blast	-osis	hypo-
cyt/o	nucle/o	-ectomy	-pathy	micro-
erythr/o	sider/o	-ic	-penia	
granul/o	splen/o	-logy	-poiesis	
hem/o	thromb/o	-lysis		
lymphaden/o	thym/o	-megaly		

1. disease of a lymph gland _____

2. excision of the thymus _____

3. enlargement of the spleen _____

4. abnormal condition of a blood clot _____

5. study of shapes (of cells) _____

6. decrease in iron _____

7. pertaining to deficient color (of red blood cells) _____

8. pertaining to small (red blood) cells _____

9. tumor of a lymph vessel _____

10. embryonic red (blood cell) _____

11. destruction of blood _____

12. pertaining to a nucleus _____

13. tumor of a gland _____

14. pertaining to without granules _____

15. formation (production) of blood _____

 Check your answers in Appendix A. Review any material that you did not answer correctly.

Correct Answers _____ X 6.67 = _____ % Score

Learning Activity 9-2
Building Medical Words

Use *thromb/o* (blood clot) to build words that mean

1. abnormal condition of a blood clot _____
2. destruction of a blood clot _____

Use *-osis* (abnormal condition; increase [used primarily with blood cells]) to build words that mean

3. abnormal increase in erythrocytes _____
4. abnormal increase in leukocytes _____
5. abnormal increase in lymphocytes _____
6. abnormal increase in reticulocytes _____

Use *-penia* (deficiency, decrease) to build words that mean

7. decrease in leukocytes _____
8. decrease in erythrocytes _____
9. decrease in thrombocytes _____
10. decrease in lymphocytes _____

Use *-poiesis* (formation, production) to build words that mean

11. production of blood _____
12. production of white blood cells _____
13. production of thrombocytes _____

Use *immun/o* (immune, immunity, safe) to build words that mean

14. specialist in the study of immunity _____
15. study of immunity _____

Build surgical words that mean

16. excision of the tonsils _____
17. removal of the thymus _____
18. removal of a lymph node _____
19. incision of the spleen _____
20. fixation of (a displaced) spleen _____

Check your answers in Appendix A. Review any material that you did not answer correctly.

Correct Answers _____ X 5 = _____ % Score

Learning Activity 9-3
Diseases and Conditions

Match the terms with the definitions in the numbered list.

anaphylaxis   hemolytic   mononucleosis   sepsis
aplastic   hemophilia   multiple myeloma   sickle cell
erythropenia   Hodgkin disease   myelogenous   SLE
graft rejection   Kaposi sarcoma   opportunistic   thrombocytopenia
hemoglobinopathy   lymphedema   sensitization   urticaria

 1. any disorder caused by abnormalities in the hemoglobin molecule _____

 2. swelling of tissue in limb(s) usually due to obstruction or disease of a lymph vessel _____
  _____

 3. chronic autoimmune inflammatory disease of collagen in the skin, joints, and internal organs
  _____

 4. anemia associated with bone marrow failure _____

 5. life-threatening allergic response _____

 6. denotes an infection that affects only those who are immunocompromised _____

 7. malignant disease of the lymph nodes characterized by Reed-Sternberg cells _____

 8. initial exposure to an allergen _____

 9. deficiency in RBCs or hemoglobin _____

10. malignancy of plasma cells in the bone marrow _____

11. infectious disorder caused by the Epstein-Barr virus _____

12. presence of bacteria or their toxins in blood _____

13. leukemia that affects granulocytes _____

14. malignancy associated with HIV _____

15. hereditary anemia found mostly in those of African descent _____

16. decrease of platelets in the circulatory system _____

17. anemia caused by destruction of erythrocytes _____

18. red itchy welts caused by an allergic reaction; also known as hives _____

19. hereditary bleeding disorder caused by deficiency in clotting factors _____

20. destruction of a transplanted organ or tissue by the recipient's immune system _____

✔ *Check your answers in Appendix A. Review any material that you did not answer correctly.*

Correct Answers _____ X 5 = _____ % Score

Learning Activity 9-4
Procedures, Pharmacology, and Abbreviations

Match the terms with the definitions in the numbered list.

ANA	homologous	PT
anticoagulants	lymphangiography	RBC
antimicrobials	lymphoscintigraphy	thrombolytics
autologous	monospot	transfusion
DIC	plasmapheresis	WBC

1. test used to diagnose bleeding disorders or excessive clotting disorders and monitor blood thinner medication _____

2. procedure that uses a contrast dye to determine blockages of the lymph vessels _____

3. serological test for infectious mononucleosis _____

4. used to prevent blood clot formation _____

5. leukocyte _____

6. transplant from a compatible donor _____

7. test that identifies antibodies that attack an individual's own cells _____

8. procedure that uses a radioactive tracer to identify the location of the sentinel node _____

9. dialysis procedure used to treat autoimmune diseases _____

10. hypercoagulation throughout the body that is life-threatening _____

11. transplant using the recipient's own stem cells _____

12. destroy bacteria, fungi, and protozoa _____

13. erythrocyte _____

14. used to dissolve blood clots _____

15. lifesaving procedure to replenish blood loss or for treatment of severe anemia _____

✓ *Check your answers in Appendix A. Review any material that you did not answer correctly.*

Correct Answers _____ X 6.67 = _____ % Score

DOCUMENTING HEALTH-CARE ACTIVITIES

This section provides practical application activities in the form of exercises to help students develop skills in documenting patient care. First, read the medical report. Then complete the activities and exercises that follow.

Documenting Health-Care Activity 9-1
Discharge Summary: Sickle Cell Crisis

General Hospital

1511 Ninth Avenue ▪ ▪ Sun City, USA 12345 ▪ ▪ (555) 802–1887

DISCHARGE SUMMARY

ADMISSION DATE: June 21, 20xx   **DISCHARGE DATE:** June 23, 20xx

CHIEF COMPLAINT: Abdominal pain

HISTORY OF PRESENT ILLNESS: This is a 46-year-old African American man who reports a history of sickle cell anemia, which typically results in abdominal cramping when he is in crisis. Upon admission, his hemoglobin was 6 g/dL which is different from his baseline of 7–8 g/dL. No history of splenectomy noted. He describes his pain as cramps in the midabdominal region. He denied any chills, fevers, nausea, vomiting, or sweats.

HOSPITAL COURSE:

Patient was admitted to a medical-surgical bed, was placed on oxygen, and given IV fluids. He received morphine and Vicodin for analgesia. Patient was given 2 units of packed red blood cells; his hemoglobin was 8 g/dL upon discharge.

An abdominal CT scan was performed and showed evidence of ileus in the small bowel with somewhat dilated small-bowel loops and also an abnormal enhancement pattern in the kidney. The patient has had no nausea or vomiting and is having regular bowel movements. He is ambulating. He even goes outside to smoke cigarettes, which he was advised not to do.

At discharge, his abdominal pain had resolved, however, he reported weakness. He was kept for an additional day for observation.

DISCHARGE DIAGNOSES:
1. Sickle cell crisis
2. Abdominal pain

DISCHARGE INSTRUCTIONS: Patient advised to follow up with his PCP for further renal function workup. Patient was encouraged to stop smoking and was provided with resources for this.

Michael R. Saadi, MD
Michael R. Saadi, MD

MRS:dp

D: 6–23–20xx; T: 6–23–20xx

Patient: Evans, Joshua	Physician: Michael R. Saadi, MD
Room #: 609 P	Patient ID#: 532657

Terminology

The terms listed in the table that follows are taken from Discharge Summary: Sickle Cell Crisis. Use a medical dictionary such as *Taber's Cyclopedic Medical Dictionary*, the appendices of this book, or other resources to define each term. Then review the pronunciation for each term and practice by reading the medical record aloud.

Term	Definition
ambulating ĂM-bū-lāt-ĭng	
analgesia ăn-ăl-JĔ-zē-ă	
anemia ă-NĔ-mē-ă	
crisis KRĪ-sĭs	
CT	
hemoglobin HĔ-mō-glō-bĭn	
ileus ĬL-ē-ŭs	
morphine MOR-fēn	
PCP	
sickle cell SĬK-ăl SĔL	
splenectomy splē-NĔK-tō-mē	
Vicodin VĪ-kō-dĭn	

Visit the Medical Terminology Systems online resource center at FADavis. com to practice pronunciation and reinforce the meanings of the terms in this medical report.

Critical Thinking

Review *Discharge Summary: Sickle Cell Crisis* to answer the questions.

1. What blood product was administered to the patient?

_____

_____

_____

2. Why was this blood product given to the patient?

_____

_____

_____

3. What medications were given to the patient for pain relief?

_____

_____

_____

4. Why was a CT scan performed on the patient?

_____

_____

_____

5. What were the three findings of the CT scan?

_____

_____

_____

6. Why should the patient see his PCP?

_____

_____

_____

Documenting Health-Care Activity 9-2

Discharge Summary: PCP and HIV

General Hospital

1511 Ninth Avenue ■ ■ Sun City, USA 12345 ■ ■ (544) 802–1887

DISCHARGE SUMMARY

ADMISSION DATE: March 5, 20xx   **DISCHARGE DATE:** March 6, 20xx

CHIEF COMPLAINT: Shortness of breath

HISTORY OF PRESENT ILLNESS: 63-year-old widowed, Caucasian woman presenting with progressive shortness of breath over the last several days. She feels easily fatigued and reports a dry cough.

PAST MEDICAL HISTORY: Significant for HIV and several episodes of diarrhea, sinusitis, thrush, and vaginal candidiasis. She has a history of unintentional 10-pound weight loss.

PROCEDURE: A chest x-ray was completed that revealed diffuse lower lobe infiltrates. A bronchoscopy with alveolar lavage was performed for further diagnostic clarification. Her antiretroviral treatment regimen was reinitiated.

DISCHARGE DIAGNOSES:
1. *Pneumocystis* pneumonia.
2. Human immunodeficiency virus infection.

DISCHARGE INSTRUCTIONS:
1. Start Bactrim antibiotic regimen to treat pneumonia. Educated to complete the entire course of medication therapy.
2. Continue antiretroviral treatment regimen.
3. Discharge to the care of her PCP, Dr. Amid Shaheen.

Michael R. Saadi, MD
Michael R. Saadi, MD

MRS:dp

D: 3–06–20xx; T: 3–06–20xx

Patient: Smart, Joann   Physician: Michael R. Saadi, MD
Room #: 540   Patient ID#: 532850

Terminology

The terms listed in the table that follows are taken from *Discharge Summary: PCP and HIV.*
Use a medical dictionary such as *Taber's Cyclopedic Medical Dictionary,* the appendices of this
book, or other resources to define each term. Then review the pronunciation for each term
and practice by reading the medical record aloud.

Term	Definition
AIDS	
alveolar lavage ăl-VĒ-ō-lăr lă-VĂZH	
antiretroviral ăn-T Ē-rě-trō-vī-rěl	
Bactrim BĂK-trĭm	
bronchoscopy brŏng-KŎS-kō-pē	
diffuse dĭ-FŪS	
HIV	
infiltrate ĬN-fĭl-trāt	
Pneumocystis **pneumonia** nū-mō-SĬS-tĭs nū-MŌ-nē-ă	
thrush THRŬSH	
vaginal candidiasis VĂJ-ĭn-ăl kăn-dĭ-DĪ-ă-sĭs	

Visit the Medical Terminology Systems online resource center at FADavis.
com to practice pronunciation and reinforce the meanings of the terms in this
medical report.

Critical Thinking

Review the medical report *Discharge Summary: PCP and HIV* to answer the questions.

1. How do you think the patient acquired the HIV infection?

_____

_____

_____

2. What four disorders in the medical history are significant for HIV?

_____

_____

_____

3. What was the x-ray finding?

_____

_____

_____

4. What antibiotic was prescribed for the pneumonia?

_____

_____

_____

5. What two procedures were performed to confirm the diagnosis of *Pneumocystis* pneumonia?

_____

_____

_____

Documenting Health-Care Activity 9-3

Constructing Chart Notes

To construct chart notes, replace the italicized and boldfaced terms in each of the two case studies with one of the listed medical terms.

arthralgia   *hematomas*   *leukocytosis*

erythropenia   *hemophilia*   *lymphadenopathy*

hemarthrosis   *hemostasis*   *splenomegaly*

hematologist

Mr. X, a 53-year-old male, presents with complaints of feeling "poorly" and not sleeping well for the past 3 months. Upon examination, the physician notes that Mr. X's gums are red and swollen. Also, there is evidence of (1) *disease in the lymph glands* under the patient's left arm and on the back of his neck. Upon palpation, the physician also notes an (2) *enlarged spleen*. The patient's CBC shows an (3) *abnormal increase of leukocytes* and a moderate (4) *decrease of erythrocytes*. The patient is referred to Dr. Jordan, a (5) *specialist in blood diseases.*

1. _____
2. _____
3. _____
4. _____
5. _____

Mr. J states that his father and uncle have (6) *"bleeder's disease."* The patient also states that he often develops (7) *large bruises* under his skin even with a minimal "bump or scrape." Today he presents with swelling and (8) *pain in his joints,* especially the knees. His present complaints are likely the result of (9) *abnormal bleeding into the joint* **cavity.** The physician prescribes an infusion of Mr. J's deficient clotting factor to (10) *control the bleeding.*

6. _____
7. _____
8. _____
9. _____
10. _____

Check your answers in Appendix A. Review any material that you did not answer correctly.

Correct Answers _____ X 10 = _____ % Score

Musculoskeletal System

Chapter Outline

Objectives

Upon completion of this chapter, you will be able to:

- Locate and describe the structures of the musculo-skeletal system.
- Describe the functional relationship between the musculoskeletal system and other body systems.
- Pronounce, spell, and build words related to the musculoskeletal system.
- Describe diseases, conditions, and procedures related to the musculoskeletal system.
- Explain pharmacology related to the treatment of musculoskeletal disorders.
- Demonstrate your knowledge of this chapter by completing the learning and documenting health-care activities.

Anatomy and Physiology

The musculoskeletal system includes muscles, bones, joints, and related structures, such as the tendons and connective tissue that function in the support and movement of body parts and organs (see Fig. 10-1).

Anatomy and Physiology Key Terms

This section introduces important terms, along with their definitions and pronunciations. The key terms are highlighted in color in the Anatomy and Physiology section. Word analyses for selected terms are also provided. Pronounce the term, and place a check mark in the box after you do so.

Term	Definition
articulation ☐ ăr-tĭk-ū-LĀ-shŭn	Place of union between two or more bones; also called *joint*
hematopoiesis ☐ hĕm-ă-tō-poy-Ē-sĭs *hemat/o:* blood *-poiesis:* formation, production	Production and development of blood cells, normally in the bone marrow
ligaments ☐ LĬG-ă-mĕnts	Connective tissue that surrounds the joint capsule to bind bones to other bones
tendons ☐ TĔN-dŭns	Connective tissue that binds muscle to bone on either side of a joint *Contraction of the muscle attached to the bone by tendon forces the bones in the joint to move.*

Pronunciation Help	Long Sound	ā — rate	ē — rebirth	ī — isle	ō — over	ū — unite
	Short Sound	ă — apple	ĕ — ever	ĭ — it	ŏ — not	ŭ — cut

Muscles

Muscle tissue is composed of contractile cells, or **fibers,** that provide movement of an organ or body part. Muscles contribute to posture, produce body heat, and act as a protective covering for internal organs. Muscles make up the bulk of the body. They have the ability to contract, relax, and return to their original size and shape. Whether muscles are attached to bones or found in internal organs and blood vessels, their primary responsibility is movement (see Table 10-1 pages 326–328.). Apparent motions provided by muscles include walking and talking. Less apparent motions include the passage and elimination of food through the digestive system, propulsion of blood through the arteries, and contraction of the bladder to eliminate urine.

There are three types of muscle tissue in the body:

• **Skeletal muscles** are attached to bones and provide the means for movement. Skeletal muscles are **voluntary muscles** that contract and relax in response to conscious thought. Because of their striped appearance on microscopic examination, they are also called **striated muscles.** Some examples of voluntary muscles are muscles that move the eyeballs, tongue, and bones.

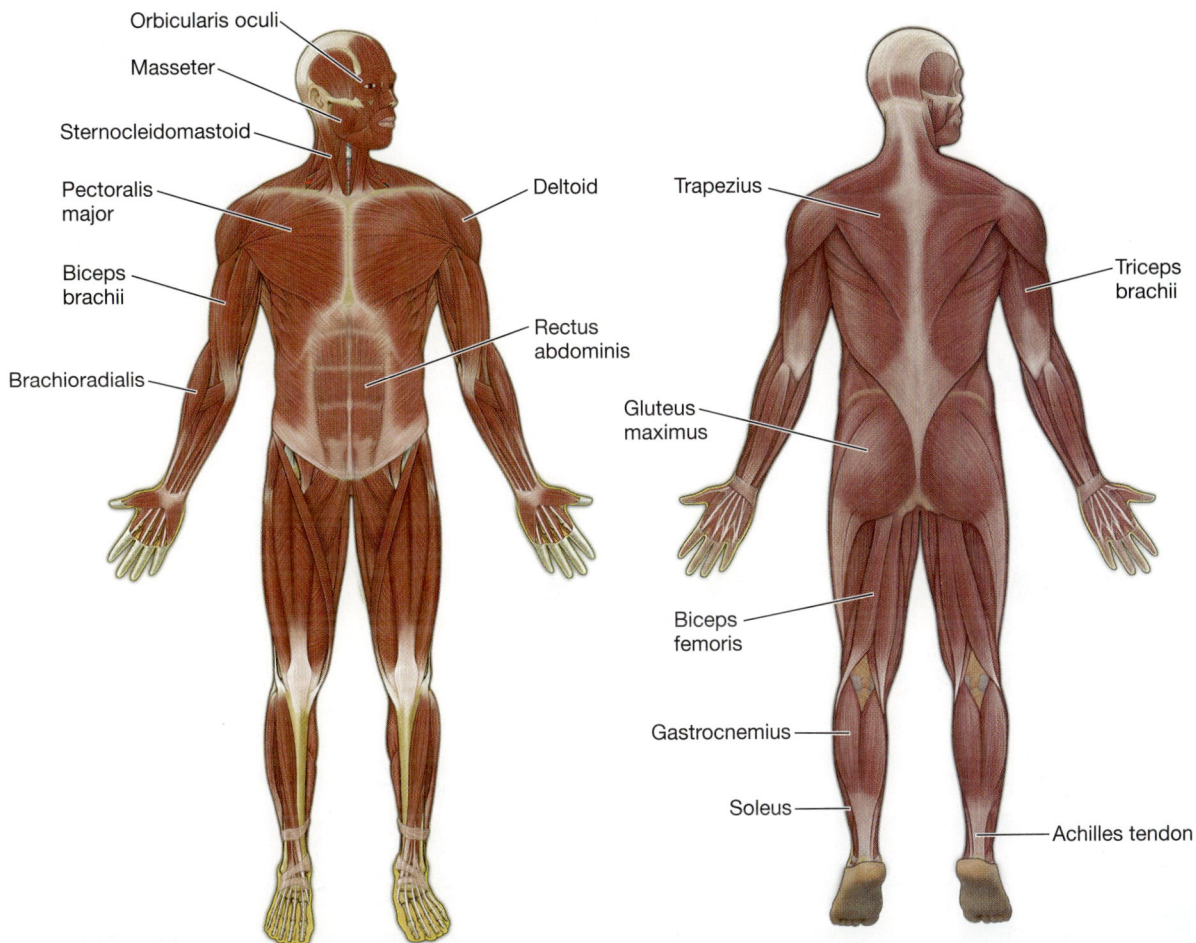

Orbicularis oculi
Masseter
Sternocleidomastoid
Pectoralis major
Biceps brachii
Brachioradialis

Deltoid
Rectus abdominis

Trapezius
Triceps brachii
Gluteus maximus
Biceps femoris
Gastrocnemius
Soleus
Achilles tendon

Figure 10-1 Selected muscles of the body.

- **Smooth muscles** are mainly responsible for assisting internal processes, such as digestion, circulation, and urination. Thus, they are called **visceral muscles.** Because their movement is not under conscious control but functions under the control of the autonomic (involuntary) nervous system, they are also known as **involuntary muscles.** Some examples of involuntary muscles are those in the digestive tract that propel food through the alimentary canal and those in the urinary system that control urination.
- **Cardiac muscle** is found only in the heart wall, where it forms the myocardium. It is striated like skeletal muscle, but it also produces rhythmic involuntary contractions like smooth muscle.

TABLE 10-1 Body Movements Produced by Muscle Action

This table lists body movements and the resulting muscle action. With the exception of rotation, these movements are in pairs of opposing functions.

Motion	Action
Adduction	Moves closer to the midline
Abduction	Moves away from the midline

Motion	Action
Flexion	Decreases the angle of a joint
Extension	Increases the angle of a joint

TABLE 10-1 Body Movements Produced by Muscle Action—cont'd

Motion	Action
Rotation	Moves a bone around its own axis

Pronation	Turns the palm downward
Supination	Turns the palm upward

Continued

TABLE 10-1 Body Movements Produced by Muscle Action—cont'd

Motion	Action
Inversion	Moves the sole of the foot inward
Eversion	Moves the sole of the foot outward

Motion	Action
Dorsiflexion	Elevates the foot
Plantar flexion	Lowers the foot (points the toes)

Anatomy Review: Muscular System

To review the anatomy of the muscular system, label the illustration using the listed terms.

Achilles tendon

biceps brachii

biceps femoris

brachioradialis

deltoid

gastrocnemius

gluteus maximus

masseter

orbicularis oculi

pectoralis major

rectus abdominis

soleus

sternocleidomastoid

trapezius

Triceps brachii

 Check your answers by referring to Figure 10–1 on page 325. Review material that you did not answer correctly.

Bones

Bones provide the framework of the body, protect internal organs, allow for movement, store calcium and other minerals, and produce blood cells within bone marrow **(hematopoiesis).** The bones of the skull protect the brain, the rib cage protects the heart and lungs, and the pelvic bones protect the developing fetus and reproductive organs. Movement is possible because bones provide points of attachment for muscles, **tendons**, and **ligaments**. As muscles contract, tendons and ligaments pull on bones and cause skeletal movement. Bones serve as a storehouse for minerals, particularly phosphorus and calcium.

Bone Types

There are four principal types of bone:

- **Short bones** are somewhat cube-shaped and are nearly equal in length and width. Examples of short bones include the bones of the wrist (carpals) and ankles (tarsals).
- **Irregular bones** include the bones that cannot be classified as short or long because of their complex shapes. Examples of irregular bones include vertebrae and the bones of the middle ear.
- **Flat bones** are exactly what their name suggests. They provide broad surfaces for muscular attachment or protection for internal organs. Examples of flat bones include bones of the skull, shoulder blades, and sternum.
- **Long bones** are found in the extremities of the body, such as the legs, arms, and fingers. The long bones have regular, well-defined shapes (see Fig. 10-2, page 331). Each long bone has three main parts:
  - The (1) **diaphysis** is the shaft, or long, main portion of a bone. It consists of **compact bone** that forms a cylinder and surrounds a central canal called the (2) **medullary cavity.** The medullary cavity is filled with "yellow bone marrow," so named because it is composed mainly of blood vessels and fatty tissue.
  - The (3) **distal epiphysis** and (4) **proximal epiphysis** (plural, **epiphyses**) are the two ends of the bones. Both ends have a somewhat bulbous shape to provide space for muscle and ligament attachments near the joints. Each epiphysis consists of three layers of tissue:
    - (5) **articular cartilage,** which is a thin outer layer of cartilage where bones meet to form joints, and the (6) **epiphyseal line (growth plate),** an area of cartilage constantly being replaced by new bone tissue as the bone grows and that is responsible for lengthening bones during childhood and adolescence and calcifies and disappears when the bone has achieved its full growth
    - thick, dense layer of hard (7) **compact bone**
    - inner layer of porous tissue called (8) **spongy** or **cancellous bone** that is less dense than compact bone and is filled with red bone marrow, so named because it is composed mainly of blood cells in various stages of development
  - The (9) **periosteum,** a dense, white, fibrous membrane, covers the remaining surface of the bone. It contains numerous blood and lymph vessels and nerves. In growing bones, the inner layer contains the bone-forming cells known as **osteoblasts.** The periosteum provides a means for bone repair and general bone nutrition. The periosteum also serves as a point of attachment for muscles, ligaments, and tendons.

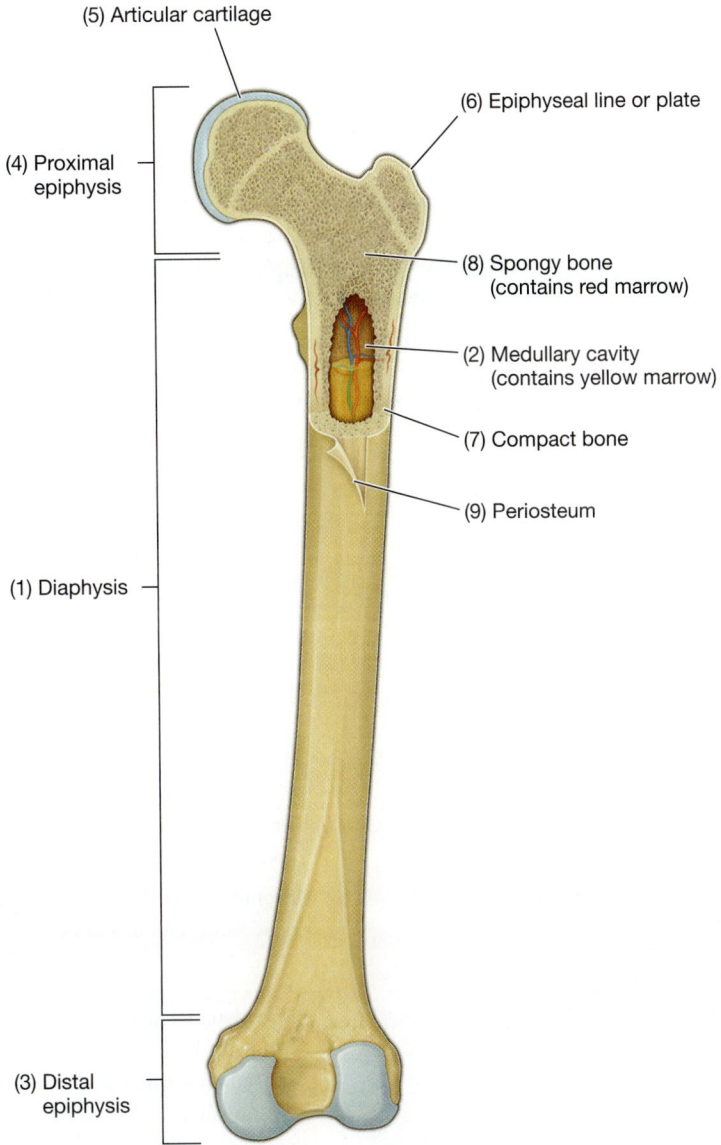

(5) Articular cartilage

(6) Epiphyseal line or plate

(4) Proximal epiphysis

(8) Spongy bone (contains red marrow)

(2) Medullary cavity (contains yellow marrow)

(7) Compact bone

(9) Periosteum

(1) Diaphysis

(3) Distal epiphysis

Figure 10-2 Longitudinal structure of a long bone.

Surface Features of Bones

Surfaces of bones are rarely smooth but consist of projections, articulating surfaces, depressions, and openings. These surfaces provide sites for muscle and ligament attachment. They also provide pathways and openings for blood vessels and nerves. Various types of projections are evident in bones, some of which serve as points of **articulation**. Table 10-2 lists common bone markings and their descriptions.

TABLE 10-2 Surface Features of Bones

This table lists the most common types of bone projections, articulating surfaces, depressions, and openings, along with the bones involved, descriptions, and examples for each. Becoming familiar with these terms will help you identify the parts of individual bones described in medical reports related to orthopedics.

Surface Type	Bone Marking	Description	Example
Projections			
• Nonarticulating surfaces	• Trochanter	• Very large, irregularly shaped process found only on the femur	• Greater trochanter of the femur
• Sites of muscle and ligament attachment	• Tubercle	• Small, rounded process	• Tubercle of the femur
	• Tuberosity	• Large, rounded process	• Tuberosity of the humerus
Articulating Surfaces			
• Projections that form joints	• Condyle	• Rounded, articulating knob	• Condyle of the humerus
	• Head	• Prominent, rounded, articulating end of a bone	• Head of the femur
Depressions and Openings			
• Sites for blood vessel, nerve, and duct passage	• Foramen	• Rounded opening through a bone to accommodate blood vessels and nerves	• Foramen of the skull through which cranial nerves pass
	• Fissure	• Narrow, slitlike opening	• Fissure of the sphenoid bone
	• Meatus	• Opening or passage into a bone	• External auditory meatus of the temporal bone
	• Sinus	• Cavity or hollow space in a bone	• Cavity of the frontal sinus containing a duct that carries secretions to the upper part of the nasal cavity

Divisions of the Skeletal System

The skeletal system of a human adult consists of 206 individual bones. For anatomical purposes, the human skeleton is divided into the axial skeleton and the appendicular skeleton (see Fig. 10-3).

Axial Skeleton

The axial skeleton is divided into three major regions: skull, rib cage, and vertebral column. It contributes to the formation of body cavities and provides protection for internal organs, such as the brain, spinal cord, and organs enclosed in the thorax. Figure 10-3 depicts the axial bones in a light tan color.

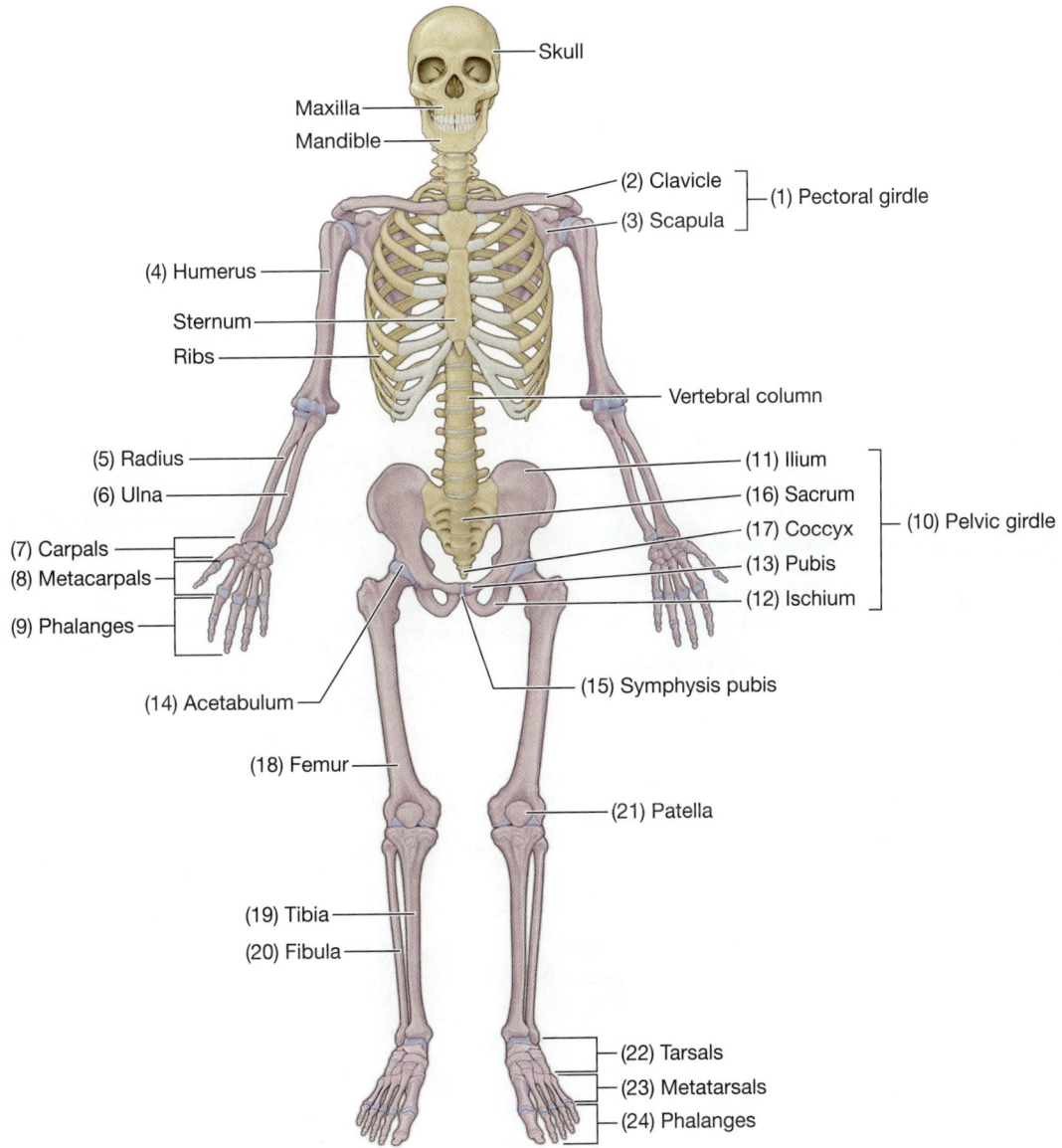

Figure 10-3 Anterior view of the axial (tan) and appendicular (blue) skeleton.

Skull

The bony structure of the skull consists of cranial bones and facial bones (see Fig. 10-4). With the exception of one facial bone, all other bones of the skull are joined together by sutures. Sutures are the lines of junction between two bones, especially of the skull, and are usually immovable.

Cranial Bones

Eight bones, collectively known as the **cranium (skull),** enclose and protect the brain and the organs of hearing and equilibrium. Cranial bones are connected to muscles to provide head movements, chewing motions, and facial expressions.

At birth, the skull is incompletely developed, with fibrous membranes connecting the cranial bones. These membranous areas are called **fontanels** or, more commonly, *soft spots*. They permit some movement between the bones that enables an infant's skull to pass more easily through the birth canal. Eventually, the fontanels close as the cranial bones grow together. The (1) **frontal bone** forms the anterior portion of the skull **(forehead)** and the roof of the bony cavities that contain the eyeballs. One (2) **parietal bone** is situated on each side of the skull just behind the frontal bone. Together they form the upper sides and roof of the cranium. Each parietal bone

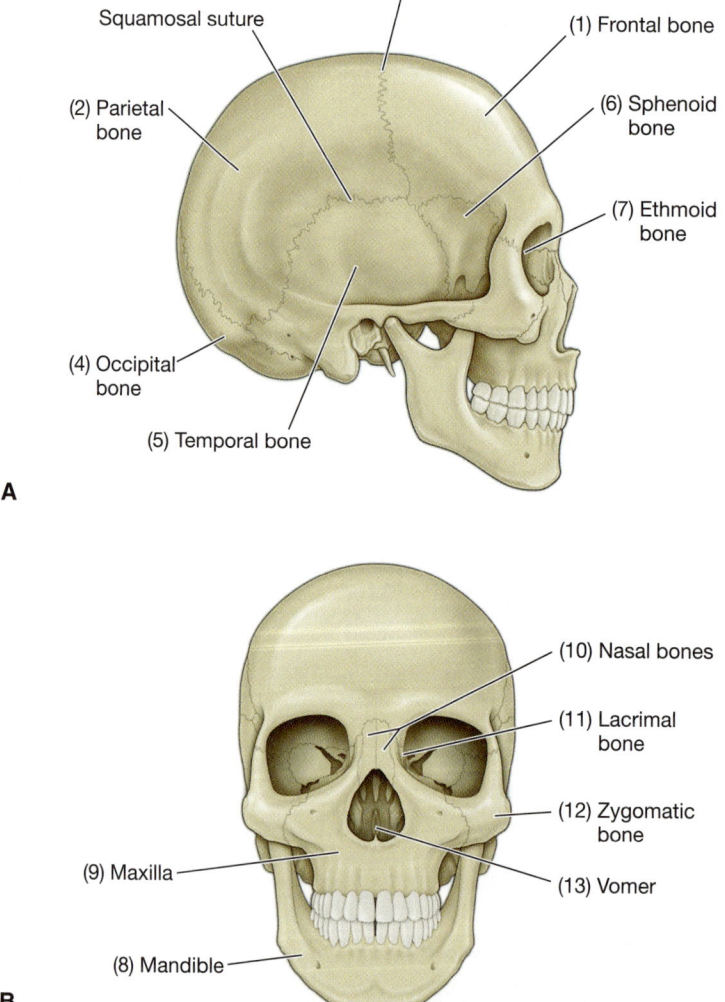

Figure 10-4 Bony structures of the skull. (A) Cranial bones. (B) Facial bones.

meets the frontal bone along the (3) **coronal suture.** A single (4) **occipital bone** forms the back and base of the skull. It contains an opening in its base through which the spinal cord passes. Two (5) **temporal bone(s),** one on each side of the skull, form part of the lower cranium. Each temporal bone has a complicated shape that contains various cavities and recesses associated with the internal ear, the essential part of the organ of hearing and balance. The temporal bone projects downward to form the **mastoid process,** which provides a point of attachment for several neck muscles. The (6) **sphenoid bone,** located at the middle part of the base of the skull, forms a central wedge that joins with all other cranial bones, holding them together. The (7) **ethmoid bone** is the anterior cranial bone located between the nasal cavity and parts of the orbits of the eyes.

Facial Bones

All facial bones, with the exception of the (8) **mandible** (lower jaw bone), are joined together by sutures and are immovable. Movement of the mandible is necessary for speaking and chewing **(mastication).** The (9) **maxillae** (singular, **maxilla**), paired upper jawbones, are fused in the midline by a suture. They form the upper jaw and **hard palate** (roof of the mouth). If the maxillary bones do not fuse properly before birth, a congenital defect called **cleft palate** results. The maxillae and mandible contain sockets for the roots of the teeth. Two thin, nearly rectangular bones, the (10) **nasal bones,** lie side by side and are fused medially, forming the shape and the bridge of the nose. Two paired (11) **lacrimal bones** are located at the corner of each eye. These thin, small bones unite to form the groove for the lacrimal sac and canals through which the tear ducts pass into the nasal cavity. The paired (12) **zygomatic bones** (cheekbones) are located on the side of the face below the eyes and form the higher portion of the cheeks below and to the sides of the eyes. The (13) **vomer** is a single, thin bone that forms the lower part of the nasal septum.

Other important structures, the **paranasal sinuses,** are cavities located within the cranial and facial bones. As their names imply, the frontal, ethmoidal, sphenoidal, and maxillary sinuses are named after the bones in which they are located (see Fig. 10-5).

Sphenoidal sinus

Frontal sinuses

Ethmoidal sinuses

Maxillary sinus

Figure 10-5 Paranasal sinuses.

Thorax

The term *thorax* refers to the entire chest. The internal organs of the thorax include the heart and lungs, which are enclosed in and protected by the **thoracic cage (rib cage)**. The thoracic cage consists of 12 pairs of ribs, all attached to the spine (see Fig. 10-6). The first seven pairs, the (1) **true ribs**, are attached directly to the (2) **sternum** by a strip of (3) **costal cartilage.** The costal cartilage of the next five pairs of ribs is not fastened directly to the sternum, so these ribs are known as (4) **false ribs.** The last two pairs of false ribs are not joined, even indirectly, to the sternum but attach posteriorly to the thoracic vertebrae. These last two pairs of false ribs are known as (5) **floating ribs.**

Vertebral Column

The vertebral column of the adult is composed of 26 bones called **vertebrae** (singular, **vertebra**). The vertebral column supports the body and provides a protective bony canal for the spinal cord. A healthy, normal spine has four curves that help make it resilient and maintain balance. The cervical and lumbar regions curve forward, whereas the thoracic and sacral regions curve backward (see Fig. 10-7 page 337).

The vertebral column consists of five regions of bones, each deriving its name from its location within the spinal column. The seven (1) **cervical vertebrae** form the skeletal framework of the neck. The first cervical vertebra, the (2) **atlas,** supports the skull. The second cervical vertebra, the (3) **axis,** makes possible the rotation of the skull on the neck. Under the cervical vertebra are 12 (4) **thoracic vertebrae,** which support the chest and serve as a point of articulation for the ribs. The next five vertebrae, the (5) **lumbar vertebrae,** are situated in the lower back area and carry most of the weight of the torso. Below this area are five sacral vertebrae, which are fused into a single bone in the adult and are referred to as the (6) **sacrum.** The tail of the vertebral column consists of four or five fragmented fused vertebrae referred to as the (7) **coccyx.**

Vertebrae are separated by flat, round structures, the (8) **intervertebral disks,** which are composed of a fibrocartilaginous substance with a gelatinous mass in the center (**nucleus pulposus**).

Figure 10-6 Thorax.

Figure 10-7 Lateral view of the vertebral column.

Appendicular Skeleton

The appendicular skeleton consists of bones of the upper and lower limbs and their girdles, which attach the limbs to the axial skeleton. The appendicular skeleton is distinguished with a blue color in Figure 10-3. The axial skeleton protects internal organs and provides central support for the body; the appendicular skeleton enables body movement. The ability to walk, run, or catch a ball is possible because of the movable joints of the limbs that make up the appendicular skeleton.

Pectoral Girdle

The (1) **pectoral (shoulder) girdle** consists of two bones, the anterior (2) **clavicle** (collarbone) and the posterior (3) **scapula** (triangular shoulder blade). The primary function of the pectoral girdle is to attach the bones of the upper limbs to the axial skeleton and provide attachments for muscles that aid upper limb movements. The paired pectoral structures and their associated muscles form the shoulders of the body.

Upper Limbs

The skeletal framework of each upper limb includes the arm, forearm, and hand. Anatomically speaking, the arm is only that part of the upper limb between the shoulder and elbow. Each **appendage** consists of the (4) **humerus** (upper arm bone) as well as the (5) **radius** and (6) **ulna,** the two bones that constitute the forearm and articulate at the elbow with the humerus. The bones of each hand include eight (7) **carpals** (wrist), five radiating (8) **metacarpals** (palm), and 10 radiating (9) **phalanges** (fingers).

Pelvic Girdle

The (10) **pelvic girdle** (hip bone) is a basin-shaped structure that attaches the lower limbs to the axial skeleton. Along with its associated ligaments, it supports the trunk of the body and provides protection for lower organs of digestion and urinary and reproductive structures.

Male and female **pelves** (singular, **pelvis**) differ considerably in size and shape but share the same basic structures. Generally, the bones of males are larger and heavier and possess larger surface markings than those of females of comparable age and physical stature. Some of the differences are attributable to the function of the female pelvis during childbearing. The female pelvis is shallower than the male pelvis but wider in all directions. The female pelvis not only supports the enlarged uterus as the fetus matures but also provides a large opening to allow the infant to pass through during birth. Regardless of these differences, the female and male pelves are divided into the (11) **ilium,** (12) **ischium,** and (13) **pubis.** These three bones fuse together in the adult to form a single hip bone called the **innominate bone.** The ilium travels inferiorly to form part of the (14) **acetabulum,** the deep socket of the hip joint, and joins the pubis. The bladder is located behind the (15) **symphysis pubis;** the rectum is in the curve of the (16) **sacrum** and (17) **coccyx.** In the female, the uterus, fallopian tubes, ovaries, and vagina are located between the bladder and the rectum.

Lower Limbs

The lower limbs support the complete weight of the erect body and are subjected to exceptional stresses, especially in running or jumping. To accommodate for these forces, the lower limb bones are stronger and thicker than comparable bones of the upper limbs.

There are three parts of each lower limb: the thigh, the leg, and the foot. The thigh consists of a single bone called the (18) **femur.** It is the largest, longest, and strongest bone in the body. The leg is formed by two parallel bones: the (19) **tibia** and the (20) **fibula.** A small triangular bone, the (21) **patella** (kneecap), is located anterior to the knee joint. The seven (22) **tarsals** (ankle bones) resemble metacarpals (wrist bones) in structure. Lastly, the bones of each foot include the (23) **metatarsals,** which consist of five small long bones numbered 1 to 5 beginning with the great toe on the medial side of the foot, and the much smaller (24) **phalanges** (toes).

Joints or Articulations

To allow for body movements, bones must have points where they meet **(articulate).** These articulating points form joints that have various degrees of mobility. The **joint capsule** contains a lubrication fluid **(synovial fluid)** that nourishes and protects the joint. The need for greater or lesser flexibility determines the type of joint in any specific location. There are three types of joints. All three types are necessary for smooth, coordinated body movements. Freely movable joints **(diarthroses)** are encased in a sleevelike extension of the periosteum, such as the hinge joints of the elbow (between the humerus and ulna). Slightly movable joints **(amphiarthroses)** are articulations between two bones connected by ligaments or elastic cartilage, such as those between the vertebrae. Immovable joints **(synarthroses)** are joints that have no mobility, such as those that constitute the sutures of the skull.

Anatomy Review: Long Bone

To review the anatomy of a typical long bone, label the illustration of the femur using the listed terms.

articular cartilage	*distal epiphysis*	*periosteum*
compact bone	*epiphyseal line or plate*	*proximal epiphysis*
diaphysis	*medullary cavity*	*spongy bone*

 Check your answers by referring to Figure 10-2 on page 331. Review material that you did not answer correctly.

Anatomy Review: Skeletal System

To review the skeletal structures, label the illustration using the listed terms.

acetabulum	humerus	pelvic girdle	sternum
carpals	ilium	phalanges	symphysis pubis
clavicle	ischium	pubis	tarsals
coccyx	metacarpals	radius	tibia
femur	metatarsals	sacrum	ulna
fibula	pectoral girdle	scapula	vertebral column

 Check your answers by referring to Figure 10–3 on page 333. Review material that you did not answer correctly.

CONNECTING BODY SYSTEMS—MUSCULOSKELETAL SYSTEM

The main function of the musculoskeletal system is to provide support, protection, and movement of body parts. Specific functional relationships between the musculoskeletal system and other body systems are summarized here.

Blood, Lymphatic, and Immune
- Muscle action pumps lymph through lymphatic vessels.
- Bone marrow provides a place for cells of the immune system to develop.

Cardiovascular
- Bone helps regulate blood calcium levels, which are important to heart function.

Digestive
- Muscles play an important role in swallowing and propelling food through the digestive tract.
- Muscles of the stomach mechanically break down food to prepare it for chemical digestion.

Endocrine
- Exercising skeletal muscles stimulates release of hormones to increase blood flow.

Female Reproductive
- Muscles are important in sexual activity and during delivery of the fetus.
- Bones provide a source of calcium during pregnancy and lactation if dietary intake is lacking or insufficient.
- The pelvis helps support the enlarged uterus during pregnancy.

Integumentary
- Involuntary muscle contractions (shivering) help regulate body temperature.

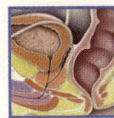

Male Reproductive
- Muscles play an important role in sexual activity.

Nervous
- Bones protect the brain and spinal cord.

Respiratory
- Muscles elevate ribs and contract the diaphragm to assist in the breathing process.

Urinary
- Bones work in conjunction with the kidneys to help regulate blood calcium levels.
- Skeletal muscles help control urine elimination.

Medical Word Elements

This section introduces combining forms, suffixes, and prefixes related to the musculoskeletal system. Word analyses are also provided. From the information provided, complete the meaning of the medical words in the right–hand column. The first one is completed for you.

Element	Meaning	Word Analysis and Meaning
Combining Forms		
Muscular System		
leiomy/o	smooth (visceral) muscle	**leiomy/**oma (lī-ō-mī-Ō-mă): *tumor of smooth muscle* *-oma:* tumor
muscul/o	muscle	**muscul/**ar (MŎS-kū-lăr):_____ *-ar:* pertaining to
my/o		**my/**oma (mī-Ō-mă): _____ *-oma:* tumor
rhabd/o	rod-shaped (striated)	**rhabd/**oid (RĂB-doyd): _____ *-oid:* resembling
rhabdomy/o	rod-shaped (striated) muscle	**rhabdomy/**oma (răb-dō-mī-Ō-mă): _____ *-oma:* tumor
Skeletal System		
Bones of the Upper Body		
brachi/o	arm	**brachi/**algia (brā-kē-ĂL-jē-ă): _____ *-algia:* pain
carp/o	carpus (wrist bone)	**carp/o/**ptosis (kăr-pŏp-TŌ-sĭs): _____ *-ptosis:* prolapse, downward displacement *Carpoptosis is commonly called* **wrist drop.**
cephal/o	head	**cephal/**ad (SĔF-ă-lăd): _____ *-ad:* toward
cervic/o	neck; cervix uteri (neck of the uterus)	**cervic/o/**dynia (sĕr-vĭ-kō-DĬN-ē-ă): _____ *-dynia:* pain *Cervicodynia is also called* **cervical neuralgia.**
clavicul/o	clavicle (collar bone)	**clavicul/**ar (klă-VĬK-ū-lăr): _____ *-ar:* pertaining to
cost/o	ribs	**cost/**ectomy (kŏs-TĔK-tō-mē): _____ *-ectomy:* excision, removal

Medical Word Elements—cont'd

Element	Meaning	Word Analysis
crani/o	cranium (skull)	**crani/o**/tomy (krā-nē-ŎT-ō-mē): _____ *-tomy:* incision
dactyl/o	fingers; toes	**dactyl**/itis (dăk-tĭl-Ī-tĭs): _____ *-itis:* inflammation

humer/o	humerus (upper arm bone)	**humer/o**/scapul/ar (hū-měr-ō-SKĂP-ū-lăr): _____
		  scapul: scapula (shoulder blade)
		  -ar: pertaining to

metacarp/o	metacarpus (hand bones)	**metacarp**/ectomy (mĕt-ă-kăr-PĔK-tō-mē): _____ *-ectomy:* excision, removal
phalang/o	phalanges (bones of the fingers and toes)	**phalang**/ectomy (făl-ăn-JĔK-tō-mē): _____ *-ectomy:* excision, removal
radi/o	radiation, x-ray; radius (lower arm bone on the thumb side)	**radi**/al (RĀ-dē-ăl): _____ *-al:* pertaining to
spondyl/o	vertebrae (backbone)	**spondyl**/itis (spŏn-dĭl-Ī-tĭs): _____ *-itis:* inflammation *The combining form* **spondyl/o** *describes diseases and conditions.*

vertebr/o		inter/**vertebr**/al (ĭn-těr-VĔRT-ĕ-brĕl): _____
		  inter-: between
		  -al: pertaining to
		The combining form **vertebr/o** *indicates anatomical terms.*

stern/o	sternum (breastbone)	**stern**/ad (STĔR-năd): _____ *-ad:* toward
thorac/o	chest	**thorac/o**/dynia (thō-răk-ō-DĬN-ē-ă): _____ *-dynia:* pain
Bones of the Lower Body		
calcane/o	calcaneum (heel bone)	**calcane/o**/dynia (kăl-kā-nē-ō-DĬN-ē-ă): _____ *-dynia:* pain
femor/o	femur (thigh bone)	**femor**/al (FĔM-or-ăl): _____ *-al:* pertaining to

Continued

Medical Word Elements—cont'd

Element	Meaning	Word Analysis
fibul/o	fibula (smaller bone of the lower leg)	**fibul/o**/calcane/al (fĭb-ū-lō-kăl-KĀ-nē-ăl): _____ *calcane:* calcaneum (heel bone) *-al:* pertaining to
ili/o	ilium (lateral, flaring portion of the hip bone)	**ili/o**/pelv/ic (ĭl-ē-ō-PĔL-vĭk): _____ *pelv:* pelvis *-ic:* pertaining to
ischi/o	ischium (lower portion of the hip bone)	**ischi/o**/dynia (ĭs-kē-ō-DĬN-ē-ă): _____ *-dynia:* pain
lumb/o	loins (lower back)	**lumb/o**/dynia (lūm-bō-DĬN-ē-ă): _____ *-dynia:* pain
metatars/o	metatarsus (foot bones)	**metatars**/algia (mĕt-ă-tăr-SĂL-jē-ă): _____ *-algia:* pain *Metatarsalgia radiates from the head of the metatarsus and worsens with weight-bearing activity or palpation.*
patell/o	patella (kneecap)	**patell**/ectomy (păt-ĕ-LĔK-tō-mē): _____ *-ectomy:* excision, removalpelv/i
pelv/i	pelvis	**pelv/i**/metry* (pĕl-VĬM-ĕt-rē): _____ *-metry:* act of measuring *Pelvimetry is routinely performed in obstetrical management.*
pelv/o		**pelv**/ic (PĔL-vĭc): _____ *-ic:* pertaining to *A woman's pelvis is usually less massive but wider and more circular than a man's pelvis.*
pod/o	foot	**pod**/iatry (pō-DĪ-ă-trē): _____ *-iatry:* medicine, treatment
pub/o	pubis (anterior part of the pelvic bone)	**pub/o**/coccyg/eal (pū-bō-k ŏk-SĬJ-ē-ăl): _____ *coccyg:* coccyx (tailbone) *-eal:* pertaining to
tibi/o	tibia (larger bone of the lower leg)	**tibi/o**/femor/al (tĭb-ē-ō-FĔM-or-ăl): _____ *femor:* femur *-al:* pertaining to

*The i in *pelv/i/metry* is an exception to the rule of using the connecting vowel *o*.

Medical Word Elements—cont'd

Element	Meaning	Word Analysis
Other		
ankyl/o	stiffness; bent, crooked	**ankyl**/osis (ăng-kĭ-LŌ-sĭs): _____ *-osis:* abnormal condition; increase (used primarily with blood cells) *Ankylosis results in immobility and stiffness of a joint. It may be the result of trauma, surgery, or disease and most commonly occurs in rheumatoid arthritis.*
arthr/o	joint	**arthr**/itis (ăr-THRĪ-tĭs): _____ *-itis:* inflammation
chondr/o	cartilage	**chondr**/itis (kŏn-DRĪ-tĭs): _____ *-itis:* inflammation
fasci/o	band, fascia (fibrous membrane supporting and separating muscles)	**fasci/o**/plasty (FĂSH-ē-ō-plăs-tē): _____ *-plasty:* surgical repair
fibr/o	fiber, fibrous tissue	**fibr**/oma (fĭ-BRŌ-mă): _____ *-oma:* tumor
kyph/o	humpback	**kyph**/osis (kī-FŌ-sĭs): _____ *-osis:* abnormal condition; increase (used primarily with blood cells)
lamin/o	lamina (part of vertebral arch)	**lamin**/ectomy (lăm-ĭ-NĔK-tō-mē): _____ *-ectomy:* excision, removal *Laminectomy is usually performed to relieve compression of the spinal cord or remove a lesion or herniated disk.*
lord/o	curve, swayback	**lord**/osis (lor-DŌ-sĭs): _____ *-osis:* abnormal condition; increase (used primarily with blood cells)
myel/o	bone marrow; spinal cord	**myel/o**/cyte (MĪ-Ĕl-ō-sīt): _____ *-cyte:* cell

orth/o	straight	**orth/o**/ped/ist (or-thō-PĒ-dĭst): _____
		  ped: foot; child
		  -ist: specialist
		
		Historically, an orthopedist corrected deformities and straightened children's bones. In today's medical practice, however, the orthopedist treats musculoskeletal disorders and associated structures in persons of all ages.

oste/o	bone	**oste**/oma (ŏs-tē-Ō-mă): _____ *-oma:* tumor *Osteomas are benign bony tumors.*

Continued

Medical Word Elements—cont'd

Element	Meaning	Word Analysis
ped/o	foot; child	**ped/o**/graph (PĔD-ō-grăf): _____ -*graph:* instrument for recording *A pedograph produces an imprint of the foot so that the gait (manner of walking) can be studied.*
scoli/o	crooked, bent	**scoli**/osis (skō-lē-Ō-sĭs): _____ -*osis:* abnormal condition; increase (used primarily with blood cells) *Scoliosis is characterized by a lateral spinal curvature.*
synov/o	synovial membrane, synovial fluid	**synov**/ectomy (sĭn-ō-VĔK-tō-mē): _____ -*ectomy:* excision, removal
ten/o	tendon	**ten/o**/desis (tĕn-ŌD-ĕ-sĭs): _____ -*desis:* binding, fixation (of a bone or joint)
tend/o		**tend/o**/plasty (TĔN-dō-plăs-tē): _____ -*plasty:* surgical repair
tendin/o		**tendin**/itis (tĕn-dĭn-Ī-tĭs): _____ -*itis:* inflammation

Suffixes

Element	Meaning	Word Analysis
-asthenia	weakness, debility	my/**asthenia** (mī-ăs-THĒ-nē-ă): _____ *my:* muscle
-clasia	to break; surgical fracture	oste/o/**clasia** (ŏs-tē-ō-KLĀ-zē-ă): _____ *oste/o:* bone *Osteoclasia is the intentional fracture of a bone to correct a deformity and is also called* **osteoclasis.**
-clast	to break; surgical fracture	oste/o/**clast** (ŎS-tē-ō-klăst): _____ *oste/o:* bone *An osteoclast is a cell that breaks down the matrix of bone. Osteoblasts and osteoclasts work together to maintain a constant bone size in adults.*
-desis	binding, fixation (of a bone or joint)	arthr/o/**desis** (ăr-thrō-DĒ-sĭs): _____ *arthr/o:* joint *This procedure immobilizes a joint to relieve intractable pain.*
-malacia	softening	chondr/o/**malacia** (kŏn-drō-măl-Ā-shē-ă): _____ *chondr/o:* cartilage *Chondromalacia is a deterioration of the articular cartilage, usually involving the patella.*
-porosis	porous	oste/o/**porosis** (ŏs-tē-ō-pŏ-RŌ-sĭs): _____ *oste/o:* bone *Osteoporosis is a disorder characterized by loss of bone density. It may cause pain, especially in the lower back, pathological fractures, loss of stature, and hairline fractures.*

Medical Word Elements—cont'd

Element	Meaning	Word Analysis
-sarcoma	malignant tumor of connective tissue	chondr/o/**sarcoma** (kŏn-drō-săr-KŌ-mă): _____ *chondr/o:* cartilage *Connective tissue is found in cartilage, fat, blood vessels, bone, nerves, and muscles.*
a-	without, not	**a**/trophy (ĂT-rō-fē): _____ *-trophy:* development, nourishment *Atrophy causes a wasting or decrease in size or physiological activity of a part of the body because of disease or other influences.*
dys-	bad; painful; difficult	**dys**/trophy (DĬS-trō-fē): _____ *-trophy:* development, nourishment
syn-	union, together, joined	**syn**/dactyl/ism (sĭn-DĂK-tĭl-ĭzm): _____ *dactyl:* fingers, toes *-ism:* condition *Syndactylism results in a fusion of two or more fingers or toes.*

Visit the Medical Terminology Systems online resource center at FADavis.com for an audio exercise of the terms in this table. Other activities are also available to reinforce content.

It is time to review medical word elements by completing Learning Activities 10–1 and 10–2.

Disease Focus

Musculoskeletal disorders include a variety of conditions that affect the muscles, bones, and joints found in neck, shoulders, wrists, back, hips, legs, knees, and feet. Pain and discomfort commonly associated with these disorders may interfere with everyday activities. These disorders are extremely common, and risk increases with age. Early diagnosis is the key to easing pain while potentially decreasing further bodily damage.

Given the different areas of the body that make up the musculoskeletal system, several other diseases can produce significant musculoskeletal signs and symptoms. These disorders include but are not limited to lower back pain, fibromyalgia, gout, osteoarthritis, rheumatoid arthritis, and tendinitis. Some of these disorders can cause mild discomfort to debilitating pain. Low back pain is the most common musculoskeletal disorder.

For diagnosis, treatment, and management of musculoskeletal disorders, the medical services of a specialist may be warranted. **Orthopedics** is the branch of medicine concerned with the prevention, diagnosis, care, and treatment of musculoskeletal disorders. The physician who specializes in the diagnosis and treatment of musculoskeletal disorders is known as an **orthopedist**. They use medical, physical, and surgical methods to restore function that has been lost as a result of musculoskeletal injury or disease. Another specialist, a **rheumatologist,** focuses on the treatment of joint diseases. Additionally, a **Doctor of Osteopathy (DO)** emphasizes the importance of proper alignment of bones, muscles, ligaments, and nerves for overall health. Osteopathic physicians, like medical doctors, combine manipulative procedures with advanced medical treatments, including prescribing medications and performing surgeries. They have the same rights, privileges, and responsibilities as the doctor of medicine (MD).

Fractures

A **fracture** is a break or crack in a bone. Fractures can range in severity from a simple hairline crack to the most serious type, where the end of the broken bone pierces through the flesh (**open fracture, compound fracture**). Fractures usually result from trauma but may also be caused by disease (**pathological fracture**). Imaging procedures confirm and determine the severity of fractures. Figure 10-8 illustrates some common types of fractures.

Treatment of fractures involves restoring the bone to its normal position (**reduction**). In a **closed reduction**, the practitioner repairs the fracture without a surgical incision of the area by aligning the bone through manual manipulation or traction. Once the practitioner reduces the fracture, the bone is immobilized using a splint, cast, or sling to maintain the position of the bone until healing occurs. In an **open reduction**, realignment of the two broken ends of the bone takes place under direct observation by exposing the fracture using surgery. Severe fractures may require the use of hardware to hold the bone together so it can heal in proper alignment. Open

Closed
Bone is broken but no open wound in skin

Open
Bone breaks through skin

Complicated
Extensive soft tissue injury such as a broken rib piercing the lung

Comminuted
Bone is crushed into several pieces

Spiral
Bone is broken into two pieces due to a twisting force applied along its axis, typically occurring when the body is in motion and one limb remains fixed in place

Impacted
Broken ends of a bone are forced into one another

Incomplete
Line of fracture does not include the whole bone

Greenstick
Bone is broken only on one side, commonly occurs mostly in children because growing bones are soft

Colles fracture
Distal radius is broken by falling onto an outstretched hand

Hairline
Small, thin crack in a bone caused by repetitive stress or overuse, often without a complete break

Figure 10-8 Types of fracture.

reduction with the use of implants such as screws, rods, or plates to hold the bone fragments in place is referred to as open reduction with **internal fixation (ORIF)** (see Fig. 10-9). Open reduction with **external fixation (OREF)** devices to treat fractures involves a metal frame (fixator) outside of the body that is typically composed of metal pins, rods, and clamps to realign the bone (see Fig. 10-10).

If the bone has a **hairline fracture**, also known as a **stress** fracture when caused by repetitive actions or overuse, no repair may be necessary, except rest and refraining from doing activities that aggravate the area until it is healed. In some cases, involving larger fractures or persistent pain, the practitioner may immobilize the area.

Figure 10-9 Open reduction with internal fixation (ORIF) of a fractured tibia with five screws.

Figure 10-10 Open reduction with external fixation (OREF) to repair a fractured tibia.

Arthritis

Arthritis, a general term for many joint diseases, is an inflammation of a joint, usually accompanied by pain, swelling, and deformity. Because of their location and constant use, joints are prone to stress injuries and inflammation. The main types of arthritis are rheumatoid arthritis and osteoarthritis.

Rheumatoid arthritis (RA), a systemic disease characterized by inflammatory changes in joints and their related structures, results in crippling deformities (see Fig. 10-11). This form of arthritis is caused by an autoimmune disease that destroys joint tissue. It occurs most commonly in women between ages 23 and 35 but can affect people of any age group. Flare-ups **(exacerbations)** of this disease are commonly associated with periods of increased physical or emotional stress. In addition to joint changes, adjacent muscles, bones, and skin atrophy. There is no specific cure, but **NSAIDs,** physical therapy, and orthopedic measures help treat less severe cases.

Osteoarthritis, also known as **degenerative joint disease (DJD),** is by far the most common form of arthritis. It is a progressive, degenerative disease that occurs when the protective cartilage at the end of the bones wears down. Pain and stiffness in the joints are the most common symptoms. The pain is commonly worse after exercise and when putting weight or pressure on the joint. Over time, the joints become stiffer and harder to move. There may also be a rubbing, grating, or crackling sound **(crepitation)** with movement of the joint. Nevertheless, some persons are asymptomatic, even though x-rays show the changes of osteoarthritis. Almost everyone has some symptoms by age 70, but these symptoms may be minor. The joints most commonly affected include the hands, knees, hips, and spine. There is a higher risk of DJD in younger athletes and overweight individuals of all ages. Playing a sport that involves direct effect on the joint (such as tennis or football), twisting (such as basketball or soccer), or throwing also increases the risk of osteoarthritis. In osteoarthritis, new bone growth **(bone spur** or **osteophyte)** commonly occurs at articular surfaces. The smallest joints at the ends of the fingers are commonly affected by spur formation that leads to the classic bony enlargement referred to as **Heberden nodes,** also known as *generalized osteoarthrosis of hand.* NSAIDs, physical therapy, and orthopedic measures are common treatments for osteoarthritis.

Proximal interphalangeal joints

Metacarpophalangeal joints

Wrist bones

Figure 10-11 Rheumatoid arthritis.

Muscular Dystrophy

Muscular dystrophy is a group of more than 30 inherited diseases that cause progressive weakness of skeletal muscles and loss of muscle mass. Some forms of muscular dystrophy also affect the heart muscle.

Symptoms of the most common variety, Duchenne muscular dystrophy, begin in childhood, usually between ages 3 and 5. These symptoms occur primarily in boys and develop rapidly. By about 12 years of age, those afflicted are unable to walk. As the disease progresses, swallowing and breathing become difficult, and a respirator is required. With other types of muscular dystrophy, symptoms may not surface until adulthood.

There is no cure for muscular dystrophy. However, medications and therapy can help manage symptoms and slow the course of the disease.

Oncology

Two major types of malignancies that affect bone are those that arise directly from bone, called **primary bone cancer,** and those that arise in another region of the body and spread (**metastasize**) to bone, called **secondary bone cancer.** Primary bone cancers are rare, but secondary bone cancers are quite prevalent. They are usually caused by malignant cells that have metastasized to the bone from the lungs, breast, or prostate.

Malignancies that originate from bone, fat, muscle, cartilage, bone marrow, and cells of the lymphatic system are called **sarcomas.** Three major types of sarcomas are fibrosarcoma, osteosarcoma, and Ewing sarcoma. **Fibrosarcoma** develops in cartilage and generally affects the pelvis, upper legs, and shoulders. Patients with fibrosarcoma are usually between ages 50 and 60. **Osteosarcoma** develops from bone tissue and generally affects the knees, upper arms, and upper legs. Patients with osteosarcoma are usually between ages 20 and 25. **Ewing sarcoma** develops from primitive nerve cells in bone marrow. It usually affects the shaft of long bones but may occur in the pelvis or other bones of the arms or legs. This disease usually affects boys between ages 10 and 20.

Signs and symptoms of sarcoma include swelling and tenderness, with a tendency toward fractures in the affected area. Magnetic resonance imaging (MRI), bone scan, and a computed tomography (CT) scan are diagnostic tests that assist in identifying bone malignancies. All malignancies, including Ewing sarcoma, are staged and graded to determine the extent and degree of malignancy. This staging helps the physician determine an appropriate treatment modality. Generally, the practitioner will use combination therapy to treat sarcomas, including chemotherapy for management of metastasis and radiation when the tumor is radiosensitive. In some cases, amputation is required.

Diseases and Conditions

This section introduces diseases and conditions of the musculoskeletal system with their meanings and pronunciations. Word analyses for selected terms are also provided.

Term	Definition
Anterior cruciate ligament (ACL) injury	ACL (one of the main ligaments of the knee) injury most commonly occurs in sports that involve sudden changes in directions, stops, or direct impact to the knee, such as in tennis, soccer, basketball, and football, and involves a partially or completely torn ligament (see Fig. 10-12). *Treatment centers around rest and physical therapy and wearing a knee brace. Depending on the severity of the tear and lifestyle of the patient, ACL reconstruction to replace the torn ligament with a graft is performed arthroscopically. ACL reconstruction is the most commonly performed orthopedic surgery.*

Femur

Anterior cruciate ligament

Lateral collateral ligament

Fibula

Tibia

Posterior cruciate ligament

Medial collateral ligament

Injured anterior cruciate ligament

Figure 10-12 Anterior cruciate ligament (ACL) injury.

Diseases and Conditions—cont'd

Term	Definition
Bakers cyst	Fluid-filled swelling that develops at the back of the knee that is commonly caused by an underlying problem with the knee joint such as a cartilage tear or arthritis; also known as a *popliteal cyst* (see Fig. 10-13).

The cyst significantly reduces the mobility of the knee joint, and as it grows and compresses surrounding nerves it causes pain, numbness, and tingling in different leg areas from the knees to the soles of the feet. Most cysts tend to heal with nonsurgical treatments or may disappear on their own without any intervention.

A   Healthy knee   B   Baker's cyst

Figure 10-13 Bakers (popliteal) cyst. (A) Healthy knee showing the synovial cavity filled with synovial fluid. (B) Flow of synovial fluid to the back of the knee forming a cyst.

Term	Definition
bunion (hallux valgus) BŬN-yŭn (HĂL-ŭks VĂL-gŭs)	Deformity in which the great toe is angled laterally toward the other toes

A bunion may cause the tissues surrounding the joint to become swollen and tender. It is a common deformity seen in women who wear pointed-toe shoes (see Fig. 10-14).

A   B

Figure 10-14 Bunion. (A) Preoperative. (B) Postoperative.

Continued

Diseases and Conditions—cont'd

Term	Definition
carpal tunnel syndrome (CTS) KĂR-păl	Painful condition resulting from compression of the median nerve within the carpal tunnel (wrist canal through which the flexor tendons and the median nerve pass)
claudication klăw-dĭ-KĀ-shŭn	Lameness, limping
contracture kŏn-TRĂK-chūr	Fibrosis of connective tissue in the skin, fascia, muscle, or joint capsule that prevents normal mobility of the related tissue or joint
crepitation krĕp-ĭ-TĀ-shŭn	Dry, grating sound or sensation caused by bone ends rubbing together, indicating a fracture or joint destruction
ganglion cyst GĂNG-lē-ŏn SĬST	Fluid-filled tumor that commonly develops along the tendons or joint of the wrists or hands that may also appear in the feet *In most instances, ganglion cysts cause no pain, require no treatment, and usually resolve spontaneously. Reasons for treatment are cosmetic or when the cyst causes pain or interferes with joint movement. Treatment involves removing the fluid or excising the cyst (see Fig. 10-15).* **Figure 10-15** Ganglion cyst of the wrist.
gout GOWT	Joint inflammation caused by uric acid crystal deposits in the joint space *Gout causes painful swelling and inflammation. Although the joint chiefly affected is the big toe, any joint may be involved.*
herniated disk (disc) HĔR-nē-āt-ĕd	Rupture of a vertebral disk's center (nucleus pulposus) through its outer edge, causing pain, numbness, or weakness in one or both legs; also called *slipped disk* or *herniated nucleus pulposus (HNP)* (see Fig. 10-16)

Diseases and Conditions—cont'd

Term	Definition

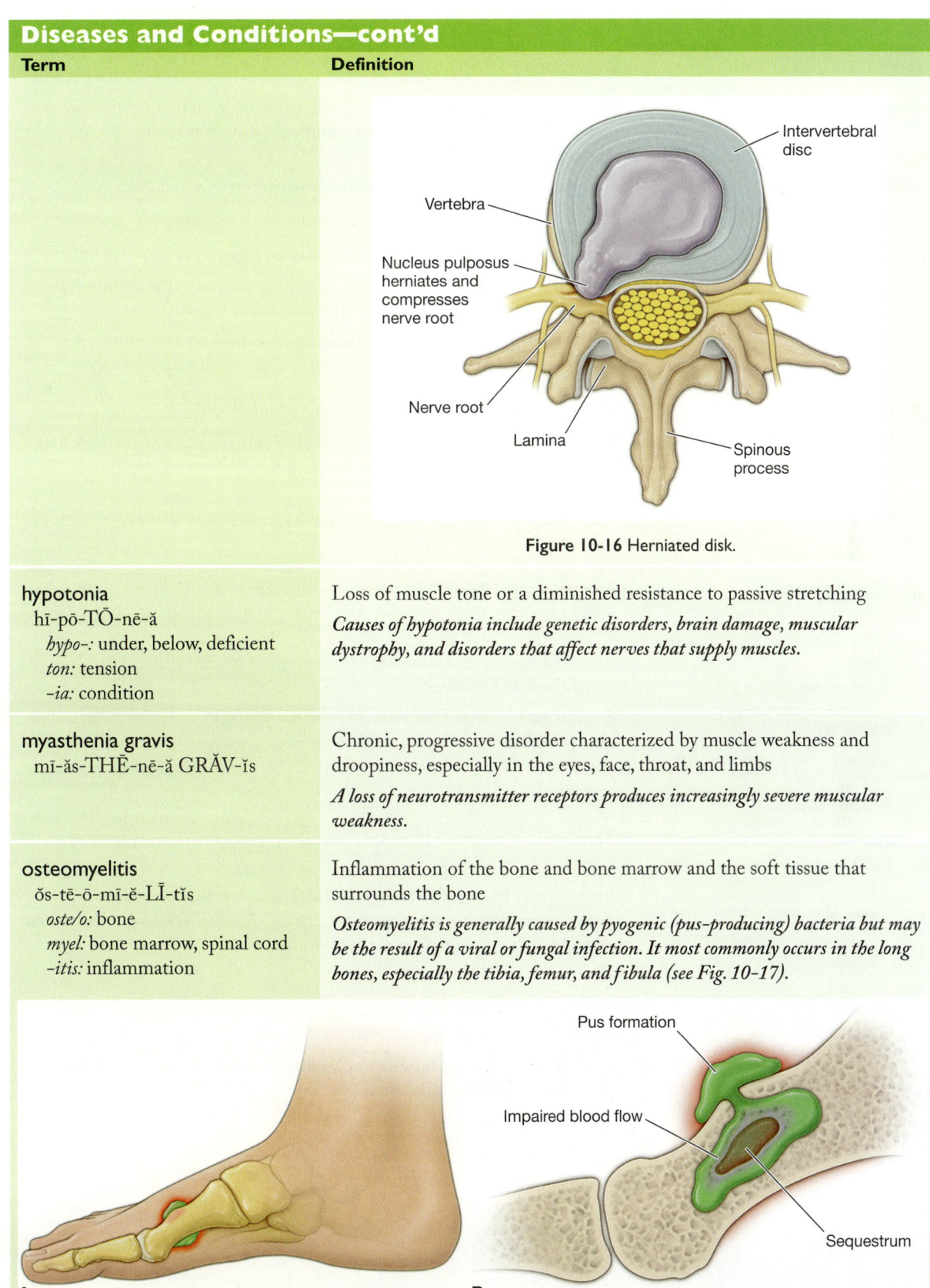

Figure 10-16 Herniated disk.

Term	Definition
hypotonia hī-pō-TŌ-nē-ă *hypo-:* under, below, deficient *ton:* tension *-ia:* condition	Loss of muscle tone or a diminished resistance to passive stretching *Causes of hypotonia include genetic disorders, brain damage, muscular dystrophy, and disorders that affect nerves that supply muscles.*
myasthenia gravis mī-ăs-THĒ-nē-ă GRĂV-ĭs	Chronic, progressive disorder characterized by muscle weakness and droopiness, especially in the eyes, face, throat, and limbs *A loss of neurotransmitter receptors produces increasingly severe muscular weakness.*
osteomyelitis ŏs-tē-ō-mī-ĕ-LĪ-tĭs *oste/o:* bone *myel:* bone marrow, spinal cord *-itis:* inflammation	Inflammation of the bone and bone marrow and the soft tissue that surrounds the bone *Osteomyelitis is generally caused by pyogenic (pus-producing) bacteria but may be the result of a viral or fungal infection. It most commonly occurs in the long bones, especially the tibia, femur, and fibula (see Fig. 10-17).*

Figure 10-17 Osteomyelitis. (A) Bone infection in the toe. (B) Blocked blood flow in the area of infection, with sequestrum (bone death) and pus formation at the infection site.

Continued

Diseases and Conditions—cont'd

Term	Definition
osteoporosis ŏs-tē-ō-por-Ō-sĭs *oste/o:* bone *-porosis:* porous	Loss of calcium and bone tissue, causing the bones to become porous, brittle, and easily fractured; most commonly seen in postmenopausal women *Prevention and treatment include calcium and vitamin D supplements, exercise, and osteoporosis medications.*
Paget disease	Chronic inflammation of bones, resulting in thickening and softening of bones, that can occur in any bone but most commonly affects the long bones of the legs, the lower spine, the pelvis, and the skull *Paget disease is most common in middle-aged and elderly adults and is also called* **osteitis deformans.**
phantom limb FĂN-tŭm	Perceived sensation after amputation of a limb that the limb still exists *The sensation that pain exists in the removed part is known as phantom limb pain.*
rickets RĬK-ĕts	Form of osteomalacia in children caused by vitamin D deficiency; also called *rachitis*
spinal curvatures	Any persistent, abnormal deviation of the vertebral column from its normal position that causes an abnormal spinal curvature (see Fig. 10-18)
scoliosis skō-lē-Ō-sĭs *scoli/o:* crooked, bent *-osis:* abnormal condition, increase (used primarily with blood cells)	Abnormal lateral curvature of the spine, either to the right or left; also called *C-shaped curvature* *Scoliosis may be congenital, caused by chronic poor posture during childhood, or the result of one leg being longer than the other. Untreated scoliosis may result in pulmonary insufficiency, back pain, sciatica, disk disease, or degenerative arthritis.*
kyphosis kī-FŌ-sĭs *kyph/o:* humpback *-osis:* abnormal condition, increase (used primarily with blood cells)	Abnormal curvature of the upper portion of the spine; also known as *humpback* or *hunchback* *Kyphosis may be caused by rheumatoid arthritis, rickets, poor posture, or chronic respiratory disease. Treatment consists of spine-stretching exercises and wearing a brace to straighten the kyphotic curve.*
lordosis lor-DŌ-sĭs *lord/o:* curve, swayback *-osis:* abnormal condition, increase (used primarily with blood cells)	Abnormal, inward curvature of a portion of the lower part of the spine; also known as *swayback* *Lordosis may be caused by obesity or excessive weight gain during pregnancy. Kyphosis and lordosis can also occur in combination with scoliosis.*

Diseases and Conditions—cont'd

Term	Definition

Figure 10-18 Spinal curvatures.

Normal   Scoliosis   Kyphosis   Lordosis

spinal stenosis
SPĪ-năl stĕ-NŌ-sĭs
spin: spine
-al: pertaining to
sten: narrowing
-osis: abnormal condition; increase (used primarily with blood cells)

Narrowing of one or more spaces within the spine that results in the nerves becoming compressed or pinched, which leads to back pain; commonly occurs in the cervical and lumbar area

Spinal stenosis usually develops slowly over time and is commonly caused by osteoarthritis or wear and tear due to the aging process (see Fig. 10–19).

Spinal cord in spinal canal

Stenosis (narrowing)

Figure 10-19 Spinal stenosis.

spondylolisthesis
spŏn-dĭ-lō-lĭs-THĒ-sĭs
spondyl/o: vertebrae (backbone)
-listhesis: slipping

Any slipping (subluxation) of a vertebra from its normal position in relationship to the one beneath it

Continued

Diseases and Conditions—cont'd

Term	Definition
spondylosis spŏn-dĭ-LŌ-sĭs *spondyl:* vertebrae (backbone) *–osis:* abnormal condition; increase (used primarily with blood cells)	Degeneration of the cervical, thoracic, and lumbar vertebrae and related tissues *Spondylosis may cause pressure on nerve roots with subsequent pain or paresthesia in the extremities.*
sprain and strain	Overstretching or tearing of ligaments (sprain) or muscle or tendon (strain) *The most common site of sprain is the ankles. The most common sites of strain are the lower back and the hamstring muscle in the back of the thigh. Initial treatment for sprains and strains includes rest, ice, compression, and elevation. Successful treatment for mild sprains and strains can occur at home. Severe sprains and strains sometimes require surgery to repair torn ligaments, muscles, or tendons.*
subluxation sŭb-lŭk-SĀ-shŭn	Partial or incomplete dislocation of one or more vertebrae
talipes equinovarus TĂL-ĭ-pēz ē-kwī-nō-VĀ-rŭs	Congenital deformity of one or both feet in which the foot is pulled downward and laterally to the side; also called *clubfoot* (see Fig. 10-20) *In talipes, the heel never rests on the ground. Treatment consists of applying casts to progressively straighten the foot and surgical correction for severe cases.*

Figure 10-20 Talipes equinovarus.

⊕ *It is time to review pathology, diseases, and conditions by completing Learning Activity 10-3.*

Diagnostic, Surgical, and Therapeutic Procedures

This section introduces diagnostic, surgical, and therapeutic procedures used to diagnose and treat musculo-skeletal disorders. Descriptions are provided, along with pronunciations and word analyses for selected terms.

Procedure	Description
Diagnostic	
Imaging	
arthrography ăr-THRŎG-ră-fē *arthr/o:* joint *-graphy:* process of recording	Series of radiographs taken after injection of contrast material into a joint cavity, especially the knee or shoulder, to outline the contour of the joint
dual-energy x-ray absorptiometry (DEXA) scan	Radiological procedure that uses low-energy x-ray absorption to measure bone mineral density (BMD) and bone loss that helps to determine the risk for osteopenia and fractures, and to diagnose osteoporosis; also called *bone density test (bone densitometry)*
discography dĭs-KŎG-ră-fē	Radiological examination of the intervertebral disk structures with injection of a contrast medium *Discography helps diagnose suspected cases of herniated disk.*
lumbosacral spinal radiography LŬM-bō-sā-krăl SPĪ-năl rā-dē-ŎG-ră-fē *lumb/o:* loins (lower back) *sacr:* sacrum *-al:* pertaining to, relating to *radi/o:* radiation, x-ray; radius (lower arm bone on thumb side) *-graphy:* process of recording	Radiography of the five lumbar vertebrae and the fused sacral vertebrae, including anteroposterior, lateral, and oblique views of the lower spine *The most common indication for lumbosacral (LS) spinal radiography is lower back pain. It helps identify or differentiate traumatic fractures, spondylosis, spondylolisthesis, and metastatic tumor.*
myelography mī-ĕ-LŎG-ră-fē *myel/o:* bone marrow; spinal cord *-graphy:* process of recording	Radiography of the spinal cord after injection of a contrast medium to identify and study spinal distortions caused by tumors, cysts, herniated intervertebral disks, or other lesions
bone scintigraphy sĭn-TĬG-ră-fē	Nuclear medicine procedure that involves intravenous injection of a radionuclide taken up into the bone *Bone scintigraphy helps detect bone disorders, especially arthritis, fractures, osteomyelitis, bone cancers, or areas of bony metastases.*
Surgical	
amputation ăm-pŭ-TĀ-shŭn	Partial or complete removal of an extremity as a result of disease, trauma, or a circulatory disorder *After removal of the extremity, the surgeon cuts a shaped flap from muscle and cutaneous tissue to cover the end of the bone and provide cushion and support for a prosthesis.*
arthrocentesis ăr-thrō-sĕn-TĒ-sĭs *arthr/o:* joint *-centesis:* surgical puncture	Puncture of a joint space using a needle to remove accumulated fluid or inject medications

Continued

Diagnostic, Surgical, and Therapeutic Procedures—cont'd

Procedure	Description
arthroclasia ăr-thrō-KLĀ-zē-ă *arthr/o:* joint *-clasia:* to break; surgical fracture	Surgical breaking of an ankylosed joint to provide movement
arthroscopy ăr-THRŌS-kō-pē *arthr/o:* joint *-scopy:* visual examination	Visual examination of the interior of a joint and its structures using a thin, flexible fiberoptic scope called an *arthroscope* (see Fig. 10-21) *The surgeon may insert other instruments through the arthroscope to scrape or cut damaged cartilage, excise tumors, remove fluid, and obtain biopsies.* **Figure 10-21** Arthroscopy (lateral view).
bone grafting GRĂFT-ĭng	Implantation or transplantation of bone tissue from another part of the body or from another person to serve as replacement for damaged or missing bone tissue
bursectomy bĕr-SĔK-tō-mē	Excision of a bursa (padlike sac or cavity found in connective tissue, usually in the vicinity of joints) *Bursectomy is commonly performed to treat chronic bursitis.*
foraminotomy fŏr-ă-mĭn-ŎT-ŏ-mē *foramin/o:* hole *-tomy:* incision	Surgical procedure to enlarge the area around a vertebra where the nerve root exits the spinal canal to relieve pressure and reduce pain on compressed nerves; also called *foraminal decompression* *Foraminotomy is a safe and effective surgery to treat nerve compression and conditions such as spinal stenosis, degenerative disk disease, and spondylolisthesis.*
laminectomy lăm-ĭ-NĔK-tō-mē *lamin:* lamina (part of vertebral arch) *-ectomy:* excision, removal	Excision of the posterior arch of a vertebra *Laminectomy is most commonly performed to relieve the symptoms of a ruptured (slipped) intervertebral disk.*

Diagnostic, Surgical, and Therapeutic Procedures—cont'd

Procedure	Description
sequestrectomy sē-kwĕs-TRĔK-tō-mē *sequester:* separation *-ectomy:* excision, removal	Excision of a sequestrum (segment of necrosed bone)
total hip replacement (THR), total hip arthroplasty (THA)	Surgical procedure to replace a hip joint damaged by a degenerative disease, commonly arthritis (see Fig. 10-22) *In THA, the femoral head and the acetabulum are replaced with a metal ball and stem (prosthesis). The stem is anchored into the central core of the femur to achieve a secure fit.*

Pelvis —
Acetabulum —
Femur —

Acetabulum cap
Femoral neck and head
Femoral shaft

A

B

Figure 10-22 Total hip replacement. (A) Left total hip replacement. (B) Radiograph showing right total hip replacement of an arthritic hip.

Continued

Diagnostic, Surgical, and Therapeutic Procedures—cont'd

Procedure	Description
vertebroplasty věr-TĒ-brō-plăs-tē *vertebr/o:* vertebrae (backbone) *-plasty:* surgical repair	Injection of medical cement through a needle that is inserted through the skin under x-ray guidance into a cracked or broken vertebrae to relieve pain and restore mobility; also called *percutaneous vertebroplasty* *Vertebroplasty is performed most often to treat a compression fracture typically caused by osteoporosis. It is considered a minimally invasive procedure and is often performed outpatient.*
Therapeutic	
bone immobilization	Procedure used to restrict movement, stabilize and protect a fracture, and facilitate the healing process
casting	Bone immobilization by application of a solid, stiff dressing formed with plaster of Paris or similar material
splinting	Bone immobilization by application of an orthopedic device to the injured body part *A splint is constructed from wood, metal, or plaster of Paris and may be moveable or immovable.*
traction	Set of mechanisms for straightening broken bones or relieving pressure on the spine and skeletal system

Pharmacology

Unlike other medications that treat specific diseases, most pharmacological agents for musculo-skeletal disorders treat symptoms (see Table 10-3). Analgesics and anti-inflammatory drugs help treat acute musculoskeletal conditions, such as strains and sprains. NSAIDs, salicylates, muscle relaxants, opioid analgesics, and narcotics commonly treat pain by anesthetizing (numbing) the area or decreasing the inflammation. NSAIDs, gold salts, and salicylates treat arthritis. Calcium supplements treat hypocalcemia.

TABLE 10-3 Drugs Used to Treat Musculoskeletal Disorders

This table lists common drug classifications used to treat musculoskeletal disorders, their therapeutic actions, and selected generic and trade names.

Classification	Therapeutic Action	Generic and Trade Names
bone resorption inhibitors	Prevent bone loss and strengthen bone affected by osteoporosis by inhibiting bone resorption and prevent fractures associated with osteoporosis	**alendronate** ăh-LĔN-drō-nāt *Fosamax* **risedronate** rīz-ĔD-rō-nāt *Actonel*
calcium supplements KĀL-sē-ŭm	Treat and prevent hypocalcemia *Over-the-counter calcium supplements are numerous and contained in many antacids to provide a secondary therapeutic effect. They help prevent osteoporosis when the normal diet is lacking adequate amounts of calcium.*	**calcium carbonate** KĀL-sē-ŭm KĀR-bŏn-āt *Calci-Mix, Tums* **calcium citrate** KĀL-sē-ŭm SĬT-rāt *Cal-Citrate 250, Citracal*
disease modifying antirheumatic drugs (DMARDs)	Slow progression of joint destruction in arthritis by inhibiting a substance that triggers inflammation *DMARDs help treat rheumatoid arthritis, psoriatic arthritis, and inflammatory diseases of the bowel, such as Crohn disease and ulcerative colitis.*	**adalimumab** ā-dăh-LĬM-yū-măb *Humira* **methotrexate** mĕth-ōh-TRĔKS-āt
muscle relaxants	Relieve muscle spasms and stiffness *Muscle relaxants also help treat muscle spasms resulting from multiple sclerosis, spinal cord injury, cerebral palsy, and stroke.*	**cyclobenzaprine** sī-klō-BĔN-ză-prēn *Flexeril* **methocarbamol and aspirin** mĕth-ō-KĀR-bă-mōl *Robaxin*
nonsteroidal anti-inflammatory drugs (NSAIDs) nŏn-STĒR-oyd-ăl ăn-tē-ĭn-FLĂM-ă-tō-rē	Decrease pain and suppress inflammation *NSAIDs help treat acute musculoskeletal conditions, such as sprains and strains, and inflammatory disorders, including rheumatoid arthritis, osteoarthritis, bursitis, gout, and tendinitis.*	**ibuprofen** ī-bū-PRō-fĕn *Advil, Motrin* **naproxen** nă-PRŎK-sĕn *Aleve, Naprosyn*
salicylates săl-ĬS-ĭl-ātz	Relieve mild-to-moderate pain and reduce inflammation *Salicylates have anti-inflammatory abilities and alleviate pain. Aspirin (acetylsalicylic acid) is the oldest drug in this classification that is used to treat arthritis.*	**aspirin** ĀS-pĕr-ĭn *Acuprin, Aspergum, Bayer Aspirin* **magnesium salicylate** măg-NĒ-zē-ŭm să-LĬS-ĭ-lāt *Magan, Mobidin*
vitamin D analogs	Fat-soluble vitamins that facilitate the absorption and utilization of calcium to improve bone strength and structure. *Vitamin D is commonly found in combination with calcium.*	**cholecalciferol (vitamin D$_3$)** kōl-ĕ-kăl-SĬ-fĕr-ōl *Maximum D$_3$* **ergocalciferol (vitamin D$_2$)** ĕr-gō-kăl SĬ-fĕr-ōl *Drisdol*

Abbreviations

This section introduces musculoskeletal–related abbreviations and their meanings.

Abbreviation	Meaning	Abbreviation	Meaning
ACL	anterior cruciate ligament	IV	intravenous
BMD	bone mineral density	L1, L2, and so on	first lumbar vertebra, second lumbar vertebra, and so on
C1, C2, and so on	first cervical vertebra, second cervical vertebra, and so on	MRI	magnetic resonance imaging
CTS	carpal tunnel syndrome	NSAIDs	nonsteroidal anti-inflammatory drugs
DEXA, DXA	dual-energy x-ray absorptiometry	OREF	open reduction external fixation
DJD	degenerative joint disease	ORIF	open reduction internal fixation
DMARDs	disease modifying antirheumatic drugs	RA	rheumatoid arthritis; right atrium
DO, D. O.	doctor of osteopathy	THA	total hip arthroplasty
HNP	herniated nucleus pulposus (herniated disk)	THR	total hip replacement

It is time to review procedures, pharmacology, and abbreviations by completing Learning Activity 10-4.

LEARNING ACTIVITIES

The activities that follow provide a review of the musculoskeletal system terms introduced in this chapter. Complete each activity and review your answers to evaluate your understanding of the chapter.

Medical Language Lab
Turning terminology into language

Visit the Medical Language Laboratory at medicallanguagelab.com. Use it to enhance your study and reinforcement of this chapter with the flash card activity. We recommend that you complete the flash card activity before starting Learning Activities 10-1 and 10-2.

Learning Activity 10-1
Medical Word Elements

Use the listed elements to build medical words. You may use elements more than once.

Combining Forms		**Suffixes**		**Prefixes**
ankyl/o	*fasci/o*	*-algia*	*-oma*	*a-*
arthr/o	*leiomy/o*	*-ar*	*-osis*	*dys-*
brachi/o	*lumb/o*	*-centesis*	*-pathy*	*syn-*
cephal/o	*oste/o*	*-clast*	*-plasty*	
chondr/o	*patell/o*	*-desis*	*-porosis*	
crani/o	*synov/o*	*-ism*	*-tome*	
dactyl/o		*-itis*	*-trophy*	
		-malacia		

1. without nourishment or development _____

2. tumor of smooth muscle _____

3. pain in the arm _____

4. pertaining to the patella (knee cap) _____

5. softening of cartilage _____

6. binding or fixation of a joint _____

7. abnormal condition of (being) bent or crooked _____

8. instrument to incise (cut) the skull _____

9. porous bone _____

10. inflammation of a joint _____

11. pertaining to the lower back _____

12. bad nourishment _____

13. inflammation of the synovial membrane _____

14. condition of joined fingers or toes _____

15. surgical puncture of a joint _____

16. inflammation of fingers or toes _____

17. cell that breaks down bone _____

18. headache _____

19. tumor of cartilage _____

20. surgical repair of the fascia _____

Check your answers in Appendix A. Review any material that you did not answer correctly.

Correct Answers _____ X 5 = _____% Score

Learning Activity 10-2
Building Medical Words

Use *oste/o* (bone) to build words that mean

1. bone cells _____
2. malignant tumor of the bone _____
3. disease of bones and joints _____
4. beginning or formation of bones _____

Use *cervic/o* (neck) to build words that mean

5. pain in the neck _____
6. pertaining to the neck and arm _____
7. pertaining to the neck and face _____

Use *myel/o* (bone marrow; spinal cord) to build words that mean

8. tumor of bone marrow _____
9. sarcoma of bone marrow (cells) _____
10. bone marrow cell _____
11. resembling bone marrow _____

Use *stern/o* (sternum) to build words that mean

12. pertaining to above the sternum _____
13. resembling the breastbone _____

Use *arthr/o* (joint) or *chondr/o* (cartilage) to build words that mean

14. embryonic cell that forms cartilage _____
15. incision of a joint _____
16. inflammation of bones and joints _____

Use *pelv/i* (pelvis) to build a word that means

17. instrument for measuring the pelvis _____

Use *my/o* (muscle) to build words that mean

18. twitching of a muscle _____
19. weakness of the muscle _____
20. rupture of a muscle _____

Build surgical words that mean

21. excision of one or more of the phalanges (bones of a finger or toe) _____

22. incision of the thorax (chest wall) _____

23. excision of a vertebra _____

24. binding of a joint _____

25. repair of muscle (tissue) _____

✓ *Check your answers in Appendix A. Review material that you did not answer correctly.*

Correct Answers _____ X 4 = _____% Score

Learning Activity 10-3
Diseases and Conditions

Match the terms with the definitions in the numbered list.

ankylosis	*ganglion cyst*	*myasthenia gravis*	*scoliosis*
bunion	*gout*	*necrosis*	*sequestrum*
carpal tunnel	*greenstick fracture*	*osteoporosis*	*spondylitis*
chondrosarcoma	*hypotonia*	*phantom limb*	*spondylolisthesis*
claudication	*kyphosis*	*pyogenic*	*subluxation*
comminuted fracture	*muscular dystrophy*	*rickets*	*talipes*
Ewing			

1. incomplete or partial dislocation _____
2. softening of the bones caused by vitamin D deficiency _____
3. slipped vertebrae _____
4. limping _____
5. disease causing degeneration of muscles _____
6. congenital deformity of the foot, which is twisted out of shape or position _____
7. part of necrosed bone that has become separated from surrounding tissue _____
8. neuromuscular disorder characterized by weakness _____
9. painful condition caused by compression of the median nerve within the wrist canal _____
10. joint capsule tumor, commonly found in the wrist _____
11. loss of muscular tonicity; diminished resistance of muscles to passive stretching _____
12. type of sarcoma that attacks the shafts rather than the ends of long bones _____
13. bone that is partially bent and partially broken and occurs in children _____
14. exaggeration of the thoracic curve of the vertebral column; humpback _____
15. disease caused by a decrease in bone density that occurs in the elderly _____
16. deviation of the spine to the right or left _____
17. cartilaginous sarcoma _____
18. describes a bone that has splintered into pieces _____
19. inflammation of the vertebrae _____
20. accumulation of uric acid, usually in the big toe _____
21. lateral deviation of the great toe as it turns in toward the second toe (angulation), which may cause the surrounding joint to become swollen _____
22. pertaining to formation of pus _____
23. death of cells, tissues, or organs _____
24. stiffening and immobility of a joint _____
25. perceived sensation after amputation that the limb still exists _____

✓ *Check your answers in Appendix A. Review material that you did not answer correctly.*

Correct Answers _____ X 4 = _____% Score

Learning Activity 10-4
Procedures, Pharmacology, and Abbreviations

Match the terms with the definitions in the numbered list.

ACL	*bone scintigraphy*	*foraminotomy*	*ORIF*
amputation	*calcium supplements*	*laminectomy*	*relaxants*
arthrodesis	*closed reduction*	*myelography*	*sequestrectomy*
arthrography	*CTS*	*NSAIDs*	*THA*
arthroscopy	*DXA scan*	*OREF*	*vertebroplasty*

1. treats and prevents hypocalcemia _____
2. surgical realignment of a bone fracture followed by external stabilization devices _____
3. procedure performed on spinal compression fractures that consists of an injection of medical cement through a needle under guided imaging _____
4. enlargement of the area around a vertebra where the nerve root exits the spinal canal to relieve pain on compressed nerves _____
5. a main ligament of the knee _____
6. imaging of the spinal cord after injection of a contrast medium _____
7. surgical bone realignment with inserted metal pins, rods, and screws _____
8. radiography to measure the density of bones to diagnose osteopenia and osteoporosis _____
9. painful disorder of the wrist due to compression of the median nerve _____
10. excision of the posterior arch of a vertebra _____
11. imaging of a joint after injection of a radiopaque substance _____
12. surgical binding or immobilizing of a joint _____
13. partial or complete removal of a limb _____
14. total hip replacement _____
15. relieve mild to moderate pain and reduce inflammation _____
16. visual examination of a joint's interior, especially the knee _____
17. excising a segment of necrosed bone _____
18. nuclear procedure in which the radionuclide is injected intravenously to detect arthritis _____
19. relieve muscle spasms and stiffness _____
20. manipulative treatment to realign bone fractures without a surgical incision _____

Check your answers in Appendix A. Review material that you did not answer correctly.

Correct Answers _____ X 5 = _____ % Score

DOCUMENTING HEALTH-CARE ACTIVITIES

This section provides practical application activities in the form of exercises to help students develop skills in documenting patient care. First, read the medical report. Then complete the activities and exercises that follow.

Documenting Health-Care Activity 10-1
Operative Report: Right Knee Arthroscopy and Medial Meniscectomy

---

General Hospital

1511 Ninth Avenue ■ ■ Sun City, USA 12345 ■ ■ (555) 802–1887

OPERATIVE REPORT

Date: August 14, 20xx   Physician: Robert L. Mead, MD
Patient: Jay, Elizabeth   Patient ID#: 20798

PREOPERATIVE DIAGNOSIS: Tear, medial meniscus, right knee.

POSTOPERATIVE DIAGNOSIS: Tear, medial meniscus, right knee.

CLINICAL HISTORY: This 42-year-old woman has jogged an average of 25 miles each week for the past 10 years. She has persistent posteromedial right knee pain with occasional effusions. The patient has an MRI-documented medial meniscal tear.

PROCEDURE: Right knee arthroscopy and medial meniscectomy.

ANESTHESIA: General.

COMPLICATIONS: None.

OPERATIVE SUMMARY: Examination of the knee under anesthesia showed a full range of motion, no effusion, no instability, and negative Lachman and negative McMurray sign tests. Arthroscopic evaluation showed a normal patellofemoral groove and normal intracondylar notch with normal ACL and PCL, some anterior synovitis, and a normal lateral meniscus and lateral compartment to the knee. The medial compartment of the knee showed an inferior surface, posterior and midmedial meniscal tear that was flipped up on top of itself. This was resected, and then the remaining meniscus was contoured back to a stable rim. A sterile dressing was applied.

Patient was taken to the postanesthesia care unit in stable condition.

Robert L. Mead, MD
Robert L. Mead, MD

rlm:bg

D: 8–14–20xx; T: 8–14–20xx

Terminology

The terms listed in the table that follows are taken from *Operative Report: Right Knee Arthroscopy and Medial Meniscectomy.* Use a medical dictionary such as *Taber's Cyclopedic Medical Dictionary,* the appendices of this book, or other resources to define each term. Then review the pronunciation for each term and practice by reading the medical record aloud.

Term	Definition
ACL	
arthroscopy ăr-THRŎS-kō-pē	
effusions ĕ-FŪ-zh ŭnz	
intracondylar ĭn-tră-KŎN-dĭ-lăr	
Lachman test	
McMurray sign test	
meniscectomy mĕn-ĭ-SĔK-tō-mē	
patellofemoral păh-TĔL-ō-fĕm- ĕ-răl	
MRI	
PCL	
synovitis sĭn-ō-VĪ-tĭs	

Visit the Medical Terminology Systems online resource center at FADavis. com to practice pronunciation and reinforce the meanings of the terms in this medical report.

Critical Thinking

Review *Operative Report: Right Knee Arthroscopy and Medial Meniscectomy* to answer the questions.

1. Describe the meniscus and identify its location.

_____

_____

_____

2. What is the probable cause of the tear in the patient's meniscus?

_____

_____

_____

3. What does normal ACL and PCL refer to in the report?

_____

_____

_____

4. Explain the McMurray sign test.

_____

_____

_____

5. Why was the surgery performed even though the Lachman and McMurray tests were negative (normal)?

_____

_____

_____

Documenting Health-Care Activity 10-2

Emergency Department Report: Oblique Spiral Fracture of Left Tibia

---

General Hospital

☐ **1511 Ninth Avenue**   ☐ **Sun City, USA 12345**   ☐ **(555) 802–1887**

EMERGENCY DEPARTMENT REPORT

DATE OF ADMISSION: June 17, 20XX

TIME REGISTERED: 4:55 pm

PATIENT NAME: Harrison R. Jefferson

PHYSICIAN: Alex Hirsch, D.O.

CHIEF COMPLAINT: Left lower extremity injury

HISTORY OF PRESENT ILLNESS: This is a 6-year-old Caucasian boy with no significant past medical history presenting to the ED after an injury to his left lower extremity earlier this afternoon. He was in a standing, stationary position with his bike at the bottom of a hill when another biker lost control and ran into his left lower extremity. Patient is unable to weight bear. Ibuprofen taken 2 hours ago provided mild relief of his pain; pain 7/10.

CURRENT MEDICATIONS: Ibuprofen as needed.

ALLERGIES: No known drug allergies.

VITAL SIGNS: Pulse: 80 and regular; R: 16; T: 98.6°F; BP: 110/68.

PHYSICAL EXAMINATION: Swelling and erythema noted in the distal left lower extremity. Tender to palpation. Sensation intact. Skin is intact, no lacerations appreciated. Range of motion intact at the left knee but limited with dorsiflexion and plantarflexion of the left ankle. Dorsalis pedis pulse is regular and normal strength.

DIAGNOSTIC STUDIES: X-ray tibia fibular left, minimum 2 views.

IMPRESSION: AP and lateral views of the left tibia-fibula demonstrate oblique spiral fracture of the distal tibial diaphysis with minimal displacement.

PLAN: Patient fitted with a splint with soft cast. Proper care of the splint was discussed with the patient and his mother. Patient is to return to the ER if he notices any throbbing, numbness, tingling, loss of sensation or capillary refill that is not relieved by removing or loosening the splint. An orthopedic referral has been made; patient is to call to schedule an appointment in 3–5 days.

DISPOSITION: Patient is in stable condition and appropriate to be discharged to home.

Alex Hirsch, D.O.
Alex Hirsch, D.O.

ah:rm

Terminology

The terms listed in the table that follows are taken from Emergency *Department Report: Oblique Spiral Fracture of Left Tibia.* Use a medical dictionary such as *Taber's Cyclopedic Medical Dictionary,* the appendices of this book, or other resources to define each term. Then review the pronunciation for each term and practice by reading the medical record aloud.

Term	Definition
AP	
diaphysis dī-ĂF-ĭ-sĭs	
dorsalis pedis DOR-săl-ĭs PĔD-ĭs	
dorsiflexion DOR-sĭ-flĕk-shŭn	
fibular FĬB-ū-lăr	
oblique spiral fracture FRĂK-chŭr	
plantar flexion PLĂN-tăr flĕk-shŭn	
tibia TĬB-ē-ă	

Visit the Medical Terminology Systems online resource center at FADavis. com to practice pronunciation and reinforce the meanings of the terms in this medical report.

Critical Thinking

Review *Emergency Department Report: Oblique Spiral Fracture of Left Tibia* to answer the questions.

1. What findings on physical examination showed limited range of motion?

2. What medication was the patient taking for pain, and did it provide relief?

3. What were the findings of the x-rays?

4. How was the injured site stabilized?

5. Under what conditions should the patient seek medical help?

Constructing Chart Notes

To construct chart notes, replace the italicized and boldfaced terms in each of the
two scenarios with one of the listed medical terms.

clavicle   *open fracture*   *osteoporosis*

comminuted   *orthopedist*   *pathological fractures*

femur   *osteopenia*   *spondylalgia*

kyphosis

Mr. L, a 30-year-old male, was brought to the ED after a head-on car collision. X-rays
revealed a minor (1) **splintered** fracture of the right (2) **collarbone**. The more serious injury
was a (3) **broken bone protruding through the skin surface** with laceration of the surrounding
soft tissue of the right thigh. Mr. L was immediately prepped for a surgical reduction of the
right (4) **thigh bone**. Dr. Michaels, the (5) **specialist in treating bone disorders**, will undertake
management of this patient.

1. _____

2. _____

3. _____

4. _____

5. _____

Mrs. P's previous surgical history shows an appendectomy at age 10 and a hysterectomy
with the removal of the ovaries and fallopian tubes at age 35. She has a history of (6) *a*
decrease in bone minerals. She is stooped over with a prominent (7) **humpback** and complains of (8) **pain in the vertebrae**. The results of her DEXA scan show (9) **porous bones**.
She is at risk for (10) **bone fractures related to disease**.

6. _____

7. _____

8. _____

9. _____

10. _____

Check your answers in Appendix A. Review any material that you did not answer correctly.

Correct Answers _____ X 10 = _____ % Score

Urinary System

Chapter Outline

Objectives

Upon completion of this chapter, you will be able to:

- Locate and describe urinary structures.
- Describe the functional relationship between the urinary system and other body systems.
- Pronounce, spell, and build words related to the urinary system.
- Describe diseases, conditions, and procedures related to the urinary system.
- Explain pharmacology related to the treatment of urinary disorders.
- Demonstrate your knowledge of this chapter by completing the learning and documenting health-care activities.

Anatomy and Physiology

The urinary system consists of two kidneys, two ureters, the urinary bladder, and the urethra. The kidneys perform the primary functions of the urinary system, while the other structures primarily serve as pathways and storage sites. The primary function of the urinary system is regulation of the extracellular fluids of the body (primarily plasma and tissue fluid). The kidneys remove waste products from plasma as they form urine. Urine, containing waste products, passes from the kidneys via the ureters to the urinary bladder for temporary storage before it is excreted from the body through the urethra.

Anatomy and Physiology Key Terms

This section introduces important urinary system terms and their definitions. The key terms are highlighted in color in the Anatomy and Physiology section. Word analyses for selected terms are also provided. Pronounce the term and place a check mark in the box after you do so.

Term	Definition
electrolyte □ ē-LĚK-trō-līt	Mineral salt of the body that carries an electrical charge and regulates nerve impulses, muscle contraction, hydration, and blood pH *The major electrolytes of the body include sodium, chloride, potassium, magnesium, calcium, phosphate, and bicarbonate.*
filtrate □ FĬL-trāt	Fluid that passes from the blood through the capillary walls of the glomeruli into Bowman capsule *Filtrate is similar to plasma but with less protein. Urine is formed from filtrate.*
nitrogenous waste □ nī-TRŎJ-ĕn-ŭs	Product of protein metabolism that includes urea, uric acid, creatine, creatinine, and ammonia
peristaltic wave □ pĕr-ĭ-STĂL-tĭk	Sequence of rhythmic contraction of smooth muscles of a hollow organ to force material forward and prevent backflow
peritoneum □ pĕr-ĭ-tō-NĒ-ŭm	Serous membrane that lines the abdominopelvic cavity and covers most of the organs within the cavity
pH	Symbol that expresses the alkalinity or acidity of a solution *A solution with a pH of 7.0 is neutral, greater than 7.0 is alkaline, and less than 7.0 is acidic.*
plasma □ PLĂZ-mă	Liquid portion of blood that is filtered by the nephrons to remove dissolved wastes

Pronunciation Help	Long Sound	ā — rate	ē — rebirth	ī — isle	ō — over	ū — unite
	Short Sound	ă — apple	ĕ — ever	ĭ — it	ŏ — not	ŭ — cut

Macroscopic Structures

The macroscopic structures that make up the urinary system include two kidneys, two ureters, a bladder, and a urethra (see Fig. 11-1). They regulate the composition of extracellular fluids (blood and tissue fluid) by removing harmful products from the body—especially **nitrogenous wastes** and excess **electrolytes**—while retaining beneficial products required by the body. Nitrogenous products are toxic, and the kidneys must continuously eliminate them or death will occur within a few days. Equally important is the proper balance of electrolytes, which are essential for brain

Figure 11-1 Urinary structures, including a cross section of the kidney.

function, nerves, muscles, and tissue repair. Along with regulating the composition of extracellular fluids, the kidneys also secrete the hormone **erythropoietin.** This hormone acts on bone marrow to stimulate production of red blood cells when blood oxygen levels are low.

The (1) **left and right kidneys,** each about the size of a fist, are located in the abdominal cavity slightly above the waistline. The location of the kidneys is **retroperitoneal** because they are located outside of the **peritoneum.** A concave medial border gives the kidney its beanlike shape. In the cross section, two distinct areas are visible: an outer area, the (2) **renal cortex,** and a middle area, the (3) **renal medulla.** These structures contain portions of the microscopic filtering units of the kidney, the **nephrons.** Near the medial border is the (4) **hilum** (or **hilus**), an opening through which the (5) **renal artery** enters and the (6) **renal vein** exits the kidney. After the kidneys remove waste products during urine formation, the filtered blood leaves the kidney by way of the renal vein. Urine, now carrying waste products, enters the (7) **renal pelvis,** a hollow cavity formed where the (8) **ureter** merges with the kidney. Each ureter is a slender tube approximately 10 inches to 12 inches long. They carry urine in **peristaltic waves** to the bladder. These waves keep urine flowing toward the bladder, rather than regurgitating back into the kidney during urination when bladder pressure increases. Urine enters the bladder at the (9) **ureteral orifice.** The (10) **urinary bladder,** an expandable hollow organ, acts as a temporary reservoir for urine. The bladder has small folds called **rugae** that expand as the bladder fills. At its base, the two openings of the ureters and the urethra form a triangular area called the **trigone** that leads into the (11) **urethra,** a tube that discharges urine from the bladder. The length of the urethra is approximately 1.5 inches in women and about 7 to 8 inches in men. In the male, the urethra passes through the prostate gland and the penis. During urination **(micturition),** the body expels urine through an opening in the urethra, the (12) **urinary meatus.**

Microscopic Structures

Microscopic examination of kidney tissue reveals the presence of approximately 1 million **nephrons.** These microscopic structures maintain homeostasis by continually adjusting and regulating the composition, volume, and **pH** of blood **plasma** and tissue fluid. Substances removed by nephrons include nitrogenous wastes, excess electrolytes, and many other products that exceed the amount tolerated by the body. Each nephron includes a renal corpuscle and a renal tubule (see Fig. 11-2). The **renal corpuscle** is composed of a tuft of capillaries called the (1) **glomerulus** and a modified, enlarged extension of the renal tubule known as the (2) **Bowman (glomerular) capsule** that surrounds the glomerulus. A larger (3) **afferent arteriole** carries blood to the glomerulus, and a smaller (4) **efferent arteriole** carries blood from the glomerulus. The difference in the size of these vessels provides the needed pressure to force fluids and soluble material from blood plasma into the Bowman capsule. These substances, now called **filtrate**, resemble plasma except that the amount of protein in filtrate is less than that found in plasma.

The efferent arteriole passes behind the renal corpuscle to form the (5) **peritubular capillaries,** a network of capillaries that surround the renal tubule. The renal tubule consists of four sections: the (6) **proximal convoluted tubule,** followed by the narrow (7) **loop of Henle,** then the larger (8) **distal tubule** and, finally, the (9) **collecting tubule.** The collecting tubule transports formed urine to the renal pelvis for excretion by the kidneys.

The nephron performs three physiological functions as it produces urine:

1. **Filtration** occurs in the renal corpuscle as water, electrolytes, sugar, and other small molecules in blood plasma in the afferent tubule pass into the Bowman capsule to form filtrate.
2. **Reabsorption** begins as filtrate travels through the long, twisted pathway of the tubule. Most of the water and some of the electrolytes and amino acids from the tubule reenter the circulating blood through the peritubular capillaries.
3. **Secretion** is the final stage of urine formation. The peritubular capillaries actively secrete waste products, such as ammonia, uric acid, and metabolic products of medications, into the renal tubules for removal in urine.

Urine leaves the collecting tubule and enters the renal pelvis. From there, urine passes to the bladder for temporary storage until urination takes place.

Figure 11-2 Nephron with its associated blood vessels.

Anatomy Review: Urinary Structures

Label the illustration using the listed terms.

hilum	*renal medulla*	*right kidney*	*urethra*
left kidney	*renal pelvis*	*ureteral orifice*	*urinary bladder*
renal artery	*renal vein*	*ureters*	*urinary meatus*
renal cortex			

Adrenal
(suprarenal
glands)

Inferior vena cava

Abdominal aorta

Prostate gland
(in males)

Renal pyramid

Inferior
vena cava

*Check your answers by referring to Figure 11–1 on page 381. Review material that you did
not answer correctly.*

Anatomy Review: Nephron

Label the illustration using the listed terms.

afferent arteriole

Bowman capsule

collecting tubule

distal tubule

efferent arteriole

glomerulus

loop of Henle

peritubular capillary

proximal convoluted tubule

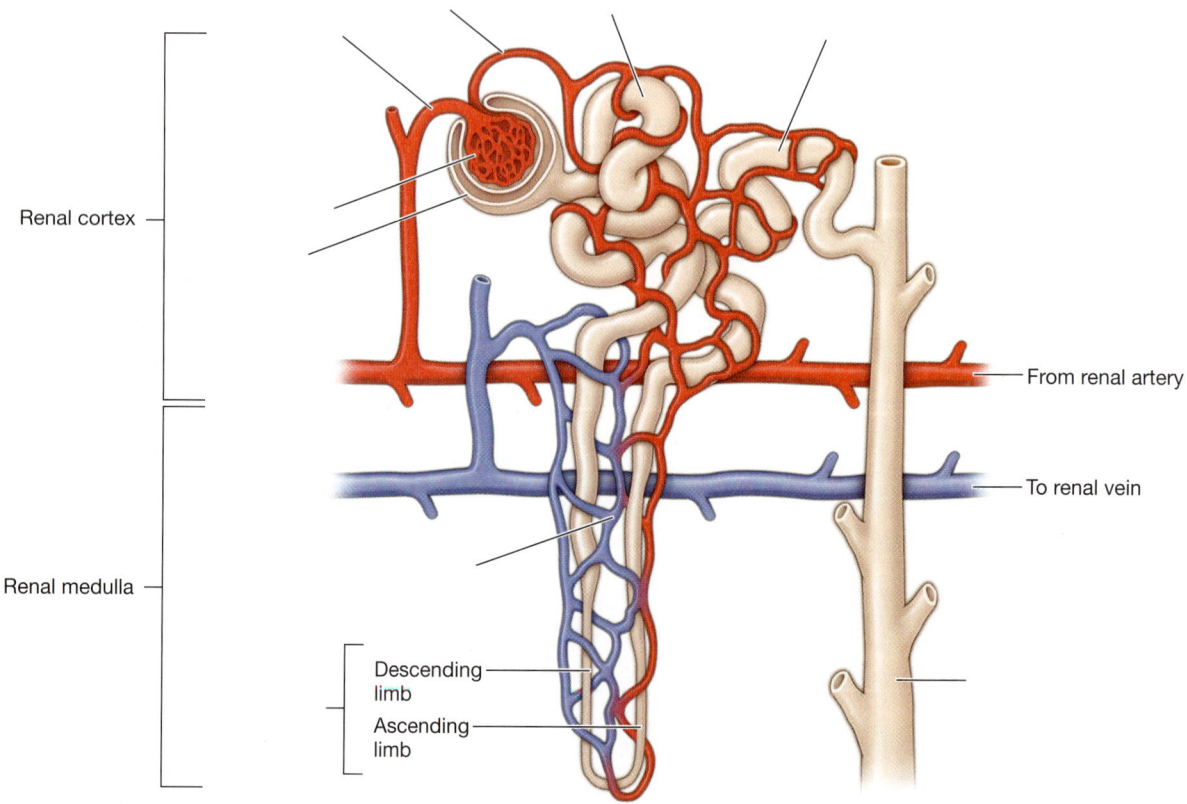

Renal cortex

Renal medulla

From renal artery

To renal vein

Descending limb

Ascending limb

Check your answers by referring to Figure 11-2 on page 382. Review material that you did not answer correctly.

CONNECTING BODY SYSTEMS—URINARY SYSTEM

The main function of the urinary system is to regulate extracellular fluids of the body. Specific functional relationships between the urinary system and other body systems are summarized here.

Blood, Lymphatic, and Immune
- The urinary system filters plasma, thereby regulating the composition, quantity, and quality of blood plasma and lymph.
- The urinary system retains needed products and integrates them back into plasma as it removes products that are excessive or toxic to the body.

Cardiovascular
- The urinary system helps regulate essential electrolytes needed for contraction of the heart.

Digestive
- The urinary system aids in removing glucose from the blood when excessive amounts are consumed.
- The urinary system removes excessive fluids absorbed from the gastrointestinal (GI) tract.

Endocrine
- The urinary system regulates electrolyte and fluid balance, which is essential for hormone transport in the blood.
- The urinary system produces erythropoietin, a hormone synthesized mainly in the kidneys to stimulate bone marrow production of blood cells.

Female Reproductive
- The urinary system aids in removing waste products produced by the fetus in the pregnant woman.

Integumentary
- The urinary system compensates for extracellular fluid loss resulting from hyperhidrosis by regulating fluid loss during urine production.
- The urinary system adjusts electrolytes, especially potassium and sodium, in response to their loss through sweating.

Male Reproductive
- The urinary system shares the urethra with the male reproductive system for delivery of semen.

Musculoskeletal
- The urinary system works in conjunction with bone tissue to maintain a constant calcium level.

Nervous
- The urinary system regulates sodium, potassium, and calcium, which are the electrolytes responsible for the transmission of nervous stimuli.

Respiratory
- The urinary system assists the lungs in regulating the acid–base balance of the body.

Medical Word Elements

This section introduces combining forms, suffixes, and prefixes related to the urinary system. Word analyses are also provided. From the information provided, complete the meaning of the medical words in the right-hand column. The first one is completed for you.

Element	Meaning	Word Analysis
Combining Forms		
albumin/o	albumin, protein	**albumin/**oid (ăl-BŪ-mĭ-noyd): *resembling albumin* *-oid:* resembling
azot/o	nitrogenous compounds	**azot/**emia (ăz-ō-TĒ-mē-ă): _____ *-emia:* blood condition *Azotemia results when the kidneys fail to excrete nitrogenous compounds, such as urea, creatinine, and other waste compounds containing nitrogen.*
bacteri/o	bacteria (singular, bacterium)	**bacteri/**uria (băk-tē-rē-Ū-rē-ă): _____ *-uria:* urine
cyst/o	bladder	**cyst/o/**scope (SĬST-ō-skōp): _____ *-scope:* instrument for examining
vesic/o		**vesic/o/**cele (VĚS-ĭ-kō-sēl): _____ *-cele:* hernia, swelling *With a vesicocele, also called* **cystocele,** *the bladder herniates into the vaginal wall, causing incomplete emptying of the bladder.*
glomerul/o	glomerulus	**glomerul/o/**pathy (glō-měr-ū-LŎP-ă-thē): _____ *-pathy:* disease

kal/i*	potassium (an electrolyte)	**kal/i/**ur/esis (kă-lē-ū-RĒ-sĭs): _____
		  ur: urine
		  -esis: condition

keton/o	ketone bodies (acids and acetones)	**keton/**uria (kē-tō-NŪ-rē-ă): _____ *-uria:* urine *Ketonuria is commonly found in diabetes mellitus, starvation, and excessive dieting.*
lith/o	stone, calculus	**lith/o/**tripsy (LĬTH-ō-trĭp-sē): _____ *-tripsy:* crushing
meat/o	opening, meatus	**meat/o/**tomy (mē-ă-TŎT-ō-mē): _____ *-tomy:* incision *A meatotomy relieves stenosis of the urethra by enlarging the urethral opening, which may be inhibiting the proper passage of urine or semen.*

*The *i* in *kal/i* is an exception to the rule of using the connecting vowel *o.*

Medical Word Elements—cont'd

Element	Meaning	Word Analysis
nephr/o	kidney	**nephr/o**/pexy (NĔF-rō-pĕks-ē): _____ *-pexy:* fixation (of an organ)
ren/o		**ren**/al (RĒ-năl): *-al:* pertaining to
noct/o	night	**noct**/uria (nok-TŪ-rē-ă): _____ *-uria:* urine *Nocturia is associated with prostate disease, urinary tract infection (UTI), and uncontrolled diabetes.*
olig/o	scanty	**olig**/uria (ŏl-ĭg-Ū-rē-ă): _____ *-uria:* urine *Oliguria is usually caused by fluid and electrolyte imbalances, renal lesions, or urinary tract obstruction.*
py/o	pus	**py**/uria (pī-Ū-rē-ă): _____ *-uria:* urine *Pyuria is associated with bacterial infections of the urinary tract.*
pyel/o	renal pelvis	**pyel/o**/plasty (PĪ-ĕ-lō-plăs-tē): _____ *-plasty:* surgical repair
ur/o	urine, urinary tract	**ur/o**/lith (Ū-rō-lĭth): _____ *-lith:* stone, calculus
ureter/o	ureter	**ureter**/ectasis (ū-rē-tĕr-ĔK-tă-sĭs): _____ *-ectasis:* dilation, expansion
urethr/o	urethra	**urethr/o**/stenosis (ū-rē-thrō-stĕn-Ō-sĭs): _____ *-stenosis:* narrowing, stricture
Suffixes		
-genesis	forming; producing; origin	lith/o/**genesis** (lĭth-ō-JĔN-ĕ-sĭs): _____ *lith/o:* stone, calculus
-iasis	abnormal condition (produced by something specified)	lith/**iasis** (lĭth-Ī-ă-sĭs): _____ *lith/o:* stone, calculus
-uria	urine	poly/**uria** (pŏl-ē-Ū-rē-ă): _____ *poly:* many, much *Polyuria is generally considered the excretion of over 2.5 L in 24 hours.*

Continued

Medical Word Elements—cont'd

Element	Meaning	Word Analysis
Prefixes		
dia-	through, across	**dia**/lysis (dī-ĂL-ĭ-sĭs): _____ *-lysis:* separation; destruction; loosening *Renal dialysis is a procedure that uses a membrane to separate and selectively remove waste products from the blood when the kidneys are unable to complete this function.*

retro-	backward, behind	**retro**/peritone/al (rĕt-rō-pĕr-ĭ-tō-NĒ-ăl): _____
		  peritone: peritoneum
		  -al: pertaining to

Visit the Medical Terminology Systems online resource center at FADavis.com for an audio exercise of the terms in this table. Other activities are also available to reinforce content.

 It is time to review medical word elements by completing Learning Activities 11-1 and 11-2.

Disease Focus

Causes of urinary system disorders include congenital anomalies, infectious diseases, trauma, and conditions that secondarily involve the urinary structures. Asymptomatic urinary diseases are commonly found when a routine urinalysis identifies abnormalities. When symptoms are present, they usually include changes in urination pattern, changes in output, or pain during urination **(dysuria).** Endoscopic tests, radiological evaluations, and laboratory tests that evaluate renal function typically identify disorders of the urinary system.

For diagnosis, treatment, and management of urinary disorders, the medical services of a specialist may be warranted. **Urology** is the branch of medicine concerned with urinary disorders and diseases of the male reproductive system. The physician who specializes in diagnosis and treatment of genitourinary disorders is known as a **urologist.** However, the branch of medicine concerned specifically with diseases of the kidney, electrolyte imbalance, renal transplantation, and dialysis therapy is **nephrology.** Physicians who practice in this specialty are called **nephrologists.**

Glomerulonephritis

Glomerulonephritis is an inflammation of the glomerular membrane in the nephrons, causing it to become "leaky" **(permeable).** Red blood cells and protein, which normally remain in blood, pass through the inflamed glomerular membrane and enter the tubule. Urinalysis reveals protein in the urine **(proteinuria),** blood in the urine **(hematuria),** and bacteria in the urine **(bacteruria),** indicators of infection or inflammation. Other signs and symptoms include high blood pressure **(hypertension),** edema, and impaired renal function.

Causes of glomerulonephritis include bacterial endocarditis, viral infections, and autoimmune diseases. Another cause of glomerular inflammation is a reaction to the toxins produced by pathogenic bacteria, especially streptococci that have recently infected another part of the body, usually strep throat. Most patients with acute glomerulonephritis associated with a streptococcal infection recover with no lasting kidney damage. Because most forms of glomerulonephritis are a consequence of another disorder, treatment of the underlying cause is important in the management of this disease.

Nephrolithiasis

Stones **(calculi)** may form in any part of the urinary tract **(urolithiasis),** but most arise in the kidney **(nephrolithiasis)** (see Fig. 11-3). They form when certain substances, such as calcium,

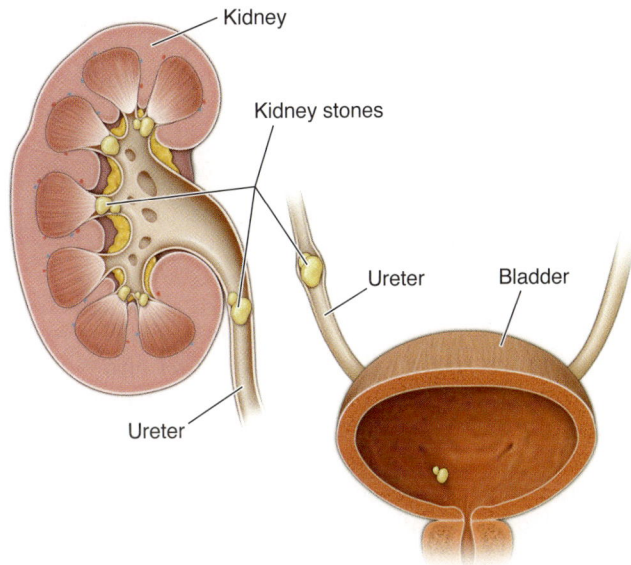

Figure 11-3 Nephrolithiasis with renal calculus traveling in the ureter and obstructing the flow of urine into the bladder.

uric acid, and oxalate, in the urine become highly concentrated and crystallize into solid masses. As the stones become larger, they commonly lodge in the ureters (**ureterolithiasis**), causing an intense, throbbing pain (**colic**). Because urine has difficulty passing into the bladder, it flows backward (**refluxes**) into the renal pelvis, causing it to dilate.

Treatment approach depends largely on the location and size of calculi. One type of treatment includes pulverizing the calculi using concentrated ultrasound shock waves generated from a machine outside the body (**extracorporeal shock-wave lithotripsy [ESWL]**; see Fig. 11-4[A]). The smaller pieces of stone can then pass through the urinary system and be expelled during urination (see Fig. 11-4[B]). For larger sized stones and patients who have contraindication to ESWL, an alternative minimally invasive surgery is available. In this procedure, the surgeon makes a small incision through the skin to create an opening into the kidney to remove the stone (**percutaneous nephrolithotomy [PCNL]**). If the stone is large, the surgeon breaks it into smaller fragments using an ultrasonic or electrohydraulic probe (**lithotriptor**) to remove the smaller fragments more easily. The surgeon may also insert a **nephrostomy** tube to drain urine from the kidney during the healing process and to expel any remaining pieces of pulverized stones. **Retrograde intrarenal**

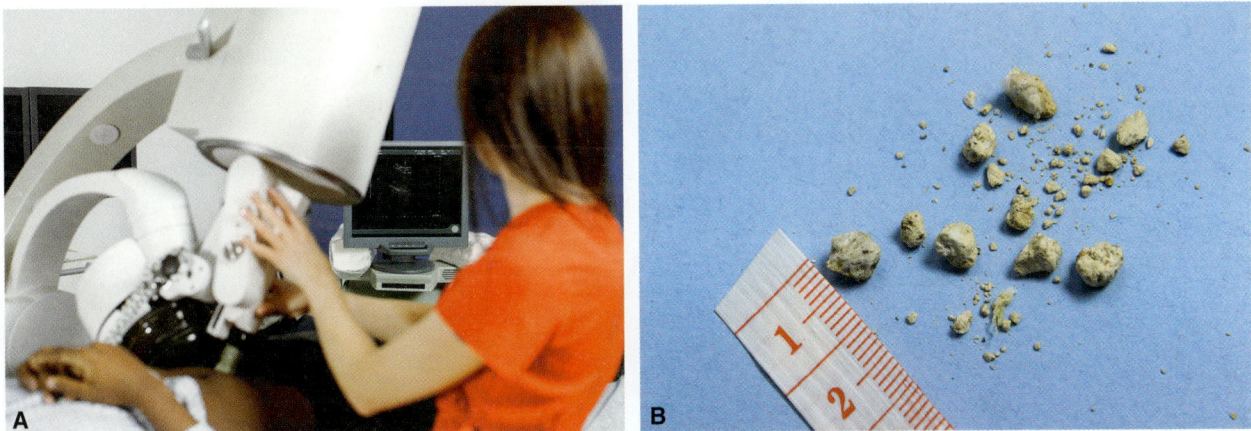

Figure 11-4 (A) Extracorporeal shock wave lithotripsy (ESWL). The physician views the digital screen to determine the kidney stones' location and then adjusts the position of the lithotripter. (B) Kidney stones after ESWL intervention (scale in centimeters).

surgery (**RIRS**) is a minimally invasive surgical procedure employed when the size or location of the calculi (**nephroliths**) makes other treatments, such as ESWL or PCNL, impractical or less effective. A flexible ureteroscope is inserted through the urethra until it reaches the kidney. The ureteroscope is equipped with a camera and specialized tools, such as a laser fiber or pneumatic lithotripter, which break up the calculi into smaller pieces. These pieces are then either extracted using a small basket-like device or flushed out through the urinary tract (see Fig. 11-5).

Acute Tubular Necrosis

In **acute tubular necrosis (ATN),** the tubular portion of the nephron is injured after the ingestion of toxic drugs (**nephrotoxic ATN**) or by a decrease in blood supply (**ischemic ATN).** Circulatory collapse, severe hypotension, hemorrhage, dehydration, or other disorders that affect blood supply are the common causes of ischemic ATN. Because specific signs and symptoms are not associated with ATN, the diagnosis relies on a positive history of risk factors. Nonspecific signs and symptoms of ATN commonly include scanty urine production (**oliguria**), fluid retention, mental apathy, nausea, vomiting, and increased blood levels of calcium (**hypercalcemia**). When tubular damage is not severe, the disorder is usually reversible.

Oncology

Bladder cancer in the United States is the fourth most common cancer in men. There are different types of bladder cancer with **urothelial carcinoma** (or transitional cell carcinoma) as the

Figure 11-5 Retrograde intrarenal surgery (RIRS) with flexible ureteroscopy for kidney stone treatment.

most common. Most urothelial carcinomas are nonmuscle invasive bladder cancers (NMIBC) and remain in the bladder inner lining. But some bladder tumors are more invasive and metastasize to surrounding tissue. Smoking and tobacco use is the biggest risk factor for bladder cancer.

Signs and symptoms of bladder cancer include hematuria, frequency, dysuria, and abdominal or back pain. Diagnostic tests include cystoscopy with biopsy of suspicious lesions and urine cytology, in which malignant cells appear in a urine sample.

Treatment depends on the type, stage, and grade of the malignancy. In the early stages when the malignancy is confined to the bladder lining, the practitioner employs an electric current or high-energy laser using a device passed through the urethra **(transurethral resection of bladder tumor [TURBT])** to destroy malignant tissue. Advanced cancers require the removal of the bladder **(cystectomy)**. Surgery combined with treatments that stimulate the immune response **(biological therapy; immunotherapy)**, chemotherapy delivered intravenously or directly into the bladder **(intravesical)**, and radiation therapy are other treatment options.

Renal cell carcinoma (RCC) is the most common type of kidney cancer in adults. It originates in the cells lining the tubules responsible for filtration of waste products to form urine **(nephrons)**. RCC typically occurs in adults aged 50 to 70 years old. Often there are no symptoms in its early stages and it can spread to lymph nodes, lungs, liver, and bones, leading to further complications. Treatment depends on the stage of the cancer and the overall health of the person. Surgery is the primary treatment for localized RCC and may involve partial or total removal of the affected kidney **(nephrectomy)**. Metastatic RCC treatment may include radiation, chemotherapy, immunotherapy, or a combination of these.

Diseases and Conditions

This section introduces diseases and conditions of the urinary system, along with their meanings and pronunciations. Word analyses for selected terms are also provided.

Term	Definition

anuria
ăn-Ū-rē-ă
  an-: without, not
  uria: urine
	Absence of urine production or output
	Anuria may be obstructive, in which there is blockage proximal to the bladder, or unobstructive, which is caused by severe damage to the nephrons of the kidneys.

azoturia
ăz-ō-TŪ-rē-ă
  azot: nitrogenous compounds
  -uria: urine
	Increase of nitrogenous substances, especially urea, in urine

bladder neck obstruction (BNO)	Blockage at the base of the bladder that reduces or prevents urine from passing into the urethra *Causes of BNO include an enlarged prostate, bladder stones, bladder tumors, and tumors in the pelvic cavity.*

Continued

Diseases and Conditions—cont'd

Term	Definition
cystocele SĬS-tō-sēl *cyst/o:* bladder *-cele:* hernia, swelling	Prolapsing or downward displacement of the bladder due to weakening of the supporting tissues between the bladder and vagina (see Fig. 11-6) *Cystocele is commonly the result of vaginal childbirth, frequent straining with constipation, or lifting of heavy objects.*

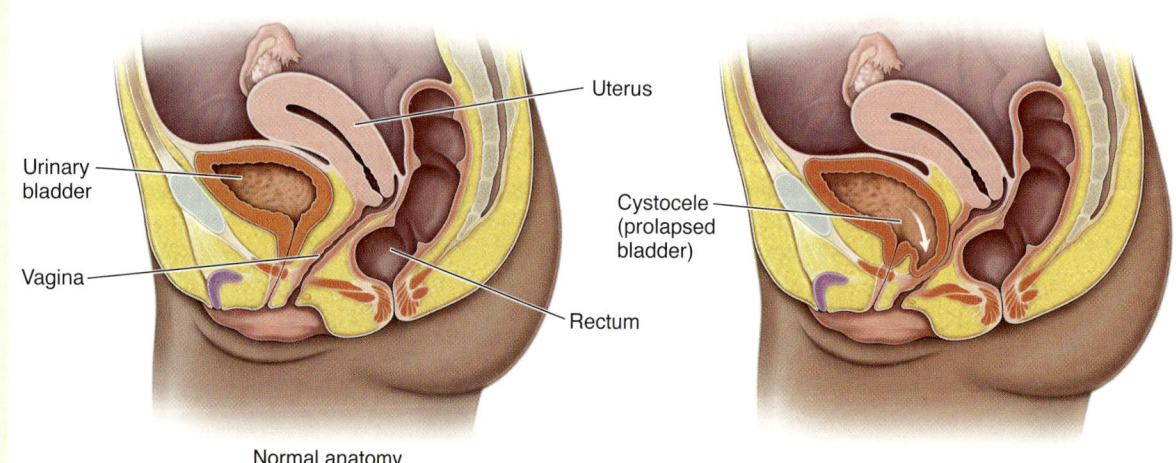

Normal anatomy

Figure 11-6 Cystocele.

Term	Definition
diuresis dī-ū-RĒ-sĭs *di-:* double *ur:* urine *-esis:* condition	Increased formation and secretion of urine
end-stage renal disease (ESRD) RĒ-năl *ren:* kidney *-al:* pertaining to	Any type of kidney disease in which there is little or no remaining kidney function, requiring the patient to undergo dialysis or kidney transplant for survival *The two most common causes of ESRD are diabetes and hypertension.*
enuresis ĕn-ū-RĒ-sĭs *en-:* in, within *ur:* urine *-esis:* condition	Involuntary discharge of urine particularly during sleep; also called *bedwetting* or *nocturnal enuresis*
fistula FĬS-tū-lă	Abnormal passage from a hollow organ to the surface or from one organ to another *The most common type of urinary fistula is vesicovaginal fistula, in which a passage forms between the bladder and vagina. Its causes include previous pelvic surgery, such as hysterectomy; difficult, prolonged labor; and reduced blood supply to the area.*

Diseases and Conditions—cont'd

Term	Definition

hydronephrosis
hī-drō-nĕf-RŌ-sĭs
hydr/o: water
nephr: kidney
-osis: abnormal condition; increase (used primarily with blood cells)

Abnormal dilation of the renal pelvis and the calyces of one or both kidneys caused by pressure from accumulated urine that cannot flow past an obstruction in the urinary tract

The causes of hydronephrosis are enlargement of the prostate, urethral strictures, and calculi that lodge in the ureter. When dilation affects the ureter, it is called **hydroureter** *(see Fig. 11-7).*

Figure 11-7 Hydronephrosis and hydroureter.

incontinence

Inability to control the excretion of urine; also refers to the inability to control feces, or both

overflow

Urinary incontinence that occurs when the bladder doesn't empty and dribbling or frequent leaking occurs

Overflow incontinence can be caused by an obstruction to the bladder outlet such as an enlarged prostate, weak bladder muscles, or nerve damage from spinal cord injuries or diabetes.

stress

Urinary incontinence due to weakened pelvic floor muscles that occurs when exercising, laughing, coughing, or sneezing

Stress incontinence occurs more often in women due to weakened pelvic floor muscles from pregnancy and childbirth.

Continued

Diseases and Conditions—cont'd

Term	Definition
interstitial cystitis (IC) ĭn-tĕr-STĬSH-ăl sĭs-TĪ-tĭs *cyst:* bladder *-itis:* inflammation	Chronic inflammation of the bladder wall that is not caused by bacterial infection and is not responsive to conventional antibiotic therapy; also called *painful bladder syndrome* *Two common symptoms include urinary frequency and bladder or pelvic pain ranging from mild to severe. Medications and physical therapy may help some patients, but other patients are unresponsive to treatment.*
nephrotic syndrome nĕ-FRŎT-ĭk SĬN-drōm *nephr/o:* kidney *-tic:* pertaining to	Loss of large amounts of plasma protein, usually albumin, through urine due to an increased permeability of the glomerular membrane *Hypoproteinemia, edema, and hyperlipidemia are commonly associated with nephrotic syndrome.*
neurogenic bladder nū-rō-JĔN-ĭk *neur/o:* nerve *gen:* forming, producing, origin *-ic:* pertaining to	Impairment of bladder control as a result of brain, spinal cord, or nerve damage *Because the nervous system controls how the bladder stores and empties urine, neurogenic bladder leads to incontinence, difficulty in urinating, or the inability to urinate.*
polycystic kidney disease (PKD) pŏl-ē-SĬS-tĭk *poly:* many, much *cyst:* bladder *-ic:* pertaining to	Inherited disease in which sacs of fluid called *cysts* develop in the kidneys *If cysts increase in number or size or if they become infected, kidney failure may result. Dialysis or kidney transplant may be necessary for renal failure caused by PKD (see Fig. 11-8).*

Polycystic kidney   Normal kidney

Figure 11-8 Polycystic kidney disease shown on the left kidney with right healthy kidney.

Term	Definition
pyelonephritis pī-ĕ-lō-nĕ-FRĪ-tĭs *pyel/o:* renal pelvis *nephr:* kidney *-itis:* inflammation	Infection of the kidney, usually the result of an infection that begins in the urethra or bladder and ascends the ureters to the kidney *Pyelonephritis requires prompt attention to avoid permanent damage to the kidneys and to keep infection from spreading to the bloodstream.*

Diseases and Conditions—cont'd

Term	Definition
renal hypertension RĒ-năl *ren:* kidney *al:* pertaining to	High blood pressure caused by a narrowing or obstruction in the renal arteries; also called *renovascular hypertension* *The most common cause is atherosclerosis. Treatment includes antihypertensive medication. Severe narrowing (stenosis) of the renal artery may require angioplasty with stent insertion to keep the artery open for adequate blood flow.*
urgency ĔR-jĕn-sē	Sensation of the need to void immediately; also called *overactive bladder* *Urinary urgency commonly occurs in urinary tract infection (UTI).*
urinary tract infection (UTI) Ū-rĭ-nār-ē *urin:* urine; urinary tract *-ary:* pertaining to	An infection, typically of bacterial origin, in any part of the urinary tract, including the kidneys (acute pyelonephritis), bladder (cystitis), or urethra (urethritis) *Dysuria, although a symptom associated with numerous conditions, is commonly associated with UTI, especially cystitis and urethritis.*
vesicoureteral reflux (VUR) vĕs-ĭ-kō-ū-RĒ-tĕr-ăl RĒ-flŭks *vesic/o:* bladder *ureter:* ureter *-al:* pertaining to	Disorder caused by the failure of urine to pass through the ureters to the bladder, usually as a result of impairment of the valve between the ureter and bladder (vesicouretral junction), or the bladder not being able to empty fully; most often occurs in infants and children *VUR may result in hydronephrosis and raises the risk of UTIs.*
Wilms tumor VĬLMZ	Rapidly developing malignant tumor of the kidney that usually occurs in children; also called *nephroblastoma* *Diagnosis of Wilms tumor is established by an excretory urogram with tomography. The tumor is well encapsulated in the early stage but may metastasize to other sites, such as the lymph nodes and lungs, at later stages.*

 It is time to review pathology, diseases, and conditions by completing Learning Activity 11-3.

Diagnostic, Surgical, and Therapeutic Procedures

This section introduces diagnostic, surgical, and therapeutic procedures used to diagnose and treat urinary disorders. Descriptions are provided, along with pronunciations and word analyses for selected terms.

Procedure	Description
Diagnostic	
Clinical	
electromyography (EMG) ē-lĕk-trō-mī-ŎG-ră-fē *electr/o:* electricity *my/o:* muscle *-graphy:* process of recording	Measures the contraction of muscles that control urination using electrodes placed in the rectum and urethra *EMG determines whether incontinence results from weak muscles or other causes.*

Continued

Diagnostic, Surgical, and Therapeutic Procedures—cont'd

Procedure	Description

Endoscopic

cystoscopy (cysto)
sĭs-TŎS-kō-pē
cyst/o: bladder
-scopy: examination

Examination of the urinary bladder for evidence of pathology, to obtain biopsies of tumors or other growths, or to remove polyps

In cystoscopy, the practitioner inserts a catheter into the hollow channel in the cystoscope to collect tissue samples or introduce contrast media during radiography (see Fig. 11-9).

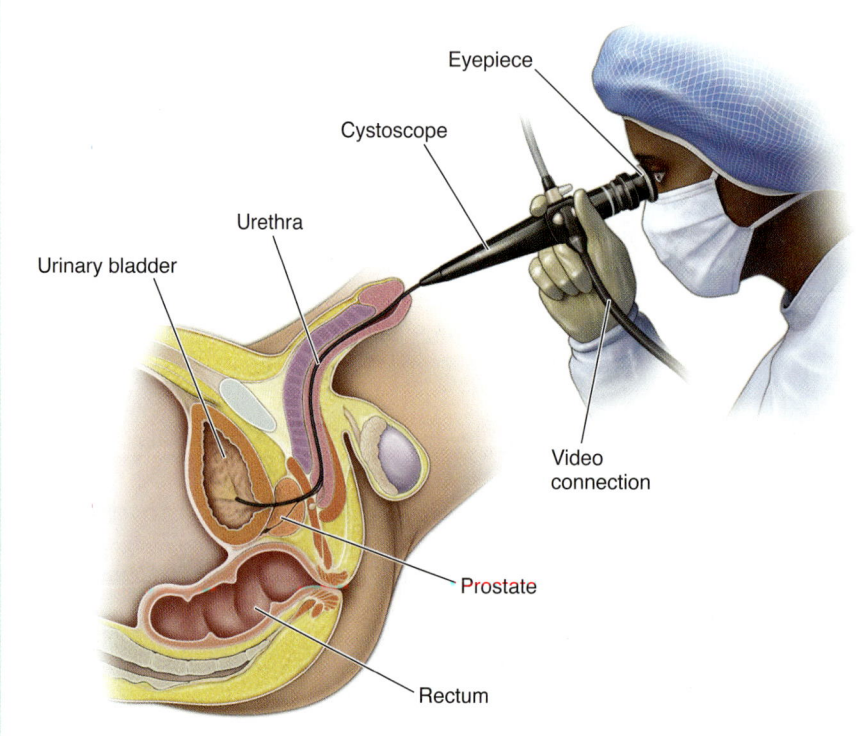

Eyepiece

Cystoscope

Urethra

Urinary bladder

Video connection

Prostate

Rectum

Figure 11-9 Cystoscopy.

Laboratory

blood urea nitrogen (BUN)
ū-RĒ-ă NĪ-trō-jĕn

Test that determines the amount of nitrogen in blood that comes from urea, a waste product of protein metabolism

Because the kidneys clear urea from the bloodstream, the BUN test helps evaluate kidney function.

serum creatinine
SĒ-rŭm krē-ĂT-ĭn-ēn

Test performed on blood to measure the amount of creatinine, a waste product of muscle metabolism that indicates kidney function

creatinine clearance
krē-ĂT-ĭn-ēn

Test to measure the level of creatinine filtered by the kidneys that consists of 24-hour urine collection with a blood sample to estimate the glomerular filtration rate (GFR) and evaluate kidney function

Creatinine clearance is an important test in assessing kidney function and in monitoring the effectiveness of kidney disease treatment.

Diagnostic, Surgical, and Therapeutic Procedures—cont'd

Procedure	Description
culture and sensitivity (C&S)	Test that determines the causative organism of an infection and identifies how the organism responds to various antibiotics *The practitioner may order a urine C&S test when a patient has chronic bladder infections or one that is unresponsive to treatment.*
urinalysis (UA) ū-rĭ-NĂL-ĭ-sĭs	Urine screening test that includes physical observation, chemical tests, and microscopic evaluation *UA not only provides information on the urinary structures but may also be the first indicator of such system disorders as diabetes and liver and gallbladder disease.*
Imaging	
bladder ultrasound (US)	A noninvasive, painless test that uses high-frequency soundwaves to produce images of the bladder before and after urination to check for urinary retention (see Fig. 11-10) *During the examination, the practitioner directs sound waves into the bladder area and records images on a monitor.* Figure 11-10 Ultrasonogram of the bladder. This scan is performed at the bedside. It may be used instead of catheterization after the patient urinates to determine the amount of urine remaining in the bladder.

computerized tomography urogram (CT urogram)
tō-MŎG-ră-fē
  tom/o: to cut, slice
  -graphy: process of recording
  ur/o: urine
  -gram: record, writing
	Imaging using intravenous (IV) contrast with x-rays and computerized technology to view the urinary system
	
	CT urograms are the primary diagnostic tool for detecting urinary system calculi and perirenal infections and have replaced intravenous pyelography (IVP). CT urograms provide better visualization of the kidneys, ureters, and bladder for a clearer picture and more accurate diagnosis.

Continued

Diagnostic, Surgical, and Therapeutic Procedures—cont'd

Procedure	Description
intravenous pyelography (IVP) ĭn-tră-VĒ-nŭs pī-ĕ-LŎG-ră-fē *intra-:* in, within *ven:* vein *-ous:* pertaining to *pyel/o:* renal pelvis *-graphy:* process of recording	Imaging of the urinary tract after IV injection of a contrast medium; also called *excretory urography* *IVP is being used less frequently and has been replaced with more advanced imaging techniques, in particular CT urography (described above).*
kidneys, ureters, bladder (KUB)	X-ray to assess the organs of the urinary system to determine their location, size, and shape and to identify obstructions and calculi formation; also called *flat plate of the abdomen* *KUB is often performed as an initial test to diagnose the cause of abdominal pain.*
renal nuclear scan RĒ-năl *ren:* kidney *-al:* pertaining to	Nuclear imaging test using a radioactive substance (tracer) injected intravenously to produce images of the kidneys *Renal nuclear scan evaluates the structure and function of the kidneys. It determines the size, shape, and position of the kidneys. It also determines the amount of blood filtered through the kidneys and evaluates kidney transplant to identify signs of rejection.*
voiding cystourethrography (VCUG) sĭs-tō-ū-rē-THRŎG-ră-fē *cyst/o:* bladder *urethr/o:* urethra *-graphy:* process of recording	X-ray with contrast medium of the bladder and urethra performed before, during, and after voiding *VCUG helps determine the cause of repeated bladder infections or stress incontinence and identifies congenital or acquired structural abnormalities of the bladder and urethra.*

Diagnostic, Surgical, and Therapeutic Procedures—cont'd

Procedure	Description
Surgical	
kidney transplant	Replacement of a diseased kidney with one that is supplied by a compatible donor (usually a family member or a cadaver who donated the kidney before death) *The surgeon usually places the kidney below the diseased one for ease in attaching it to existing blood vessels. The diseased kidney usually remains in place unless there is concern that it will cause infection, uncontrolled hypertension, or reflux to the kidneys (see Fig. 11-11).*

Diseased kidneys

Transplanted kidney

Transplanted ureter

Urinary bladder

Figure 11-11 Kidney transplant with typical positioning of the kidney beneath the diseased kidney.

Continued

Diagnostic, Surgical, and Therapeutic Procedures—cont'd

Procedure	Description
nephrostomy ně-FRŎS-tō-mē *nephr/o:* kidney *–stomy:* forming an opening (mouth)	Opening created between the skin and kidney to drain urine through a tube to a collecting receptacle outside the body when the ureters are unable to do so *Besides providing for urine drainage, nephrostomy may help access the kidney, evaluate kidney function, or deliver medications (see Fig. 11-12).*

Figure 11-12 Percutaneous nephrostomy with a nephrostomy tube exiting through the skin.

Diagnostic, Surgical, and Therapeutic Procedures—cont'd

Procedure	Description

ureteral stent placement
ū-RĒ-tĕr-ăl

   ureter: ureter
   -al: pertaining to

Insertion of a thin, narrow tube into the ureter to prevent or treat obstruction of urine flow from the kidney

Indwelling stents require constant monitoring because they may lead to infections, blockages, or stone formation. To avoid complications, they must be removed or changed periodically (see Fig. 11-13).

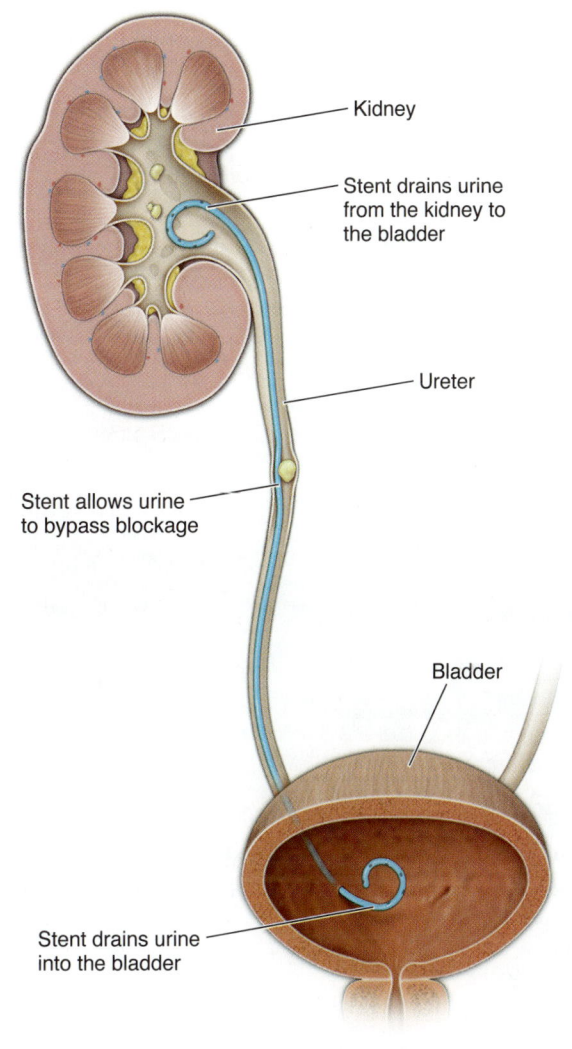

Kidney

Stent drains urine from the kidney to the bladder

Ureter

Stent allows urine to bypass blockage

Bladder

Stent drains urine into the bladder

Figure 11-13 Ureteral stent placement.

Continued

Diagnostic, Surgical, and Therapeutic Procedures—cont'd

Procedure	Description
Therapeutic	

catheterization (Cath)
kăth-ĕ-tĕr-ĭ-ZĀ-shŭn

Insertion of a catheter (hollow flexible tube) into a body cavity or organ to instill a substance or remove fluid, most commonly through the urethra into the bladder to drain urine

Catheters are available as two basic types: a straight catheter, which is used only for immediate drainage, and a Foley catheter, which is used for short-term and long-term (indwelling) drainage. An inflated balloon keeps the catheter in place (see Fig. 11-14).

Figure 11-14 Urinary catheterization with a Foley catheter.

dialysis
dī-ĂL-ĭ-sĭs
  dia-: through, across
  -lysis: separation; destruction; loosening

Filtering procedure used to remove fluid and waste products from the blood and correct for electrolyte imbalances

Dialysis allows patients with kidney failure a chance to live productive lives.

Diagnostic, Surgical, and Therapeutic Procedures—cont'd

Procedure	Description
hemodialysis hē-mō-dī-ĂL-ĭ-sĭs *hem/o:* blood *dia-:* through, across *-lysis:* separation; destruction; loosening	Dialysis in which an artificial kidney machine receives waste-filled blood through direct access of a catheter or fistula into the bloodstream and filters it using a solution called a *dialysate* and then returns the dialyzed (clean) blood to the patient's bloodstream (see Fig. 11-15)

Blood with waste products

Dialyzer

Dialysate lines

Filtered clean blood

Access

Figure 11-15 Hemodialysis. Blood from the access containing waste products flows into the dialyzer, where impurities and excess fluid are drawn into the dialysis solution. Filtered, cleansed blood is then returned through the secondary access line and into the bloodstream.

peritoneal dialysis pĕr-ĭ-tō-NĒ-ăl *peritone:* peritoneum *-al:* pertaining to *dia-:* through, across *-lysis:* separation; destruction; loosening	Dialysis that uses the peritoneum as a filter to remove waste products from the blood through infusion of dialysate via an abdominal catheter (see Fig. 11-16) *Peritoneal dialysis is less restrictive on the patient than hemodialysis because it allows for self-treatment at home or while on trips.*

A

B

Figure 11-16 Peritoneal dialysis. (A) Patient connecting abdominal catheter to tubing of dialysate solution. (B) Dialysate solution flows into the peritoneal cavity where waste products and excess fluids pass from the blood vessels in the peritoneal membrane into the dialysate for a prescribed period of time. The secondary empty bag (right side) will then be lowered to allow the used dialysate, now containing waste products and excess fluid, to drain out of the peritoneal cavity.

Pharmacology

Pharmacological agents used to treat urinary tract disorders include antibiotics, diuretics, antidiuretics, urinary antispasmodics, and potassium supplements, which are commonly taken concurrently with diuretics to counteract potassium depletion (see Table 11-1).

TABLE 11-1 Drugs Used To Treat Urinary Disorders

This table lists common drug classifications used to treat urinary disorders, their therapeutic actions, and selected generic and trade names.

Classification	Therapeutic Action	Generic and Trade Names
antibiotics ăn-tĭ-bī-ŎT-ĭks	Treat bacterial infections of the urinary tract by acting on the bacterial membrane or one of its metabolic processes *The type of antibiotic prescribed depends on the infecting organism and the type and extent of infection.*	**ciprofloxacin** sĭp-rō-FLŎX-ă-sĭn *Cipro* **sulfamethoxazole/trimethoprim** sŭl-fă-mĕth-ŎX-ă-zol trī-MĔTH-ō-prĭm *Bactrim*
antispasmodics ăn-tĭ-spăz-MŎT-ĭks	Decrease spasms in the urethra and bladder by relaxing the smooth muscles lining their walls, thus allowing normal emptying of the bladder *Bladder spasms can result from such conditions as UTIs and catheterization.*	**tolterodine** tōl-TĔR-ō-dēn Detrol LA **solifenacin** sōl-ĭ-FĔN-ă-sĭn *Vesicare*
diuretics dī-ū-RĔT-ĭks	Promote and increase the excretion of urine *Diuretics are grouped by their action and are used to treat edema, hypertension, heart failure, and various renal and hepatic diseases.*	**furosemide** fū-RŌ-sĕ-mīd *Lasix* **spironolactone** spī-rō-nō-LĂK-tōn *Aldactone*
potassium supplements pō-TĂS-ē-ŭm	Replace potassium after depletion caused by diuretics *Dietary sources of potassium are usually not sufficient to replace potassium loss caused by diuretics.*	**potassium chloride** pō-TĂS-ē-ŭm KLŌ-rīd *K-Tab, Kaon Cl*

Abbreviations

This section introduces urinary system–related abbreviations and their meanings.

Abbreviation	Meaning	Abbreviation	Meaning
ATN	acute tubular necrosis	PCNL	percutaneous nephrolithotomy
BNO	bladder neck obstruction	pH	symbol for degree of acidity or alkalinity
BUN	blood urea nitrogen	PKD	polycystic kidney disease
C&S	culture and sensitivity	RCC	renal cell carcinoma
cath	catheterization	RIRS	retrograde intrarenal surgery
CT urogram	computed tomography urogram	TURBT	transurethral resection of bladder tumor
cysto	cystoscopy	UA	urinalysis
EMG	electromyogram, electromyography	UP	ureteropelvic
ESRD	end-stage renal disease	US	ultrasound; ultrasonography
ESWL	extracorporeal shock-wave lithotripsy	UTI	urinary tract infection
IC	interstitial cystitis	VCUG	voiding cystourethrography
IVP	intravenous pyelogram; intravenous pyelography	VUR	vesicoureteral reflux
NMIBC	nonmuscle invasive bladder cancers		

It is time to review procedures, pharmacology, and abbreviations by completing Learning Activity 11-4.

LEARNING ACTIVITIES

The activities that follow provide a review of the urinary system terms introduced in this chapter. Complete each activity and review your answers to evaluate your understanding of the chapter.

Medical Language Lab
Turning terminology into language

Visit the Medical Language Laboratory at medicallanguagelab.com. Use it to enhance your study and reinforcement of this chapter with the flash card activity. We recommend that you complete the flash card activity before starting Learning Activities 11-1 and 11-2.

Learning Activity 11-1
Medical Word Elements

Use the listed elements to build medical words. You may use the elements more than once.

Combining Forms		Suffixes		Prefixes
azot/o	pyel/o	-cele	-plasty	an-
cyst/o	ureter/o	-ectasis	-sclerosis	dia-
glomerul/o		-emia	-scopy	olig-
hemat/o		-genesis	-tome	
lith/o		-gram	-tripsy	
meat/o		-lysis	-uria	
nephr/o		-pathy		

1. (x-ray) record of the bladder _____

2. hernia of the kidney _____

3. surgical repair of the renal pelvis _____

4. without (producing) urine _____

5. disease of the glomerulus _____

6. process of examining the bladder _____

7. separation across (a membrane) _____

8. blood in the urine _____

9. (producing) scanty urine _____

10. dilation of the ureters _____

11. instrument to cut (enlarge) the meatus _____

12. nitrogenous compounds in the blood _____

13. forming (producing) stones _____

14. crushing of a stone _____

15. disease of the kidney _____

Check your answers in Appendix A. Review any material that you did not answer correctly.

Correct Answers _____ X 6.67 = _____ % Score

Learning Activity 11-2
Building Medical Words

Use *nephr/o* (kidney) to build words that mean

1. enlargement of the kidney _____
2. abnormal condition of pus in the kidney _____
3. stone in the kidney _____

Use *pyel/o* (renal pelvis) to build words that mean

4. inflammation of the renal pelvis and kidney _____
5. disease of the renal pelvis _____

Use *ureter/o* (ureter) to build words that mean

6. dilation of a ureter _____
7. calculus in a ureter _____
8. pain in the ureters _____

Use *cyst/o* (bladder) to build words that mean

9. inflammation of the bladder _____
10. instrument to view the bladder _____
11. hernia of the bladder _____

Use *vesic/o* (bladder) to build words that mean

12. herniation of the bladder _____
13. pertaining to the bladder and urethra _____

Use *urethr/o* (urethra) to build words that mean

14. narrowing or stricture of the urethra _____
15. surgical repair of the urethra _____

Use *ur/o* (urine, urinary tract) to build words that mean

16. study of the urinary tract _____
17. disease of the urinary tract _____

Use the suffix *-uria* (urine) to build words that mean

18. difficult or painful urination _____
19. blood in the urine _____
20. protein in the urine _____

Build surgical words that mean

21. surgical repair of the ureters _____

22. excision of the bladder _____

23. suture of the urethra _____

24. forming a mouth in the renal pelvis _____

25. fixation of the bladder _____

Check your answers in Appendix A. Review material that you did not answer correctly.

Correct Answers _____ X 4 = _____ % Score

Learning Activity 11-3
Diseases and Conditions

Match the terms with the definitions in the numbered list.

anuria	enuresis	nephrolithiasis	pyelonephritis
azotemia	fistula	nephropyosis	reflux
colic	hydronephrosis	nephrotic syndrome	urgency
cystocele	incontinence	neurogenic bladder	urolithiasis
diuresis	interstitial cystitis	polycystic	Wilms tumor

1. need to void immediately _____
2. abnormal passage from a hollow organ to the surface or between organs _____
3. increased formation and secretion of urine _____
4. absence of urine production _____
5. nitrogenous wastes in the blood _____
6. abnormal condition of the kidneys due to water (urine reflux) _____
7. abnormal condition of a stone in any part of the urinary tract _____
8. chronic inflammation of the bladder wall _____
9. abrupt pain in stomach or bowels _____
10. inflammation of the kidney and renal pelvis _____
11. herniation of the bladder _____
12. involuntary discharge of urine _____
13. kidney disease characterized by the presence of fluid-filled sacs _____
14. loss of bladder control due to brain or nerve damage _____
15. formation of pus in the kidney _____
16. loss of plasma protein due to increased permeability of the glomerulus _____
17. involuntary discharge of urine while sleeping _____
18. backflow of urine into the kidney _____
19. rapidly developing malignant neoplasm of the kidney _____
20. abnormal condition of stones in the kidneys _____

Check your answers in Appendix A. Review any material that you did not answer correctly.

Correct Answers _____ X 5 = _____ % Score

Learning Activity 11-4

Procedures, Pharmacology, and Abbreviations

Match the terms with the definitions in the numbered list.

bladder US	*EMG*	*potassium*
C&S	*ESWL*	*RCC*
creatinine clearance	*hemodialysis*	*renal nuclear scan*
CT urogram	*nephrostomy*	*stent placement*
diuretics	*peritoneal*	*UA*

1. primary diagnostic tool for detecting urinary system calculi and perirenal infections _____

2. measures the contraction of urinary muscles _____

3. laboratory test to estimate the glomerular filtration rate and evaluate kidney function _____

4. the most common type of kidney cancer in adults _____

5. laboratory test that identifies and evaluates the effect of an antibiotic on an organism _____

6. drugs used to promote the excretion of urine _____

7. positioning of a tube in the ureter to treat obstruction of urine flow _____

8. noninvasive procedure used to pulverize urinary or bile stones _____

9. dialysis of toxic substances by perfusing the abdominopelvic cavity _____

10. imaging that uses a tracer to produce images of the kidney _____

11. dialysis of toxic products by shunting blood from the body _____

12. opening created in the kidney to drain urine to an outside receptacle _____

13. imaging that uses sound waves to evaluate urine retention _____

14. supplement used to treat or prevent the hypokalemia commonly associated with the use of diuretics _____

15. test that includes physical observation as well as chemical and microscopic evaluation of urine _____

✓ *Check your answers in Appendix A. Review material that you did not answer correctly.*

Correct Answers _____ X 6.67 = _____ % Score

DOCUMENTING HEALTH-CARE ACTIVITIES

This section provides practical application activities in the form of exercises to help students develop skills in documenting patient care. First, read the medical report. Then complete the activities and exercises that follow.

Documenting Health-Care Activity 11-1
Operative Report: Cystoscopy With Cystolithotripsy

General Hospital

1511 Ninth Avenue ■ ■ Sun City, USA 12345 ■ ■ (555) 802–1887

OPERATIVE REPORT

Date: May 14, 20xx   Physician: Elmer Augustino, MD
Patient: Motch, Edwin   Patient: ID#: 48778

PREOPERATIVE DIAGNOSIS: Hematuria with left ureterocele and ureterocele calculus.

POSTOPERATIVE DIAGNOSIS: Hematuria with left ureterocele and ureterocele calculus.

OPERATION: Cystoscopy, transurethral incision of ureterocele, extraction of stone, and cystolithotripsy.

ANESTHESIA: General.

COMPLICATIONS: None.

PROCEDURE: Patient was prepped and draped and placed in the lithotomy position. The urethra was calibrated with ease using a #26 French Van Buren urethral sound. A #24 resectoscope was inserted with ease. The prostate and bladder appeared normal, except for the presence of a left ureterocele, which was incised longitudinally; a large calculus was extracted from the ureterocele. There was minimal bleeding and no need for fulguration. The stone was crushed with the Storz stone-crushing instrument, and the fragments were evacuated. The bladder was emptied and the procedure terminated.

Patient tolerated the procedure well and was transferred to the postanesthesia care unit.

Elmer Augustino, MD
Elmer Augustino, MD

ea:bg

D: 5–14–20xx
T: 5–14–20xx

Terminology

The terms listed in the table that follows are taken from *Operative Report: Cystoscopy With Cystolithotripsy*. Use a medical dictionary such as *Taber's Cyclopedic Medical Dictionary*, the appendices of this book, or other resources to define each term. Then review the pronunciation for each term and practice by reading the medical record aloud.

Term	Definition
calculus KĂL-kū-lŭs	
cystolithotripsy sĭs-tō-LĬTH-ō-trĭp-sē	
cystoscope SĬST-ō-skōp	
fulguration fŭl-gŭ-RĀ-shŭn	
hematuria hē-mă-TŪ-rē-ă	
resectoscope rē-SĔK-tō-skōp	
transurethral trăns-ū-RĒ-thrăl	
ureterocele ū-RĒ-tĕr-ō-sēl	
urethral sound ū-RĒ-thrăl	

Visit the Medical Terminology Systems online resource center at FADavis.com to practice pronunciation and reinforce the meanings of the terms in this medical report.

Critical Thinking

Review *Operative Report: Cystoscopy With Cystolithotripsy* to answer the questions.

1. What were the findings from the resectoscopy?

_____

_____

_____

2. What were the name and size of the urethral sound used in the procedure?

_____

_____

_____

3. What is the function of the urethral sound?

_____

_____

_____

4. In what direction was the ureterocele incised?

_____

_____

_____

5. Was fulguration required? Why or why not?

_____

_____

_____

Operative Report: Extracorporeal Shock-Wave Lithotripsy

General Hospital

1511 Ninth Avenue ■ ■ Sun City, USA 12345 ■ ■ (555) 802–1887

OPERATIVE REPORT

Date: April 1, 20xx   Physician: Elmer Augustino, MD
Patient: Marino, Julius   Room: 7201

PREOPERATIVE DIAGNOSIS: Left renal calculus.

POSTOPERATIVE DIAGNOSIS: Left renal calculus.

PROCEDURE: Extracorporeal shock-wave lithotripsy, cystoscopy with double-J stent removal.

INDICATION FOR PROCEDURE: This 69-year-old male had undergone ESWL on 5/15/xx, with double-J stent placement to allow stone fragments to pass from the calyx to the bladder. At that time, approximately 50% of a partial staghorn calculus was fragmented. He now presents for the fragmenting of the remainder of the calculus and removal of the double-J stent.

ANESTHESIA: General.

COMPLICATIONS: None.

OPERATIVE TECHNIQUE: Patient was brought to the lithotripsy unit and placed in the supine position on the lithotripsy table. After induction of anesthesia, fluoroscopy was used to position the patient in the focal point of the shock waves. Being well positioned, he was given a total of 4,000 shocks with a maximum power setting of 3.0. After confirming complete fragmentation via fluoroscopy, the patient was transferred to the cystoscopy suite.

Patient was placed in the dorsal lithotomy position and draped and prepped in the usual manner. A cystoscope was inserted into the bladder through the urethra. Once the stent was visualized, it was grasped with the grasping forceps and removed as the scope was withdrawn.

Patient tolerated the procedure well and was transferred to recovery.

Elmer Augustino, MD
Elmer Augustino, MD

ea:bg

D: 4–1–20xx;
T: 4–1–20xx

Terminology

The terms listed in the table that follows are taken from *Operative Report: Extracorporeal Shock-Wave Lithotripsy.* Use a medical dictionary such as *Taber's Cyclopedic Medical Dictionary,* the appendices of this book, or other resources to define each term. Then review the pronunciation for each term and practice by reading the medical record aloud.

Term	Definition
calculus KĂL-kū-lŭs	
calyx KĀ-lĭx	
cystoscope SĬST-ō-skōp	
cystoscopy sĭs-TŎS-kō-pē	
dorsal lithotomy DOR-săl lĭth-ŎT-ō-mē	
ESWL	
extracorporeal ĕks-tră-kor- POR-ē-ăl	
fluoroscopy floo-or-ŎS-kō-pē	
lithotripsy LĬTH-ō-trĭp-sē	
shock-wave	
staghorn calculus STĂG-horn KĂL-kū-lŭs	
stent STĔNT	

Visit the Medical Terminology Systems online resource center at FADavis. com to practice pronunciation and reinforce the meanings of the terms in this medical report.

Critical Thinking

Review *Operative Report: Extracorporeal Shock-Wave Lithotripsy* to answer the questions.

1. What previous procedures were performed on the patient?

_____

_____

_____

_____

2. Why is the current procedure being performed?

_____

_____

_____

_____

3. What imaging technique was used for positioning the patient to ensure that the shock waves would strike the calculus?

_____

_____

_____

_____

4. In what position was the patient placed in the cystoscopy suite?

_____

_____

_____

_____

5. How was the double-J stent removed?

_____

_____

_____

_____

Constructing Chart Notes

To construct chart notes, replace the italicized and boldfaced terms in each of the two case studies with one of the listed medical terms.

glomerulonephritis	*oliguria*	*pyelectasis*
hematuria	*prognosis*	*pyuria*
hypertension	*proteinuria*	*ureterolithiasis*
lithotripsy		

Mr. J complains of intense pain in the abdomen and the side of the back with fever and chills. Urinalysis reveals (1) ***blood in the urine,*** uric acid crystals, and (2) ***pus in the urine.*** Radiology examination shows (3) ***the presence of a stone in the ureter.*** Because of its size, urine is unable to pass to the bladder, causing (4) ***dilation of the renal pelvis.*** It appears unlikely that the stone will pass through his urinary system. Because of its size and location, an ultrasound procedure will be used to (5) ***crush the stone.***

1. _____
2. _____
3. _____
4. _____
5. _____

Mr. K was diagnosed with strep throat. Although he is on antibiotics, the infection is still present. Mr. K now presents with (6) ***diminished urine output,*** (7) ***elevated blood pressure,*** and (8) ***protein in the urine.*** The physician explained that the toxins from the strep infection caused (9) ***inflammation of the glomerulus,*** impairing kidney function. The doctor's (10) ***anticipated outcome of this disease*** is full recovery once the strep infection is addressed and resolved.

6. _____
7. _____
8. _____
9. _____
10. _____

✅ *Check your answers in Appendix A. Review any material that you did not answer correctly.*

Correct Answers _____ X 10 = _____ % Score

Female Reproductive System

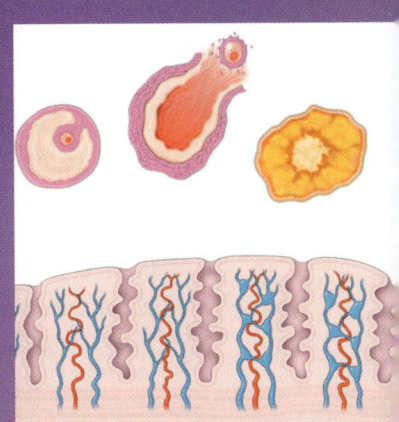

Chapter Outline

Objectives

Upon completion of this chapter, you will be able to:

- Locate and describe the structures of the female reproductive system.
- Describe the functional relationship between the female reproductive system and other body systems.
- Pronounce, spell, and build words related to the female reproductive system.
- Describe diseases, conditions, and procedures related to the female reproductive system.
- Explain pharmacology related to the treatment of female reproductive disorders.
- Demonstrate your knowledge of this chapter by completing the learning and documenting health-care activities.

Anatomy and Physiology

The female reproductive system is designed to produce and transport ova (female sex cells), discharge ova from the body if fertilization does not occur, and nourish and provide a place for the developing fetus throughout pregnancy if fertilization occurs. The female reproductive system also produces the female sex hormones estrogen and progesterone, which play an important role in the reproductive process. These hormones are responsible for the development of secondary sex characteristics, such as breast development and regulation of the menstrual cycle.

Anatomy and Physiology Key Terms

This section introduces important terms, along with their definitions and pronunciations. The key terms are highlighted in color in the Anatomy and Physiology section. Word analyses for selected terms are also provided. Pronounce the term and place a check mark in the box after you do so.

Term	Definition
external genitalia ☐ jĕn-ĭ-TĀL-ē-ă	Sex, or reproductive, organs visible on the outside of the body; also called *genitals* *The external female genitalia are also called the **vulva**. Male genitalia include the penis, scrotum, and testicles.*

gestation ☐
jĕs-TĀ-shŭn
  gest: pregnancy
  -ation: process (of)
	Length of time from conception to birth
	
	The human gestational period typically extends approximately 280 days from the last menstrual period. Gestation (pregnancy) of less than 36 weeks is considered premature.

lactation ☐
lăk-TĀ-shŭn
  lact: milk
  -ation: process (of)
	Production and release of milk by mammary glands

libido ☐ lĭ-BĒ-dō	Psychological and physical drive for sexual activity
orifice ☐ OR-ĭ-fĭs	Opening that is an entrance or outlet of any body cavity

Pronunciation Help						
	Long Sound	ā — rate	ē — rebirth	ī — isle	ō — over	ū — unite
	Short Sound	ă — apple	ĕ — ever	ĭ — it	ŏ — not	ŭ — cut

Female Reproductive Structures

The female reproductive system is composed of the internal organs of reproduction and the **external genitalia** (see Fig. 12-1). The internal organs include the (1) **ovaries,** (2) **fallopian tubes,** (3) **uterus,** and (4) **vagina.** The **external genitalia** are collectively known as the **vulva.** Included in these structures are the (5) **labia minora,** (6) **labia majora,** (7) **clitoris,** (8) **Bartholin glands,** and **mons pubis,** an elevation of adipose tissue covered by skin and coarse pubic hair that cushions the **pubis (pubic bone).** The area between the vaginal **orifice** and the anus is known as the **perineum.**

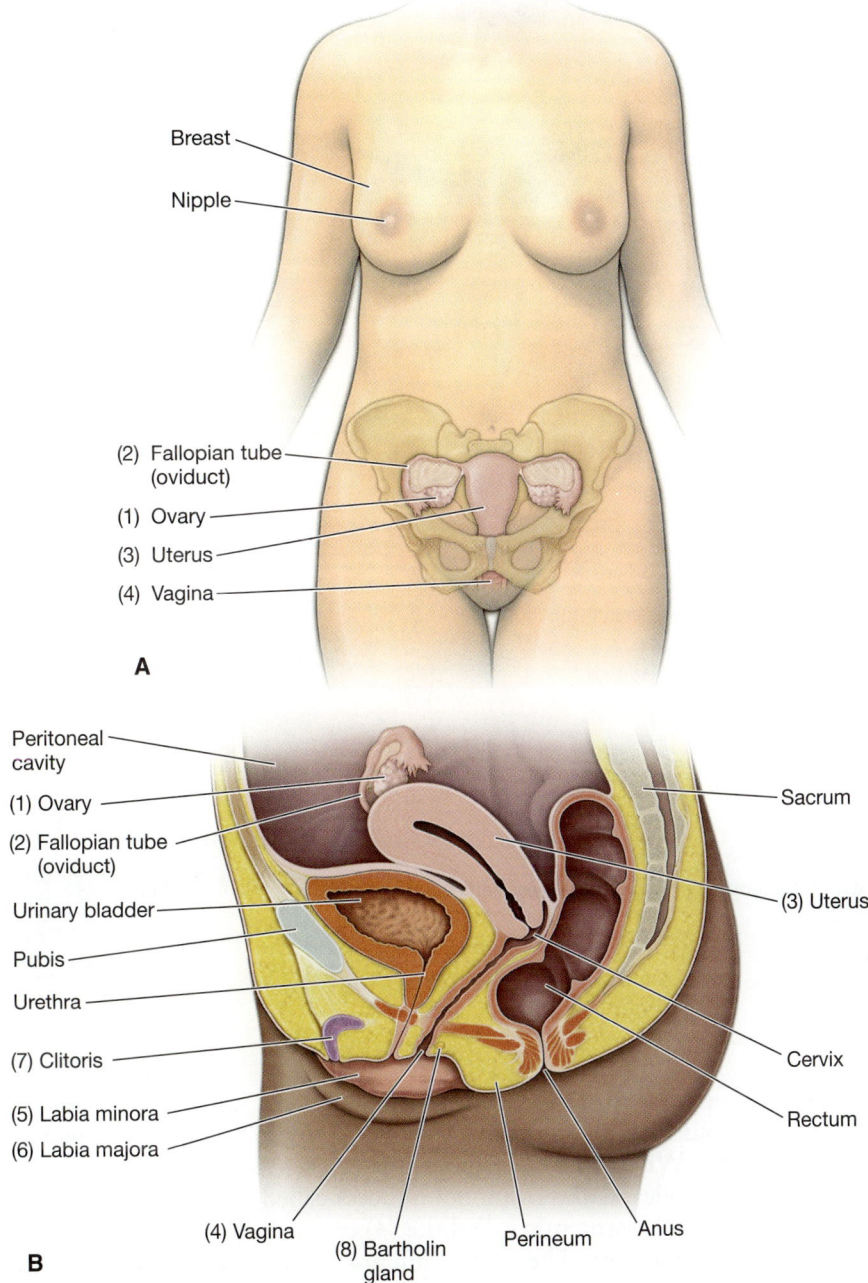

Figure 12-1 Female reproductive system. (A) Anterior view. (B) Lateral view showing the organs within the pelvic cavity.

Female Reproductive Organs

The female reproductive organs include the ovaries, fallopian tubes, uterus, and vagina. They are designed to produce female reproductive cells **(ova),** transport the cells to the site of fertilization, provide a favorable environment for a developing fetus through pregnancy and childbirth, and produce female sex hormones. Hormones play a key role in the female reproductive system by influencing **libido** and supporting vital stages of the reproductive process, including preconception, conception, fertilization, and **gestation** (see Fig. 12-2).

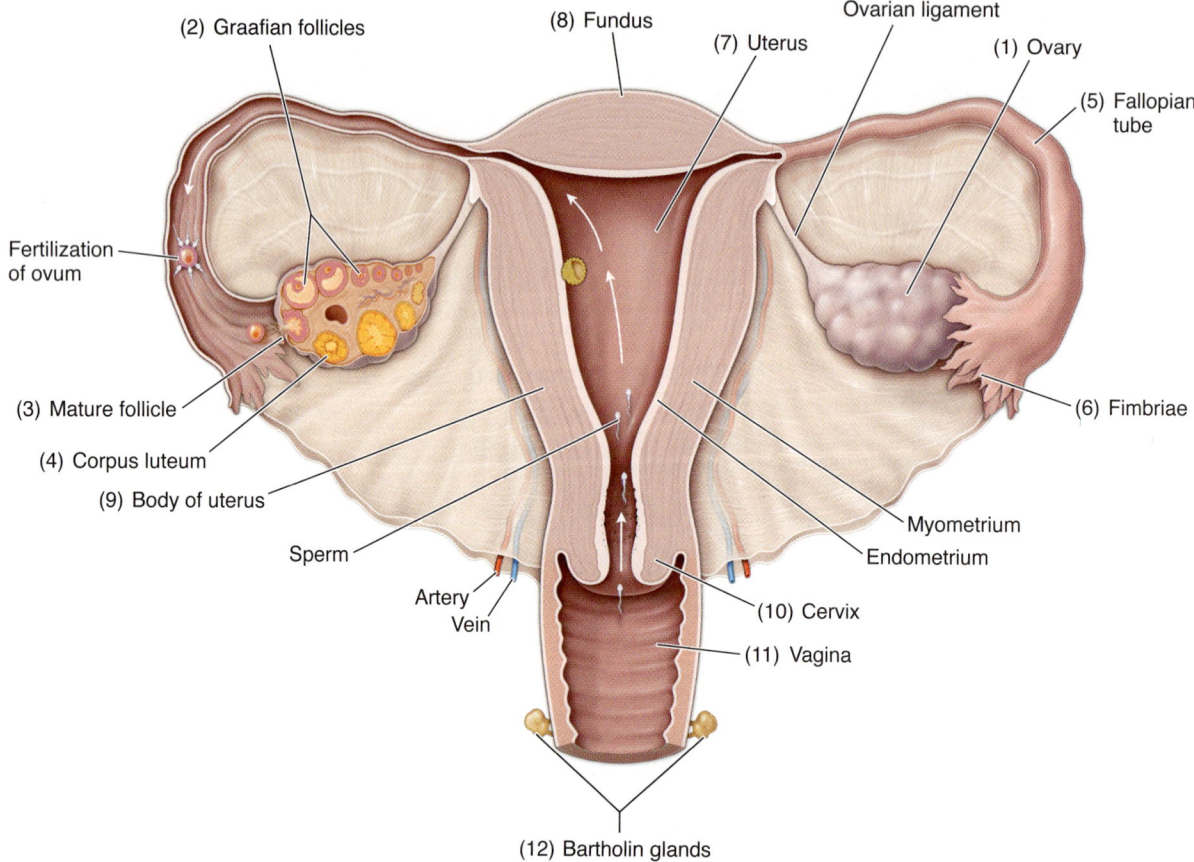

Figure 12-2 Anterior view of the female reproductive system with the developing follicles shown in the cross section of the right ovary.

Ovaries

The (1) **ovaries** are almond-shaped glands located in the pelvic cavity, one on each side of the uterus. Each ovary contains thousands of tiny, saclike structures called (2) **graafian follicles,** each containing an ovum. When an ovum ripens, the (3) **mature follicle** moves to the surface of the ovary, ruptures, and releases the ovum in a process called **ovulation.** After ovulation, the empty follicle transforms into a structure called the (4) **corpus luteum,** a small yellow mass that secretes estrogen and progesterone. The corpus luteum degenerates at the end of a nonfertile cycle. Estrogen and progesterone influence the menstrual cycle and menopause. They also prepare the uterus for implantation of the fertilized egg, help maintain pregnancy, promote growth of the placenta, and play an important role in development of secondary sex characteristics (see Chapter 14, Endocrine System).

Fallopian Tubes

Two (5) **fallopian tubes (oviducts, uterine tubes)** extend laterally from superior angles of the uterus. The (6) **fimbriae** are fingerlike projections that create wavelike currents in fluid surrounding the ovary to move the ovum into the uterine tube. If the egg unites with a spermatozoon, the male reproductive cell, fertilization (or conception) takes place. The fertilized egg then continues its journey to the uterus, where it implants on the uterine wall. If conception does not occur, the ovum disintegrates within 48 hours and is discharged through the vagina.

Uterus and Vagina

The (7) **uterus** contains and nourishes the embryo from the time the fertilized egg is implanted until the fetus is born. It is a muscular, hollow structure shaped like an inverted pear and is located in the pelvic area between the bladder and rectum. The uterus normally tilts forward (**anteflexion**) in the pelvic cavity and consists of three parts: the (8) **fundus,** the upper, rounded part; the (9) **body,** the central part; and the (10) **cervix,** also called the **neck of the uterus** or **cervix uteri,** the inferior constricted portion that opens into the vagina.

The (11) **vagina** is a muscular tube that extends from the cervix to the exterior of the body. Its lining consists of folds of mucous membrane that give the organ an elastic quality. During sexual excitement, the vaginal orifice is lubricated by secretions from (12) **Bartholin glands.** In addition to serving as the organ of sexual intercourse and receptor of semen, the vagina discharges menstrual flow. It also acts as a passageway for the delivery of the fetus. The **clitoris,** located anterior to the vaginal orifice, is composed of erectile tissue that is richly innervated with sensory endings. The clitoris is similar in structure to the penis in the male, but it is smaller and has no urethra. The area between the vaginal orifice and the anus is known as the **perineum.** During childbirth, this area may be surgically incised (**episiotomy**) to enlarge the vaginal opening for delivery.

Mammary Glands

Although mammary glands (breasts) are present in both sexes, they function only in females (see Fig. 12-3). The breasts are not directly involved in reproduction but become important after delivery. Their biological role is to secrete milk for the nourishment of the newborn, a process called **lactation.** Breasts begin to develop during puberty as a result of periodic stimulation of the ovarian hormones estrogen and progesterone and are fully developed by age 16. Estrogen is responsible for the development of (1) **adipose tissue,** which enlarges the size of the breasts until they reach full maturity. Breast size is primarily determined by the amount of fat around the glandular tissue but is not indicative of functional ability. Each breast is composed of 15 to 20 lobules of milk-producing glands that are drained by a (2) **lactiferous duct,** which opens on the tip of the raised (3) **nipple.** Circling the nipple is a border of slightly darker skin called the (4) **areola.** During pregnancy, the breasts enlarge and remain so until lactation ceases. At menopause, breast tissue begins to atrophy.

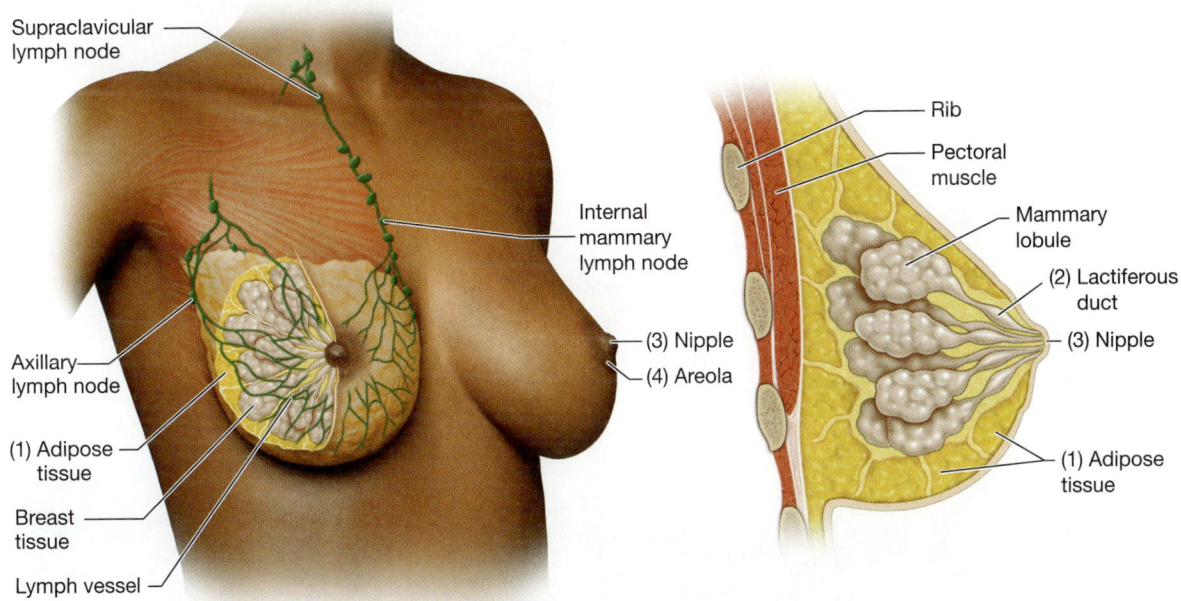

Figure 12-3 Structure of mammary glands.

Menstrual Cycle

Menarche, the initial menstrual period, occurs at puberty (about age 12), and menstruation continues for approximately 40 years, except during pregnancy. The menstrual cycle consists of a series of phases, during which the uterine endometrium changes as it responds to changing levels of ovarian hormones (see Table 12-1). The duration of the menstrual cycle is approximately 28 days (see Fig. 12-4).

TABLE 12-1 Phases of the Menstrual Cycle

This table outlines the changes involved during the typical 28-day menstrual cycle.

Phase	Description
Menstrual Days 1–5	Uterine endometrium sloughs off because of hormonal stimulation, a process accompanied by bleeding. The detached tissue and blood are discharged through the vagina as menstrual flow.
Ovulatory Days 6–14	When menstruation ceases, the endometrium begins to thicken as new tissue is rebuilt. As the estrogen level rises, several ova begin to mature in the graafian follicles, usually with only one ovum reaching full maturity. At about the 14th day of the cycle, the graafian follicle ruptures, releasing the egg, a process called *ovulation.* The egg then leaves the ovary and travels down the fallopian tube toward the uterus.
Postovulatory Days 15–28	The empty graafian follicle fills with a yellow material and is now called the *corpus luteum.* Secretions of estrogen and progesterone by the corpus luteum stimulate the building of the endometrium in preparation for implantation of an embryo. If fertilization does not occur, the corpus luteum begins to degenerate as estrogen and progesterone levels decrease.* With decreased hormone levels, the uterine lining begins to shed, the menstrual cycle starts over again, and the first day of menstruation begins.

*Some women experience a loose grouping of symptoms called **premenstrual syndrome (PMS).** These symptoms usually occur about 5 days after the decrease in hormone levels and include nervous tension, irritability, headaches, breast tenderness, and a feeling of depression.

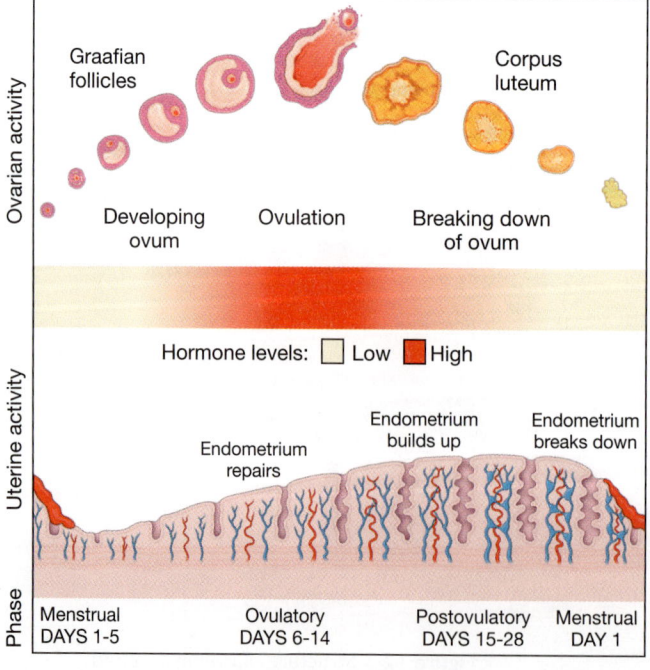

Figure 12-4 Menstrual cycle.

Pregnancy

During pregnancy, the uterus changes its shape, size, and consistency. It increases greatly in size and muscle mass; houses the growing placenta, which nourishes the embryo-fetus; and expels the fetus after gestation. To prepare to serve as the birth canal at the end of pregnancy, the vaginal canal elongates as the uterus rises in the pelvis. The mucosa thickens, secretions increase, and the vascularity and elasticity of the cervix and vagina become more pronounced.

The average pregnancy (gestation) lasts approximately 9 months and is followed by childbirth (parturition). Up to the third month of pregnancy, the product of conception is referred to as the *embryo*. From the third month to the time of birth, the unborn offspring is referred to as the *fetus*.

Pregnancy also causes enlargement of the breasts, sometimes to the point of pain. Many other changes occur throughout the body to accommodate the development and birth of the fetus. Toward the end of gestation, the myometrium begins to contract weakly at irregular intervals. At this time, the full-term fetus is usually positioned head down within the uterus.

Labor and Childbirth

Labor is the physiological process by which the fetus is expelled from the uterus. Labor occurs in three stages. The first is the **stage of dilation,** which begins with uterine contractions and terminates when there is complete dilation of the cervix (10 cm). The second is the **stage of expulsion,** the time from complete cervical dilation to birth of the baby. The last stage is the **placental stage** or **afterbirth.** This stage begins shortly after childbirth when the uterine contractions discharge the placenta from the uterus (see Fig. 12-5, page 426.).

Menopause

Menopause is the cessation of ovarian activity and diminished hormone production that occurs at about age 50. Menopause is usually diagnosed if absence of menses (**amenorrhea**) has persisted for 1 year. The period during which symptoms of approaching menopause occur is known as the **change of life** or the **climacteric.**

Many women experience hot flashes and vaginal drying and thinning (**vaginal atrophy**) as estrogen levels fall. Although **hormone replacement therapy (HRT)** has become more controversial, it is still used to treat vaginal atrophy and porous bones (**osteoporosis**), and it is believed to play a role in heart attack prevention. Restraint in prescribing estrogens for long periods in all menopausal women arises from concern that there is an increased risk that long-term usage will induce neoplastic changes in estrogen-sensitive aging tissue.

(1) Labor begins, membranes intact

(2) Effacement of cervix, which is now partially dilated

(3) When head reaches floor of pelvis, it rotates

(4) Extension of the cervix allows head to pass through

(5) Delivery of head, head rotates to realign itself with body

(6) Delivery of shoulders

(7) Delivery of infant is complete, uterus begins to contract

(8) Umbilical cord is cut, external massage to uterus continues to stimulate contractions, and placenta is delivered

Figure 12-5 Sequence of labor and childbirth.

Anatomy Review: Female Reproductive Structures (Lateral View)

To review the anatomy of the female reproductive system, label the illustration using the listed terms.

Bartholin gland

cervix

clitoris

fallopian tube

labia majora

labia minora

ovary

perineum

uterus

vagina

Peritoneal cavity

Urinary bladder

Pubis

Urethra

Sacrum

Rectum

Anus

 Check your answers by referring to Fig. 12-1 on page 421. Review material that you did not answer correctly.

Anatomy Review: Female Reproductive Structures (Anterior View)

To review the anatomy of the female reproductive system, label the illustration using the listed terms.

Bartholin glands	*fertilization of ovum*	*ovarian ligament*
body of the uterus	*fimbriae*	*ovary*
cervix	*fundus of uterus*	*uterus*
corpus luteum	*graafian follicles*	*vagina*
fallopian tube	*mature follicle*	

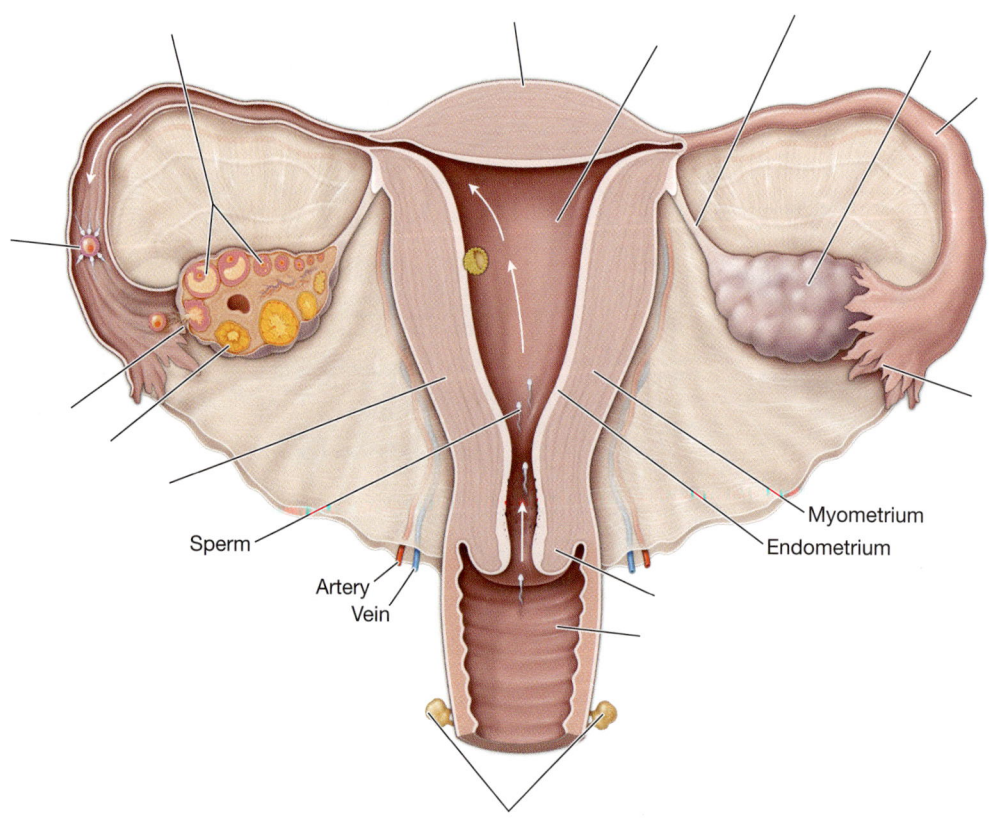

Sperm

Artery

Vein

Myometrium

Endometrium

 Check your answers by referring to Fig. 12–2 on page 422. Review material that you did not answer correctly.

CONNECTING BODY SYSTEMS—FEMALE REPRODUCTIVE SYSTEM

The main function of the female reproductive system is to produce hormones and to provide structures that support fertilization and development of a developing fetus. It also provides very limited support to the functions of other body systems. These limited functional relationships are summarized here.

Blood, Lymphatic, and Immune
- The female immune system has special mechanisms that inhibit destruction of sperm cells.
- The female reproductive tract secretes enzymes and other substances that inhibit entry of pathogens into the internal reproductive structures.

Cardiovascular
- Estrogens lower blood cholesterol levels and promote cardiovascular health in premenopausal women.

Digestive
- Estrogens have an effect on the metabolic rate.

Endocrine
- Estrogens provide a feedback mechanism that influences pituitary function.
- Estrogens assist in the production of human chorionic gonadotropin (HCG) hormone.

Integumentary
- Female hormones affect growth and distribution of body hair.
- Female hormones influence the activity of sebaceous glands.
- Female hormones influence skin texture and fat distribution.

Male Reproductive
- The female reproductive system provides the ovum needed to make fertilization by sperm possible.

Musculoskeletal
- Estrogen influences muscle development and size.
- Estrogen influences bone growth, maintenance, and closure of epiphyseal plates.

Nervous
- Estrogen affects central nervous system development and sexual behavior.
- Estrogen provides antioxidants that have a neuroprotective function.

Respiratory
- Sexual arousal and pregnancy produce changes in the rate and depth of breathing.
- Estrogen is believed to provide a beneficial effect on the alveoli of the lungs.

Urinary
- Kidneys dispose of nitrogenous wastes and maintain the homeostatic mechanisms of the mother and fetus.

Medical Word Elements

This section introduces combining forms, suffixes, and prefixes related to the female reproductive system. From the information provided, complete the meaning of the medical words in the right-hand column. The first one is completed for you.

Element	Meaning	Analysis
Combining Forms		
amni/o	amnion (amniotic sac)	**amni/o**/centesis (ăm-nē-ō-sĕn-TĒ-sĭs): *surgical puncture of the amniotic sac* *-centesis:* surgical puncture *Amniocentesis is performed under ultrasound guidance using a needle and syringe to remove amniotic fluid.*
cervic/o	neck; cervix uteri (neck of the uterus)	**cervic**/itis (sĕr-vĭ-SĪ-tĭs): _____ *-itis:* inflammation
colp/o	vagina	**colp/o**/scopy (kŏl-PŎS-kō-pē): _____ *-scopy:* visual examination
vagin/o		**vagin**/itis (văj-ĭn-Ī-tĭs): _____ *-cele:* hernia, swelling *Vaginitis is usually caused by infection.*
galact/o	milk	**galact/o**/poiesis (gă-lăk-tō-poy-Ē-sĭs): _____ *-poiesis:* formation, production
lact/o		**lact/o**/gen (LĂK-tō-jĕn): _____ *-gen:* forming, producing, origin *The term* **lactogen** *refers to any substance that stimulates milk production, such as a hormone.*
gynec/o	woman, female	**gynec/o**/logist (gī-nĕ-KŎL-ō-jĭst): _____ *-logist:* specialist in the study of
hyster/o	uterus (womb)	**hyster**/ectomy (hĭs-tĕr-ĔK-tō-mē): _____ *-ectomy:* excision, removal

metri/o		endo/**metri**/al (ĕn-dō-MĒ-trē-ăl): _____
		  endo-: in, within
		  -al: pertaining to

uter/o		**uter/o**/vagin/al (ū-tĕr-ō-VĂJ-ĭ-năl): _____
		  vagin/o: vagina
		  -al: pertaining to

mamm/o	breast	**mamm/o**/gram (MĂM-ō-grăm): _____ *-gram:* record, writing
mast/o		**mast/o**/pexy (MĂS-tō-pĕks-ē): _____ *-pexy:* fixation (of an organ) *Mastopexy is reconstructive cosmetic surgery performed to affix sagging breasts in a more elevated position, commonly improving their shape.*

Medical Word Elements—cont'd

Element	Meaning	Word Analysis
men/o	menses, menstruation	**men/o**/rrhagia (měn-ō-RĀ-jē-ă): _____ *-rrhagia:* bursting forth (of) *Menorrhagia refers to an excessive amount of menstrual bleeding that lasts longer than 7 days.*
metr/o	uterus (womb); measure	**metr/o**/ptosis (mē-trō-TŌ-sĭs): _____ *-ptosis:* prolapse, downward displacement
nat/o	birth	pre/**nat**/al (prē-NĀ-tăl): _____ *pre-:* before, in front *-al:* pertaining to
oophor/o	ovary	**oophor**/oma (ō-ŏf-ō-RŌ-mă): _____ *-oma:* tumor
ovari/o		**ovari/o**/rrhexis (ō-vă-rē-ō-RĔK-sĭs): _____ *-rrhexis:* rupture
perine/o	perineum (area between the scrotum [or vulva in the female] and anus)	**perine/o**/rrhaphy (pĕr-ĭ-nē-OR-ă-fē): _____ *-rrhaphy:* suture *Perineorrhaphy repairs an episiotomy or a laceration that occurs during delivery of the fetus.*
salping/o	tube (usually fallopian or eustachian [auditory] tubes)	**salping/o**/plasty (săl-PĬNG-gō-plăs-tē): _____ *-plasty:* surgical repair
Suffixes		
-arche	beginning	men/**arche** (měn-ĂR-kē): _____ *men:* menses, menstruation
-cyesis	pregnancy	pseudo/**cyesis** (soo-dō-sī-Ē-sĭs): _____ *pseudo-:* false *Pseudocyesis is a condition in which a woman develops bodily changes consistent with pregnancy when she is not pregnant.*
-gravida	pregnant woman	multi/**gravida** (mŭl-tĭ-GRĂV-ĭ-dă): _____ *multi-:* many, much *The term gravida may be followed by numbers that indicate the number of pregnancies, such as gravida 1 and gravida 2 or gravida I, gravida II, and so forth.*

Continued

Medical Word Elements—cont'd

Element	Meaning	Word Analysis
-para	to bear (offspring)	nulli/**para** (nŭl-ĬP-ă-ră): _____ _nulli-:_ none *The term para followed by a Roman numeral or preceded by a Latin prefix (such as primi-, quadri-, and so forth) designates the number of times a pregnancy has culminated in a single or multiple birth. For example, para I and primipara refer to a woman who has given birth for the first time. Whether the births were multiple (twins, triplets) is irrelevant.*
-salpinx	tube (usually fallopian or eustachian [auditory] tubes)	hem/o/**salpinx** (hē-mŌ-SĂL-pĭnks): _____ _hem/o:_ blood *Hemosalpinx is also called hematosalpinx.*
-tocia	childbirth, labor	dys/**tocia** (dĭs-TŌ-sē-ă): _____ _dys-:_ bad; painful; difficult
-version	turning	retro/**version** (rĕt-rō-VĔR-shŭn): _____ _retro-:_ backward, behind *Retroversion of the uterus occurs in one of every four otherwise healthy women.*

Prefixes

Element	Meaning	Word Analysis
ante-	before, in front of	**ante**/version (ăn-tē-VĔR-zhŭn): _____ _-version:_ turning
dys-	bad; painful; difficult	**dys**/men/o/rrhea (dĭs-mĕn-ō-RĒ-ă): _____ _men/o:_ menses, menstruation _-rrhea:_ discharge, flow
endo-	in, within	**endo**/metr/itis (ĕn-dō-mē-TRĪ-tĭs): _____ _metr:_ uterus (womb); measure _-itis:_ inflammation
multi-	many, much	**multi**/para (mŭl-TĬP-ă-ră): _____ _-para:_ to bear (offspring)
post-	after	**post**/nat/al (pōst-NĀ-tăl): _____ _nat:_ birth _-al:_ pertaining to
primi-	first	**primi**/gravida (prī-mĭ-GRĂV-ĭ-dă): _____ _-gravida:_ pregnant woman

Visit the Medical Terminology Systems online resource center at FADavis.com for an audio exercise of the terms in this table. Other activities are also available to reinforce content.

It is time to review medical word elements by completing Learning Activities 12-1 and 12-2.

Disease Focus

Female reproductive disorders may be caused by infection, injury, or hormonal dysfunction. Although some disorders may be mild and correct themselves over time, others, such as those caused by infection, may require medical attention. Pain, itching, lesions, and discharge are signs and symptoms commonly associated with sexually transmitted diseases and must not be ignored. Other common problems of the female reproductive system are related to hormonal dysfunction that may cause menstrual disorders.

As a preventive measure, a woman should undergo pelvic examination regularly throughout life. This diagnostic procedure helps identify many pelvic abnormalities and diseases. Cytological and bacteriological specimens are usually obtained at the time of examination.

Gynecology (GYN) is the branch of medicine concerned with diseases of the female reproductive organs and breasts. **Obstetrics (OB)** is the branch of medicine that manages the health of a woman and her fetus during pregnancy and childbirth. It also includes the **puerperium,** which is the period of adjustment after childbirth during which the reproductive organs of the mother return to their normal, nonpregnant state. Generally, this period lasts 6 to 8 weeks and ends with the first ovulation and the return of normal menstruation. Because of the obvious overlap between gynecology and obstetrics, many practices include both specialties. The physician who simultaneously practices these specialties is called an **obstetrician/gynecologist (OB/GYN).**

Endometriosis

Endometriosis is the presence of functional endometrial tissue in areas outside the uterus (see Fig. 12-6). The ectopic tissue is usually confined to the pelvic area but may appear anywhere in the abdominopelvic cavity. Like normal endometrial tissue, the ectopic endometrium responds to the hormonal fluctuations of the menstrual cycle. The endometrial tissue can cause superficial lesions or deep nodules, or can bind to surrounding organs and tissue (**adhesions**) causing scar tissue, pain, and infertility. When endometriosis affects the ovaries, chocolate cysts (**ovarian endometriomas, endometriotic cysts**) filled with menstrual blood may develop. Treatment for endometriosis includes pain relief and hormone therapy to suppress the menstrual cycle. Some cases may involve surgical removal of the ectopic endometrial tissue or hysterectomy.

Figure 12-6 Endometriosis.

Pelvic Inflammatory Disease

Pelvic inflammatory disease (PID) is a general term for inflammation of the uterus, fallopian tubes, ovaries, and adjacent pelvic structures. It is usually caused by bacterial infection, but other organisms may be implicated. These disease-producing organisms **(pathogens)** generally enter through the vagina during coitus, induced abortion, childbirth, or the postpartum period. As an ascending infection, the pathogens spread from the vagina and cervix to the upper structures of the female reproductive tract. Untreated gonorrhea and chlamydia cause most cases of PID. Other causes include abortion, childbirth, and pelvic procedures.

The symptoms of PID can vary and may include lower abdominal pain, vaginal discharge, fever, nausea, and vomiting. If diagnosed at an early stage, PID can be treated easily and effectively with antibiotics. If left untreated, it can lead to more serious, long-term complications including infertility.

Oncology

The two most common forms of cancer involving the female reproductive system are breast cancer and cervical cancer.

Breast Cancer

Breast cancer, also called **carcinoma of the breast,** is the most common diagnosed malignancy, and the second cause of cancer death of women in the United States. This disease appears to be associated with a family history of breast cancer, increasing age, excess body weight, the use of HRT, alcohol consumption, and physical inactivity. Women who have never had children **(nulliparous)** or those who have had an early onset of the first menstrual period **(menarche)** or late onset of menopause are also more likely to develop breast cancer. Because this type of malignancy is highly responsive to treatment when detected early, women are urged to practice breast self-examination (BSE) monthly and to receive an annual screening **mammogram** beginning at age 40. Those with a family history of breast or ovarian cancer and inherited genetic mutations, such as **BRCA1** and **BRCA2**, need to follow the guidelines of their physician. Many breast malignancies are detected by the patient. Routine screening, early detection, and treatment have contributed to a decline in mortality rates over the past 35 years.

Treatment depends on the type and the stage of cancer, family history, and personal preference. Surgical removal **(mastectomy)** is often the first line of treatment. After mastectomy, one or a combination of the following are implemented: radiation, chemotherapy, hormone therapy, targeted drug therapy, and immunotherapy.

Cervical Cancer

Cancer of the cervix is most frequently diagnosed in women between ages 35 and 44 but can occur at any age. The primary cause is the **human papillomavirus (HPV)**, which is spread from one person to another during skin to skin contact including oral, vaginal, and anal sex. There are 150 strains of HPV, and some cause warts **(papillomas)**. Different types of HPV cause warts on different body parts including the hands, feet, lips, tongue, and genitals **(condylomata)** (see Fig. 12-7). Other strains, especially HPV-16 and HPV-18, are considered high risk because they can cause changes in cervical cells that may lead to cancer. Other risk factors include multiple sexual partners, smoking, and a weakened immune system.

The **Pap test,** a cytological examination, can detect cervical cancer before the disease becomes clinically evident. This test can identify precancerous cells **(dysplasia)** before they change into cancer. Annual Pap screening is essential for early detection and treatment because symptoms of stage I cervical cancer are often absent (see Fig. 12-8). Abnormal cervical cytology routinely calls for **colposcopy,** which can detect the presence and extent of preclinical lesions requiring biopsy and histological examination. Treatment of cervical cancer consists of surgery, radiation, chemotherapy, targeted drug therapy, and immunotherapy.

Figure 12-7 Genital warts (condylomata). (From Williams PD, Hopper LS: *Understanding medical-surgical nursing,* ed 7, 2022, Williams & Hopper, p. 878, Fig. 44.3 [Condylomata, commonly known as genital warts].)

Figure 12-8 Stages of cervical cancer development.

Diseases and Conditions

This section introduces diseases and conditions of the female reproductive system, along with their meanings and pronunciations. Word analyses for selected terms are also provided.

Term	Definition
Female Reproductive System	
atresia ă-TRĒ-zē-ă	Congenital absence or closure of a normal body opening, such as the vagina
candidiasis kăn-dĭ-DĪ-ă-sĭs	Fungal infection caused by *Candida albicans* that is a common cause of vaginal infections in women, characterized by a curdy or cheeselike discharge and extreme itching; also referred to as a *vaginal yeast infection* *Candidiasis is a common condition and can be treated with over-the-counter antifungal cream or ointment. Candidiasis occurring in the oral cavity and on the tongue is called thrush.*

Continued

Diseases and Conditions—cont'd

Term	Definition
choriocarcinoma kō-rē-ō-kăr-sĭ-NŌ-mă *chori/o:* chorion *carcin:* cancer *-oma:* tumor	Malignant neoplasm of the uterus or at the site of an ectopic pregnancy *Although its actual cause is unknown, choriocarcinoma is a rare tumor that may occur after pregnancy or abortion.*
dyspareunia dĭs-pă-RŪ-nē-ă	Pain during sexual intercourse *Dyspareunia is not always related to an underlying condition but may be caused by insufficient lubrication, irritation, or psychological issues such as a history of sexual abuse.*
endocervicitis ĕn-dō-sĕr-vĭ-SĪ-tĭs *endo-:* in, within *cervic:* neck; cervix uteri (neck of the uterus) *-itis:* inflammation	Inflammation of the mucous lining of the cervix uteri *Endocervicitis is usually chronic, commonly as a result of infection, and accompanied by cervical erosion.*
fibrocystic breast disease fĭ-brō-SĬS-tĭk	Presence of single or multiple cysts that are palpable in the breasts *The cysts are benign and fairly common but must be observed carefully for change and growth with a possible biopsy to differentiate from carcinoma of the breast. In most cases, no treatment is necessary.*
menstrual disorders MĔN-stroo-ăl *menstru/o:* monthly discharge of blood *-al:* pertaining to	Abnormal condition in the menstrual cycle; also called *dysfunctional uterine bleeding (DUB)* *Menstrual irregularities can be caused by a variety of conditions, including pregnancy, hormonal imbalances, infections, malignancies, diseases, trauma, and certain medications.*
amenorrhea ă-mĕn-ō-RĒ-ă *a-:* without, not *men/o:* menses; menstruation *-rrhea:* discharge, flow	Absence of a menstrual period in a woman of reproductive age *Normal causes of amenorrhea include pregnancy and lactation (breastfeeding). Outside of reproductive years, absence of menses occurs during childhood and after menopause.*
dysmenorrhea dĭs-mĕn-ō-RĒ-ă *dys-:* bad; painful; difficult *men/o:* menses; menstruation *-rrhea:* discharge, flow	Cramps or painful menstruation *Dysmenorrhea includes menstrual periods that are accompanied by sharp, intermittent pain or dull, aching pain—usually in the pelvis or lower abdomen.*
menorrhagia mĕn-ō-RĀ-jē-ă *men/o:* menses; menstruation *-rrhagia:* bursting forth (of)	Abnormally heavy, prolonged menstrual period *In early life, menorrhagia may be caused by endocrine disturbances; in later life, it is usually a result of inflammatory diseases, fibroids, or tumors.*
metrorrhagia mē-trō-RĀ-jē-ă *metr/o:* uterus (uterus); measure *-rrhagia:* bursting forth (of)	Irregular uterine bleeding between menstrual periods or after menopause *Metrorrhagia is usually symptomatic of disease, including benign or malignant uterine tumors. It is considered one of the most serious menstrual disorders. Thus, early diagnosis and treatment are warranted.*

Diseases and Conditions—cont'd

Term	Definition
oligomenorrhea ŏl-ĭ-gō-měn-ō-RĒ-ă *olig/o:* scanty *men/o:* menses, menstruation *-rrhea:* discharge, flow	Abnormally light or infrequent menstrual periods *Causes of oligomenorrhea include a side effect of birth control pills, hormonal imbalances, excessive exercise, and ovarian cysts.*
premenstrual syndrome (PMS) prē-MĚN-stroo-ăl SĬN-drōm	Symptoms that occur between ovulation and the onset of menstruation *PMS symptoms include such physical symptoms as breast tenderness, back pain, abdominal cramps, headache, and changes in appetite and the psychological symptoms of anxiety, depression, and unrest.*
ovarian cysts	A globular sac filled with fluid or semisolid material that develops in or on the ovary
polycystic ovarian syndrome (PCOS) *poly:* many, much *cyst:* bladder *-ic:* pertaining to	Hormonal imbalance in women of reproductive age that occurs when the ovaries produce abnormally high levels of androgens with characteristic symptoms of irregular menstrual cycles, excess hair growth (hirsutism), and acne; enlarged ovaries containing small follicle cysts with immature eggs may or may not be present on ultrasound (US) *PCOS is a common cause of infertility and may also increase the risk of other health conditions such as diabetes and hypertension (see Fig. 12-9).* **Figure 12-9** Ultrasound with arrows pointing to multiple ovarian cysts of an ovary with polycystic ovarian syndrome (PCOS).
sterility stěr-ĬL-ĭ-tē	Inability of the female to become pregnant or the male to impregnate the female

Continued

Diseases and Conditions—cont'd

Term	Definition

uterine fibroids
Ū-tĕr-ĭn FĪ-broyds
  fibr: fiber, fibrous tissue
  -oids: resembling
	Benign tumors composed of muscle and fibrous tissue that develop in the uterus; also called *fibromyomas, leiomyomas,* or *myomas.*
	
	Myomectomy or hysterectomy may be indicated if the fibroids grow too large, causing such symptoms as metrorrhagia, pelvic pain, and menorrhagia (see Fig. 12-10).
	
	Figure 12-10 Surgical removal of multiple fibroids (myomectomy) from the wall of the uterus.

Obstetrics

Term	Definition
abortion (AB) ă-BOR-shŭn	Termination of pregnancy before the embryo or fetus is capable of surviving on its own *Abortions are spontaneous or induced (deliberate). A spontaneous abortion (SAB) occurs without any apparent cause and is also called a* **miscarriage.** *A woman undergoes an induced abortion when she elects to end pregnancy because her health is endangered (therapeutic abortion) or for some other personal reason.*
abruptio placentae ă-BRŬP-shē-ō plă-SĔN-tē	Premature separation of the placenta from the uterine wall before the third stage of labor; also called *placental abruption* *Abruptio placentae results in uterine hemorrhage and threatens the life of the mother. It also disrupts blood flow and oxygen through the umbilical cord and threatens the life of the fetus.*
breech presentation	Common abnormality of delivery in which the fetal buttocks or feet present first rather than the head

Diseases and Conditions—cont'd

Term	Definition
Down syndrome DOWN SĬN-drōm	Genetic condition in which there is an extra copy of chromosome 21 (trisomy), altering physical and mental development of the child; also called *trisomy 21* *Symptoms vary and can range from mild to severe. However, children with Down syndrome have a widely recognized appearance.*
ectopic pregnancy ĕk-TŎP-ĭk PRĔG-năn-sē	Pregnancy in which the fertilized ovum becomes implanted on any tissue other than the lining of the uterine cavity *Types of ectopic pregnancy include abdominal pregnancy, ovarian pregnancy, and tubal pregnancy (see Fig. 12-11).*

Figure 12-11 Ectopic pregnancy. (A) Tubal pregnancy. (B) Other sites of ectopic pregnancy.

Continued

Diseases and Conditions—cont'd

Term	Definition
gestational hypertension jĕs-TĀ-shŭn-ăl hī-pĕr-TĔN-shŭn	High blood pressure that begins in the latter part of pregnancy, usually after 20 weeks *Gestational hypertension may develop into preeclampsia if untreated.*
preeclampsia prē-ĕ-KLĂMP-sē-ă	Gestational hypertension characterized by edema and proteinuria, which left untreated, may progress to eclampsia *Treatment includes bedrest and blood pressure monitoring.*
eclampsia ĕ-KLĂMP-sē-ă	Convulsive form of gestational hypertension that is a medical emergency and life-threatening to the mother and baby *Treatment includes bedrest, blood pressure monitoring, and antiseizure medication.*
placenta previa plă-SĔN-tă PRĒ-vē-ă	Obstetric complication in which the placenta is attached close to or covers the cervical canal and that results in bleeding during labor when the cervix dilates *Placenta previa is a leading cause of vaginal bleeding (spotting) that may lead to other complications. It may also necessitate a cesarean delivery.*

It is time to review pathology, diseases, and conditions by completing Learning Activity 12-3.

Diagnostic, Surgical, and Therapeutic Procedures

This section introduces diagnostic, surgical, and therapeutic procedures used to diagnose and treat female reproductive disorders. Descriptions are provided, along with pronunciations and word analyses for selected terms.

Procedure	Description
Diagnostic	
amniocentesis ăm-nē-ō-sĔn-TĒ-sĭs *amni/o:* amnion (amniotic sac) *-centesis:* surgical puncture	Transabdominal puncture of the amniotic sac under ultrasound guidance using a needle (with the needle's position verified by US on a monitor screen) and syringe to remove amniotic fluid (see Fig. 12-12) *Chemical and cytological studies of the sample obtained in amniocentesis detect genetic and biochemical disorders and fetal maturity. The procedure also enables transfusion of blood to the fetus and instillation of drugs for treating the fetus.*

Figure 12-12 Amniocentesis.

BRCA1 and BRCA2	Genetic test performed on a blood sample to indicate the genetic mutations of *BRCA* (breast cancer) genes, which significantly increase the risk of developing breast and ovarian cancer
breast biopsy	Obtaining a sample of breast tissue for examination under the microscope to determine whether it is cancerous or benign
fine needle aspiration (FNA)	Use of a thin needle to withdraw cells or fluid from a breast lump *FNA is most often done if the suspicious area is likely to be a cyst.*

Continued

Diagnostic, Surgical, and Therapeutic Procedures—cont'd

Procedure	Description
image guided	Use of ultrasound (US), magnetic resonance imaging (MRI), or a mammogram, to locate abnormal tissue or tumor, and to then guide a large needle to the area of biopsy; also called an *image-guided core needle biopsy* (CNB) (see Fig. 12-13)

Figure 12-13 Image-guided core needle biopsy utilizing ultrasound (US).

surgical	Surgical removal of all or part of an abnormal breast mass that can be an **incisional biopsy** to remove part of the abnormal mass, or an **excisional biopsy** to remove the entire mass (tumor) with the edge **(margin)** of normal breast tissue around the tumor
chorionic villus sampling (CVS) kor-ē-ŎN-ĭk VĬL-ŭs SĂM-plĭng	Sampling of placental tissues for prenatal diagnosis of potential genetic defects *CVS involves insertion of a catheter into the uterus to obtain the sample. The advantage of CVS over amniocentesis is that it can be undertaken in the first trimester of pregnancy.*

Diagnostic, Surgical, and Therapeutic Procedures—cont'd

Procedure	Description

colposcopy
kŏl-PŎS-kō-pē
    colp/o: vagina
    -scopy: visual examination
	Visual examination of the vagina and cervix with an optical magnifying instrument (colposcope) (see Fig. 12-14)
	
	Colposcopy is used chiefly to identify areas of cervical dysplasia in women with abnormal Papanicolaou tests and as an aid in biopsy or excision procedures, including cautery, cryotherapy, and loop electrosurgical excision.
	
	A
	
	B
	
	Figure 12-14 Colposcopy. (A) Woman in dorsal lithotomy position for examination. (B) Colposcope illuminating the cervix for biopsy. (From *Simplified*, ed 7, p. 381, Fig. 8-18.)

cordocentesis kor-dō-sĕn-TĒ-sĭs	Diagnostic prenatal test in which a sample of the baby's blood is removed from the umbilical cord for testing; also called *percutaneous umbilical blood sampling (PUBS)* *Cord blood is evaluated in the laboratory to identify hemolytic diseases or genetic abnormalities.*

Continued

Diagnostic, Surgical, and Therapeutic Procedures—cont'd

Procedure	Description
endometrial biopsy ĕn-dō-MĒ-trē-ăl BĪ-ŏp-sē *endo-:* in, within *metri:* uterus (womb); measure *-al:* pertaining to	Removal of a sample of uterine endometrium for microscopic study *Endometrial biopsy is commonly used in fertility assessment to confirm ovulation and as a diagnostic tool to determine the cause of dysfunctional and postmenopausal bleeding.*
insufflation ĭn-sŭ-FLĀ-shŭn	Delivery of pressurized air or gas into a cavity, chamber, or organ to allow visual examination, remove an obstruction, or apply medication *Insufflation increases the distance between structures so that the physician can see more clearly and better diagnose possible disorders.*
Papanicolaou (Pap) test pă-pă-NĪ-kō-lŏw	An exfoliative cytology test to detect abnormal cells that are scraped from the cervix, usually obtained during routine pelvic examination (see Fig. 12-15) *A Pap test is commonly used to screen for and diagnose cervical cancer. It may also be used to evaluate cells from any organ, such as the pleura and peritoneum, to detect changes that indicate malignancy.*

A   B

Figure 12-15 Papanicolaou (Pap) test. (A) Insertion of speculum to expand the vaginal walls and reveal the cervix. (B) Cervix is exposed to obtain cells for Pap test. (From Dillon PM: *Nursing health assessment,* ed 2, Philadelphia, 2007, F.A. Davis, pp. 634–635, with permission.)

Procedure	Description
pelvimetry pĕl-VĬM-ĕ-trē *pelv/i:* pelvis *-metry:* act of measuring	Measurement of pelvic dimensions to determine whether the head of the fetus will be able to pass through the bony pelvis to allow vaginal delivery *Pelvimetry is performed manually, by x-ray, or by ultrasound, depending on the stage of the pregnancy. The size of the pelvic outlet determines whether or not the baby is delivered vaginally or by cesarean section.*
pregnancy test	Test performed on urine or blood to detect human chorionic gonadotropin (HCG), a hormone produced by the body when pregnant

Diagnostic, Surgical, and Therapeutic Procedures—cont'd

Procedure	Description
sentinel lymph node biopsy (SLNB)	Biopsy to determine whether cancer has spread beyond the primary breast tumor to a nearby lymph node, where a dye or radioactive tracer is injected near the tumor and flows through the lymphatic vessels to identify the node to be removed for examination *The first node identified by the dye is the most likely node where cancer is to spread (sentinel node). If cancer is absent in the sentinel node, it is highly unlikely that it has spread to other lymph nodes, and no further lymph node surgery will be needed.*

Imaging

Procedure	Description
hysterosalpingography (HSG) hĭs-tĕr-ō-săl-pĭn-GŎG-ră-fē *hyster/o:* uterus (womb) *salping/o:* tube (usually fallopian or eustachian [auditory] tube) *-graphy:* process of recording	Radiography and, usually, fluoroscopy of the uterus and uterine tubes (oviducts) after injection of a contrast medium *HSG helps determine pathology in the uterine cavity, evaluate tubal patency, and determine the cause of infertility.*
mammography măm-ŎG-ră-fē *mamm/o:* breast *-graphy:* process of recording	Radiographic examination of the breast to screen for breast cancer; takes two-dimensional (2D) images *Mammography detects tumors, cysts, and microcalcifications and may help locate a malignant lesion (see Fig. 12-16).* **Figure 12-16** Mammography. One breast at a time is compressed between two plates for x-ray imaging to detect abnormal growths and breast cancer.
digital breast tomosynthesis (DBT)	Technologically advanced imaging technique that builds on 2D mammography by capturing multiple images of the breast from different angles and reconstructing them into a 3D image to produce a more reliable image that is better at detecting cancer, especially in dense breast tissue; also called *3D mammography* *The breast is positioned similarly to traditional mammography. DBT is being used more often in conjunction with 2D mammography as part of routine breast cancer screening.*

Continued

Diagnostic, Surgical, and Therapeutic Procedures—cont'd

Procedure	Description

ultrasonography (US)
ŭl-tră-sŏn-ŎG-ră-fē

    ultra-: excess, beyond
    son/o: sound
    -graphy: process of recording

Radiographic procedure in which a small transducer passed over the skin transmits high-frequency sound waves (ultrasound) that bounce off body tissues and are then recorded to produce an image of an internal organ or tissue

Pelvic US is used to evaluate the female reproductive organs and fetus during pregnancy (see Fig. 12-17).

Figure 12-17 Fetal ultrasound. (A) Ultrasound (US) on a pregnant patient. (B) Monitor screen showing sonogram of the developing fetus.

Diagnostic, Surgical, and Therapeutic Procedures—cont'd

Procedure	Description
transvaginal ultrasonography (TVUS) trănz-VĂJ-ĭ-năl ŭl-tră-sōn-ŎG-ră-fē *trans-:* through, across *vagin:* vagina *-al:* pertaining to	US of the pelvic area performed with a probe inserted into the vagina, which provides sharper images of pathological and normal structures within the pelvis

Surgical

cerclage sĕr-KLĂZH	Suturing of the cervix to prevent it from dilating prematurely during pregnancy, thus decreasing the chance of a spontaneous abortion or preterm birth *Cerclage is sometimes referred to as the purse-string procedure. The sutures are removed before delivery.*
cesarean section (C-section) sē-SĀR-ē-ăn	Incision of the abdomen and uterus to remove the fetus; also called *C-section* *C-section is most commonly used in the event of cephalopelvic disproportion, presence of sexually transmitted disease, fetal distress, and breech presentation.*
conization kŏn-ĭ-ZĀ-shŭn	Excision of a cone-shaped piece of tissue, such as mucosa of the cervix, for histological examination
cryosurgery krī-ō-SĔR-jĕr-ē	Process of freezing tissue to destroy cells; also called *cryocautery* *Cryosurgery is used for chronic cervical infections and erosions because offending organisms may be entrenched in cervical cells and glands. The process destroys these infected areas; in the healing process, normal cells are replenished.*

Continued

Diagnostic, Surgical, and Therapeutic Procedures—cont'd

Procedure	Description
dilation and curettage (D&C) dī-LĂ-sh ŭn, kū-r ĕ-TĂZH	Widening of the cervical canal with a dilator and scraping of the uterine endometrium with a curette *D&C obtains a sample for cytological examination of tissue, controls abnormal uterine bleeding, and treats incomplete abortion (see Fig. 12-18).*

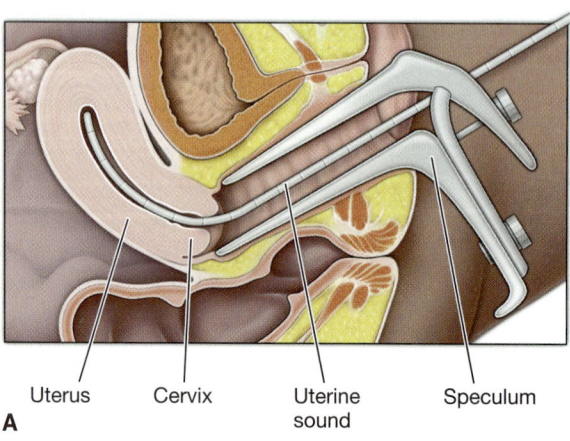

Uterus   Cervix   Uterine sound   Speculum

A

Cervical dilator

B

C Serrated curet

Figure 12-18 Dilation and curettage. (A) Examination of the uterine cavity with a uterine sound. (B) Dilation of the cervix with a series of cervical dilators. (C) Curettage (scraping) of the uterine lining with a serrated uterine curet.

Diagnostic, Surgical, and Therapeutic Procedures—cont'd

Procedure	Description
episiotomy ĕ-pĭs-ē-ŎT-ō-mē *episi/o:* vulva *-tomy:* incision	Surgical incision of the perineum to enlarge the vaginal opening for obstetrical purposes during the birth process *Episiotomy is used to aid a difficult delivery and prevent rupture of tissues.*
hysterectomy hĭs-tĕr-ĔK-tō-mē *hyster:* uterus (womb) *-ectomy:* excision, removal	Excision of the uterus (see Fig. 12-19) *Indications for hysterectomy include abnormalities of the uterus and cervix (cancer, severe dysfunctional bleeding, large or bleeding fibroid tumors, prolapse of the uterus, or severe endometriosis). The surgical approach may be laparoscopic, abdominal, vaginal, or robotic-assisted surgery (RAS).*

Subtotal hysterectomy
(cervix not removed)

Total hysterectomy
(cervix removed)

**Total hysterectomy
plus bilateral
salpingo-oophorectomy**

Figure 12-19 Hysterectomy.

robotic-assisted	Hysterectomy where small incisions are made into the abdomen for robotic arm entry; the surgeon controls robotic arms with a computer while viewing the images on a monitor (see Fig. 4-14)
subtotal	Hysterectomy in which the cervix, ovaries, and fallopian tubes remain
total	Hysterectomy in which the cervix is removed but the ovaries and fallopian tubes remain; also called *complete hysterectomy*
total plus bilateral salpingo-oophorectomy bī-LĂT-ĕr-ăl săl-pĭng-gō-ō-ŏf-ō-RĔK-tō-mē *bi-:* two *later:* side, to one side *-al:* pertaining to *salping/o:* tube (usually the fallopian or eustachian [auditory] tube) *oophor:* ovary *-ectomy:* excision, removal	Total (complete) hysterectomy, including removal of the uterus, cervix, fallopian tubes, and ovaries

Continued

Diagnostic, Surgical, and Therapeutic Procedures—cont'd

Procedure	Description
laparoscopy lăp-ăr-ŎS-kō-pē *lapar/o:* abdomen *-scopy:* visual examination	Procedure performed through small incisions in the abdomen to visualize and operate on the abdominopelvic cavity using a thin flexible tube (laparoscope) with a camera and light that provides high-definition images on a monitor (see Fig. 12-20) *Laparoscopy has become a standard technique for many surgical procedures on the female reproductive organs including hysterectomy, removal of tumors, cysts and endometrial tissue, and tubal ligation. The smaller incisions produce minimal scarring, reduce the risk of infection, and decrease postoperative pain and recovery time versus an open abdominal incision.*

Figure 12-20 Laparoscopy. (A) Trocars are placed through small abdominal incisions for the entry of the laparoscope and surgical instruments. (B) The surgeon views the images on the screen as he manipulates the instruments through the trocars to perform the removal of uterine fibroids (myomectomy).

Diagnostic, Surgical, and Therapeutic Procedures—cont'd

Procedure	Description
lumpectomy lŭm-PĔK-tō-mē	Excision of a small primary breast tumor (or "lump") and some of the normal tissue that surrounds it (see Fig. 12-21A) *In lumpectomy, lymph nodes may also be removed because they are located within the breast tissue taken during surgery. Typically, the patient will undergo radiation therapy after lumpectomy.*

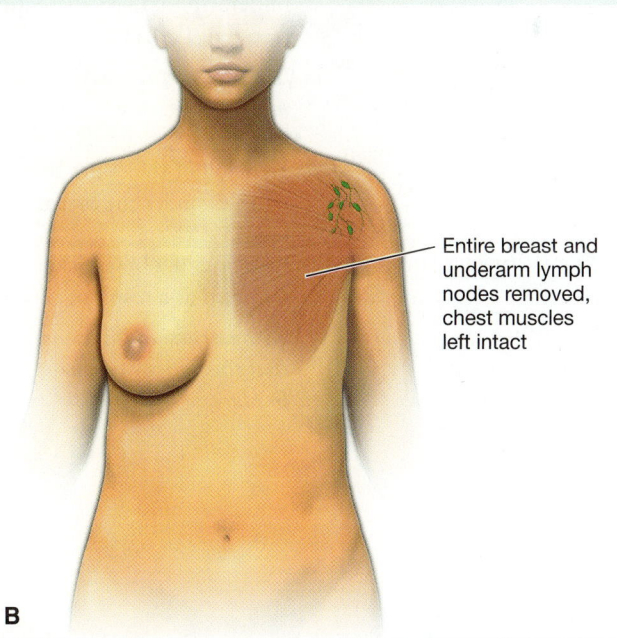

Figure 12-21 Lumpectomy and mastectomy. (A) Lumpectomy with the primary tumor in red and the surrounding tissue removed in pink. (B) Modified radical mastectomy.

Continued

Diagnostic, Surgical, and Therapeutic Procedures—cont'd

Procedure	Description
mammoplasty MĂM-ō-plăs-tē *mamm/o:* breast *-plasty:* surgical repair	Surgical reconstruction of the breast(s) to change the size, shape, or position
augmentation	Insertion of a breast prosthesis (filled with silicone gel or saline) beneath the skin or beneath the pectoralis major muscle *Augmentation surgery increases breast size or replaces a breast that has been surgically removed.*
reduction	Breast reduction to reduce the size of a large, pendulous breast *Breast reduction may be performed in conjunction with mastopexy, a surgery to uplift a sagging breast.*
mastectomy măs-TĔK-tō-mē *mast:* breast *-ectomy:* excision, removal	Removal of the breast
total (simple)	Excision of the entire breast, nipple, areola, and the involved overlying skin *In total mastectomy, lymph nodes are removed only if they are included in the breast tissue being removed.*
modified radical	Excision of the entire breast, including the lymph nodes in the underarm (axillary dissection) but with the chest muscles left intact (see Fig. 12-21B) *Most women who have mastectomies today have modified radical mastectomies.*
radical	Excision of the entire breast, all underarm lymph nodes, and the chest wall muscles under the breast
reconstructive breast surgery	Creation of a breast-shaped mound to replace a breast that has been removed as a result of cancer or other disease *Reconstruction is commonly possible immediately after mastectomy so that the patient awakens from anesthesia with a breast mound already in place.*

Diagnostic, Surgical, and Therapeutic Procedures—cont'd

Procedure	Description
tissue (skin) expansion	Common breast reconstruction technique in which a balloon expander is inserted beneath the skin and chest muscle, saline solution is gradually injected to increase size, and the expander is then replaced with a more permanent implant (see Fig. 12-22, below.)

Figure 12-22 Tissue expander for breast reconstruction.

Continued

Diagnostic, Surgical, and Therapeutic Procedures—cont'd

Procedure	Description
transverse rectus abdominis muscle (TRAM) flap	Surgical creation of a skin flap using skin and fat from the lower half of the abdomen, which is passed under the skin to the breast area; the abdominal tissue (flap) is then shaped into a natural-looking breast and sutured into place (see Fig. 12-23)

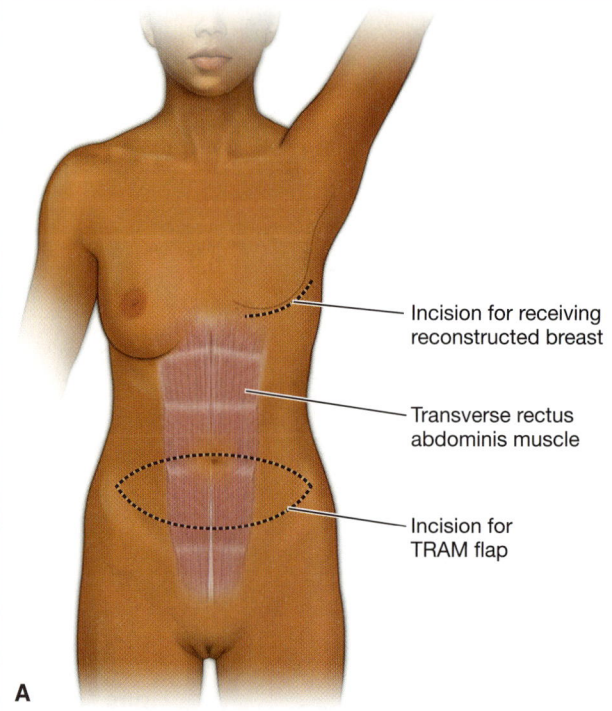

Incision for receiving reconstructed breast

Transverse rectus abdominis muscle

Incision for TRAM flap

A

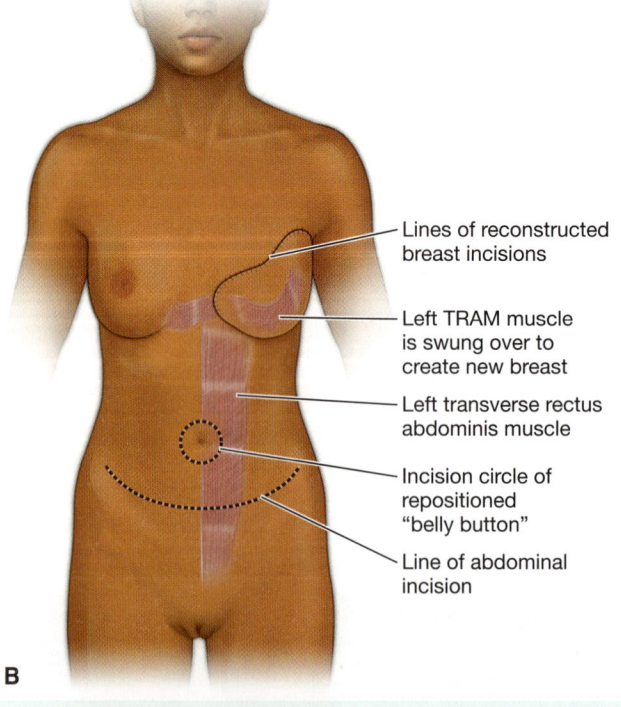

Lines of reconstructed breast incisions

Left TRAM muscle is swung over to create new breast

Left transverse rectus abdominis muscle

Incision circle of repositioned "belly button"

Line of abdominal incision

B

Figure 12-23 Transverse rectus abdominis muscle (TRAM) flap. (A) After mastectomy. (B) Process of TRAM reconstruction.

Diagnostic, Surgical, and Therapeutic Procedures—cont'd

Procedure	Description
tubal ligation TŪ-băl lī-GĀ-shŭn	Procedure that ties (ligates) the fallopian tubes to prevent pregnancy *Tubal ligation is a form of sterilization surgery usually performed laparoscopically.*

Therapeutic

Procedure	Description
Human papillomavirus (HPV) vaccine PĂP-ĭl-ō-mă-VĪ-rŭs	Vaccination that protects against the most common, high-risk strains of HPV to prevent cervical cancer *The American Cancer Society recommends health-care providers to routinely offer the HPV series to boys and girls between the ages of 9 and 12, before sexual activity begins. The vaccination is given in a series and is approved for ages 9 to 45 years of age.*
intrauterine device (IUD) ĭn-tră-Ū-tĕr-ĭn	Small, T-shaped device inserted by a physician inside the uterus to prevent pregnancy *Two types of modern IUDs are available: a copper IUD, which releases copper particles to prevent pregnancy, and a hormonal IUD, which releases the hormone progestin to prevent pregnancy.*

Pharmacology

Hormone replacement therapy (HRT) is the use of synthetic or natural estrogens or a combination of estrogen and progestin to replace the decline or lack of natural hormones, a condition that accompanies hysterectomy and menopause (see Table 12-2). Estrogen may be administered orally, transdermally, by injection, or as a topical cream (to treat vaginal symptoms only). Other hormones, including oxytocics and prostaglandins, are used for obstetrical applications. In addition, pharmacological agents are available for birth control and family planning. These agents include oral contraceptives, implants, and spermicides.

TABLE 12-2 Drugs Used to Treat Obstetrical and Gynecological Disorders

This table lists common drug classifications used to treat obstetric and gynecological disorders, along with their therapeutic actions and selected generic and trade names.

Classification	Therapeutic Action	Generic and Trade Names
antifungals ăn-tĭ-FŬNG-găls	Treat vaginal yeast infection by altering the yeast cell membrane or interfering with a metabolic process *Most antifungals used to treat vaginal yeast infections are applied topically as ointments, suppositories, or vaginal tablets. Fluconazole is used orally.*	fluconazole flū-KŎN-ă-zōl *Diflucan* miconazole mī-KŎN-ă-zōl *Monistat*
aromatase inhibitors ă-RŌ-mă-tās	Treat hormone receptor-positive (ER-positive) breast cancer by reducing the amount of estrogen in the body by inhibiting the enzyme aromatase	anastrozole ăn-ĂS-trō-zōl *Arimidex* letrozole LĔT-rō-zōl *Femara*

(continued)

TABLE 12-2 Drugs Used to Treat Obstetrical and Gynecological Disorders—cont'd

Classification	Therapeutic Action	Generic and Trade Names
estrogens ĔS-trō-jĕns	Treat symptoms of menopause (hot flashes, vaginal dryness, fatigue) through hormone replacement therapy (HRT); may be given orally or topically; topical use may decrease risks *Long-term use of estrogen has been linked with an increased risk of thrombophlebitis and breast and endometrial cancers.*	**conjugated estrogens (oral only)** KŎN-jū-gā-tĕd ĔS-trō-jĕnz *Cenestin, Premarin* **estradiol** ĕs-tră-DĪ-ŏl *Estrace (oral), Climara (topical)*
oral contraceptives kŏn-tră-SĔP-tĭvs	Synthetic hormones used to prevent pregnancy and treat menstrual disorders *Oral contraceptives, or birth control pills, contain a combination of estrogen and progestin and are highly effective in preventing pregnancy if taken as directed.*	**desogestrel/ethinyl estradiol** dĕz-ō-JĔS-trăl, ĔTH-ĭ-nĭl ĕs-tră-DĪ-ŏl *Desogen, Ortho-Cept* **ethinyl estradiol/norgestrel** ĔTH-ĭ-nĭl ĕs-tră-DĪ-ŏl, nor-JĔS-trĕl *Lo/Ovral-28*
oxytocics ŏk-sē-TŌ-sĭks	Induce labor at term by increasing the strength and frequency of uterine contractions *Oxytocics are also used during the postpartum period to control bleeding after the expulsion of the placenta.*	**oxytocin** ŏk-sē-TŌ-sĭn *Pitocin*
prostaglandins PRŎS-tă-glănd-ĭns	Terminate pregnancy *Large doses of certain prostaglandins can cause the uterus to contract strongly enough to spontaneously abort a fetus.*	**dinoprostone** dī-nō-PRŎS-tōn *Prostin E2, Cervidil* **mifepristone** mī-fĕ-PRĬS-tōn *Mifeprex*
selective estrogen receptor modulators (SERMs)	Treat and reduce the risk of breast cancer by blocking estrogen from binding to breast cancer cells and preventing their growth; slows bone loss and reduces the risk of osteoporosis	**tamoxifen** tă-MŎX-ĭ-fĕn *Novadex, Soltamox* **raloxifene** RĂ-lŏx-ĭ-fĕn *Evista*
spermicides SPĔR-mĭ-sīds	Chemically destroy sperm by creating a highly acidic environment in the uterus *Spermicides are available in foam, gel, and suppository forms. They are used within the female vagina for contraception. When used alone, spermicides have a higher failure rate than other methods of birth control.*	**nonoxynol 9, octoxynol 9** nŏn-ŎK-sĭ-nŏl, ŏk-TŎKS-ĭ-nŏl *Semicid, Koromex, Ortho-Gynol*

Abbreviations

This section introduces female reproductive–related abbreviations and their meanings.

Abbreviation	Meaning	Abbreviation	Meaning
AB	abortion	LMP	last menstrual period
AUB	abnormal uterine bleeding	OB	obstetrics
BRCA	breast cancer	OCPs	oral contraceptive pills
BSE	breast self-examination	Pap	Papanicolaou (test)
CA	cancer	para 1, 2, 3 and so on	unipara, bipara, tripara (number of viable births)
CNB	core needle biopsy	PCOS	polycystic ovarian syndrome
C-section, CS	cesarean section	PID	pelvic inflammatory disease
CVS	chorionic villus sampling	PMS	premenstrual syndrome
D&C	dilatation (dilation) and curettage	PUBS	percutaneous umbilical blood sampling
DBT	digital breast tomosynthesis	SAB	spontaneous abortion
DUB	dysfunctional uterine bleeding	SERMs	selective estrogen receptor modulators
FNA	fine needle aspiration	SLNB	sentinel lymph node biopsy
GYN	gynecology	STI	sexually transmitted infection
HPV	human papilloma virus	TRAM	transverse rectus abdominis muscle (flap)
HRT	hormone replacement therapy	TVUS	transvaginal ultrasonography
HSG	hysterosalpingography	US	ultrasound
IUD	intrauterine device		

It is time to review procedures, pharmacology, and abbreviations by completing Learning Activity 12–4.

LEARNING ACTIVITIES

The activities that follow provide a review of the female reproductive system terms introduced in this chapter. Complete each activity and review your answers to evaluate your understanding of the chapter.

Medical Language Lab
Turning terminology into language

Visit the Medical Language Laboratory at medicallanguagelab.com. Use it to enhance your study and reinforcement of this chapter with the flash card activity. We recommend that you complete the flash card activity before starting Learning Activities 12-1 and 12-2.

Learning Activity 12-1
Medical Word Elements

Use the listed elements to build medical words. You may use the elements more than once.

Combining Forms		Suffixes		Prefixes	
amni/o	men/o	-al	-plasty	dys-	primi-
cervic/o	nat/o	-arche	-poiesis	multi-	pseudo-
colp/o	oophor/o	-centesis	-rrhaphy	pre-	
galact/o	perine/o	-cyesis	-rrhexis		
hem/o	salping/o	-ectomy	-salpinx		
hyster/o		-gravida	-scopy		
		-itis	-tocia		
		-para			

1. surgical repair of a fallopian tube _____
2. pertaining to (the time) before birth _____
3. difficult childbirth _____
4. rupture of the uterus _____
5. excision of the ovary _____
6. inflammation of the cervix uteri (neck of the uterus) _____
7. surgical puncture of the amnion (amniotic sac) _____
8. suture of the perineum _____
9. visual examination of the vagina _____
10. pregnant woman (for the) first (time) _____
11. false pregnancy _____
12. blood in a fallopian tube _____
13. to bear many (offspring) _____
14. beginning of menses or menstruation _____
15. formation or production of milk _____

Check your answers in Appendix A. Review any material that you did not answer correctly.

Correct Answers _____ X 6.67 = _____ % Score

Learning Activity 12-2
Building Medical Words

Use *gynec/o* (woman, female) to build words that mean

  1. study of disease (specific to) women _____

  2. physician who specializes in diseases of the female _____

Use *cervic/o* (neck; cervix uteri) to build words that mean

  3. inflammation of the cervix, uteri, and vagina _____

  4. pertaining to the cervix, uteri, and bladder _____

Use *colp/o* (vagina) to build words that mean

  5. instrument used to examine the vagina _____

  6. visual examination of the vagina _____

Use *vagin/o* (vagina) to build words that mean

  7. inflammation of the vagina _____

  8. herniation of the vagina _____

Use *hyster/o* (uterus) to build words that mean

  9. myoma of the uterus _____

10. disease of the uterus _____

11. radiography of the uterus and oviducts _____

Use *mast/o* (breast) to build words that mean

12. fixation of the breast _____

13. removal of the breast _____

Use *uter/o* (uterus) to build words that mean

14. herniation of the uterus _____

15. relating to the uterus and cervix _____

16. pertaining to the uterus and bladder _____

Use *oophor/o* (ovary) to build words that mean

17. tumor of an ovary _____

18. inflammation of an ovary and oviduct _____

Use *salping/o* (fallopian tube) to build words that mean

19. herniation of a fallopian tube _____
20. radiography of uterine tubes _____

Build surgical words that mean

21. fixation of (a displaced) ovary _____
22. excision of the uterus and ovaries _____
23. suturing the perineum _____
24. excision of the uterus, oviducts, and ovaries _____
25. puncture of the amnion (amniotic sac) _____

Check your answers in Appendix A. Review any material that you did not answer correctly.

Correct Answers _____ X 4 = _____ % Score

Learning Activity 12-3
Diseases and Conditions

Match the terms with the definitions in the numbered list.

breech	*dyspareunia*	*fibroids*	*primigravida*
candidiasis	*dystocia*	*gestation*	*primipara*
choriocarcinoma	*eclampsia*	*menarche*	*pyosalpinx*
condylomata	*endometriosis*	*metrorrhagia*	*retroversion*
Down syndrome	*fibrocystic disease*	*oligomenorrhea*	*sterility*

1. infrequent menstrual flow _____

2. woman who has had one pregnancy that has resulted in a viable offspring _____

3. average pregnancy; approximately 9 months _____

4. inability of the female to become pregnant _____

5. uterus that is tipped backward from its normal position _____

6. condition of benign cysts that are palpable in the breasts _____

7. difficult labor or childbirth _____

8. genital warts caused by the human papillomavirus _____

9. trisomy 21 _____

10. functional endometrial tissue outside the uterus _____

11. occurrence of pain during sexual intercourse _____

12. irregular uterine bleeding between menstrual periods _____

13. beginning of menstrual function _____

14. benign uterine tumor composed of muscle and fibrous tissue _____

15. accumulation of pus in a uterine tube _____

16. abnormal delivery in which fetal buttocks or feet present first rather than the head _____

17. most serious form of toxemia during pregnancy _____

18. malignant neoplasm of the uterus or at the site of an ectopic pregnancy _____

19. fungal infection caused by *Candida albicans* _____

20. woman during her first pregnancy _____

✔ *Check your answers in Appendix A. Review any material that you did not answer correctly.*

Correct Answers _____ X 5 = _____ % Score

Learning Activity 12-4

Procedures, Pharmacology, and Abbreviations

Match the terms with the definitions in the numbered list.

amniocentesis	cryosurgery	IUD	Pap test
antifungals	DBT	laparoscopy	PCOS
cerclage	episiotomy	lumpectomy	PID
chorionic villus sampling	estrogens	OCPs	prostaglandins
cordocentesis	FNA	oxytocins	tubal ligation

1. excision of a small primary breast tumor _____

2. 3D mammography _____

3. puncture of the amniotic sac to remove amniotic fluid for biochemical and cytological study _____

4. drugs used to treat vaginal yeast infections _____

5. abnormally high levels of androgens with enlarged ovaries containing small follicle cysts with immature eggs _____

6. diagnostic test in which a sample of baby's blood is removed from the umbilical cord for testing _____

7. suturing the cervix to prevent it from dilating prematurely during pregnancy _____

8. tying uterine tubes to prevent pregnancy _____

9. freezing tissue to destroy cells _____

10. examination of the abdominal cavity using an endoscope _____

11. incision of the perineum to facilitate childbirth _____

12. inflammation of the uterus, fallopian tubes, ovaries, and adjacent pelvic structures, usually caused by bacterial infection _____

13. test to detect chromosomal abnormalities that can be done earlier than amniocentesis _____

14. hormone replacement to reduce adverse symptoms of menopause _____

15. agents used to induce labor and rid the uterus of an unexpelled placenta or a fetus that has died _____

16. birth control pills taken orally _____

17. birth control method in which an object is placed inside the uterus to prevent pregnancy _____

18. withdrawal of cells or fluid from a breast lump for biopsy with a small fine needle _____

19. cytological study of tissue to detect cancer cells _____

20. agents used to terminate pregnancy _____

✓ *Check your answers in Appendix A. Review material that you did not answer correctly.*

Correct Answers _____ X 5 = _____ % Score

DOCUMENTING HEALTH-CARE ACTIVITIES

This section provides practical application activities in the form of exercises to help students develop skills in documenting patient care. First, read the medical report. Then complete the activities and exercises that follow.

Documenting Health-Care Activity 12-1
SOAP Note: Primary Herpes 1 Infection

Progress Notes

O'Malley, Roberta   09/01/xx

S: This 24-year-old patient started having some sore areas around the labia, both rt and lt side. She stated that the last few days she started having a brownish discharge. She has pruritus and pain of her vulvar area with adenopathy, p.m. fever, and blisters. Apparently, her partner had a cold sore and they had oral-genital sex. Patient has been using condoms since last seen in April. She has not missed any OCPs. LMP 5/15/xx.

O: Patient has what looks like herpes lesions and ulcers all over vulva and introitus area. Rt labia appears as an ulcerlike lesion; it appears to be almost like an infected follicle. Speculum inserted, a brown discharge noted. GC screen, chlamydia screen, and genital culture obtained. Wet prep revealed monilial forms. Viral culture obtained from the ulcerlike lesion on the right labia.

A: Primary herpes 1 infection; will rule out other infectious etiologies.

P: Patient advised to return next week for consultation with Dr. Abdu.

Joanna Masters, MD.
Joanna Masters, MD

JM:st

Terminology

The terms listed in the table that follows are taken from *SOAP Note: Primary Herpes 1 Infection.* Use a medical dictionary such as *Taber's Cyclopedic Medical Dictionary,* the appendices of this book, or other resources to define each term. Then review the pronunciation for each term and practice by reading the medical record aloud.

Term	Definition
adenopathy ăd-ĕ-NŎP-ă-thē	
chlamydia klă-MĬD-ē-ă	
GC screen	
herpes lesions HĔR-pēz LĒ-zhŭnz	
introitus ĭn-TRŌ-ĭ-tŭs	
labia LĀ-bē-ă	
LMP	
monilial mō-NĬL-ē-ăl	
OCPs	
pruritus proo-RĪ-tŭs	
OCPs	
R/O	
vulvar VŬL-văr	
wet prep	

Visit the Medical Terminology Systems online resource center at FADavis. com to practice pronunciation and reinforce the meanings of the terms in this medical report.

Critical Thinking

Review *SOAP Note: Primary Herpes 1 Infection* to answer the questions.

1. Did the patient have any discharge? If so, describe it.

_____

_____

_____

2. What type of discomfort did the patient experience around the vulvar area?

_____

_____

_____

3. Has the patient been taking her oral contraceptive pills regularly?

_____

_____

_____

4. Where was the viral culture obtained?

_____

_____

_____

5. Even though the patient's partner used a condom, how do you think the patient became infected with herpes?

_____

_____

_____

Preoperative Consultation: Menometrorrhagia

Physician Center

2422 Rodeo Drive ■ ■ Sun City, USA 12345 ■ ■ (555)788–2427

Preoperative Consultation

Mazza, Rosemary   July 2, 20xx

CHIEF COMPLAINT: Dysmenorrhea and night sweats.

HISTORY OF PRESENT ILLNESS: Patient is a 43-year-old gravida 2, para 1 with multiple small uterine fibroids, irregular menses twice a month, family history of ovarian cancer, benign endometrial biopsy, normal Pap, normal mammogram, and normal thyroid function tests. Negative cervical cultures. She has completed childbearing and desires to control irregular, heavy, prolonged menstrual periods.

SURGICAL HISTORY: Cesarean section, therapeutic abortion, and cholecystectomy.

ASSESSMENT: This is a patient with menometrorrhagia who declines palliative treatment and desires definitive treatment in the form of a hysterectomy.

PLAN: The plan is to perform a laparoscopic assisted vaginal hysterectomy because the patient has essentially no uterine prolapse and desires her ovaries to be taken out. She desires to start on Premarin in the postoperative period. She has been counseled concerning the risks of surgery, including injury to bowel or bladder, infection, and bleeding. She voices understanding and agrees to the plan to perform a laparoscopic assisted vaginal hysterectomy and bilateral salpingo-oophorectomy.

Julia Masters, MD
Julia Masters, MD

JM:st

Terminology

The terms listed in the table that follows are taken from *Preoperative Consultation: Menometrorrhagia.* Use a medical dictionary such as *Taber's Cyclopedic Medical Dictionary*, the appendices of this book, or other resources to define each term. Then review the pronunciation for each term and practice by reading the medical record aloud.

Term	Definition
ablation ăb-LĀ-shŭn	
benign bē-NĬN	
cesarean section sĕ-SĀR-ē-ăn	
cholecystectomy kō-lē-sĭs-TĔK-tō-mē	
dysmenorrhea dĭs-mĕn-ō-RĒ-ă	
endometrial biopsy ĕn-dō-MĒ-trē-ăl BĪ-ŏp-sē	
fibroids FĪ-broyds	
gravida 2 GRĂV-ĭ-dă	
hysterectomy hĭs-tĕr-ĔK-tō-mē	
laparoscopic lăp-ă-rō-SKŎP-ĭk	
mammogram MĂM-ō-grăm	
menometrorrhagia mĕn-ō-mĕt-rō-RĀ-jē-ă	
palliative PĂL-ē-ā-tĭv	

Continued

Term	Definition
para 1 PĂR-ă	
postoperative pōst-ŎP-ĕr-ă-tĭv	
Premarin PRĔM-ă-rĭn	
salpingo- oophorectomy săl-pĭng-gō-ō- ŏf-ō-RĔK-tō-mē	
therapeutic abortion thĕr-ă-PŪ-tĭk ă-BOR-shŭn	
thyroid function test THĪ-royd	

Visit the Medical Terminology Systems online resource center at FADavis.com to practice pronunciation and reinforce the meanings of the terms in this medical report.

Critical Thinking

Review the medical record *Preoperative Consultation: Menometrorrhagia* to answer the questions.

1. How many pregnancies did this patient have? How many viable infants did she deliver?

2. What is a therapeutic abortion?

3. Why did the physician propose to perform a hysterectomy?

4. What are the advantages of laparoscopic surgery?

5. Does the surgeon plan to remove one or both ovaries and fallopian tubes?

6. What is the purpose of the Premarin?

Constructing Chart Notes

To construct chart notes, replace the italicized and boldfaced terms in each of the two case studies with one of the listed medical terms.

dysmenorrhea	menopause	needle biopsy
gravida 3, para 3	menorrhagia	nullipara
mammography	metrorrhagia	uterine fibroids
menarche		

Ms. T is a 32-year-old female who presents at our office with complaints of bleeding. Her past reproductive history includes (1) *three pregnancies resulting in three live births.* She is now experiencing (2) *midcycle bleeding* and complains of (3) *excessively heavy periods,* commonly with blood clots. The patient further complains of (4) *severe cramps, headache, and tension* during her period. She is scheduled for a complete pelvic examination and a transvaginal ultrasound to establish the diagnosis of (5) *benign tumors of the uterus.*

1. _____
2. _____
3. _____
4. _____
5. _____

Mrs. D presents with a complaint of a small lump in her right breast and is concerned that this may be cancer. Her mother and sister are both cancer survivors. Besides a family history of the disease, she has several risk factors, including (6) *never giving birth* and early (7) *onset of menstruation.* She admits that she went through the (8) *change of life* 3 years ago at age 53. She is scheduled for (9) *breast x-ray* and (10) *an examination of a small piece of tissue obtained using a needle,* which will be performed under ultrasound guidance.

6. _____
7. _____
8. _____
9. _____
10. _____

✓ *Check your answers in Appendix A. Review any material that you did not answer correctly.*

Correct Answers _____ X 10 = _____ % Score

Male Reproductive System

Chapter Outline

Objectives

Upon completion of this chapter, you will be able to:

- Locate and describe the structures of the male reproductive system.
- Describe the functional relationship between the male reproductive system and other body systems.
- Pronounce, spell, and build words related to the male reproductive system.
- Describe diseases, conditions, and procedures related to the male reproductive system.
- Explain pharmacology related to the treatment of male reproductive disorders.
- Demonstrate your knowledge of this chapter by completing the learning and documenting health-care activities.

Anatomy and Physiology

The male reproductive system produces, maintains, and transports sperm, the male sex cell required for fertilization of the female egg. It is also responsible for developing and maintaining male secondary sex characteristics (see Fig. 13-1).

Anatomy and Physiology Key Terms

This section introduces important terms, along with their definitions and pronunciations. The key terms are highlighted in color in the Anatomy and Physiology section. Word analyses for selected terms are also provided. Pronounce the term and place a check mark in the box after you do so.

Term	Definition
gamete ☐ GĂM-ēt	Reproductive cell (ovum or sperm) that contains one-half of the chromosomes required to produce an offspring of the species
libido ☐ lĭ-BĒ-dō	Psychological and physical drive for sexual activity
semen ☐ SĒ-mĕn	Fluid containing sperm and secretions from the prostate and other structures of the male reproductive system; also called *seminal fluid*
sphincter ☐ SFĬNGK-tĕr	Ringlike muscle that opens and closes a body opening to allow or restrict passage through the structure
testosterone ☐ tĕs-TŎS-tĕr-ōn	Androgenic hormone responsible for the development of the male sex organs, including the penis, testicles, scrotum, and prostate *Testosterone plays a key role in development of secondary sex characteristics such as increased muscle mass, body and facial hair growth, and thickening of vocal cords.*

Pronunciation Help	Long Sound	ā — rate	ē — rebirth	ī — isle	ō — over	ū — unite
	Short Sound	ă — apple	ĕ — ever	ĭ — it	ŏ — not	ŭ — cut

Male Reproductive Structures

The primary male reproductive organ consists of two (1) **testes** (singular, **testis**) located in the (2) **scrotum,** an external sac lying behind and below the penis. The muscular wall of the scrotum allows for the control of temperature of the testes. It moves the testes closer to the body for warmth and farther from the body for cooling. The testes produce the hormone **testosterone**, which enables development of secondary sex characteristics, including the growth of facial and body hair, deepening of the voice, increased muscle mass, and so forth. It also plays an important role in **libido**. Within the testes are numerous small tubes that twist and coil to form (3) **seminiferous tubules,** which produce sperm, the male **gamete**. Lying over the superior surface of each testis is a single, tightly coiled tube called the (4) **epididymis**. This structure stores sperm after it leaves the seminiferous tubules. The epididymis is the first duct through which sperm passes after its production in the testes. During ejaculation, the epididymis contracts, expelling sperm into the

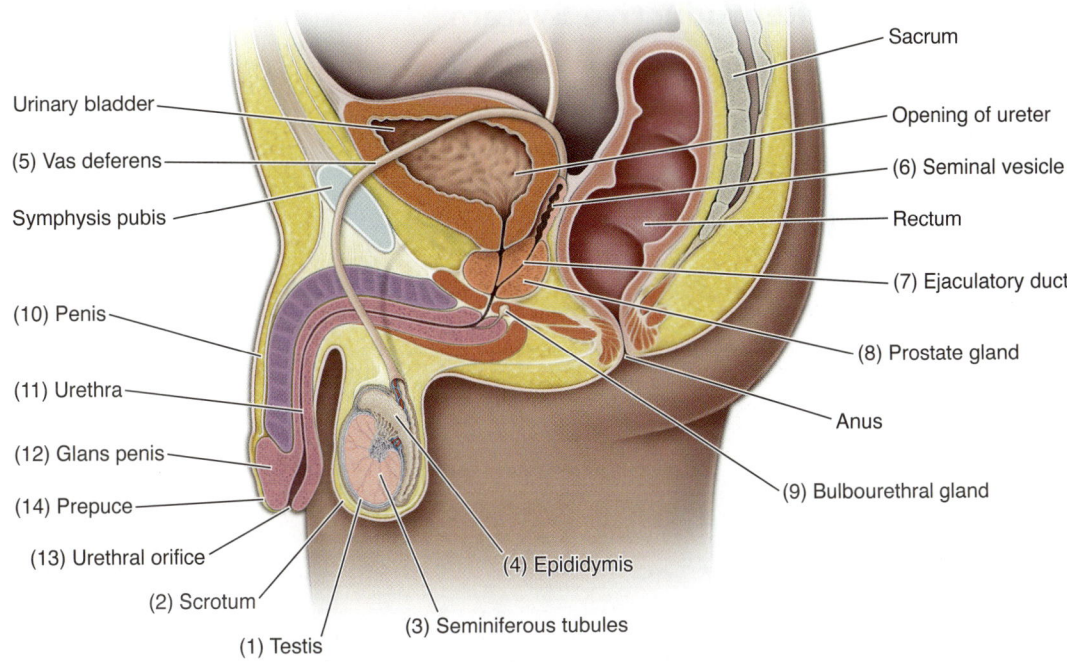

Urinary bladder

(5) Vas deferens

Symphysis pubis

(10) Penis

(11) Urethra

(12) Glans penis

(14) Prepuce

(13) Urethral orifice

(2) Scrotum

(1) Testis

(3) Seminiferous tubules

(4) Epididymis

Sacrum

Opening of ureter

(6) Seminal vesicle

Rectum

(7) Ejaculatory duct

(8) Prostate gland

Anus

(9) Bulbourethral gland

Figure 13-1 Midsagittal section of the male reproductive structures shown through the pelvic cavity.

(5) **vas deferens** (**seminal duct** or **ductus deferens**), a narrow tube that passes through the inguinal canal into the abdominal cavity. The vas deferens extends over the top and down the posterior surface of the bladder, where it joins the (6) **seminal vesicle.** The seminal vesicle contains nutrients that support sperm viability and produces approximately 60% of the **semen** (seminal fluid) that is ultimately ejaculated during sexual intercourse (**coitus**). The union of the vas deferens with the duct from the seminal vesicle forms the (7) **ejaculatory duct.** The ejaculatory duct joins to the urethra as it passes at an angle through the (8) **prostate gland,** a triple-lobed organ fused to the base of the bladder. The prostate gland secretes a thin, alkaline substance that accounts for about 30% of seminal fluid. Its alkalinity helps protect sperm from the acidic environments of the male urethra and the female vagina. Two pea-shaped structures, the (9) **bulbourethral (Cowper) glands**, are located below the prostate and are connected by a small duct to the urethra. The bulbourethral glands provide additional alkaline fluid that neutralizes any residual acidity in the male urethra to further assist in sperm viability. The (10) **penis** is the male organ of copulation. It is cylindrical and composed of erectile tissue that becomes rigid and erect upon sexual arousal. The penis encloses the (11) **urethra** that expels both **semen** and urine from the body. During ejaculation, the **sphincter** at the base of the bladder closes, stopping urine from being expelled with semen while also preventing semen from entering the bladder. The enlarged tip of the penis, the (12) **glans penis,** contains the (13) **urethral orifice (meatus)**, through which urine and semen exit the body. The glans penis contains a number of highly sensitive nerve endings. A movable hood of skin, the (14) **prepuce (foreskin),** covers the glans penis.

Anatomy Review: Male Reproductive System

To review the anatomy of the male reproductive system, label the illustration using the listed terms.

bulbourethral gland	*prepuce*	*testis*
ejaculatory duct	*prostate gland*	*urethra*
epididymis	*scrotum*	*urethral orifice*
glans penis	*seminal vesicle*	*vas deferens*
penis	*seminiferous tubules*	

Urinary bladder

Symphysis pubis

Sacrum

Opening of ureter

Rectum

Anus

 Check your answers by referring to Figure 13-1 on page 473. Review material that you did not answer correctly.

CONNECTING BODY SYSTEMS—MALE REPRODUCTIVE SYSTEM

The main function of the male reproductive system is to enable sexual reproduction. Specific functional relationships between the male reproductive system and other body systems are discussed here.

Blood, Lymphatic, and Immune
- The male reproductive system secretes testosterone into the extracellular fluids of the blood, lymphatic, and immune system for delivery throughout the body.
- The male reproductive system relies on increased blood supply to support the erectile tissue needed for copulation.

Cardiovascular
- Male hormones are transported throughout the body by the vascular system.
- Increased heart rate maintains the sexual excitement needed for ejaculation.

Digestive
- The male reproductive structures rely on a continuous supply of food and nourishment for proper functioning of the organs of reproduction.
- Male reproductive activities require food and nourishment for sexual behavior.

Endocrine
- The gonads produce hormones that provide feedback to influence pituitary function.
- Hormones produce and regulate the development of secondary sex characteristics.

Female Reproductive
- The male reproductive structures produce and deliver sperm, the cell that provides one-half of the genetic complement required for the development of a fetus.
- The male organs of reproduction work in conjunction with the female reproductive system to enable fertilization of the ovum.

Integumentary
- Male hormones produce facial and body hair growth consistent with maleness.

Musculoskeletal
- Male hormones produce skeletal and muscular structures consistent with a larger body frame than that normally found in females.

Nervous
- The male reproductive structures rely on the nervous system to innervate the organs responsible for copulation.
- Mature male reproductive activities are regulated by the emotional aspects of the nervous system, especially the brain.

Respiratory
- The male reproductive system relies on the increased respiratory activity required for sexual activity.
- The male organs of reproduction require a constant supply of oxygen and the removal of waste gases for healthy functioning.
- The male reproductive system causes laryngeal changes, resulting in a deepening of the voice.

Urinary
- The male reproductive system and the urinary system share common structures.
- Waste substances produced by the male reproductive organs are removed by the urinary system.

Medical Word Elements

This section introduces combining forms, suffixes, and prefixes related to the male reproductive system. Word analyses are also provided. From the information provided, complete the meaning of the medical words in the right-hand column. The first one is completed for you.

Element	Meaning	Word Analysis
Combining Forms		
andr/o	male	**andr/o**/gen/ic (ăn-drō-JĔN-ĭk): *pertaining to maleness* *gen:* forming, producing, origin *-ic:* pertaining to *Androgenic hormones include all natural or synthetic compounds that stimulate or maintain male characteristics. The most common androgenic hormone is testosterone.*
balan/o	glans penis	**balan/o**/plasty (BĂL-ă-nō-plăs-tē): _____ *-plasty:* surgical repair
crypt/o	hidden	**crypt**/orchid/ism (krĭpt-OR-kĭd-ĭzm): _____ *orchid:* testis (plural, testes) *-ism:* condition *Cryptorchidism, also called* **cryptorchism,** *is the failure of the testes to descend into the scrotum and is usually a congenital disorder.*
epididym/o	epididymis	**epididym/o**/tomy (ĕp-ĭ-dĭd-ĭ-MŎT-ō-mē): _____ *-tomy:* incision
genit/o	genitalia	**genit/o**/urin/ary (jĕn-ĭ-tō-ŪR-ĭ-nār-ē): _____ *-urin:* urine, urinary tract *-ary:* pertaining to
gonad/o	gonads, sex glands	**gonad/o**/pathy (gŏn-ă-DŎP-ă-thē): _____ *-pathy:* disease
gon/o	seed (ovum or spermatozoon)	**gon/o**/rrhea (gŏn-ō-RĒ-ă): _____ *-rrhea:* discharge, flow *Characteristic of gonorrhea is a discharge of pus, mistakenly believed to be sperm in the early days of medicine.*
olig/o	scanty	**olig/o**/sperm/ia (ŏl-ĭ-gō-SPĔR-mē-ă): _____ *sperm:* spermatozoa, sperm cells *-ia:* condition *Oligospermia is a low concentration of sperm in the semen and may be a cause of male infertility.*
orch/o	testis (plural, testes)	**orch**/itis (or-KĪ-tĭs): _____ *-itis:* inflammation *A common cause of orchitis in young males is a mumps infection.*
orchi/o		**orchi**/algia (or-kē-ĂL-jē-ă): _____ *-algia:* pain
orchid/o		**orchid/o**/rrhaphy (or-kĭ-DOR-ă-fē): _____ *-rrhaphy:* suture

Medical Word Elements—cont'd

Element	Meaning	Word Analysis
test/o		**test**/algia (tĕs-TĂL-jē-ă): _____ *-algia:* pain
perine/o	perineum (area between scrotum [or vulva in the female] and anus)	**perine**/al (pĕr-ĭ-NĒ-ăl): _____ *-al:* pertaining to
prostat/o	prostate gland	**prostat/o**/megaly (prŏs-tă-tō-MĔG-ă-lē): _____ *-megaly:* enlargement
spermat/o	spermatozoa, sperm cells	**spermat/o**/cele (spĕr-MĂT-ō-sēl): _____ *-cele:* hernia, swelling *A spermatocele is usually an epididymal cyst, commonly containing sperm.*
sperm/o		**sperm**/ic (SPĔR-mĭk): _____ *-ic:* pertaining to
varic/o	dilated vein	**varic/o**/cele (VĂR-ĭ-kō-sēl): _____ *-cele:* hernia, swelling *Varicocele is a dilation of the veins of the spermatic cord, the structure that supports the testicles.*
vas/o	vessel; vas deferens; duct	**vas**/ectomy (văs-ĔK-tō-mē): _____ *-ectomy:* excision, removal *Bilateral vasectomy is a surgical procedure to produce sterility in the male.*
vesicul/o	seminal vesicle	**vesicul**/itis (vĕ-sĭk-ū-LĪ-tĭs): _____ *-itis:* inflammation

Suffixes

Element	Meaning	Word Analysis
-cide	killing	sperm/i/**cide** (SPĔR-mĭ-sīd): _____ *sperm/i:* spermatozoa, sperm cells *Spermicide is also called* **spermaticide.**
-genesis	forming, producing, origin	spermat/o/**genesis** (spĕr-măt-ō-JĔN-ĕ-sĭs): _____ *spermat/o:* sperm
-ism	condition	an/orch/**ism** (ăn-OR-kĭzm): _____ *an-:* without, not *orch:* testis (plural, testes) *Anorchism is the congenital or acquired absence of one or both testes.*
-spadias	slit, fissure	hypo/**spadias** (hī-pō-SPĀ-dē-ăs): _____ *hypo-:* under, below *Hypospadias is a congenital defect in which the urethra opens on the underside of the glans penis instead of the tip.*

Continued

Medical Word Elements—cont'd

Element	Meaning	Word Analysis
Prefixes		
brachy-	short	**brachy**/therapy (brăk-ē-THĔR-ă-pē): _____ –*therapy:* treatment *In brachytherapy, radioactive seeds are implanted directly into the malignant tissue.*
epi-	above, upon	**epi**/spadias (ĕp-ĭ-SPĀ-dē-ăs): _____ –*spadias:* slit, fissure

Visit the Medical Terminology Systems online resource center at FADavis.com for an audio exercise of the terms in this table. Other activities are also available to reinforce content.

It is time to review medical word elements by completing Learning Activities 13-1 and 13-2.

Disease Focus

Diseases of the male reproductive system include reproductive disorders, congenital abnormalities, diseases and infections, and various types of cancers. Signs and symptoms commonly include pain, especially during urination, erectile dysfunction, and loss of libido. Performance of a complete evaluation of the genitalia, reproductive history, and past and present genitourinary infections and disorders is necessary to identify disorders associated with male reproductive structures.

For diagnosis, treatment, and management of male reproductive disorders, the medical services of a specialist may be warranted. **Urology** is the branch of medicine concerned with the male reproductive system and urinary disorders in males and females. The physician who specializes in diagnosis and treatment of genitourinary disorders is known as a **urologist.**

Sexually Transmitted Infections

Sexually transmitted infections (STIs), also called **sexually transmitted diseases (STDs),** include any contagious disease acquired during sexual activity with an infected partner. In the United States, the widespread occurrence of STIs is regarded as epidemic. The Centers for Disease Control estimates that there are nearly 20 million new STIs annually, and half of these are among young adults between 15 and 24 years old. Because genital warts, genital herpes, and trichomonas infections are not routinely reported, the current statistics of STIs capture only a fraction of the actual number of these cases. Many STIs can lead to severe reproductive problems, including sterility and infertility in males and females and ectopic pregnancy, preterm delivery, and infection transmitted to the newborn during delivery in females. In addition, many STIs increase the risk of acquiring HIV infection (see Chapter 9 for a discussion of HIV infection).

Gonorrhea

Gonorrhea is caused by the bacterium *Neisseria gonorrheae.* It involves the mucosal surface of the genitourinary tract and can also involve the rectum and pharynx. This disease spreads through sexual intercourse and through orogenital and anogenital contact. The most common symptoms of gonorrhea include pain on urination (**dysuria**) and a white discharge (**leukorrhea**). Left untreated, the disease may infect the bladder (**cystitis**) and inflame joints (**arthritis**). In males, gonorrhea can cause epididymitis that leads to infertility or scarring inside the urethra, making urination difficult. Many women are asymptomatic; however, when symptoms are present, they include a vaginal discharge or pelvic pain. Scars may develop in the reproductive tubes and cause infertility. The organism can infect the eyes of the newborn during vaginal delivery, leading to blindness.

As a precaution, physicians administer silver nitrate in the eyes of all newborns immediately after delivery as a preventive measure to ensure that this infection does not occur. Both sex partners require treatment for gonorrhea because the infection can recur. The usual treatment is antibiotics.

Chlamydia

Chlamydia, caused by infection with the bacterium *Chlamydia trachomatis*, is the most prevalent and one of the most damaging STIs in the United States. It is called the "silent disease" because symptoms are commonly absent or mild, and the disease remains untreated until there is irreversible damage to the reproductive structures. If symptoms are present, males produce a whitish discharge from the penis. Inflammation of epididymis (**epididymitis**) can cause pain and swelling in the scrotum. In women, there is a mucopurulent discharge and inflammation of the cervix uteri (**cervicitis**). During the birth process, chlamydia may spread to the newborn baby and cause conjunctivitis or pneumonia. Antibiotics are effective in treating chlamydia infections. Screening for other STIs is important because chlamydia places the individual at higher risk of having other STIs, including gonorrhea and HIV.

Syphilis

Although less common than gonorrhea, syphilis is the more serious of the two diseases. It is caused by the bacterium *Treponema pallidum*. If left untreated, syphilis may become a chronic, infectious, multisystemic disease.

Syphilis manifests in three distinct stages. In primary syphilis, a painless sore called a **chancre,** appears 3 to 90 days after exposure (see Fig. 13-2). In secondary syphilis, a body rash that commonly occurs on the palms of the hands and soles of the feet appears 4 to 10 weeks after exposure (see Fig. 13-3). A latency period of several years usually follows when sign and symptoms

Figure 13-2 Syphilis chancre. (From Lewis SL, Ruff Dirksen S, McLean Heltkemper M, Bucher L: *Understanding medical-surgical nursing*, ed 9, 2013, F.A. Davis, p. 876, Fig. 44.1.)

Figure 13-3 Secondary stage of syphilis. (A) Cutaneous eruptions of syphilis on the hands and wrist. (B) Syphilis rash on the bottom of the feet.

are absent or very mild; however, the individual is still infectious. Tertiary syphilis develops 3 to 15 years after exposure when the disease spreads throughout the body, especially in the nervous and cardiovascular systems. Early treatment with antibiotics is very effective. Timely identification and treatment are essential to halt the disease's advancement and its associated complications, which encompass vision impairment, stroke, psychiatric disorders, and ultimately, mortality.

Genital Herpes

Although genital herpes and oral herpes are caused by the herpes simplex virus (HSV), genital herpes is associated with type 2 (HSV-2), and oral herpes is associated with type 1 (HSV-1). Regardless, both forms can cause oral and genital infections through oral-genital sexual activity. Genital herpes causes red, blisterlike, painful lesions in the genital area that closely resemble fever blisters or cold sores that appear on the lips and around the mouth (see Fig. 13-4). Fluid in the blisters in genital herpes is highly infectious and contains the active virus. However, this disease is communicable even when the blisters are not present through a phenomenon called *viral shedding*. In men, lesions appear on the glans, foreskin, or penile shaft. In females, lesions appear in the vaginal area, buttocks, and thighs. Individuals with a herpes infection may have only one episode or may have repeated attacks that usually lessen in severity over the years. The disease may spread to a baby during the birth process and, although rare, may lead to death of the infant. Antiviral medication can relieve pain and discomfort during an outbreak by healing the sores more quickly. However, there is no cure available for this disease.

Genital Warts

Genital warts (**condylomata**, **condylomas**) are caused by one or more of the many different human papillomavirus (HPV) strains. The warts may be very small and barely visible or may be large and appear in clusters. HPV can spread from one person to another during skin-to-skin contact and does not require sexual activity. The warts can also spread from one part of the body to another. In males, the lesions commonly appear on the penis or around the rectum. In females, the lesions commonly appear on the vulva, in the vagina, or on the cervix (see Fig. 12-7).

Some high-risk strains of HPV are associated with anal and penile cancer in males and vaginal and cervical cancer in females. Females diagnosed with high-risk strains of HPV require regular Pap smears. HPV vaccines are available and protect against the high-risk strains. To be effective, young adults require vaccination before they begin engaging in sexual activity.

Many warts disappear without treatment, but there is no way to determine which ones will resolve. When treatment is required, the usual method is surgical excision or freezing the wart.

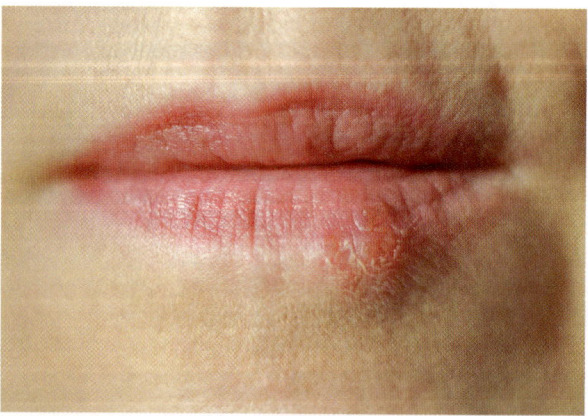

Figure 13-4 Herpes simplex virus type 1 (HSV-1).

Trichomoniasis

Trichomoniasis, caused by the protozoan *Trichomonas vaginalis*, affects males and females but symptoms are more common in females. When symptoms are present in males, they include irritation inside the penis, mild discharge, or slight burning during urination (**dysuria**) or ejaculation. In women, trichomonas causes vaginitis, urethritis, and cystitis with discomfort during urination or intercourse. Often there is a frothy, yellow-green vaginal discharge with a strong odor and irritation or itching of the vulva. Both sexual partners require treatment because reinfection is possible.

Oncology

Prostate cancer is one of the most common forms of cancer among men, second only to skin cancer. With early diagnosis and treatment, the prognosis for long-term survival is excellent.

In the United States, men younger than age 50 rarely develop prostate cancer. However, the incidence dramatically increases with age. Early presymptomatic tests include a blood test for prostate-specific antigen (PSA) and periodic digital rectal examination (DRE). In early stages of prostate cancer, symptoms include dysuria, frequency of urination, loss of bladder control, and hematuria. As prostate cancer progresses, symptoms include blood in the semen, erectile dysfunction, and numbness or pain in the pelvis.

Once diagnosed, oncologists stage and grade prostate cancer to determine appropriate forms of therapy. Very early stages of prostate cancer may not require medical intervention, and many men may never need any further treatment. Nevertheless, active surveillance with blood tests, digital rectal examinations, and possibly biopsies with follow-up is required.

Surgery and radiation therapy are common treatments for prostate cancer. For malignancy confined only to the prostate, surgery that removes the entire prostate, seminal vesicles, and surrounding lymph nodes (**radical prostatectomy**) provides the best treatment option. Because testosterone fuels the growth of prostate cancer, hormone therapy, called **androgen-deprivation therapy (ADT),** is important in the management of the disease. Removal of both testes (**bilateral orchiectomy, castration**) blocks testosterone but is permanent and irreversible, and many men opt for drug therapy. Drug therapy that includes antiandrogenic agents and hormones that deplete the body of testicular hormones (**combined hormonal therapy**) is part of this form of treatment.

Testicular Cancer

Testicular cancer is relatively rare compared with other types of cancer but is the most common cancer in males aged 15 to 35. There are certain risk factors that increase the likelihood of developing this cancer that include being born with an undescended testicle (**cryptorchidism**), and a family history of testicular cancer.

Prevention primarily involves awareness and testicular self-examination (TSE). This can be done by the individual in front of a mirror to first inspect the appearance of the testicle for any changes such as enlargement, and then to feel for any lumps. Any abnormality that is detected should be followed up with prompt medical evaluation.

Treatment for testicular cancer depends on the type and stage but commonly involves surgery to remove the affected testicle (orchiectomy), radiation, and chemotherapy.

Diseases and Conditions

This section introduces diseases and conditions of the male reproductive system with their meanings and pronunciations. Word analyses for selected terms are also provided.

Term	Definition
benign prostatic hyperplasia (BPH) bē-NĪN prŏs-TĂT-ĭk hī-pĕr-PLĀ-zē-ă *prostat:* prostate *–ic:* pertaining to *hyper-:* excessive, above normal *–plasia:* formation, growth	Enlargement of the prostate, commonly associated with aging, narrows the urethra and leads to urinary symptoms including frequency, hesitancy, nocturia, and urinary retention (see Fig. 13-5) *Urine that remains in the bladder commonly becomes a breeding ground for bacteria, causing cystitis and, ultimately, nephritis.*

Bladder

Prostate gland

Ureter

Healthy prostate

Urine

Benign prostate hyperplasia (BPH)

Figure 13-5 Benign prostatic hyperplasia (BPH).

balanitis băl-ă-NĪ-tĭs *balan:* glans penis *–itis:* inflammation	Inflammation of the skin covering the glans penis, caused by bacteria, fungi, or a virus *Uncircumcised men with poor personal hygiene are prone to this disorder.*
erectile dysfunction (ED) ĕ-RĔK-tĭl	Repeated inability to initiate or maintain an erection sufficient for sexual intercourse *Any disorder that causes injury to the nerves or impairs blood flow in the penis has the potential to cause ED.*

Diseases and Conditions—cont'd

Term	Definition
hypogonadism hī-pō-GŌ-năd-ĭzm *hypo-:* under, below, deficient *gonad:* gonads, sex glands *-ism:* condition	Decrease or lack of hormones normally produced by the gonads *Hypogonadism involves a lack of testosterone, which plays a key role in masculinization and development during puberty.*
hypospadias hī-pō-SPĀ-dē-ăs *hypo-:* under, below, deficient *-spadias:* slit, fissure	Congenital abnormality in which the opening of the male urethra is on the undersurface of the penis instead of at its tip
Peyronie disease	Condition characterized by the development of scar tissue and curvature in the penis *Peyronie disease may cause pain and make sexual intercourse difficult and can lead to erectile dysfunction.*
phimosis fĭ-MŌ-sĭs *phim:* muzzle *-osis:* abnormal condition; increase (used primarily with blood cells)	Stenosis or narrowing of foreskin so that it cannot be retracted over the glans penis
priapism PRĬ-ă-pĭzm	Prolonged, commonly painful erection of the penis, which occurs without sexual stimulation *Priapism is associated with sickle cell disease, leukemia, spinal cord injury, and as an adverse effect of drugs used to treat ED. Prompt treatment is necessary to prevent permanent tissue damage that could result in ED or disfigurement of the penis.*
prostatitis prŏs-tă-TĪ-tĭs *prostat:* prostate *-itis:* inflammation	Acute or chronic inflammation of the prostate *Prostatitis is commonly caused by a urinary tract infection or a sexually transmitted infection.*
sterility stĕr-ĬL-ĭ-tē	Inability to produce offspring *In the male, sterility is the inability to fertilize the ovum.*
testicular abnormalities tĕs-TĬK-ū-lăr	Any of the various disorders that affect the testes (see Fig. 13-6)

anorchism
   ăn-OR-kĭzm
    an-: without, not
    orch: testis (plural, testes)
    -ism: condition
	Absence of one or both testicles; also called *anorchia* or *anorchidism*
	Treatment includes androgen (male hormone) supplementation, testicular prosthetic implantation, and psychological support.

Continued

Diseases and Conditions—cont'd

Term	Definition
epididymitis ĕp-ĭ-dĭd-ĭ-MĪ-tĭs *epididym:* epididymis *-itis:* inflammation	Inflammation of the epididymis (see Fig. 13-6[A]) *Epididymitis is most common in males between ages 14 and 35 and is usually associated with STIs, especially gonorrhea and chlamydia.*
hydrocele HĪ-drō-sēl *hydr/o:* water *-cele:* hernia, swelling	Swelling of the sac surrounding the testes that is typically harmless (see Fig. 13-6[B]) *Hydrocele in a neonate usually resolves without treatment within a year. In men and young males, it is commonly caused by inflammation or injury to the scrotum.*
orchitis or-KĪ-tĭs *orch:* testis (plural, testes) *-itis:* inflammation	Painful swelling of one or both testes, commonly associated with mumps that develop after puberty (see Fig. 13-6[C]) *Other causes of orchitis include infection of the epididymis or STIs.*
spermatocele spĕr-MĂT-ō-sēl *spermat/o:* spermatozoa, sperm cells *-cele:* hernia, swelling	Abnormal, fluid-filled sac that develops in the epididymis and may or may not contain sperm; also called *spermatic cyst* (see Fig. 13-6[D])
testicular mass tĕs-TĬK-ū-lăr	New tissue growth that appears on one or both testes and may be malignant or benign (see Fig. 13-6[E])
testicular torsion tĕs-TĬK-ū-lăr TOR-shŭn	Spontaneous twisting of a testicle within the scrotum, leading to a decrease in blood flow to the affected testicle (see Fig. 13-6[F]) *Testicular torsion is a medical emergency because interruption of blood supply may permanently damage the testicle.*
varicocele VĂR-ĭ-kō-sēl *varic/o:* dilated vein *-cele:* hernia, swelling	Swelling and distention of veins of the spermatic cord, somewhat resembling varicose veins of the legs (see Fig. 13-6[G]) *Some varicoceles cause sterility as a result of low sperm production or poor sperm quality. Varicoceles can be treated surgically.*

A. Epididymitis   **B.** Hydrocele   **C.** Orchitis   **D.** Spermatocele   **E.** Testicular mass   **F.** Testicular torsion   **G.** Varicocele

Figure 13-6 Testicular abnormalities.

 It is time to review pathology, diseases, and conditions by completing Learning Activity 13-3.

Diagnostic, Surgical, and Therapeutic Procedures

This section introduces diagnostic, surgical, and therapeutic procedures used to treat and diagnose male reproductive disorders. Descriptions are provided along with pronunciations and word analyses for selected terms.

Procedure	Description
Diagnostic	
Clinical	
digital rectal examination (DRE) DĬJ-ĭt-ăl RĔK-tăl	Screening test in males that evaluates the size and consistency of the prostate (see Fig. 13-7) *In males and females, DRE helps assess the rectal wall surface for lesions and evaluates abnormalities of the pelvic area.* Figure 13-7 Digital rectal examination.
Laboratory	
prostate-specific antigen (PSA) PRŎS-tāt spĕ-SĬF-ĭk ĂN-tĭ-jĕn	Blood test used to detect prostatic disorders, especially prostate cancer; also called *tumor marker test* *PSA is a substance produced by the prostate and found in small quantities in blood. The blood level is elevated in prostatitis, benign prostatic hyperplasia, and tumors of the prostate.*
semen analysis SĒ-mĕn ă-NĂL-ĭ-sĭs	Test that analyzes a semen sample for volume, sperm count, motility, and morphology to evaluate fertility or verify sterilization after a vasectomy

Continued

Diagnostic, Surgical, and Therapeutic Procedures—cont'd

Procedure	Description
testosterone tĕs-TŎS-tă-rōn	Blood test to measure the level of testosterone, the main sex hormone in males, to detect multiple conditions in males and females, including infertility
Imaging	
prostate-specific membrane antigen (PSMA) positron emission tomography (PET) scan	PSMA PET scan is a highly sensitive imaging technique that uses a radiotracer pharmaceutical injected into the bloodstream followed by PET imaging to detect areas of cancer cell growth; used in the diagnosis, staging, and monitoring of prostate cancer *PSMA is a protein that is expressed on the surface of prostate cancer cells. The radiotracer binds specifically to the PSMA on cancer cells. The PET scan then detects the radiation emitted and produces three-dimensional (3D) images that pinpoint the location and extent of prostate cancer and its metastasis.*
scrotal ultrasound (US) SKRŌ-tăl ŬL-tră-sownd	Imaging procedure using sound waves to assess the contents of the scrotum, including the testicles, epididymis, and vas deferens; also called *testicular ultrasound* *Scrotal US helps to diagnose neoplasms, causes of infertility, and structural abnormalities in the testicles.*
transrectal ultrasound (TRUS) biopsy of the prostate trăns-RĔK-tăl ŬL-tră-sownd BĪ-ŏp-sē PRŎS-tāt *trans:* across, through *rect:* rectum *-al:* pertaining to	Imaging procedure using soundwaves emitted by a probe inserted through the rectum to serve as a guide for biopsy of the prostate when prostate specific antigen (PSA) and digital rectal exam (DRE) are abnormal (see Fig. 13-8)

Figure 13-8 Transrectal ultrasound and needle biopsy of the prostate.

Diagnostic, Surgical, and Therapeutic Procedures—cont'd

Procedure	Description
Surgical	
circumcision sĕr-kŭm-SĬ-zhŭn	Removal of the foreskin, or fold of skin covering the tip (glans) of the penis *Circumcision is usually performed on infant males for religious or social reasons.*
laser of the prostate	Use of concentrated light to generate precise and intense heat to destroy excess prostate tissue, primarily for treatment of BPH *Laser surgery provides a minimally invasive option compared with treatments such as transurethral resection of the prostate (TURP) or open prostatectomy. Employing an endoscope inserted through the urethra, lasers target and remove prostate tissue, alleviating urinary symptoms associated with BPH while minimizing risks and hastening recovery. The choice of laser type takes into account factors such as the patient's health, prostate size, and the surgeon's proficiency.*
Green Light	Laser surgery that utilizes a high-energy green laser to vaporize and remove excess prostate tissue; also called *photoselective vaporization of the prostate (PVP)* *Green Light laser is used for moderate to severe BPH with larger prostates and for those at higher risk for bleeding complications.*
holmium	Laser surgery that utilizes a holmium laser to remove excess prostate tissue causing urinary obstruction; also called *holmium laser enucleation of the prostate (HoLEP)*
thulium	Laser surgery that utilizes a thulium laser to remove excess prostate tissue that enables effective tissue ablation while minimizing thermal damage to surrounding tissue; also called *thulium laser enucleation of the prostate (ThuLEP)* *ThuLEP is one of the newest technologies and is considered the most effective BPH treatment that can be performed on prostates of any size with reduced risk of complications compared with other laser procedures.*
orchiopexy or-kē-ō-PĔK-sē *orchi/o:* testis (plural, testes) *-pexy:* fixation (of an organ)	Fixation of the testes in the scrotum *Orchiopexy is performed for undescended testicles (cryptorchidism), usually before age 2, or for correction of testicular torsion.*
prostatectomy prŏs-tă-TĔK-tō-mē *prostat:* prostate *-ectomy:* excision, removal	Removal of all (radical) or part (simple) of the prostate *Several types of prostatectomy procedures are available depending on the extent and reason for removal. Laparoscopic prostatectomy and robotic-assisted laparoscopic prostatectomy (RALP) are becoming more common because they have better results with fewer complications and faster recovery time.*

Continued

Diagnostic, Surgical, and Therapeutic Procedures—cont'd

Procedure	Description

transurethral resection of the prostate (TURP)
trăns-ū-RĒ-thrăl rē-SĔK-shŭn, PRŎS-tāt
 	
  trans: across, through
  urethr: urethra
  -al: pertaining to
	Excision of prostate tissue by inserting a special endoscope (resectoscope) through the urethra and into the bladder to remove small pieces of tissue from the prostate gland (see Fig. 13-9)
	
	The resectoscope is fitted with an electrically activated wire loop that removes tissue when dragged over the site and cauterizes it to minimize bleeding.

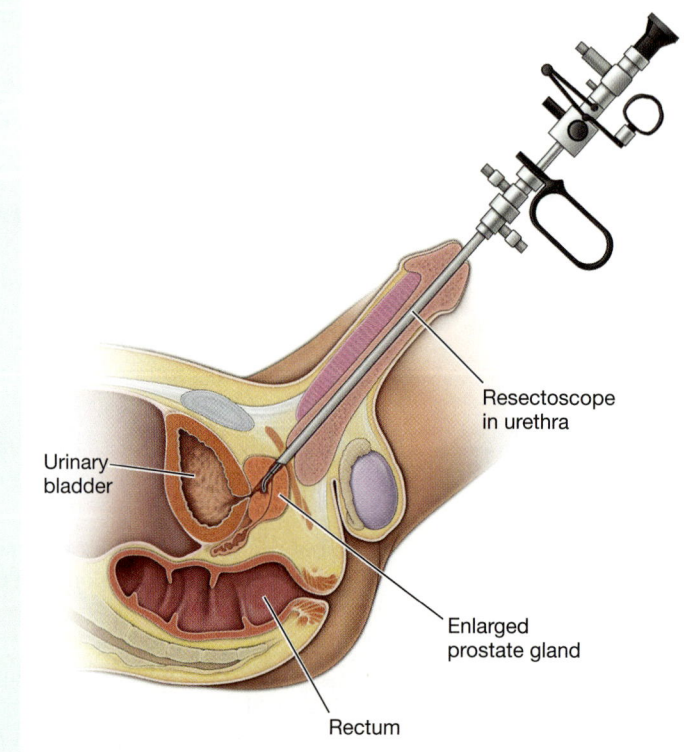

Resectoscope in urethra

Urinary bladder

Enlarged prostate gland

Rectum

Figure 13-9 Transurethral resection of the prostate (TURP).

Diagnostic, Surgical, and Therapeutic Procedures—cont'd

Procedure	Description
transurethral microwave thermotherapy (TUMT) *therm/o:* heat *therapy:* treatment	Treatment for BPH that employs microwave energy to heat a specialized catheter and destroy excess prostate tissue (see Fig. 13-10) 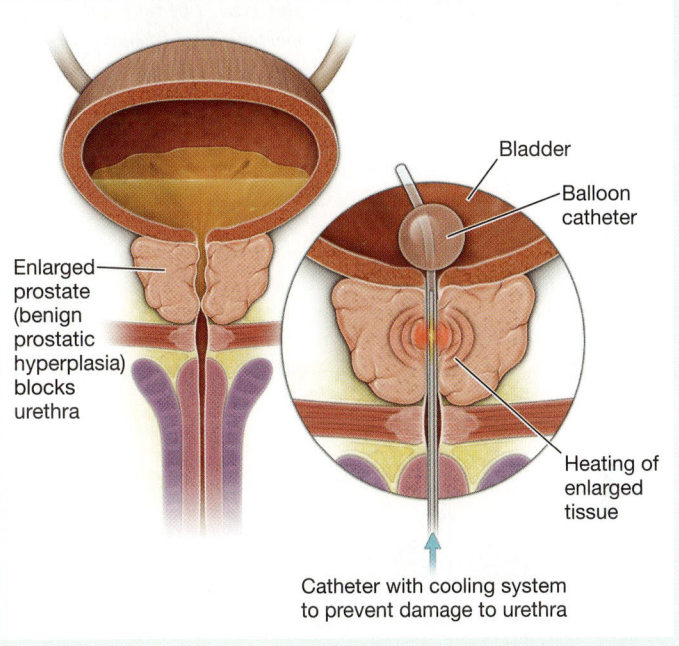 **Figure 13-10** Transurethral microwave thermotherapy (TUMT).
urethroplasty ū-RĒ-thrō-plăs-tē *urethr/o:* urethra *-plasty:* surgical repair	Reconstruction of the urethra to relieve stricture or narrowing *Urethroplasty relieves pain and discomfort experienced during voiding and reduces the risk of contracting orchitis, prostatitis, and urinary tract infections.*

Continued

Diagnostic, Surgical, and Therapeutic Procedures—cont'd

Procedure	Description
vasectomy văs-ĔK-tō-mē *vas:* vessel; vas deferens; duct *-ectomy:* excision, removal	Removal of all or a segment of the vas deferens for male sterilization *Vasectomy reversal (vasovasostomy) rejoins the two segments of the vas deferens. The reversal has the greatest chance of producing a pregnancy if performed within 3 years of the vasectomy. After 10 years, the success rate for producing pregnancy is less than 30% (see Fig. 13-11).*

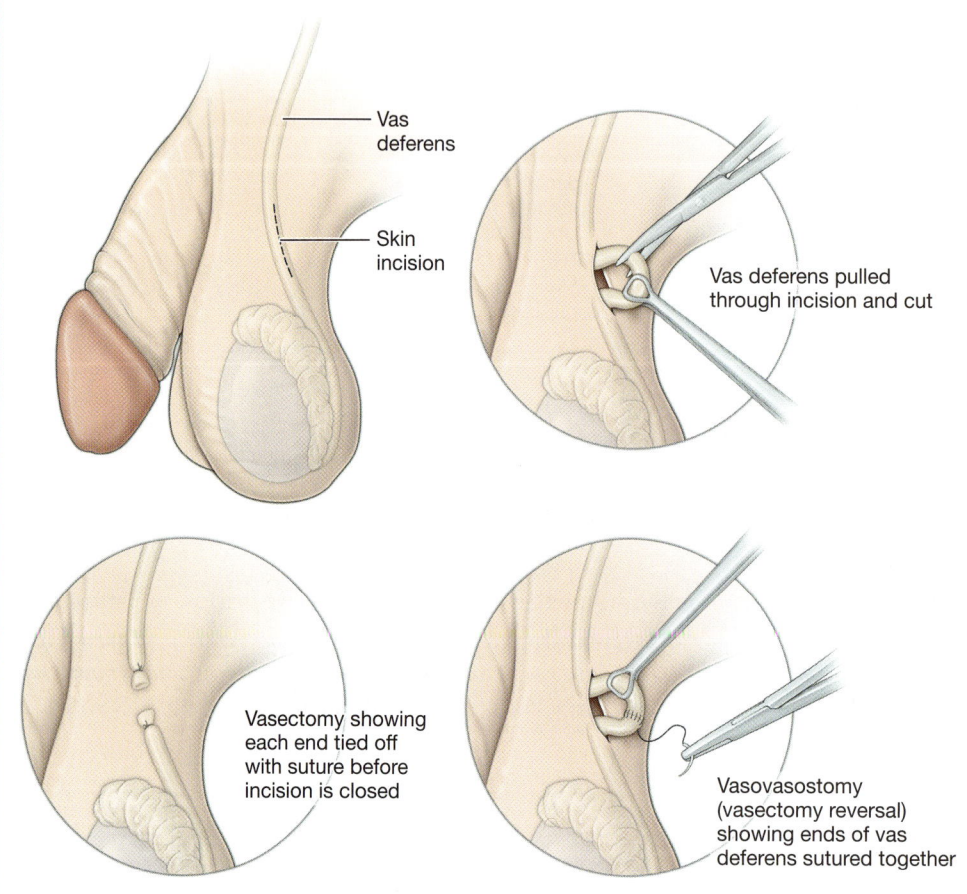

Figure 13-11 Vasectomy and vasovasostomy.

Diagnostic, Surgical, and Therapeutic Procedures—cont'd

Procedure	Description
Therapeutic	

brachytherapy of the prostate
brăk-ē-THĔR-ă-pē
brachy: short (distance)
-therapy: treatment

A type of internal radiation therapy that involves placing radioactive material directly into or near the prostate gland to deliver targeted radiation to cancer cells while sparing much of the surrounding healthy tissue

low-dose-rate (LDR)

Radioactive seeds that emit low levels of radiation are permanently implanted in the prostate through an incision in the perineum and remain indefinitely as the radiation gradually weakens and becomes inactive

LDR is usually performed in a single outpatient session with a relatively quick recovery time. There's a small risk of exposing others to radiation for a short time after the procedure. Patients are advised to follow safety precautions around children and pregnant women (see Fig. 13–12).

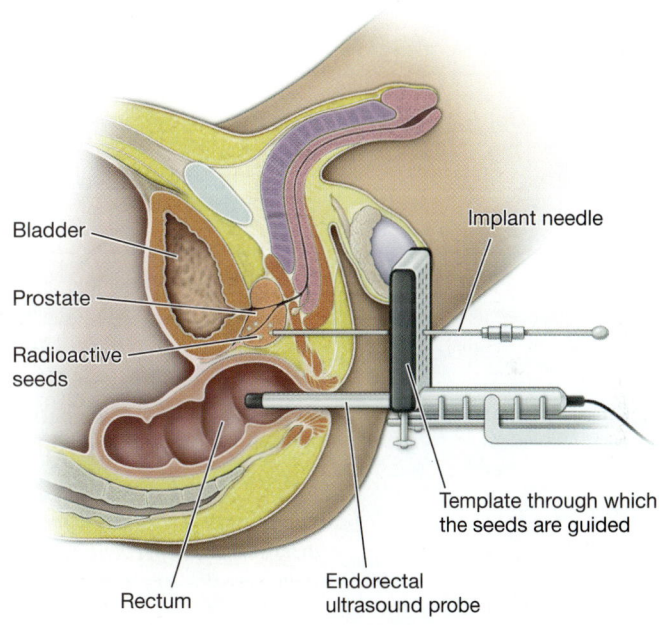

Bladder

Prostate

Radioactive seeds

Rectum

Implant needle

Template through which the seeds are guided

Endorectal ultrasound probe

Figure 13-12 Low-dose-rate (LDR) brachytherapy of the prostate.

high-dose-rate (HDR)

Thin catheters that deliver a high dose of radiation are placed in the prostate temporarily through an incision in the perineum and then removed after a few minutes

HDR is typically delivered over 1–2 days with one to four treatment sessions, Because the radioactive material is inserted and removed during each treatment session, it reduces concerns about long-term radiation exposure.

Continued

Diagnostic, Surgical, and Therapeutic Procedures—cont'd

Procedure	Description
cryotherapy of the prostate krī-ō-THĔR-ă-pē PRŎS-tāt *cry/o:* cold *-therapy:* treatment	Freezing of the prostate, causing cancer cells to die (see Fig. 13-13) *Cryotherapy is used in early stages of prostate cancer or when prostate cancer has returned after other types of treatments failed.* **Figure 13-13** Cryosurgery of the prostate.
external beam radiation therapy (EBRT)	Procedure in which the patient is positioned at a distance from the radiation source, which is then directed at the prostate; also called *external beam therapy (EBT)* or *teletherapy* *EBRT may also be performed before surgery to reduce the size of the tumor or after surgery to prevent recurrence of the tumor. EBRT is usually given five days a week over several weeks and performed outpatient.*

Pharmacology

Several classes of drugs are used to treat conditions of the male reproductive system, including antiviral and antibiotic agents to treat diseases and infections. In addition, hormones help treat hypogonadism and some reproductive disorders (see Table 13-1).

TABLE 13-4 Drugs Used to Treat Disorders of the Male Reproductive System

This table lists common drug classifications used to treat male reproductive disorders, their therapeutic actions, and selected generic and trade names.

Classification	Therapeutic Action	Generic and Trade Names
alpha-1 blockers ĂL-fă	Block alpha-1 receptors in the prostate and bladder, relaxing muscles and improving urine flow in BPH	**tamsulosin** tăm-SŪ-lō-sĭn *Flomax* **terazosin** tĕr-Ā-zō-sĭn *Hytrin*
androgens ĂN-drō-jĕnz	Increase testosterone levels *Androgens, administered topically or intramuscularly, help correct hormone deficiency in hypogonadism and treat delayed puberty in males.*	**testosterone base** tĕs-TŎS-tĕr-ōn *Androderm, Testim* **testosterone cypionate** tĕs-TŎS-tĕr-ōn SĬP-ē-ō-nāt *Depo-testosterone*
antiandrogens ăn-tĭ-ĂN-drō-jĕnz	Suppress the production of androgen *Antiandrogens may stop the growth of certain types of cancer cells and may help treat prostate cancer. Some antiandrogens in combination with alpha-1 blockers help treat BPH.*	**dutasteride** doo-TĂS-tĭr-īd *Avodart* **flutamide** FLOO-tă-mīd *Eulexin*
anti-impotence agents ăn-tĭ-ĬM-pō-tĕnts	Treat erectile dysfunction (impotence) by increasing blood flow to the penis, resulting in an erection *Anti-impotence drugs should not be used by patients with coronary artery disease or hypertension.*	**sildenafil citrate** sĭl-DĔN-ă-fĭl SĬT-răt *Viagra* **vardenafil** văr-DĔN-ă-fĭl *Levitra*
antivirals ăn-tĭ-VĪ-rălz	Treat viral disorders by inhibiting the development of the offending virus *Antivirals do not have the ability to destroy a virus. They are used to treat recurrent herpes in adults and lesions associated with chickenpox and shingles.*	**acyclovir** ā-SĪ-klō-vēr *Zovirax* **famciclovir** făm-SĪ-klō-vēr *Famvir*

Abbreviations

This section introduces abbreviations related to the male reproductive system, along with their meanings.

Abbreviation	Meaning	Abbreviation	Meaning
ADT	androgen deprivation therapy	PSA	prostate-specific antigen
BPH	benign prostatic hyperplasia; benign prostatic hypertrophy	PSMA	prostate-specific membrane antigen
DRE	digital rectal examination	PVP	photoselective vaporization of the prostate
EBRT	external beam radiation therapy	RALP	robotic-assisted laparoscopic prostatectomy
EBT	external beam therapy	STD	sexually transmitted disease
ED	erectile dysfunction; emergency department	STI	sexually transmitted infection
HDR	high-dose-rate	ThuLEP	thulium laser enucleation of the prostate
HIV	human immunodeficiency virus	TRUS	transrectal ultrasound
HoLEP	holmium laser enucleation of the prostate	TSE	testicular self-examination
HPV	human papillomavirus	TUMT	transurethral microwave thermotherapy
HSV	herpes simplex virus	TURP	transurethral resection of the prostate
LDR	low-dose-rate	US	ultrasound; ultrasonography

⊕ *It is time to review procedures, pharmacology, and abbreviations by completing Learning Activity 13–4.*

LEARNING ACTIVITIES

The activities that follow provide a review of the male reproductive system terms introduced in this chapter. Complete each activity and review your answers to evaluate your understanding of the chapter.

Visit the Medical Language Laboratory at medicallanguagelab.com. Use it to enhance your study and reinforcement of this chapter with the flash card activity. We recommend that you complete the flash card activity before starting Learning Activities 13-1 and 13-2.

Learning Activity 13-1
Medical Word Elements

Use the listed elements to build medical words. You may use these elements more than once.

Combining Forms		Suffixes		Prefixes
andr/o	scrot/o	-ary	-ism	an-
balan/o	sperm/i	-cele	-itis	dys-
epididym/o	urin/o	-ectomy	-megaly	epi-
genit/o	varic/o	-gen	-plasty	hypo-
gonad/o	vas/o	-graphy	-spadias	oligo-
orch/o	vesicul/o	-ia	-uria	
prostat/o				

1. scanty sperm (formation) _____

2. swelling of a dilated vein _____

3. excision of the epididymis _____

4. pertaining to genitals and the urinary tract _____

5. excision of a gonad _____

6. condition without testes _____

7. enlargement of the prostate _____

8. surgical repair of the scrotum _____

9. fissure on the dorsum (of the penis) _____

10. process of recording the seminal vesicle _____

11. inflammation of the glans penis _____

12. forming or producing a male _____

13. difficult or painful urination _____

14. excision of the vas deferens _____

15. condition of deficiency (in hormones) of the sex glands _____

Check your answers in Appendix A. Review any material that you did not answer correctly.

Correct Answers _____ X 6.67 = _____ % Score

Learning Activity 13-2
Building Medical Words

Use *orchid/o* (testis [plural, testes]) to build words that mean

1. removal of the testi _____
2. prolapse or downward displacement of the testes _____

Use *balan/o* (glans penis) to build words that mean

3. flow or discharge of the glans penis _____
4. hernia, swelling of the glans penis _____

Use *spermat/o* to build words that mean

5. sperm cell _____
6. embryonic sperm (cell) _____
7. swelling or hernia (containing) sperm _____

Use *prostat/o* to build words that mean

8. inflammation of the prostate and bladder _____
9. discharge of the prostate _____
10. enlargement of the prostate _____
11. stone or calculus of the prostate _____

Use the suffix *-spadias* (slit, fissure) to build words that mean

12. fissure under (ventrum of the penis) _____
13. fissure above (dorsum of the penis) _____

Use *vesicul/o* (seminal vesicle) to build words that mean

14. inflammation of the seminal vesicle _____
15. process of recording the seminal vesicle _____

Use *gonad/o* (gonads, sex glands) to build words that mean

16. disease of the gonads _____
17. hormone that stimulates the gonads _____

Build surgical words that mean

18. excision of (a segment of the) vas deferens _____
19. surgical repair of the scrotum _____
20. treatment using cold (freezing) methods _____

Check your answers in Appendix A. Review any material that you did not answer correctly.

Correct Answers _____ X 5 = _____ % Score

Learning Activity 13-3
Diseases and Conditions

Match the terms with the definitions in the numbered list.

anorchidism	*condyloma*	*hydrocele*	*phimosis*
balanitis	*cryptorchidism*	*hyperplasia*	*priapism*
BPH	*epididymitis*	*hypospadias*	*sterility*
chancre	*gynecomastia*	*leukorrhea*	*testicular torsion*
chlamydia	*herpes*	*Peyronie disease*	*varicocele*

1. growth of breast tissue in males _____
2. STI that causes blister-like lesions in the genital area _____
3. failure of the testicles to descend into the scrotum before birth _____
4. condition of the absence of (one or both) testicles _____
5. stenosis of the foreskin so that it cannot be drawn over the glans _____
6. characterized by the development of scar tissue and curvature in the penis _____
7. swelling and distention of the spermatic cord veins _____
8. twisting of the testicle within the scrotum _____
9. wart located in the genital area _____
10. condition where the urethra opens on the underside of the penis _____
11. inflammation of the glans penis _____
12. persistent, painful erection lasting more than 4 hours _____
13. excessive formation or growth (of tissue) _____
14. fluid in the sac surrounding the testes, causing swelling in the scrotum _____
15. inability to produce offspring _____
16. inflammation of the epididymis _____
17. common STI called the *silent disease* because symptoms are mild or absent _____
18. syphilitic lesion found in primary syphilis _____
19. excessive tissue formation in the prostate gland _____
20. white discharge commonly associated with gonorrhea _____

✅ *Check your answers in Appendix A. Review any material that you did not answer correctly.*

Correct Answers _____ X 5 = _____ % Score

Learning Activity 13-4

Procedures, Pharmacology, and Abbreviations

Match the terms with the definitions in the numbered list.

androgens	circumcision	PSA	TUMT
antiandrogens	cryosurgery	RALP	TURP
antivirals	holmium	scrotal	urethroplasty
BPH	HPV	semen analysis	vasectomy
brachytherapy	orchiopexy	TSE	vasovasostomy

1. treatment for benign prostatic hyperplasia that employs microwave energy to destroy excess prostate tissue _____

2. the type of laser used for the HoLEP procedure of the prostate _____

3. a self-practice that can detect early testicular cancer _____

4. oncology procedure of the prostate using radioactive "seeds" _____

5. laparoscopy using robotic assistance for prostatectomy _____

6. test used to evaluate fertility or verify sterilization after vasectomy _____

7. agents used to increase testosterone levels _____

8. US procedure to assess the testicles, epididymis, and vas deferens for abnormalities _____

9. freezing technique used to destroy cancer _____

10. male sterilization procedure _____

11. surgical repair of the urethra to relieve a stricture or narrowing _____

12. reversal of a vasectomy _____

13. agents that suppress the production of an androgen _____

14. excision of the prostate through the urethra _____

15. blood test to detect prostate disorders, especially cancer _____

16. medications used to treat recurrent herpes _____

17. fixation of the testes in the scrotum _____

18. removal of the foreskin from the glans _____

19. virus causing genital warts _____

20. nonmalignant enlargement of the prostate that is usually associated with aging _____

✓ *Check your answers in Appendix A. Review any material that you did not answer correctly.*

Correct Answers _____ X 5 = _____ % Score

DOCUMENTING HEALTH-CARE ACTIVITIES

This section provides practical application activities in the form of exercises to help students develop skills in documenting patient care. First, read the medical report. Then complete the activities and exercises that follow.

Documenting Health-Care Activity 13-1

Consultation Report: Benign Prostatic Hyperplasia

General Hospital

1511 Ninth Avenue ■ ■ Sun City, USA 12345 ■ ■ (555) 802–1887

Patient: Smith, Milton
Birthdate: 05/10/xx

Consulting Physician: Richard Apper, MD
Patient ID#: 23–3444

CONSULTATION

DATE: 03/04/xx

REASON FOR CONSULTATION: Benign prostatic hyperplasia.

HISTORY OF PRESENT ILLNESS: This 82-year-old white male was admitted 03/04/xx for left inguinal hernia repair and ventral hernia repair. The patient has been seen by this provider in the past and is currently on Proscar. He had a Foley catheter in place postoperatively, which was removed this a.m., and since then the patient has complained of dysuria, frequency, and a feeling of incomplete emptying with weak stream. The patient recently voided 300 cc and then 250 cc again. He feels that he may have to void now. He denies incontinence, nocturia, and hematuria but has had microscopic hematuria. The patient has a history of urinary hesitancy, weak stream, and voiding every 2–3 hours. He has no history of any calculi or genitourinary malignancies. History of urinary tract infection with catheter in the past.

PAST MEDICAL HISTORY: Benign prostatic hyperplasia and hyperlipidemia.

PAST SURGICAL HISTORY: Right inguinal hernia repair x3, lysis of adhesions, ventral hernia repair.

SOCIAL HISTORY: Smokes ½ ppd.

MEDICATIONS: Lipitor, Proscar, Demerol, and Darvocet.

ALLERGIES: No known drug allergies.

PHYSICAL EXAMINATION: Afebrile and vital signs are stable. Urine output is good. Abdomen is soft, and there is suprapubic tenderness. The incision overlies the bladder area, and it is difficult to assess for bladder distention. Digital examination reveals a 4- to 5-cm prostate without nodules.

IMPRESSION: This is an 82-year-old white male with questionable urinary retention. Will hold on postvoid residual check because patient is voiding well. Send a urinalysis and culture and sensitivity. Will pass a catheter if he has any difficulty voiding.

Richard Apper, MD
Richard Apper, MD

RC:kan

D: 03/04/xx; T: 03/04/xx

Terminology

The terms listed in the table that follows are taken from *Consultation Report: Benign Prostatic Hyperplasia*. Use a medical dictionary such as *Taber's Cyclopedic Medical Dictionary*, the appendices of this book, or other resources to define each term. Then review the pronunciation for each term and practice by reading the medical record aloud.

Term	Definition
adhesions ăd-HĒ-zhŭnz	
benign bē-NĪN	
calculi KĂL-kū-lī	
catheter KĂTH-ĕ-tĕr	
culture and sensitivity KŬL-tūr, sĕn-sĭ-TĬV-ĭ-tē	
dysuria dīs-Ū-rē-ă	
hematuria hē-mă-TŪ-rē-ă	
hernia HĔR-nē-ă	
hesitancy HĔS-ĭ-tăn-sē	
hyperlipidemia hī-pĕr-lĭp-ĭ-DĒ-mē-ă	
hyperplasia hī-pĕr-PLĀ-zē-ă	
incontinence ĭn-KŎNT-ĭn-ĕns	

Continued

Term	Definition
lysis LĪ-sĭs	
malignancies mă-LĬG-năn-sēz	
nocturia nŏk-TŪ-rē-ă	
suprapubic soo-pră-PŪ-bĭk	

Visit the *Medical Terminology Systems* online resource center at FADavis.com to practice pronunciation and reinforce the meanings of the terms in this medical report.

Critical Thinking

Review *Consultation Report: Benign Prostatic Hyperplasia* to answer the questions.

1. What is the reason for the present admission?

2. What occurred when the physician removed the Foley catheter?

3. What did the patient's previous history indicate regarding these symptoms?

4. Why was it difficult to assess for bladder distention?

5. Was there a definitive diagnosis identified in the impression?

6. What procedure will the physician perform if the patient has difficulty voiding?

Chart Note: Acute Epididymitis

Homer, Aaron **April 1, 20xx**

DOB: 6/15/XX

CC: Patient is a 31-year-old male presenting with the chief complaint of severe left-sided groin pain, scrotal pain, and urethritis.

HISTORY OF PRESENT ILLNESS: Patient reports symptoms have developed over the last 2 days. He is sexually active, heterosexual, and says he had two sexual partners within the last month, the most recent being 4 days ago. Patient notes a clear urethral discharge.

PHYSICAL EXAMINATION: The patient is uncircumcised, and the prepuce is easily retractable. There are no observable lesions on the glans or shaft, and there is no balanitis. The urethral meatus is normal. A clear discharge is expressed upon compression of the glans, and swabs are obtained for testing. The testes are descended bilaterally, smooth, and without masses. There is moderate pain and tenderness of the left testicle, which is alleviated with elevation of the testicles. There is no evidence of torsion of the spermatic cord. The scrotum is erythematous, and there is a left-sided hydrocele. The left epididymis is palpable, with significant induration and tenderness. The right epididymis is normal and nontender. No inguinal or femoral hernia is felt. There is enlargement of the left inguinal lymph nodes. Rectal examination reveals mild prostatic hyperplasia and tenderness. Urinalysis is positive for leukocytes and bacteria.

IMPRESSION: Acute epididymitis.

Plan: Laboratory tests for chlamydia, gonorrhea, and prostate-specific antigen. Administer intravenous antibiotics, prescribe oral antibiotics and analgesics.

Julia Halm, MD
Julia Halm, MD

D: 04–01–20xx; T: 04–01–20xx

bcg

Terminology

The terms listed in the table that follows are taken from *Chart Note: Acute Epididymitis*. Use a medical dictionary such as *Taber's Cyclopedic Medical Dictionary*, the appendices of this book, or other resources to define each term. Then review the pronunciation for each term and practice by reading the medical record aloud.

Term	Definition
balanitis băl-ă-NĪ-tĭs	
erythematous ĕr-ĭ-THĔM-ă-tŭs	
hydrocele HĪ-drō-sēl	
hyperplasia hī-pĕr-PLĀ-zē-ă	
induration ĬN-dū-rā-shŭn	
inguinal ĬNG-gwĭ-năl	
meatus mē-Ā-tŭs	
prepuce PRĒ-pūs	
prostate-specific antigen PRŎS-tāt, ĂN-tĭ-jĕn	
scrotal SKRŌ-tăl	
torsion TOR-shŭn	

Visit the Medical Terminology Systems online resource center at FADavis. com to practice pronunciation and reinforce the meanings of the terms in this medical report.

Critical Thinking

Review Chart Note: Acute Epididymitis to answer the questions.

1. What were the complaints of the patient?

_____

_____

_____

2. What procedure did the physician perform regarding the urethral discharge?

_____

_____

_____

3. What information does the chart note provide regarding the left testicle?

_____

_____

_____

4. How does the chart note describe the left epididymis?

_____

_____

_____

5. What did the rectal examination reveal?

_____

_____

_____

Constructing Chart Notes

To construct chart notes, replace the italicized and boldfaced terms in each of the two case studies with one of the listed medical terms.

asymptomatic	leukorrhea	prostatomegaly
benign	meatus	pruritus
digital rectal examination	orchialgia	PSA
dysuria		

Mr. R is a sexually active junior at State College. For the last 6 weeks, he was aware of a slight (1) **white discharge** from the tip of the penis but ignored this symptom. He now complains of (2) **pain upon urination,** (3) **intense itching** around the tip of the penis, and (4) **pain in the testicles.** Suspecting chlamydia, the physician will confirm his diagnosis with a swab taken from the urethral (5) **opening** and a urine test for the presence of chlamydia. In the meantime, the patient will begin a regimen of oral antibiotics and will return for a retest in 2 weeks. He was instructed on the benefits of condom use and advised to refrain from sexual activity until his infection resolves.

1. _____
2. _____
3. _____
4. _____
5. _____

Mr. L is a 68-year-old male who presents for his annual checkup. His blood test shows a slight elevation of the (6) **prostate tumor marker** test. During the (7) **manual examination of his lower rectum,** there was no evidence of nodules or lumps on the prostate gland. However, Dr. P noted a slight (8) **enlargement of the prostate gland.** Because Mr. L has (9) **no symptoms** related to the urinary system, his diagnosis is noted as a (10) **nonmalignant** enlargement of the prostate. The patient was advised to have a follow-up examination in 6 months.

6. _____
7. _____
8. _____
9. _____
10. _____

Check your answers in Appendix A. Review any material that you did not answer correctly.

Correct Answers _____ X 10 = _____ % Score

Endocrine System

Objectives

Upon completion of this chapter, you will be able to:

- Locate and describe the structures of the endocrine system.
- Describe the functional relationship between the endocrine system and other body systems.
- Pronounce, spell, and build words related to the endocrine system.
- Describe diseases, conditions, and procedures related to the endocrine system.
- Explain pharmacology related to the treatment of endocrine disorders.
- Demonstrate your knowledge of this chapter by completing the learning and documenting health-care activities.

Anatomy and Physiology

The primary function of the endocrine system is to produce specialized chemicals called **hormones** that directly enter the bloodstream and travel to specific tissues or organs of the body called **targets.** Some hormonal actions cause short-term changes, such as a faster heartbeat or sweaty palms during a panic situation. Others control long-term changes, such as bone and muscle development. Still other hormones help maintain continuous body functions, such as a balance of body fluids and a normal metabolism. The endocrine system also maintains an internal state of equilibrium in the body **(homeostasis)** so that all body systems function effectively. The ductless glands of the endocrine system include the **pituitary, thyroid, parathyroid, adrenal, pancreatic, pineal,** and **thymus** glands and the **ovaries** and **testes** (see Fig. 14-1).

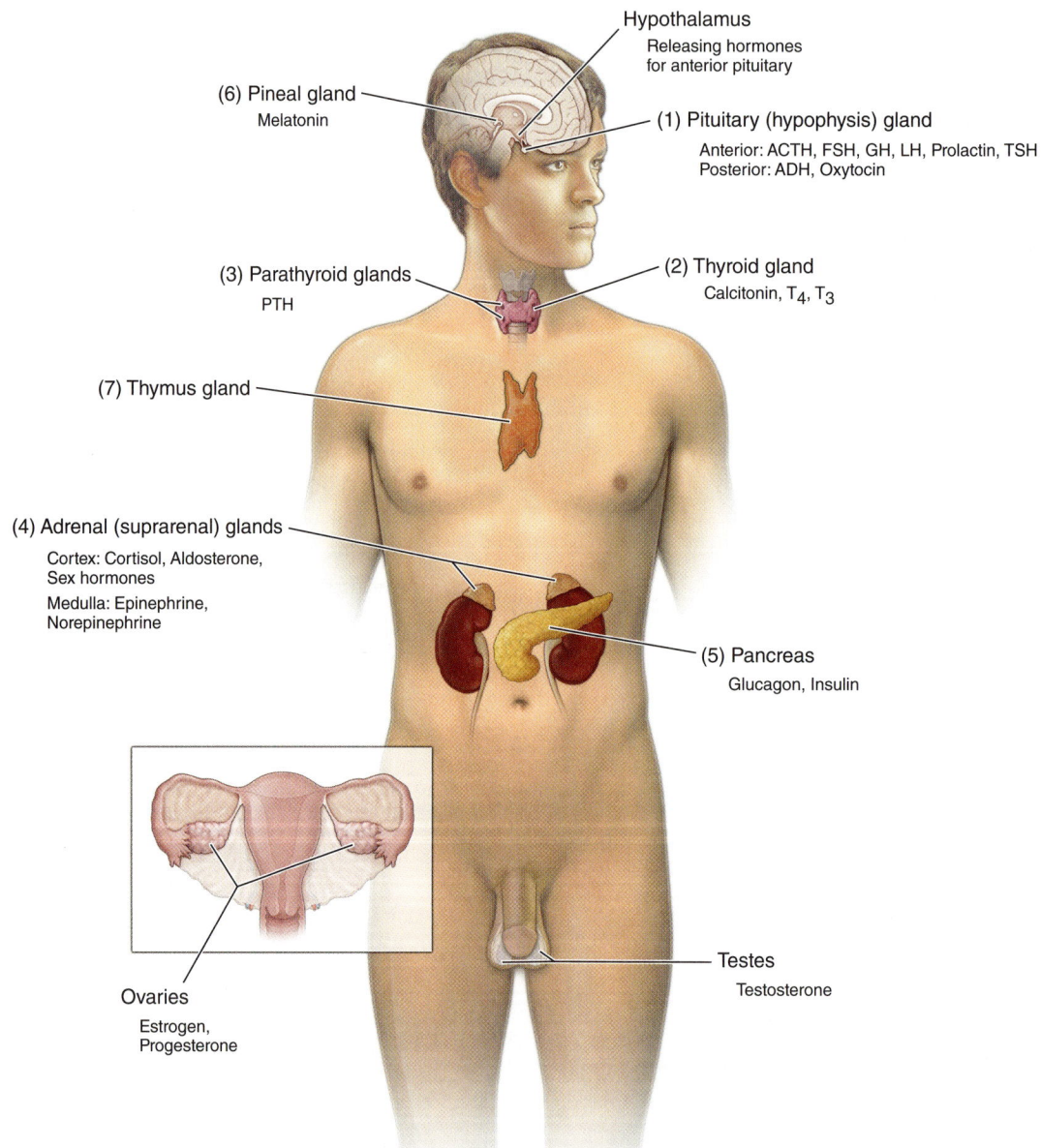

Hypothalamus
Releasing hormones
for anterior pituitary

(6) Pineal gland
Melatonin

(1) Pituitary (hypophysis) gland
Anterior: ACTH, FSH, GH, LH, Prolactin, TSH
Posterior: ADH, Oxytocin

(3) Parathyroid glands
PTH

(2) Thyroid gland
Calcitonin, T_4, T_3

(7) Thymus gland

(4) Adrenal (suprarenal) glands
Cortex: Cortisol, Aldosterone,
Sex hormones
Medulla: Epinephrine,
Norepinephrine

(5) Pancreas
Glucagon, Insulin

Ovaries
Estrogen,
Progesterone

Testes
Testosterone

Figure 14-1 Locations of major endocrine glands.

Although hormones travel throughout the body in blood and lymph, they affect only the target tissues or organs that have specific receptors for the hormone. Once bound to the receptor, the hormone initiates a specific biological effect. For example, thyroid-stimulating hormone (TSH) binds to receptors on cells of the thyroid gland, causing it to secrete thyroxine. However, it does not bind to cells of the ovaries because ovarian cells do not have TSH receptors. Some hormones, such as insulin and thyroxine, have many target organs. Other hormones, such as calcitonin and some pituitary gland hormones, have only one or a few target organs. In general, hormones regulate growth, metabolism, reproduction, energy level, and sexual characteristics.

Anatomy and Physiology Key Terms

This section introduces important terms, along with their definitions and pronunciations. The key terms are highlighted in color in the Anatomy and Physiology section. Word analyses for selected terms are also provided. Pronounce the term and place a check mark in the box after you do so.

Term	Definition
antagonistic ☐ ăn-TĂG-ō-nĭst-ĭk	Acting in opposition; mutually opposing
electrolytes ☐ ē-LĔK-trō-līts	Salts and minerals that conduct electrical impulses in the body *Electrolytes control the fluid balance of the body and are important in muscle contraction, energy generation, and almost every major biochemical reaction in the body. Common human electrolytes are sodium chloride, potassium, calcium, and sodium bicarbonate.*
glucagon ☐ GLOO-kă-gŏn	Hormone produced by pancreatic alpha cells that stimulates the liver to change stored glycogen (a starch form of sugar) to glucose *Glucagon opposes the action of insulin. It is used to reverse hypoglycemic reactions in insulin shock.*
glucose ☐ GLOO-kōs	Simple sugar that is the end product of carbohydrate digestion *Glucose is found in many foods, especially fruits, and is a major source of energy for living organisms. Analysis of blood glucose levels is an important diagnostic test in diabetes and other disorders.*
sympathomimetic ☐ sĭm-pă-thō-mĭm-ĔT-ĭk	Agent that mimics the effects of the sympathetic nervous system, the division of the nervous system that increases the "fight or flight" response *Epinephrine and norepinephrine are sympathomimetic hormones because they produce effects that mimic those brought about by the sympathetic nervous system.*

Pronunciation Help	Long Sound	ā — rate	ē — rebirth	ī — isle	ō — over	ū — unite
	Short Sound	ă — apple	ĕ — ever	ĭ — it	ŏ — not	ŭ — cut

Pituitary Gland

Refer to Figure 14-1 on page 510 to identify the location and function of the endocrine glands. The (1) **pituitary gland,** or **hypophysis,** is a pea-sized organ located at the base of the brain. It is known as the **master gland** because it regulates many body activities and stimulates other glands to secrete their own specific hormones (see Fig. 14-2). The pituitary gland consists of two distinct portions, an anterior lobe **(adenohypophysis)** and a posterior lobe **(neurohypophysis).** The anterior lobe, triggered by the action of the hypothalamus, produces at least six hormones. The posterior lobe stores and secretes two hormones produced by the hypothalamus: antidiuretic hormone (ADH) and oxytocin. These hormones are released into the bloodstream as needed (see Table 14-1).

Thyroid Gland

The (2) **thyroid gland** is the largest gland of the endocrine system. An H-shaped organ located in the neck just below the larynx, this gland is composed of two large lobes that are separated by a strip of tissue called an **isthmus.** Thyroid hormone (TH) is the body's major metabolic hormone.

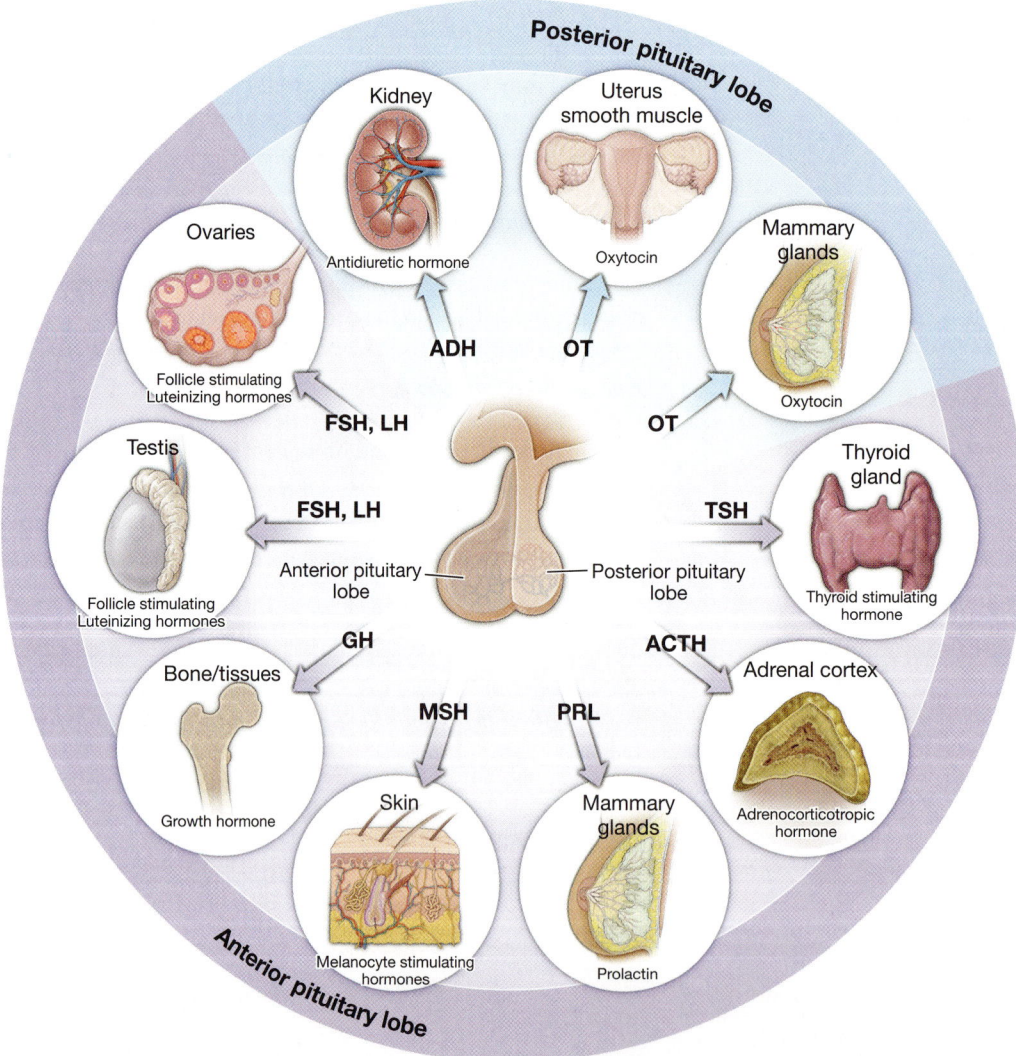

Figure 14-2 Hormones secreted by the anterior and posterior pituitary gland, along with target organs.

TABLE 14-1 Pituitary Hormones

This table identifies pituitary hormones, their target organs and functions, and associated disorders.

Hormone	Target Organ and Functions	Disorders
Anterior Pituitary Hormones (Adenohypophysis)		
Adrenocorticotropic hormone (ACTH)	• Adrenal cortex—promotes secretion of corticosteroids, especially cortisol	• Hyposecretion is rare. • Hypersecretion causes Cushing disease.
Follicle-stimulating hormone (FSH)	• Ovaries—in females, stimulates egg (ova) production; increases secretion of estrogen • Testes—in males, stimulates sperm production	• Hyposecretion causes failure of sexual maturation. • Hypersecretion has no known significant effects.
Growth hormone (GH) or somatotropin	• Regulates growth of bone, muscle, and other body tissues • Increases use of fats for energy	• Hyposecretion during childhood and puberty causes pituitary dwarfism. • Hypersecretion during childhood and puberty causes gigantism; hypersecretion during adulthood causes acromegaly.
Luteinizing hormone (LH)	• Ovaries—in females, promotes ovulation; stimulates production of estrogen and progesterone • Testes—in males, promotes secretion of testosterone	• Hyposecretion in nursing mothers causes poor lactation. • Hyposecretion causes failure of sexual maturation. • Hypersecretion has no known significant effects.
Prolactin (PRL)	• Breast—in conjunction with other hormones, promotes lactation	• Hypersecretion in nursing mothers causes excessive secretion of milk (galactorrhea).
Thyroid-stimulating hormone (TSH) or thyrotropin	• Thyroid gland—stimulates secretion of thyroid hormones	• Hyposecretion in infants causes cretinism; hyposecretion in adults causes myxedema. • Hypersecretion causes Graves disease, which results in exophthalmos.
Posterior Pituitary Hormones (Neurohypophysis)		
Antidiuretic hormone (ADH)	• Kidney—increases water reabsorption (water returns to the blood)	• Hyposecretion causes diabetes insipidus (DI). • Hypersecretion causes syndrome of inappropriate antidiuretic hormone (SIADH).
Oxytocin (OT)	• Uterus—stimulates uterine contractions; initiates labor • Breast—promotes milk secretion from the mammary glands	• Unknown

TH increases the rate of oxygen consumption and, thus, the rate at which carbohydrates, proteins, and fats are metabolized. TH is actually two active iodine-containing hormones: **thyroxine (T_4)** and **triiodothyronine (T_3)**. T_4 is the major hormone secreted by the thyroid; most T_3 is formed at the target tissues by conversion of T_4 to T_3. Except for the adult brain, spleen, testes, uterus, and the thyroid gland itself, TH affects virtually every cell in the body. TH also influences growth hormone and plays an important role in maintaining blood pressure (see Table 14-2).

TABLE 14-2 Thyroid Hormones

This table identifies thyroid hormones, their functions, and associated disorders.

Hormone	Target Organs and Functions	Disorders
Calcitonin	• Regulates calcium levels in the blood in conjunction with parathyroid hormone • Decreases the reabsorption of calcium and phosphate from bones to blood	• The most significant effects are exerted in childhood when bones are growing and changing dramatically in mass, size, and shape. • At best, calcitonin is a weak hypocalcemic agent in adults.
Thyroxine (T_4) and triiodothyronine (T_3)	• Increases energy production from all food types • Increases rate of protein synthesis	• Hyposecretion in infants causes cretinism; hyposecretion in adults causes myxedema. • Hypersecretion causes Graves disease, which results in exophthalmos.

Parathyroid Glands

The (3) **parathyroid glands** consist of at least four separate glands located on the posterior surface of the lobes of the thyroid gland. The only hormone known to be secreted by the parathyroid glands is parathyroid hormone (PTH). PTH helps to regulate calcium balance by stimulating three target organs: bones, kidneys, and intestines (see Table 14-3). Because of PTH stimulation, calcium and phosphates are released from bones, increasing concentration of these substances in blood. Calcium that is necessary for the proper functioning of body tissues is then made available in the bloodstream. At the same time, PTH enhances the absorption of calcium and phosphates from foods in the intestine, causing a rise in blood levels of calcium and phosphates. PTH causes the kidneys to conserve blood calcium and increase the excretion of phosphates in urine.

TABLE 14-3 Parathyroid Hormones

This table identifies the target organs and functions of the parathyroid hormone and associated disorders.

Hormone	Target Organ and Functions	Disorders
Parathyroid hormone (PTH)	• Bones—increases the reabsorption of calcium and phosphate from bone to blood • Kidneys—increases calcium absorption and phosphate excretion • Small intestine—increases absorption of calcium and phosphate	• Hyposecretion causes tetany. • Hypersecretion causes osteitis fibrosa cystica.

Adrenal Glands

The (4) **adrenal glands** are paired organs covering the superior surface of the kidneys. Because of their location, the adrenal glands are also known as **suprarenal glands.** Each adrenal gland is divided into two sections, each having its own structure and function. The outer adrenal cortex makes up the bulk of the gland, and the adrenal medulla makes up the inner portion. Although these regions are not sharply divided, they represent distinct glands that secrete different hormones.

Adrenal Cortex

The adrenal cortex secretes three types of steroid hormones:

1. **Mineralocorticoids,** mainly aldosterone, are essential to life. These hormones act mainly through the kidneys to maintain the balance of **electrolytes** (sodium and potassium) in the body. More specifically, aldosterone causes the kidneys to conserve sodium and excrete potassium (K). At the same time, it promotes water conservation by reducing urine output.
2. **Glucocorticoids,** mainly cortisol, influence the metabolism of carbohydrates, fats, and proteins. The glucocorticoid with the greatest activity is **cortisol.** It helps regulate the concentration of **glucose** in the blood, protecting against low blood glucose levels between meals. Cortisol also stimulates the breakdown of fats in adipose tissue and releases fatty acids into the blood. The increase in fatty acids causes many cells to use relatively less glucose.
3. **Sex hormones,** including androgens, estrogens, and progestins, help maintain secondary sex characteristics, such as development of the breasts in females and distribution of body hair in adults.

Adrenal Medulla

The cells of the adrenal medulla secrete two closely related hormones: epinephrine **(adrenaline)** and norepinephrine (**noradrenaline**). Both hormones are activated when the body responds to crisis situations, and they are considered **sympathomimetic** agents because they produce effects that mimic those brought about by the sympathetic nervous system. Because hormones of the adrenal medulla merely intensify activities set into motion by the sympathetic nervous system, their deficiency does not cause dysfunction.

Of the two hormones, epinephrine is secreted in larger amounts. In the physiological response to stress, epinephrine is responsible for maintaining blood pressure and cardiac output, dilating airways, and raising blood glucose levels. All of these functions are useful for frightened, traumatized, injured, or sick persons. Norepinephrine reduces the diameter of blood vessels in the periphery (vasoconstriction), thereby raising blood pressure (see Table 14-4).

TABLE 14-4 Adrenal Hormones

This table identifies adrenal hormones, their target organs and functions, and associated disorders.

Hormone	Target Organ and Functions	Disorders
Adrenal Cortex Hormones		
Glucocorticoids (mainly cortisol)	• Body cells—promote gluconeogenesis; regulate metabolism of carbohydrates, proteins, and fats; and help depress inflammatory and immune responses	• Hyposecretion causes Addison disease. • Hypersecretion causes Cushing syndrome.
Mineralocorticoids (mainly aldosterone)	• Kidneys—increase blood levels of sodium and decrease blood levels of potassium in the kidneys	• Hyposecretion causes Addison disease. • Hypersecretion causes aldosteronism.
Sex hormones (any of the androgens, estrogens, or related steroid hormones produced by the ovaries, testes, and adrenal cortices)	• In females, possibly responsible for female libido and source of estrogen after menopause (otherwise, insignificant effects in adults)	• Hypersecretion of adrenal androgen in females leads to virilism (development of male secondary sex characteristics). • Hypersecretion of adrenal estrogen and progestin secretion in males leads to feminization (development of female secondary sex characteristics). • Hyposecretion has no known significant effect.
Adrenal Medullary Hormones Epinephrine and norepinephrine	• Sympathetic nervous system target organs—hormone effects mimic sympathetic nervous system activation (sympathomimetic), increase metabolic rate and heart rate, and raise blood pressure by promoting vasoconstriction	• Hyposecretion has no known significant effect. • Hypersecretion causes prolonged "fight-or-flight" reaction and hypertension.

Pancreas

The **pancreas** lies inferior to the stomach in a bend of the duodenum. It functions as an exocrine and endocrine gland. In its exocrine role, it carries digestive secretions from the pancreas to the small intestine through a large pancreatic duct. The digestive secretions assist in the breakdown of proteins, starches, and fats in the small intestine. In its endocrine role, the pancreas secretes two other hormones through the **islets of Langerhans: glucagon,** which is produced by the alpha cells, and **insulin,** which is produced by the beta cells. Both hormones play important roles in regulating blood glucose (sugar) levels:

- **Glucagon** stimulates the release of glucose from storage sites in the liver when blood glucose levels are low **(hypoglycemia),** thereby raising the blood glucose level.

- **Insulin** clears glucose molecules from the blood by promoting their storage in tissues as carbohydrates when blood glucose levels are high (**hyperglycemia**), thereby lowering the blood glucose level and enabling the cells to use glucose for energy.

Insulin and glucagon function **antagonistically**, so that normal secretion of both hormones ensures a blood glucose level that fluctuates within normal limits (see Table 14-5).

TABLE 14-5 Pancreatic Hormones

This table identifies pancreatic hormones, their target organs and functions, and associated disorders.

Hormone	Target Organ and Functions	Disorders
Glucagon	• Liver and blood—raises the blood glucose level by accelerating conversion of glycogen into glucose in the liver (glycogenolysis) and other nutrients into glucose in the liver (gluconeogenesis) and releasing glucose into blood (glycogen to glucose)	• A deficiency in glucagon may cause persistently low blood glucose levels (hypoglycemia).
Insulin	• Tissue cells—lowers blood glucose level by accelerating glucose transport into cells and the use of that glucose for energy production (glucose to glycogen)	• Hyposecretion of insulin causes diabetes mellitus. • Hypersecretion of insulin causes hyperinsulinism.

Pineal Gland

Continue to review Figure 14-1 on page 510 to examine the (6) **pineal gland**, a small organ shaped like a pine cone and located deep within the brain, just behind the thalamus. Although the exact functions of this gland have not been established, there is evidence that it secretes the hormone melatonin. It is believed that melatonin may inhibit the activities of the ovaries. When melatonin production is high, ovulation is blocked, and there may be a delay in puberty.

Thymus Gland

The (7) **thymus gland** is a butterfly-shaped gland that lies at the base of the neck and is formed mostly of lymphatic tissue. The thymus functions as part of the body's immune system (discussed in Chapter 9, Blood, Lymphatic, and Immune Systems) and part of the endocrine system. As an endocrine gland, the thymus secretes **thymosin,** which plays a role in the development of the immune response in newborns. After puberty, the lymphatic tissue gradually degenerates.

Anatomy Review: Endocrine System

To review the anatomy of the endocrine system, label the illustration using the listed terms.

adrenal (suprarenal) glands   parathyroid glands   testes

ovaries   pineal gland   thymus gland

pancreas   pituitary (hypophysis) gland   thyroid gland

 Check your answers by referring to Figure 14-1 on page 510. Review material that you did not answer correctly.

CONNECTING BODY SYSTEMS—ENDOCRINE SYSTEM

The main function of the endocrine system is to secrete hormones that have a diverse effect on cells, tissues, organs, and organ systems. Specific functional relationships between the endocrine system and other body systems are summarized here.

Blood, Lymphatic, and Immune
- Hormones from the thymus stimulate lymphocyte production.
- Glucocorticoids depress the immune response and inflammation.

Cardiovascular
- Hormones influence heart rate, contraction strength, blood volume, and blood pressure.
- Estrogen helps maintain vascular health in women.

Digestive
- Hormones help control digestive system activity.
- Hormones influence the motility and glandular activity of the digestive tract, gallbladder secretion, and secretion of enzymes from the pancreas.
- Insulin and glucagon adjust glucose metabolism in the liver.

Female Reproductive
- Hormones play a major role in the development and function of the reproductive organs.
- Hormones influence the menstrual cycle, pregnancy, parturition, and lactation.
- Sex hormones play a major role in the development of secondary sex characteristics.
- The hormone oxytocin triggers contraction of the pregnant uterus and later stimulates the release of breast milk.

Integumentary
- Hormones regulate the activity of the sebaceous glands, the distribution of subcutaneous tissue, and hair growth.
- Hormones stimulate melanocytes to produce skin pigment.
- The hormone estrogen increases skin hydration.

Male Reproductive
- Hormones play a major role in the development and function of the reproductive organs.
- Sex hormones play a major role in the development of secondary sex characteristics.
- Hormones play a role in sexual development, sex drive, and sperm production.

Musculoskeletal
- Hormone secretions influence blood flow to muscles during exercise.
- Hormones influence muscle metabolism, mass, and strength.
- Hormones from the pituitary and thyroid glands and the gonads stimulate bone growth.
- Hormones govern blood-calcium balance.

Nervous
- Several hormones play an important role in the normal maturation and function of the nervous system.
- Epinephrine and norepinephrine hormones target sympathetic nervous system activation (sympathomimetic), increase metabolic rate and heart rate, and raise blood pressure by promoting vasoconstriction.

Respiratory
- Hormones stimulate red blood cell production when the body experiences a decrease in oxygen.
- Epinephrine influences ventilation by dilating the bronchioles; epinephrine and thyroxine stimulate cell respiration.

Urinary
- Hormones regulate water and electrolyte balance in the kidneys.

Medical Word Elements

This section introduces combining forms, suffixes, and prefixes related to the endocrine system. Word analyses are also provided. From the information provided, complete the meaning of the medical words in the right-hand column. The first one is completed for you.

Element	Meaning	Word Analysis and Meaning
Combining Forms		
adren/o	adrenal glands	**adren/o**/megaly (ăd-rēn-ō-MĚG-ă-lē): enlargement of adrenal glands *-megaly:* enlargement
adrenal/o		**adrenal**/ectomy (ăd-rē-năl-ĔK-tō-mē): _____ *-ectomy:* excision, removal
calc/o	calcium	hyper/**calc**/emia (hī-pĕr-kăl-SĒ-mē-ă): _____ *hyper-:* excessive, above normal *-emia:* blood condition
crin/o	secrete	endo/**crin/o**/logy (ĕn-dō-krĭn-ŎL-ō-jē): _____ *endo-:* in, within *-logy:* study of *Endocrinology is the branch of medicine concerned with endocrine glands and hormones.*
gluc/o	sugar, sweetness	**gluc/o**/genesis (gloo-kō-JĔN-ĕ-sĭs): _____ *-genesis:* forming, producing, origin
glyc/o		hypo/**glyc**/emia (hī-pō-glī-SĒ-mē-ă): _____ *hypo-:* under, below *-emia:* blood condition *Common causes of hypoglycemia include too much insulin, excessive secretion of insulin by the islet cells of the pancreas, and dietary deficiency.*
glycos/o		**glycos**/uria (glī-kō-SŪ-rē-ă): _____ *-uria:* urine
home/o	same, alike	**home/o**/stasis (hō-mē-ō-STĀ-sĭs): _____ *-stasis:* standing still
kal/i	potassium (an electrolyte)	**kal**/emia (kă-LĒ-mē-ă): _____ *-emia:* blood condition
pancreat/o	pancreas	**pancreat/o**/tomy (păn-krē-ă-TŎT-ō-mē): _____ *-tomy:* incision
parathyroid/o	parathyroid glands	**parathyroid**/ectomy (păr-ă-thī-royd-ĔK-tō-mē): _____ *-ectomy:* excision, removal
thym/o	thymus gland	**thym**/oma (thī-MŌ-mă): _____ *-oma:* tumor *A thymoma is a rare neoplasm of the thymus gland. Treatment includes surgical removal, radiation therapy, and chemotherapy.*

Medical Word Elements—cont'd

Element	Meaning	Word Analysis
thyr/o	thyroid gland	**thyr/o**/megaly (thī-rō-MĔG-ă-lē): _____ -*megaly*: enlargement
thyroid/o		hyper/**thyroid/i**sm (hī-pĕr-THĪ-royd-ĭzm): _____ *hyper-*: excessive, above normal -*ism*: condition
toxic/o	poison	**toxic/o**/logist (tŏks-ĭ-KŎL-ō-jĭst): _____ -*logist*: specialist in the study of *Toxicologists study the effects of toxins and antidotes used for treatment of toxic disorders.*

Suffixes

Element	Meaning	Word Analysis
-crine	secrete	endo/**crine** (ĔN-dō-krĭn): _____ *endo-*: in, within
-dipsia	thirst	poly/**dipsia** (pŏl-ē-DĬP-sē-ă): _____ *poly*: many, much *Polydipsia is one of the three "polys" (along with polyphagia and polyuria) associated with diabetes.*
-gen	forming, producing, origin	andr/o/**gen** (ĂN-drō-jĕn): _____ *andr/o*: male
-toxic	pertaining to poison	thyr/o/**toxic** (thī-rō-TŎKS-ĭk): _____ *thyr/o*: thyroid gland
-uria	urine	glycos/**uria** (glī-kō-SŪ-rē-ă): _____ *glycos*: sugar, sweetness

Prefixes

Element	Meaning	Word Analysis
eu-	good	**eu**/thyr/oid (ū-THĪ-royd): _____ *thyr/o*: thyroid gland -*oid*: resembling
exo-	outside	**exo**/crine (ĔKS-ō-krĭn): _____ -*crine*: secrete *Exocrine glands (sweat and oil glands) secrete their products outwardly through excretory ducts.*
poly	many	**poly**/uria (pŏl-ē-Ū-rē-ă): _____ -*uria*: urine *Some causes of polyuria are diabetes, use of diuretics, excessive fluid intake, and hypercalcemia.*

Visit the Medical Terminology Systems online resource center at FADavis.com for an audio exercise of the terms in this table. Other activities are also available to reinforce content.

It is time to review medical word elements by completing Learning Activities 14–1 and 14–2.

Disease Focus

Disorders of the endocrine system are caused by underproduction (**hyposecretion**) or overproduction (**hypersecretion**) of hormones. Hyposecretion is most often treated with drug therapy in the form of hormone replacement. Hypersecretion is most often treated with surgery. Most hormone deficiencies result from genetic defects in the glands, surgical removal of the glands, or production of poor-quality hormones.

For diagnosis, treatment, and management of endocrine disorders, the medical services of a specialist may be warranted. **Endocrinology** is the branch of medicine concerned with endocrine glands and hormones. The physician who specializes in the diagnosis and treatment of endocrine disorders is known as an **endocrinologist**.

Thyroid Disorders

Thyroid gland disorders are common and may occur at any time during life. They may be the result of a developmental problem, injury, disease, or dietary deficiency.

Deficiency of thyroid hormone (**hypothyroidism**) that develops in infants is called **cretinism**. If not treated, this disorder leads to mental retardation, impaired growth, low body temperatures, and abnormal bone formation. Usually, these symptoms do not appear at birth because the infant has received thyroid hormones from the mother's blood during fetal development. When hypothyroidism develops during adulthood, it is known as **myxedema**. The signs and symptoms of this disease include edema, low blood levels of T_3 and T_4, weight gain, cold intolerance, fatigue, depression, muscle or joint pain, and sluggishness.

Hyperthyroidism is a condition in which the thyroid gland produces excessive amounts of thyroid hormone. The most common form is **Graves disease,** also known as **diffuse toxic goiter,** an autoimmune disorder in which the immune system produces autoantibodies that stimulate the production of excessive thyroid hormone. Another cause of hyperthyroidism is the formation of nodules on the thyroid gland known as **multinodular hyperthyroidism** or **toxic multinodular goiter.**

Signs and symptoms of hyperthyroidism include an elevated metabolic rate, abnormal weight loss, excessive perspiration, muscle weakness, and emotional instability. Additionally, the eyes are likely to protrude (**exophthalmos** or **proptosis**) due to edematous swelling in the tissues behind them. This condition is known as **thyroid eye disease** (TED; see Fig. 14-3). Simultaneously, the thyroid gland is prone to enlargement, resulting in the formation of a **goiter** (see Fig. 14-4).

Treatment for **hyperthyroidism** may involve drug therapy to block the production of thyroid hormones or surgical removal of all or part of the thyroid gland. TED treatment includes pharmacological treatment to reduce swelling and pain in the eye. Another method for treating this disorder is to administer a sufficient amount of radioactive iodine to destroy the thyroid secretory cells.

Figure 14-3 Exophthalmos caused by Graves disease.

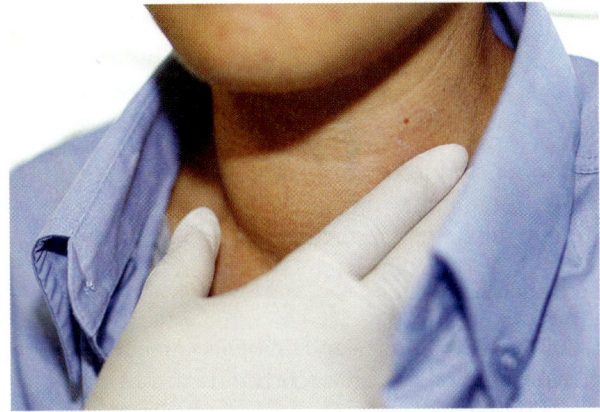

Figure 14-4 Enlargement of the thyroid gland in goiter.

Parathyroid Disorders

Dysfunction of the parathyroids is usually characterized by inadequate or excessive hormone secretion. Insufficient production of parathyroid hormone (PTH), called **hypoparathyroidism,** may be caused by primary parathyroid dysfunction or elevated blood calcium levels. This condition can result from an injury or from surgical removal of the glands, sometimes in conjunction with thyroid surgery. The primary effect of hypoparathyroidism is a decreased blood calcium level **(hypocalcemia).** Decreased calcium causes muscle twitches and spasms **(tetany).**

Excessive production of PTH, called **hyperparathyroidism,** is commonly caused by a benign tumor. The increase in PTH secretion leads to demineralization of bones **(osteitis fibrosa cystica),** making them porous **(osteoporosis)** and highly susceptible to fracture and deformity. When this condition is the result of a benign glandular tumor **(adenoma)** of the parathyroid, the tumor is removed. Excess PTH also causes calcium deposits in the kidneys, which increases the risk for kidney stone formation.

Adrenal Gland Disorders

The adrenal cortex and adrenal medulla have their own structures and functions and their own sets of associated disorders.

Adrenal Cortex

The adrenal cortex is mainly associated with Addison disease, Cushing syndrome, and aldosteronism.

Addison Disease

Addison disease, also referred to as **primary adrenal insufficiency,** is a rare disorder characterized by inadequate production of the adrenal hormones aldosterone and cortisol. The most common cause is autoimmune destruction of the adrenal cortex. Hypofunction of the adrenal cortex interferes with the body's ability to handle internal and external stress. The symptoms of Addison disease can be subtle and develop gradually. They often include muscle weakness, anorexia, nausea, vomiting, fatigue, hypoglycemia, hypotension, low blood sodium **(hyponatremia),** and high serum potassium **(hyperkalemia).** If treatment for this condition begins early (usually with adrenocortical hormone therapy), the prognosis is excellent. If untreated, the disease will continue a chronic course with progressive but relatively slow deterioration. In some patients, the deterioration may be rapid.

Treatment involves corticosteroid replacement therapy with hormones such as hydrocortisone or prednisone to replace cortisol. Mineralocorticoid replacement therapy to replace aldosterone and regulate salt and water balance may also be prescribed.

Cushing Syndrome

Cushing syndrome is a cluster of symptoms produced by excessive amounts of cortisol, adrenocorticotropic hormone (ACTH), or both circulating in the blood (see Fig. 14-5).

Causes of this excess secretion include the following:

- Long-term administration of steroid drugs (glucocorticoids) in treating such diseases as rheumatoid arthritis, lupus erythematosus, and asthma
- Adrenal tumor, resulting in excessive production of cortisol
- Cushing disease, a pituitary disorder caused by hypersecretion of ACTH from an adenoma in the anterior pituitary gland

Cushing syndrome alters carbohydrate and protein metabolism and electrolyte balance. Overproduction of mineralocorticoids and glucocorticoids causes blood glucose concentration to remain high, depleting tissue protein. In addition, sodium retention causes increased fluid in tissues, leading to edema. These metabolic changes produce weight gain and may cause structural changes, such as a moon-shaped face, grossly exaggerated head and trunk, and pencil-thin arms and legs. Other symptoms include fatigue, high blood pressure, and excessive hair growth in unusual places (**hirsutism**),

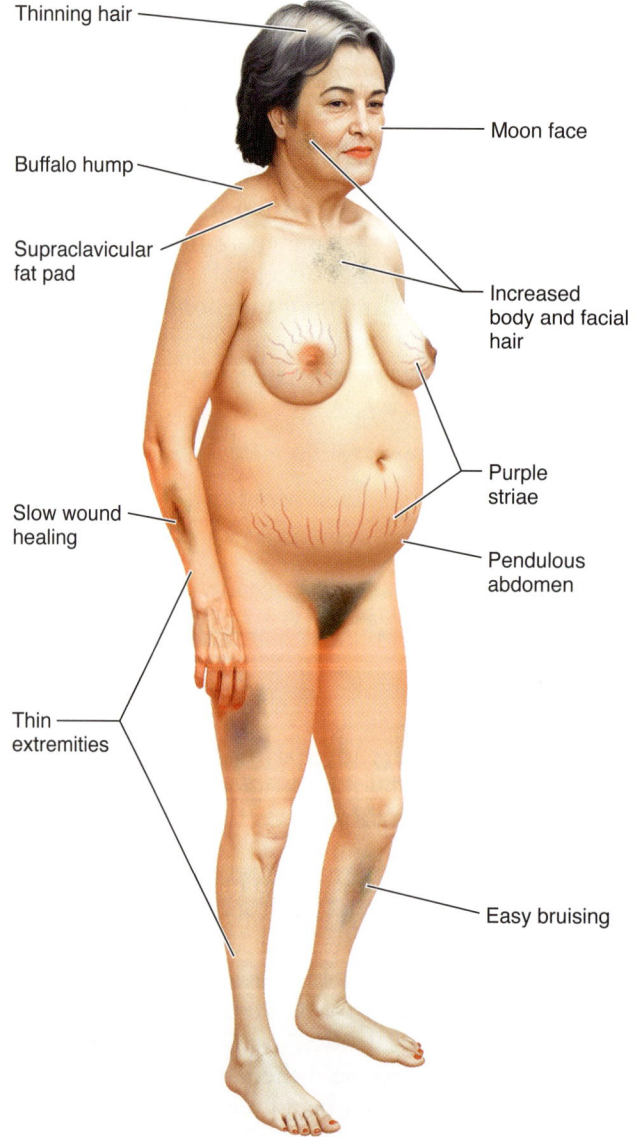

Thinning hair

Buffalo hump

Supraclavicular fat pad

Slow wound healing

Thin extremities

Moon face

Increased body and facial hair

Purple striae

Pendulous abdomen

Easy bruising

Figure 14-5 Physical manifestations of Cushing syndrome.

especially in women. The treatment goal for this disease is to restore serum cortisol to normal levels. Treatment and management of Cushing syndrome depend on the underlying cause. When the cause is a tumor of the pituitary or adrenal gland, surgical removal or radiation may be required. Medical management of symptoms such as hypertension or osteoporosis may also be necessary.

Adrenal Medulla

No specific diseases can be traced directly to a deficiency of hormones from the adrenal medulla. However, medullary tumors sometimes cause excess secretions. The most common disorder is a neoplasm known as **pheochromocytoma,** which produces excessive amounts of epinephrine and norepinephrine. Most of these tumors are encapsulated and benign. These hypersecretions produce high blood pressure, rapid heart rate, stress, fear, palpitations, headaches, visual blurring, muscle spasms, and sweating. Treatment typically involves surgical removal of the tumor.

Pancreatic Disorders

The most prevalent pancreatic disorder is **diabetes mellitus** (DM), a chronic condition marked by elevated blood sugar levels **(hyperglycemia).** The term *diabetes* typically refers to diabetes mellitus. DM is a long-term metabolic disorder that disrupts the metabolism of carbohydrates, proteins, and fats due to either inadequate insulin production or the body's inability to use insulin effectively. When body cells cannot access glucose, their main energy source, hyperglycemia develops as the body starts to break down proteins and fats for energy.

Diabetes stems from a combination of genetic, environmental, and lifestyle influences, with the specific causes differing based on the type of diabetes. DM occurs in two primary forms: type 1 and type 2.

Type 1 Diabetes

Type 1 diabetes is an autoimmune disease. It is usually diagnosed in children and young adults. In type 1 diabetes, the body does not produce a sufficient amount of insulin. Like all autoimmune diseases, it requires constant monitoring and medicating. Blood glucose levels are monitored by the patient several times a day using a **glucometer** to determine the amount of insulin needed to control blood sugar (BS) levels. The patient administers insulin injections as needed. Insulin injections are recommended to be administered in a different subcutaneous site each time to avoid injury to the tissues (see Fig. 14-6). Recent technological advances include a smartphone app (see Fig. 14-7)

Figure 14-6 Rotation sites for injection of insulin. (From Williams LS, Hopper PD: *Understanding medical-surgical nursing,* ed 4, Philadelphia, 2011, F.A. Davis, p. 922, with permission.)

Figure 14-7 This teenage girl is connecting her smartphone app to the continuous glucose monitor (CGM) system to check her blood glucose level.

synced with an insulin pump to monitor glucose levels and deliver appropriate insulin doses throughout the day and night. This avoids the patient having to stick themselves with a needle multiple times each day.

Type 2 Diabetes

In **type 2 diabetes**, either the body's cells are resistant to insulin or the pancreas is deficient in producing insulin. In both cases, the body's cells do not absorb glucose and it remains in the blood, causing hyperglycemia. Type 2 diabetes is the most common form and is distinctively different from type 1. Its onset is typically later in life; however, it has become more prevalent in children as the incidence of obesity has increased. Risk factors include a family history of diabetes and obesity. Treatment for type 2 diabetes includes exercise, diet, weight loss, and insulin or oral antidiabetic agents, if needed (see Table 14-6).

TABLE 14-6 Differences Between Type 1 and Type 2 Diabetes

*This table summarizes the differences between type 1 and type 2 diabetes.**

	Onset	**Low Blood Glucose**	**Prevention**
Type 1 diabetes	• Symptoms usually start in childhood or young adulthood. • Patients commonly seek medical attention because they experience serious symptoms associated with a high blood glucose level.	• Episodes of low blood glucose level (hypoglycemia) are common.	• Prevention is not possible.
Type 2 diabetes	• The disease is usually discovered during a routine checkup, commonly before symptoms occur. • It is commonly diagnosed in adulthood, but an increasing number of children are being diagnosed with the disease.	• There are no episodes of low blood glucose level, unless the person is taking excessive insulin or certain diabetes medicines.	• Healthy lifestyle measures to prevent or delay onset include maintaining a healthy weight, eating sensibly, and exercising regularly.

*Both types of diabetes greatly increase a person's risk for a range of serious complications. Although monitoring and managing the disease can prevent complications, diabetes remains the leading cause of blindness and kidney failure. It also continues to be a critical risk factor for heart disease, stroke, and foot or leg amputations.

Primary Diabetes Complications

The primary complication of diabetes is hyperglycemia and its direct effects on the body. **Diabetic ketoacidosis (DKA)** is a serious complication associated with diabetes, particularly type 1 diabetes, although it can also occur in type 2 diabetes under certain circumstances. Causes include a missed insulin dose, illness and infection, and severe stress. The symptoms of ketoacidosis can develop relatively quickly and typically include excessive thirst (**polydipsia**), excessive urination (**polyuria**), nausea and vomiting, fruity smelling breath, **tachypnea**, confusion, and, in severe cases, coma. Ketoacidosis requires immediate medical treatment, typically involving administration of insulin, along with fluid and electrolyte replacement to correct dehydration and electrolyte balance. Without proper treatment, ketoacidosis can be life-threatening.

Another complication, **insulin shock**, also known as *severe hypoglycemia,* occurs when BS levels drop to dangerously low levels due to an excess of insulin in the body. Immediate treatment is required to prevent serious complications, including loss of consciousness, seizures, and even death. Causes include excess insulin administration, inadequate food intake, alcohol consumption, increased physical activity, and the possible side effect of certain medications that increase hypoglycemic risk when combined with insulin therapy. Treatment is the ingestion of glucose tabs, fruit juice, regular soda, or a glucagon injection given by the patient or medical personnel.

Secondary Diabetes Complications

Secondary, or long-term complications, may occur years after the patient is diagnosed with diabetes. These include:

- Stroke
- Atherosclerosis
- Arteriosclerosis
- Eye disease
- Gastroparesis
- Nephropathy
- Neuropathy
- Diabetic foot

Figure 14-8 illustrates the secondary complications from DM. Keeping glucose levels within the normal range prevents or minimizes long-term complications.

Oncology

Oncological disorders of the endocrine system vary based on the organ involved and include pancreatic cancer, pituitary tumors, and thyroid carcinoma.

Pancreatic Cancer

Most carcinomas of the pancreas arise as epithelial tumors (**adenocarcinomas**) and make their presence known by causing obstructions and local invasion. Because the pancreas is richly supplied with nerves, pain is a prominent feature of pancreatic cancer, whether it arises in the head, body, or tail of the organ.

The prognosis in pancreatic cancer is poor, with only a 2% survival rate in 5 years. Pancreatic cancer is the fourth leading cause of cancer death in the United States. The highest incidence is among people ages 60 to 70. Its aggressive nature and lack of noticeable symptoms until it has reached an advanced stage contribute to its high mortality rate. The etiology is unknown, but cigarette smoking, exposure to occupational chemicals, a diet high in fats, and heavy coffee intake are associated with an increased incidence of pancreatic cancer.

Pituitary Tumors

Pituitary tumors are abnormal growths that develop in the pituitary gland. Some pituitary tumors cause excessive production of hormones that regulate important functions of the body. Other pituitary tumors can restrict normal function of the pituitary gland, causing it to produce lower levels of hormones. The vast majority of pituitary tumors are noncancerous (**benign**) growths

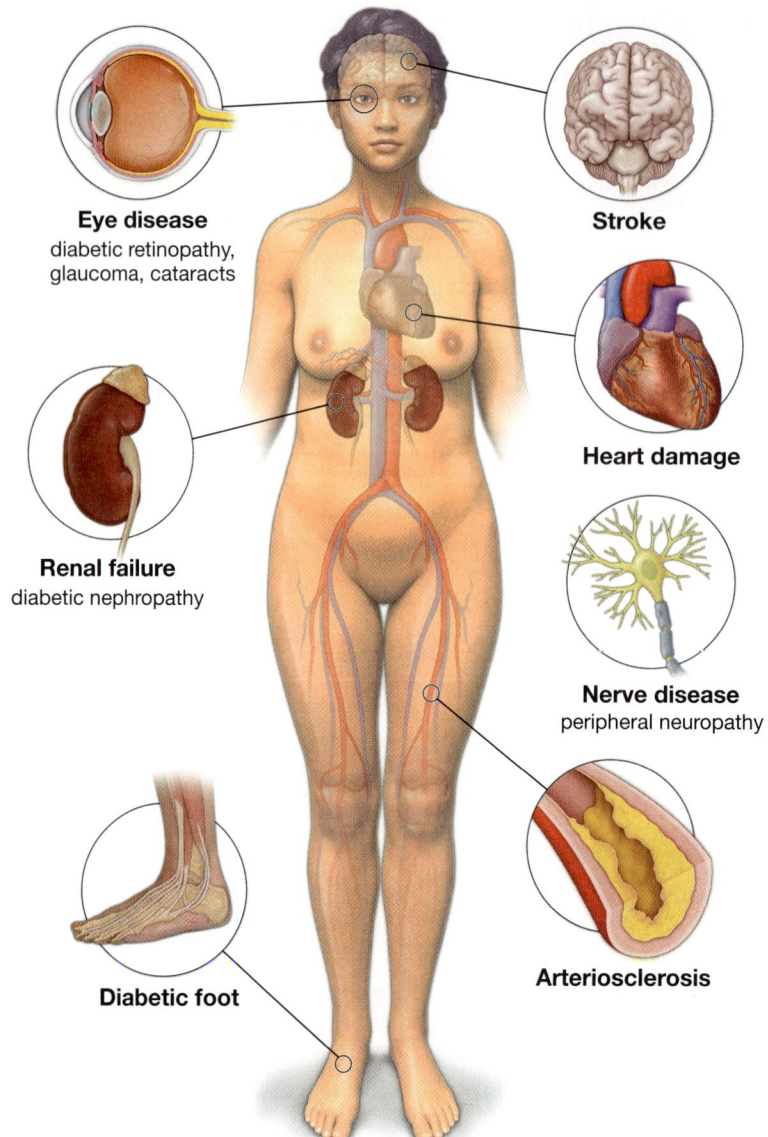

Eye disease
diabetic retinopathy,
glaucoma, cataracts

Stroke

Heart damage

Renal failure
diabetic nephropathy

Nerve disease
peripheral neuropathy

Diabetic foot

Arteriosclerosis

Figure 14-8 Secondary complications of diabetes mellitus.

known as **adenomas.** Adenomas remain confined to the pituitary gland or surrounding tissues and do not spread to other parts of the body. As the tumor grows, it can cause a variety of symptoms, including compression of nearby nerves, resulting in vision problems. Treatment involves removing the tumor, especially if it is pressing on the optic nerves, which could cause blindness. Removal of pituitary tumors commonly occurs through the nose and sphenoid sinuses (**transsphenoidal hypophysectomy**). Other treatment modalities include restoring normal hormone levels or radiation therapy to shrink the tumor. These treatments occur in combination with surgery or for patients who cannot tolerate surgery.

Thyroid Carcinoma

Cancer of the thyroid gland, or **thyroid carcinoma,** is classified according to the specific tissue that is affected. In general, however, all types share many predisposing factors, including radiation, prolonged TSH stimulation, familial disposition, and chronic goiter. The malignancy usually begins with a painless, commonly hard nodule or a nodule in the adjacent lymph nodes accompanied by an enlarged thyroid. When the tumor is large, it typically destroys thyroid tissue, which results in symptoms of hypothyroidism. Sometimes the tumor stimulates the production of thyroid hormone, resulting in symptoms of hyperthyroidism. Treatment includes surgical removal, radiation, or both.

Diseases and Conditions

This section introduces diseases and conditions of the endocrine system, along with their meanings and pronunciations. Word analyses for selected terms are also provided.

Term	Definition
aldosteronism ĂL-dă-stĕ-rĕ-nĭzm	Condition of excessive production of aldosterone that results in abnormal electrolyte levels of sodium and potassium, as well as hypertension; also known as *hyperaldosteronism* *When caused by adrenal adenoma, surgical removal is often the treatment. Other causes may be treated by medications that block the effects of aldosterone and control blood pressure and electrolyte balance.*
diabetes insipidus (DI) dī-ă-BĒ-tēz ĭn-SĬP-ĭ-dŭs	Disorder characterized by excessive thirst (polydipsia) and excessive urination (polyuria) due to inadequate production of antidiuretic hormone (ADH)

diuresis
dī-ū-RĒ-sĭs
  di–: double
  ur: urine
  -esis: condition
	Increased formation and secretion of urine
	
	Diuresis commonly occurs in diabetes. Alcohol and coffee are common diuretics that increase formation and secretion of urine.

gestational diabetes jĕs-TĀ-shŭn-ăl dī-ă-BĒ-tēz	Diabetes that develops during pregnancy (gestation) *In gestational diabetes, the blood glucose level usually returns to normal soon after delivery. However, it places the woman at risk for type 2 diabetes.*

growth hormone (GH) disorders
 	
  acromegaly
  ăk-rō-MĔG-ă-lē
    acr/o: extremity
    -megaly: enlargement
	Pituitary gland disorder that generally involves a hypersecretion or hyposecretion of GH and commonly results from a pituitary tumor
	
	Hypersecretion of GH in adults, resulting in enlargement of bones in the extremities and head (see Fig. 14-9)
	
	Treatment for acromegaly includes radiation, pharmacological agents, or surgery to remove a portion of the pituitary gland.

Figure 14-9 Acromegaly. (A) Hands. (B) Face. (From Chanson P, Sylvie S: Acromegaly, *Orphanet J Rare Dis* 3:17, 2008. Published online 2008 June 25, PMCID. © 2008 Chanson and Salenave, licensee BioMed Central Ltd.)

Continued

Diseases and Conditions—cont'd

Term	Definition
dwarfism	Hyposecretion of GH during childhood, resulting in extreme shortness in stature (final height of only 3 to 4 feet) but normal body proportions *Treatment for dwarfism includes administration of GH during childhood, before skeletal growth is complete.*
giantism	Hypersecretion of GH during childhood, resulting in abnormal increase in the length of long bones and extreme height (up to 8 feet tall) but with body proportions remaining about normal (see Fig. 14-10) *Removal of the pituitary tumor using radiation, surgery, or medications may lower GH hormone levels and control abnormal growth.* **Figure 14-10** Giantism and dwarfism. (From Williams and Hopper: *Understanding Medical-Surgical Nursing*, 7th ed. F.A. Davis, Philadelphia, 2011, p. 743, Figure 39-1.)
hirsutism HĬR-sū-tĭzm	Excessive distribution of body hair, especially in women *Common causes of hirsutism include abnormalities of androgen production, medications, and tumors.*
hypercalcemia hī-pĕr-kăl-SĒ-mē-ă *hyper-:* excessive, above normal *calc:* calcium *-emia:* blood	Condition in which the calcium level in the blood is higher than normal *The main cause of hypercalcemia is overactivity in one or more parathyroid glands. Other causes include cancer, medications, and excessive use of calcium and vitamin D supplements.*
hyperkalemia hī-pĕr-kă-LĒ-mē-ă *hyper-:* excessive, above normal *kal:* potassium (an electrolyte) *-emia:* blood	Condition in which the potassium level in the blood is higher than normal *Potassium is a critical electrolyte in the proper functioning of nerve and muscle cells, including the heart. Severe hyperkalemia requires immediate treatment because it can lead to cardiac arrest and death.*

Diseases and Conditions—cont'd

Term	Definition
hypervolemia hī-pĕr-vŏl-Ē-mē-ă *hyper-:* excessive, above normal *vol:* volume *-emia:* blood	Abnormal increase in the volume of blood plasma (liquid part of the blood and lymphatic fluid) in the body *Hypervolemia commonly results from retention of large amounts of sodium and water by the kidneys.*
hyponatremia hī-pō-nă-TRĒ-mē-ă *hypo-:* under, below, deficient *natr:* sodium (an electrolyte) *-emia:* blood	Lower than normal level of sodium in the blood *Hyponatremia is commonly caused by drinking too much water when exercising (especially in the heat), thereby diluting the amount of sodium in the blood. In the rare occurrence of Addison disease, severe hyponatremia may be present.*
insulinoma ĭn-sū-lĭn-Ō-mă *insulin:* insulin *-oma:* tumor	Tumor of the islets of Langerhans of the pancreas, causing the excessive production of insulin and leading to hypoglycemia; also called *pancreatic tumor*
obesity ō-BĒ-sĭ-tē	Abnormal accumulation of body fat, usually 20% or more of an individual's ideal body weight, or a body mass index (BMI) of 30 or higher *Obesity is associated with increased risk of illness, disability, and death. The branch of medicine that deals with the study and treatment of obesity is known as* **bariatrics** *and has become a separate medical and surgical specialty. Recent treatments also include pharmacological intervention.*
panhypopituitarism păn-hī-pō-pĭ-TŪ-ĭ-tăr-ĭzm *pan-:* all *hyp/o:* under, below, deficient *pituitar:* pituitary gland *-ism:* condition	Total pituitary impairment that brings about a progressive and general loss of hormone activity *Panhypopituitarism can lead to symptoms associated primarily with insufficiency of gonadotropins, growth hormones, and thyroid hormones.*
thyroid storm THĪ-royd *thyr:* thyroid gland *-oid:* resembling	Crisis of uncontrolled hyperthyroidism caused by the release into the bloodstream of an increased amount of thyroid hormone; also called *thyroid crisis* or *thyrotoxic crisis* *Thyroid storm is a medical emergency and, if left untreated, may be fatal.*
virilism VĬR-ĭl-ĭzm	Masculinization or development of male secondary sex characteristics in a woman

 It is time to review pathology, diseases, and conditions by completing Learning Activity 14–3.

Diagnostic, Surgical, and Therapeutic Procedures

This section introduces diagnostic, surgical, and therapeutic procedures used to diagnose and treat endocrine system disorders. Descriptions are provided, along with pronunciations and word analyses for selected terms.

Procedure	Description
Diagnostic	
Clinical	

exophthalmometry
ĕk-sŏf-thăl-MŎM-ĕ-trē
    ex-: out, out from
    ophthalm/o: eye
    -metry: act of measuring
	Measures the degree of forward displacement of the eyeball (exophthalmos) as seen in Graves disease (see Fig. 14-11)
	
	Figure 14-11 Comparison of a normal eyeball compared with the proptosis (displacement) in exophthalmus, a disorder caused by Graves disease.

Laboratory	
fasting blood sugar (FBS)	Test that measures glucose levels in a blood sample after a fast of at least 8 hours *This test helps diagnose diabetes and monitor glucose levels in patients with diabetes.*
glucose tolerance test (GTT) GLOO-kōs	Screening test in which a dose of glucose is administered and blood samples are taken at regular intervals after the dose to determine how quickly glucose is cleared from the blood *GTT is performed to diagnose prediabetes and gestational diabetes.*
glycated hemoglobin (HbA1c) test	Blood test used to diagnose and manage type 1 and type 2 diabetes; also called *glycosylated hemoglobin, hemoglobin A1c* *The HbA1c test result reflects the average blood sugar level for the past 3 months by measuring the percentage of hemoglobin (a protein in red blood cells that carries oxygen) coated with sugar (glycated).*

Diagnostic, Surgical, and Therapeutic Procedures—cont'd

Procedure	Description
insulin tolerance test (ITT) ĬN-sŭ-lĭn	Diagnostic test in which insulin is injected into the vein, causing severe hypoglycemia to assess growth hormone (GH) and cortisol reserve *The symptoms of low blood glucose will cause the release of GH and cortisol. The test measures GH and cortisol at specified intervals.*
thyroid function test (TFT) THĪ-royd	Test that detects an increase or decrease in thyroid function *The TFT measures levels of thyroid-stimulating hormone (TSH), triiodothyronine (T_4), and thyroxine (T_4).*
total calcium test KĂL-sē-ŭm	Test that measures blood calcium levels to detect bone and parathyroid disorders, malabsorption, or an overactive thyroid *Hypercalcemia can indicate primary hyperparathyroidism; hypocalcemia can indicate hypoparathyroidism.*
Imaging	
radioactive iodine uptake (RAIU) and scan rā-dē-ō-ĂK-tĭv Ī-ō-dĭn	Nuclear imaging procedure that combines a thyroid scan with an RAIU procedure to evaluate the structure and physiological functioning of the thyroid gland *The thyroid scan shows the size and shape of the thyroid gland and identifies areas of the thyroid gland that are underactive or overactive. A normal scan shows a uniform distribution of radioactive tracer throughout the thyroid gland. The RAIU measures how well the thyroid gland is able to absorb iodine from the blood (iodine uptake) and evaluates thyroid function and thyroid abnormalities, especially an overactive thyroid gland (hyperthyroidism).*
Surgical	
parathyroidectomy păr-ă-thī-royd-ĔK-tō-mē *para-:* near, beside; beyond *thyroid:* thyroid gland *-ectomy:* excision, removal	Excision of one or more of the parathyroid glands, usually to control hyperparathyroidism *Robotic-assisted techniques are employed where trained surgeons and technology are available. They offer better visualization and precise removal of parathyroid adenomas or hyperplastic glands through small incisions, often using a transaxillary approach.*
thyroidectomy thī-royd-ĔK-tō-mē *thyroid:* thyroid gland *-ectomy:* excision, removal	Excision of the entire thyroid gland (thyroidectomy), a part of it (subtotal thyroidectomy), or a single lobe (thyroid lobectomy) *Thyroidectomy is performed for goiter, tumors, or hyperthyroidism that does not respond to iodine therapy and antithyroid drugs. Robotic-assisted thyroidectomy allows for a transaxillary or retroauricular approach, avoiding a visible neck scar. The robotic arms and high-definition cameras enable precise dissection and nerve preservation.*

Continued

Diagnostic, Surgical, and Therapeutic Procedures—cont'd

Procedure	Description
transsphenoidal hypophysectomy trăns-sfē-NOY-dăl hī-pŏf-ĭ-SĔK-tō-mē	Endoscopic surgery to remove a pituitary tumor through an incision in the sphenoid sinus (transsphenoidal) without disturbing brain tissue (see Fig. 14-12) *Transsphenoidal hypophysectomy is a minimally invasive procedure that is commonly performed to remove abnormal pituitary gland tissue or pituitary tumors. It also treats Cushing syndrome resulting from a pituitary tumor.*

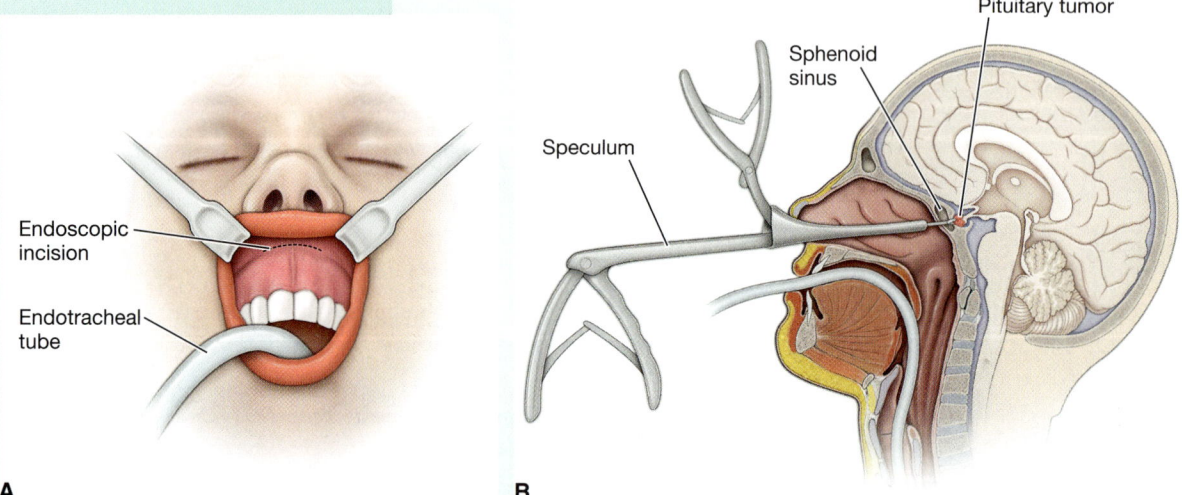

Figure 14-12 Hypophysectomy. (A) Incision made beneath the upper lip to enter the nasal cavity and gain access to the pituitary gland. (B) Insertion of a speculum and special forceps used to remove the pituitary tumor.

Therapeutic

continuous glucose monitor (CGM)	A tiny sensor placed under the skin that constantly monitors glucose levels and sends data to a transmitter, which then wirelessly forwards the readings to a smartphone app (Fig. 14-7) *Users can manually input data such as carbohydrate intake, exercise, or stress, which the app can use to make more accurate recommendations for insulin dosing. All data are recorded and can be used by the health-care provider and patient to effectively manage diabetes. It also means the patient doesn't have to puncture their skin each time they want a glucose reading.*
insulin injection therapy	Lifelong therapy using a fine needle and syringe to subcutaneously inject insulin for controlling type 1 diabetes and sometimes for type 2 *Treatment usually requires a mixture of insulin types or combinations, including long-acting and rapid-acting insulins, to keep blood glucose levels in a target range. The patient calculates insulin types and dosage by monitoring the blood glucose level throughout the day using a handheld monitor such as a glucometer.*

Diagnostic, Surgical, and Therapeutic Procedures—cont'd

Procedure	Description
insulin pump therapy	Device that delivers insulin through a catheter placed under the skin that provides continuous basal insulin and bolus doses for meals or high blood sugar corrections
	Advanced insulin pumps can communicate with the CGM and a smartphone app to adjust insulin delivery based on glucose readings. The smartphone app captures the glucose level and insulin dosing data to help inform the patient and health-care provider to effectively manage diabetes. This system is often referred to as a hybrid closed loop or an artificial pancreas system (see Fig. 14-13).

Figure 14-13 Woman wearing an insulin pump that delivers insulin through a catheter placed under the skin. It can provide continuous basal insulin and bolus doses for meals and high blood sugar readings.

Pharmacology

Common disorders associated with endocrine glands include hyposecretion and hypersecretion of hormones. When deficiencies of this type occur, the physician prescribes natural and synthetic hormones, such as insulin and thyroid agents. These agents normalize hormone levels to maintain proper functioning and homeostasis. Therapeutic agents are also available to regulate various substances in the body, such as glucose levels in patients with diabetes. Hormone replacement therapy (HRT), such as synthetic thyroid and estrogen, treats these hormone deficiencies. Although this section does not cover specific chemotherapy drugs, hormone chemotherapy drugs help treat certain cancers, such as testicular, ovarian, breast, and endometrial cancer (see Table 14-7).

TABLE 14-7 Drugs Used to Treat Endocrine Disorders

This table lists common drug classifications used to treat endocrine disorders, their therapeutic actions, and selected generic and trade names.

Classification	Therapeutic Action	Generic and Trade Names
antithyroids ăn-tĭ-THĪ-roydz	Treat hyperthyroidism by impeding the formation of T$_3$ and T$_4$ hormone *Antithyroids are administered in preparation for a thyroidectomy, in thyrotoxic crisis, and for treatment of Graves disease.*	**methimazole** mĕth-ĬM-ă-zōl *Tapazole* **strong iodine solution** Ī-ō-dĭn *Lugol's solution*
corticosteroids kor-tĭ-kō-STĔR-oydz	Replace hormones lost in adrenal insufficiency (Addison disease) *Corticosteroids are also widely used to suppress inflammation, control allergic reactions, reduce rejection in transplantation, and treat some cancers.*	**cortisone** KOR-tĭ-sōn *Cortisone acetate* **hydrocortisone** hī-drō-KOR-tĭ-sōn *A-Hydrocort, Cortef*
growth hormone replacements	Increase skeletal growth in children and growth hormone deficiencies in adults *Growth hormones increase spinal bone density and help manage growth failure in children.*	**somatropin (recombinant)** sō-mă-TRŌ-pĭn *Humatrope, Norditropin*
incretin mimetics (GLP-1 agonist)	Treatment of type 2 diabetes and weight loss in adults that is given as a weekly subcutaneous injection	**semaglutide** SĔM-ă-glū-tīd *Wegovy, Ozempic* **tirzepatide** tĭr-ZĔP-ă-tīd *Zepbound*
insulins* ĬN-sŭ-lĭns	Lower blood glucose levels by promoting its entrance into body cells and converting glucose to glycogen (a starch-storage form of glucose) *Type 1 diabetes must always be treated with insulin. Insulin can also be administered through an implanted pump, which infuses the drug continuously. Type 2 diabetes that cannot be controlled with oral antidiabetics may require insulin to maintain a normal level of glucose in the blood.*	**regular insulin** ĬN-sŭ-lĭn *Humulin R, Novolin R* **insulin aspart** ĬN-sŭ-lĭn *Novolog* **insulin glargine** ĬN-sŭ-lĭn GLĂR-jēn *Lantus*
oral antidiabetics ăn-tĭ-dī-ă-BĔT-ĭks	Treat type 2 diabetes mellitus by stimulating the pancreas to produce more insulin and decrease peripheral resistance to insulin *Antidiabetic drugs are not insulin, and they are not used in treating type 1 diabetes mellitus.*	**glipizide** GLĬP-ĭ-zīd *Glucotrol, Glucotrol XL* **metformin** mĕt-FOR-mĭn *Glucophage*
thyroid supplements	Replace or supplement thyroid hormones *Each thyroid supplement contains T$_3$, T$_4$, or a combination of both. Thyroid supplements are also used to treat some types of thyroid cancer.*	**levothyroxine** lē-vō-thī-R ŎK-sēn *Levo-T, Levoxyl, Synthroid* **liothyronine** lī-ō-THĪ-rō-nēn *Cytomel, Triostat*

*Traditionally, insulin has been derived from beef or pork pancreas. Human insulin is genetically produced using recombinant DNA techniques to avoid the potential for allergic reaction.

Abbreviations

This section introduces endocrine-related abbreviations and their meanings.

Abbreviation	Meaning	Abbreviation	Meaning
ACTH	adrenocorticotropic stimulating hormone	LH	luteinizing hormone
ADH	antidiuretic hormone	OT	oxytocin
BMI	body mass index	PRL	prolactin
CGM	continuous glucose monitor	PTH	parathyroid hormone; also called *parathormone*
DI	diabetes insipidus	RAI	radioactive iodine
DKA	diabetic ketoacidosis	RAIU	radioactive iodine uptake
DM	diabetes mellitus	SIADH	syndrome of inappropriate antidiuretic hormone
FBS	fasting blood sugar	T_3	triiodothyronine (thyroid hormone)
FSH	follicle-stimulating hormone	T_4	thyroxine (thyroid hormone)
GH	growth hormone	TED	thyroid eye disease
GTT	glucose tolerance test	TFT	thyroid function test
HbA1c	glycated hemoglobin	TH	thyroid hormone
ITT	insulin tolerance test	TSH	thyroid-stimulating hormone

It is time to review procedures, pharmacology, and abbreviations by completing Learning Activity 14-4.

LEARNING ACTIVITIES

The activities that follow provide a review of the endocrine system terms introduced in this chapter. Complete each activity and review your answers to evaluate your understanding of the chapter.

Visit the Medical Language Laboratory at medicallanguagelab.com. Use it to enhance your study and reinforcement of this chapter with the flash card activity. We recommend that you complete the flash card activity before starting Learning Activities 14-1 and 14-2.

Learning Activity 14-1
Medical Word Elements

Use the listed elements to build medical words. You may use elements more than once.

Combining Forms		Suffixes		Prefixes	
acr/o	pancreat/o	-crine	-logist	a-	poly-
adrenal/o	thym/o	-dipsia	-lysis	endo-	
calc/o	thyr/o	-emia	-megaly	exo-	
glyc/o	toxic/o	-genesis	-oma	hyper-	
kal/i		-itis		hypo-	

1. tumor of the thymus _____

2. inflammation of the pancreas _____

3. much thirst _____

4. forming or producing sugar _____

5. (glands that) secrete within (the blood) _____

6. without thirst _____

7. (glands that) secrete outward (through ducts) _____

8. blood condition of excessive sugar _____

9. destruction of the thymus _____

10. enlargement of the thyroid gland _____

11. inflammation of the adrenal glands _____

12. blood condition of below-normal calcium _____

13. blood condition of excessive potassium (an electrolyte) _____

14. enlargement of the extremities _____

15. specialist in the study of poison(s) _____

Check your answers in Appendix A. Review any material that you did not answer correctly.

Correct Answers _____ X 6.67 = _____ % Score

Learning Activity 14-2
Building Medical Words

Use *thym/o* (thymus gland) to build words that mean

1. tumor of the thymus gland _____
2. enlargement of the thymus gland _____
3. incision of the thymus gland _____

Use *kal/i* (potassium) to build words that mean

4. above normal levels of potassium in the blood _____
5. low levels of potassium in the blood _____

Use *glyc/o* (sugar) to build words that mean

6. blood condition of excessive glucose _____
7. blood condition of deficiency of glucose _____
8. forming or producing glycogen _____

Use *pancreat/o* (pancreas) to build words that mean

9. inflammation of the pancreas _____
10. destruction of the pancreas _____
11. disease of the pancreas _____

Use *thyr/o* or *thyroid/o* (thyroid gland) to build words that mean

12. inflammation of the thyroid gland _____
13. enlargement of the thyroid _____

Build surgical words that mean

14. excision of a parathyroid gland _____
15. removal of the adrenal gland _____

✔ *Check your answers in Appendix A. Review any material that you did not answer correctly.*

Correct Answers _____ X 6.67 = _____ % Score

Learning Activity 14-3
Diseases and Conditions

Match the terms with the definitions in the numbered list.

acromegaly	exophthalmic goiter	myxedema
Addison disease	glycosuria	pheochromocytoma
cretinism	hirsutism	thyroid storm
Cushing syndrome	hyperkalemia	type 1
diuresis	hyponatremia	type 2

1. abnormal enlargement of the extremities _____

2. hypothyroidism acquired in adulthood _____

3. increased excretion of urine _____

4. excessive growth of hair in unusual places, especially in women _____

5. congenital hypothyroidism _____

6. crisis of uncontrolled hyperthyroidism _____

7. caused by deficiency in the secretion of adrenocortical hormones _____

8. characterized by protrusion of the eyeballs, increased heart action, enlargement of the thyroid gland, weight loss, and nervousness _____

9. excessive amount of potassium in the blood _____

10. small chromaffin cell tumor usually located in the adrenal medulla _____

11. insulin-dependent diabetes mellitus; occurs most commonly in children and adolescents (juvenile onset) _____

12. decreased concentration of sodium in the blood _____

13. abnormal presence of glucose in the urine _____

14. metabolic disorder caused by hypersecretion of the adrenal cortex, resulting in excessive production of glucocorticoids, mainly cortisol _____

15. noninsulin-dependent diabetes mellitus; occurs later in life (maturity onset) _____

✓ *Check your answers in Appendix A. Review any material that you did not answer correctly.*

Correct Answers _____ X 6.67 = _____ % Score

Learning Activity 14-4
Procedures, Pharmacology, and Abbreviations

Match the terms with the definitions in the numbered list.

antithyroids	exophthalmometry	insulin	TED
CGM	FBS	parathyroidectomy	TFT
corticosteroids	GH	RAIU	thyroid scan
DI	GLP-1 agonists	T_3	total calcium test
DKA	GTT	T_4	transsphenoidal

1. measures circulating glucose level after a 12-hour fast _____

2. detects how quickly ingested iodine is taken into the thyroid gland _____

3. replacement hormones for adrenal insufficiency (Addison disease) _____

4. increases skeletal growth in children _____

5. nuclear imaging procedure that shows the size and shape of the thyroid gland _____

6. excision of the gland that produces PTH _____

7. ketone and acid buildup in the body from hyperglycemia _____

8. condition characterized by inadequate production of antidiuretic hormone (ADH) _____

9. drugs used in the treatment of type 2 diabetes and weight loss in adults _____

10. protrusion of the eyeball due to edematous swelling in the posterior tissues _____

11. thyroxine _____

12. device that reads the continuous glucose levels of the blood _____

13. test to determine how quickly glucose is cleared from the blood _____

14. used to treat hyperthyroidism by impeding the formation of T_3 and T_4 hormone _____

15. type of hypophysectomy to remove a pituitary tumor without disturbing brain tissue _____

16. triiodothyronine _____

17. abbreviation for a test that measures thyroid function _____

18. measures the degree of forward displacement of the eyeball as seen in Graves disease _____

19. used to detect bone and parathyroid disorders _____

20. hormone used to treat type 1 diabetes _____

Check your answers in Appendix A. Review any material that you did not answer correctly.

Correct Answers _____ X 5 = _____ % Score

DOCUMENTING HEALTH-CARE ACTIVITIES

This section provides practical application activities in the form of exercises to help students develop skills in documenting patient care. First, read the medical report. Then complete the activities and exercises that follow.

Documenting Health-Care Activity 14-1
Consultation Note: Hyperparathyroidism

Consultation Note

Day, Phyllis   **5/25/xx**   **Med Record:**   **P25882**

HISTORY OF PRESENT ILLNESS: This 66-year-old former blackjack dealer is under evaluation for hyperparathyroidism. Surgery evidently has been recommended, but there is confusion as to how urgent this is. She has a 13-year history of type 1 diabetes mellitus, a history of shoulder pain, osteoarthritis of the spine, and peripheral vascular disease with claudication. She states her 548-pack/year smoking history ended 3-1/2 years ago. Her first knowledge of parathyroid disease was about 3 years ago when laboratory findings revealed an elevated calcium level. This subsequently led to the diagnosis of hyperparathyroidism. She was further evaluated by an endocrinologist in the Lake Tahoe area, who determined that she also had hypercalciuria, although there is nothing to suggest a history of kidney stones.

IMPRESSION: Hyperparathyroidism and hypercalciuria, probably a parathyroid adenoma

PLAN: Patient advised to make a follow-up appointment with her endocrinologist.

Juan Perez, MD
Juan Perez, MD

D: 05–25–xx
T: 05–25–xx

jp:lg

Terminology

The terms listed in the table that follows are taken from *Consultation Note: Hyperparathyroidism.* Use a medical dictionary such as *Taber's Cyclopedic Medical Dictionary,* the appendices of this book, or other resources to define each term. Then review the pronunciation for each term and practice by reading the medical record aloud.

Term	Definition
adenoma ăd-ĕ-NŌ-mă	
claudication klăw-dĭ-KĀ-shŭn	
diabetes mellitus dī-ă-BĒ-tēz MĔ-lĭ-tŭs	
endocrinologist ĕn-dō-krĭn- ŎL-ō-jĭst	
hypercalciuria hī-pĕr-kăl-sē-Ū-rē-ă	
hyperparathyroidism hī-pĕr-păr-ă- THĪ-roy-dĭzm	
impression ĭm-PRĔSH-ŭn	
osteoarthritis ŏs-tē-ō-ăr-THRĪ-tĭs	
peripheral vascular disease pĕr-ĭF-ĕr-ăl VĂS-kū-lăr	

Visit the Medical Terminology Systems online resource center at FADavis. com to practice pronunciation and reinforce the meanings of the terms in this medical report.

Critical Thinking

Review *Consultation Note: Hyperparathyroidism* to answer the questions.

1. What is an adenoma?

   _____

   _____

   _____

   _____

2. What does the physician suspect caused the patient's hyperparathyroidism?

   _____

   _____

   _____

   _____

3. What type of laboratory findings revealed parathyroid disease?

   _____

   _____

   _____

   _____

4. What is hypercalciuria?

   _____

   _____

   _____

   _____

5. If the patient smoked 548 packs of cigarettes per year, how many packs did she smoke in an average day?

   _____

   _____

   _____

   _____

Documenting Health-Care Activity 14-2
SOAP Note: Diabetes Mellitus

Emergency Department Record

Date: 2/4/xx   Time Registered: 1445 hours

Patient: Pleume, Roberta   Physician: Samara Batichara, MD

Age: 68   Patient ID#: 22258

Chief Complaint: Frequent urination, increased hunger and thirst

S: This 200-pound patient was admitted to the hospital because of a 10-day history of polyuria, polydipsia, and polyphagia. She has been very nervous, irritable, and very sensitive emotionally and cries easily. During this period, she has had headaches and has become very sleepy and tired after eating. On admission, her Accu-Chek was 540 mg/dL. Family history is significant in that both parents and two sisters have type 1 diabetes.

O: Physical examination was essentially negative. The abdomen was difficult to evaluate because of morbid obesity.

A: Diabetes mellitus; obesity, exogenous.

P: Patient admitted to the hospital for further evaluation.

Samara Batichara, MD
Samara Batichara, MD

D: 02–04-xx
T: 02–04-xx

sb:lb

Terminology

The terms listed in the table that follows are taken from SOAP Note: Diabetes Mellitus.
Use a medical dictionary such as *Taber's Cyclopedic Medical Dictionary,* the appendices of this
book, or other resources to define each term. Then review the pronunciation for each term
and practice by reading the medical record aloud.

Term	Definition
Accu-chek ĂK-ū-ch ĕk	
morbid obesity MOR-bĭd ō-BĒ-sĭ-tē	
obesity, exogenous ō-BĒ-sĭ-tē, ĕks-ŎJ-ĕ-nŭs	
polydipsia pŏl-ē-DĬP-sē-ă	
polyphagia pŏl-ē-FĀ-jē-ă	
polyuria pŏl-ē-Ū-rē-ă	

Visit the Medical Terminology Systems online resource center at FADavis.
com to practice pronunciation and reinforce the meanings of the terms in this
medical report.

Critical Thinking

Review SOAP Note: Diabetes Mellitus to answer the questions.

1. How long has this patient been experiencing voracious eating?

_____

_____

_____

_____

2. Was the patient's obesity a result of overeating or a metabolic imbalance?

_____

_____

_____

_____

3. Why did the doctor experience difficulty in examining the patient's abdomen?

_____

_____

_____

_____

4. Was the patient's blood glucose above or below normal on admission?

_____

_____

_____

_____

5. What is the reference range for fasting blood glucose?

_____

_____

_____

_____

Documenting Health-Care Activity 14-3
Constructing Chart Notes

To construct chart notes, replace the italicized and boldfaced terms in each of the scenarios with one of the listed medical terms.

bradycardia	*hypopnea*	*polyphagia*
constipation	*lethargy*	*polyuria*
glycosuria	*polydipsia*	*triiodothyronine and thyroxine*
hyperglycemia		

Ms. H, a 20-year-old nursing student, presents with complaints of (1) *excessive thirst*, (2) *excessive urination*, and (3) *excessive hunger*. She has headaches and occasional blurred vision. Because of her training as a health-care provider, she recognizes that these symptoms are associated with diabetes. She is further concerned because her mother and sister have diabetes. Her laboratory tests indicate (4) *high blood sugar* and (5) *sugar in the urine*. She will be seen by Dr. M for a more complete workup, and he will begin management of her condition.

1. _____
2. _____
3. _____
4. _____
5. _____

Ms. C, a 56-year-old female, presents with complaints of (6) *lack of energy*, (7) *difficulty passing stool*, and "always feeling cold." Although she has decreased appetite, she has slowly gained 12 lb over the last 2 years. Her hair appears thin and brittle. Her physical examination was unremarkable except for a (8) *slow heart rate* and (9) *shallow breathing*. The physician schedules her for a CBC, metabolic blood panel, lipid panel, and (10) T_3 *and* T_4 tests.

6. _____
7. _____
8. _____
9. _____
10. _____

✓ *Check your answers in Appendix A. Review any material that you did not answer correctly.*

Correct Answers _____ X 10 = _____ % Score

Nervous System

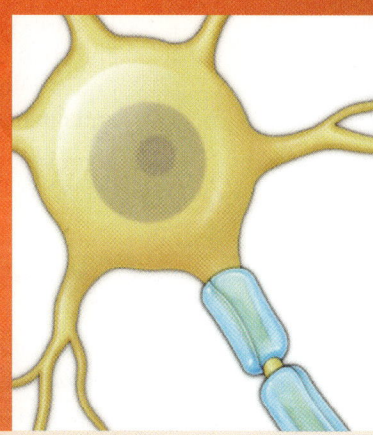

Chapter Outline

Objectives

Upon completion of this chapter, you will be able to:

- Locate and describe the structures of the nervous system.
- Describe the functional relationship between the nervous system and other body systems.
- Pronounce, spell, and build words related to the nervous system.
- Describe diseases, conditions, and procedures related to the nervous system.
- Explain pharmacology related to the treatment of nervous and mental disorders.
- Demonstrate your knowledge of this chapter by completing the learning and documenting health-care activities.

Anatomy and Physiology

The nervous system is one of the most complicated systems of the body in structure and function. It senses physical and chemical changes in the internal and external environments, processes them, and then responds to maintain homeostasis. The nervous system coordinates, regulates, and integrates voluntary activities, such as walking and talking, and involuntary activities, such as digestion and circulation. The entire neural network of the body relies on the transmission of electrochemical impulses that travel from one area of the body to another. The speed at which this transmission occurs is almost instantaneous, thus providing an immediate response to change.

Anatomy and Physiology Key Terms

This section introduces important terms, along with their definitions and pronunciations. The key terms are highlighted in color in the Anatomy and Physiology section. Word analyses for selected terms are also provided. Pronounce the term and place a check mark in the box after you do so.

Term	Definition
afferent ☐ ĂF-ĕr-ĕnt	Carry or move inward or toward a central structure *In the nervous system, afferent impulses carry sensory information from the body to the central nervous system (CNS). These include impulses such as pain, temperature, and proprioception.*
blood–brain barrier	Protective mechanism that regulates the passage of substances from the bloodstream into the brain, allowing essential nutrients while blocking potentially harmful substances from entering delicate brain tissue
efferent ☐ ĔF-ĕ-rĕnt	Carry or move away from a central structure *In the nervous system, efferent impulses travel away from the central nervous system to muscles, glands, or other effectors, resulting in a response or action.*
limbic system ☐ LĬM-bĭk	Complex neural system located beneath the cerebrum that controls basic emotions and drives and plays an important role in memory *The limbic system is primarily related to survival and emotions such as fear, anger, and pleasure (food and sexual behavior).*
neurilemma ☐ nū-rĭ-LĔM-ă	Outermost layer of the Schwann cell that surrounds the myelin sheath on axons in the peripheral nervous system (PNS) *The neurilemma aids in peripheral nerve regeneration after injury by providing a pathway for axonal regrowth.*
ventricle ☐ VĔN-trĭk-l *ventr:* belly, belly side *-icle:* minute, small	Organ chamber or cavity that receives or holds fluid *Cerebrospinal fluid is produced within the ventricles of the brain, then circulates around the brain and spinal cord, and is eventually reabsorbed back into the bloodstream.*

Pronunciation Help	Long Sound	ā — rate	ē — rebirth	ī — isle	ō — over	ū — unite
	Short Sound	ă — apple	ĕ — ever	ĭ — it	ŏ — not	ŭ — cut

Cellular Structure of the Nervous System

Despite its complexity, the nervous system is composed of only two principal cell types: neurons and glial cells, or neuroglia. Together, neurons and glial cells constitute the nervous tissue of the body.

Neurons

Neurons transmit information through electrical and chemical impulses, or signals. Depending on the direction in which they transmit information, neurons and nerves are classified as **afferent** (when the impulse moves toward the brain or spinal cord) or **efferent** (when the impulse moves away from the brain or spinal cord). The three major structures of the neuron are the cell body, axon, and dendrites (see Fig. 15-1). The (1) **cell body** is the enlarged structure of the neuron that contains the (2) **nucleus** of the cell and various organelles. Its branching cytoplasmic projections are (3) **dendrites** that carry impulses to the cell body and (4) **axons** that carry impulses from the cell body. Dendrites resemble tiny branches on a tree, providing additional surface area for receiving impulses from other neurons. Axons are threadlike extensions of nerve cells that transmit impulses to dendrites of other neurons, muscles, or glands at specialized junctions called **synapses** (see Fig. 15-1B).

Axons possess a white, lipoid covering called a (5) **myelin sheath.** This covering acts as an electrical insulator that reduces the possibility of an impulse stimulating adjacent nerves. It also accelerates impulse transmission through the axon. On nerves in the **peripheral nervous system (PNS),** the myelin sheath is formed by a glial cell called a (6) **Schwann cell** that wraps tightly around the axon. Its exterior surface forms a thin tube called the (7) **neurilemma,** or **neurolemma.**

Figure 15-1 Neuron. (A) Schwann cell. (B) Synapse.

The neurilemma acts as a protective coat for peripheral neurons. If the neurilemma covering remains intact after an injury to the nerve, it forms a tube that provides a pathway for possible neuron regeneration after injury.

Oligodendrocytes, rather than Schwann cells, are glial cells that form the myelin sheath covering the axons in the CNS. Oligodendrocytes do not produce neurilemma, and this is one reason that injury or damage to neurons located in the CNS is much more challenging to repair. The short, unmyelinated spaces between adjacent segments of the myelin sheath are called (8) **nodes of Ranvier.** These nodes help speed the transmission of impulses down the axon.

The functional connection between two neurons or between a neuron and its effector organ (muscle or gland) is a gap or space called a (9) **synaptic cleft.** Impulses must travel from the (10) **axon terminal** of one neuron, the presynaptic neuron, to the dendrite of the next neuron, the postsynaptic neuron, or to its effector organ, by crossing this space. The impulse within the transmitting axon causes chemical substances called (11) **neurotransmitters** to be released into and diffused across the synaptic cleft to bind to receptors on the postsynaptic neuron membrane. If the postsynaptic neuron receives enough excitatory input, it may generate its own impulse, continuing the signal transmission process. The termination of a signal occurs when neurotransmitter molecules are removed from the synaptic cleft through various mechanisms such as reuptake, enzymatic degradation, or diffusion. Once the neurotransmitter molecules are removed from the synaptic cleft, the postsynaptic neuron returns to its resting state until it receives another signal.

Glial Cells

Glial cells, also known as **neuroglia,** are nonneuronal cells that provide support and protection to neurons. They play essential roles in supporting the structure and function of neurons, aiding in neural development, and engaging in tasks like neuronal repair and immune defense within the nervous system. The five major types of glial cells are Schwann cells (Fig. 15-1A), astrocytes, oligodendrocytes, microglia, and ependymal cells (see Fig. 15-2).

Oligodendrocyte

Microglia

Endymal cells

Astrocyte

Figure 15-2 Glial cells of the central nervous system (CNS).

Schwann cells produce myelin on the axons of neurons in the PNS. **Astrocytes** are star-shaped glial cells that provide three-dimensional mechanical support for neurons and regulate the chemical environment of the brain by taking up excess neurotransmitters. They also contribute to the blood–brain barrier by forming tight sheaths around the capillaries of the brain.

Oligodendrocytes, also called **oligodendroglia,** are responsible for developing myelin on the axons of neurons in the CNS. **Microglia,** the smallest of the glial cells, act as the primary immune defense in the CNS, protecting against pathogens and removing damaged cells and debris through their phagocytic properties. **Ependymal cells** are ciliated cells that line the fluid-filled cavities of the CNS, especially the **ventricles** of the brain. They assist in the production and circulation of cerebrospinal fluid (CSF).

Nervous System Divisions

The two major divisions of the nervous system are the central nervous system and the peripheral nervous system (see Fig. 15-3). The central nervous system consists of all nervous tissue located in the brain and spinal cord. The peripheral nervous system includes all nervous tissue located outside the central nervous system and is divided into two main components: the somatic and the autonomic nervous systems.

Central Nervous System

The **central nervous system (CNS)** consists of the brain and spinal cord. It is the primary control center and responsible for processing information, coordinating actions, and transmitting signals to all parts of the body. Its nervous tissue consists of **white matter** and **gray matter.** Bundles of axons and their white lipoid myelin sheaths constitute white matter, forming tracts or pathways that facilitate the transmission of signals between different regions of the brain and spinal cord. Unmyelinated fibers, dendrites, and nerve cell bodies make up the gray matter of the brain and spinal cord. Gray matter serves as the primary site for integrating and processing neural signals.

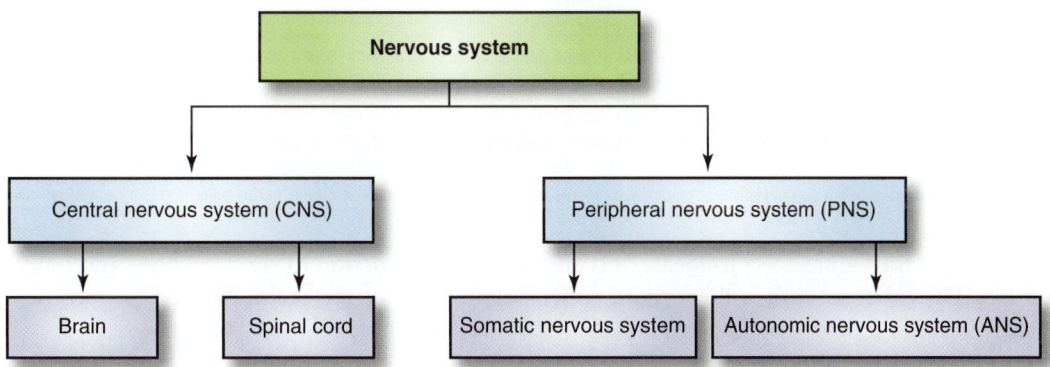

Figure 15-3 Major divisions of the nervous system.

Brain

In addition to being one of the largest organs of the body, the brain is highly complex in structure and function. It integrates almost every physical and mental activity of the body and is the center for memory, emotion, thought, judgment, reasoning, and consciousness. The brain can be divided into lobes that are named by the bones that lie directly above them. Figure 15-4 contains the lobes of the brain and their location and functions.

The brain's four primary structures include the:

• Cerebrum
• Cerebellum
• Diencephalon
• Brainstem

Parietal lobe
Perception
Object classification
Spelling
Knowledge of numbers
Spatial perception

Frontal lobe
Thinking
Problem solving
Emotions
Behavioral control
Decision making

Occipital lobe
Vision
Color determination
Face recognition
Object recognition

Broca area
Language expression

Temporal lobe
Hearing
Language
Memory

Cerebellum
Balance
Coordination

Brain stem
Heartbeat
Breathing
Blood pressure
Swallowing

Figure 15-4 Lobes of the brain and their function (left lateral view)

Cerebrum

Follow along with Figure 15-5 to locate and understand the function of the structures and lobes of the brain. The (1) **cerebrum** is the largest, uppermost portion of the brain. Major functions of the cerebrum include sensory perception and interpretation, language, voluntary movement, and memory. It consists of two hemispheres divided by a deep groove called the **longitudinal fissure.** The fissure does not completely separate the hemispheres. A structure called the (2) **corpus callosum** joins these hemispheres, permitting communication between the right and left sides of the brain. The left side of the brain is adept at tasks involving logic, analytical thinking, reasoning, language, and numbers. The right side of the brain is adept at expressive and creative tasks, intuition, music, and art. Each hemisphere consists of lobes: (3) **frontal,** (4) **parietal,** (5) **temporal,** and (6) **occipital.**

The cerebral surface consists of numerous folds, or convolutions, called **gyri.** The gyri are separated by furrows, or fissures, called **sulci**. A thin layer called the **cerebral cortex** covers the entire cerebrum and is composed of gray matter. Most information processing occurs in the cerebral cortex. White matter is also present, forming connections within the cerebrum and with other parts of the brain.

There are other crucial components of the cerebrum including the basal ganglia, cerebral ventricles, and the limbic system. The basal ganglia is involved in motor control, reward processing, and procedural learning. The ventricles are fluid-filled cavities within the cerebrum that produce and circulate cerebrospinal fluid (CSF).

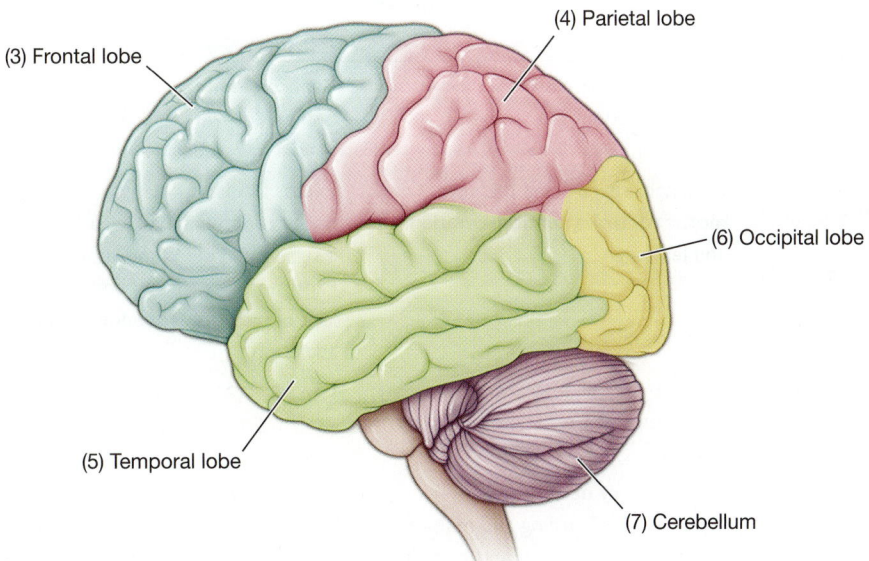

Figure 15-5 Brain structures.

Deep within the brain, just under the cerebral hemispheres, is a primitive "emotional brain" called the **limbic system** (see Fig. 15-6). The limbic system is essential for survival and works in conjunction with the "thinking brain." It regulates behaviors like rage, fear, and anger, as well as emotional facets such as appetite, pleasure, and sexual activity. Mental and emotional disorders are commonly the result of an imbalance of brain chemicals (neurotransmitters) or electrical activity in the limbic system. Table 15-1 describes the main neurotransmitters of the brain.

Cerebellum

The second largest structure of the brain, the (7) **cerebellum,** occupies the posterior portion of the skull. Most functions of the cerebellum involve movement, posture, or balance. When the cerebrum initiates muscular movement, the cerebellum coordinates and refines it.

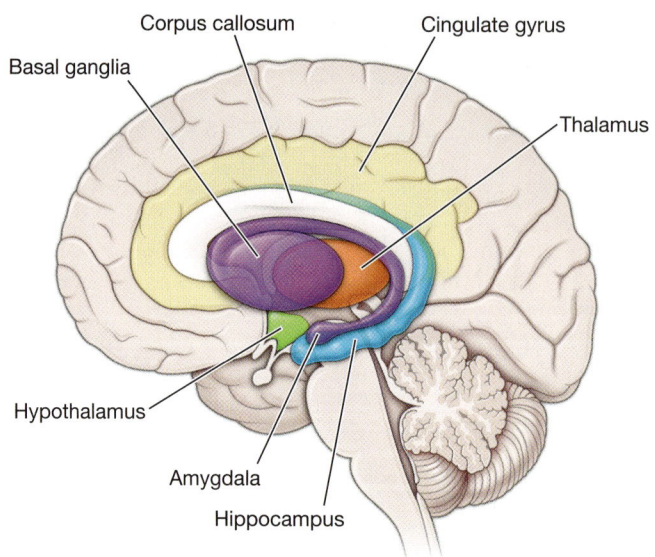

Basal ganglia
Corpus callosum
Cingulate gyrus
Thalamus
Hypothalamus
Amygdala
Hippocampus

Figure 15-6 Limbic system.

TABLE 15-1 Neurotransmitters

Neurotransmitter	Function	Clinical Significance
Acetylcholine (Ach)	Role in learning, memory, thought, and muscle function	Reduced levels are linked to Alzheimer disease; dysfunction with Ach receptors (AchR) plays a role in myasthenia gravis (MG).
Dopamine (DA)	Influences reward and pleasure, motor control, attention, emotion, and learning	Excess DA is associated with positive symptoms of schizophrenia (hallucinations); lack of DA plays a significant role in movement disorders such as Parkinson disease and depressive disorders with lack of pleasure (anhedonia); plays a large role in addiction.
Gamma-Aminobutyric Acid (GABA)	An inhibitory neurotransmitter; has effects on sleep, muscle tone, and anxiety	Low levels can cause anxiety, pain, and seizures.
Glutamate	An excitatory neurotransmitter; important for learning and memory, neural communication, and synaptic growth	Oversupply can lead to seizures; dysregulation is implicated in the cognitive symptoms of schizophrenia.
Norepinephrine (NE)	Important role in arousal, attention, and fight or flight stress response	Lack of NE contributes to difficulties with focus seen in ADHD; excess amounts can lead to hypertension (HTN) and excessive stress response.
Serotonin (5-HT)	Influences sleep, mood, anxiety, sensory perception, and memory	Deficits in 5-HT can lead to depression and anxiety.

Diencephalon

Continue with Figure 15-5 to locate the (8) **diencephalon** (also called the **interbrain**), composed of many smaller structures, including the thalamus and the hypothalamus. The (9) **thalamus** acts as a relay station for sensory information, passing signals from sensory receptors, except olfactory stimuli, throughout the body to the cerebral cortex. In addition, the thalamus plays a role in regulating consciousness, sleep, and alertness. The (10) **hypothalamus** regulates involuntary activities to maintain homeostasis, including body temperature and the sleep-wake cycle. Other key functions include controlling appetite and thirst, managing emotional responses, endocrine hormone balance, and emotional responses and behaviors.

Brainstem

The **brainstem** is composed of three structures: the (11) **midbrain** (also called the **mesencephalon**) separates the cerebrum from the brainstem, and the (12) **pons**, or "bridge," connects the midbrain to the (13) **medulla oblongata**, which attaches to the spinal cord. In general, the brainstem is a pathway for impulse conduction between the brain and spinal cord. The brainstem is the origin of 10 of the 12 pairs of cranial nerves and controls many vital functions necessary for survival, including respiration, blood pressure, and heart rate. The brainstem is the site that controls the beginning of life (initiation of the heartbeat in a fetus) and the end of life (cessation of respiration and heart activity).

Spinal Cord

The **spinal cord** transmits sensory impulses from the body to the brain and motor impulses from the brain to the muscles and organs of the body. The sensory nerve tracts are called **ascending tracts** because the direction of the impulse is upward to the brain. Conversely, motor nerve tracts are called **descending tracts** because they carry impulses in a downward direction to muscles and organs. A cross-sectional view of the spinal cord reveals an inner area of gray matter composed of cell bodies and dendrites and an outer area of white matter composed of myelinated tissue of the ascending and descending tracts (see Fig. 15-7).

The entire spinal cord is located within the spinal cavity of the vertebral column, with spinal nerves exiting between the intervertebral spaces throughout almost the entire length of the

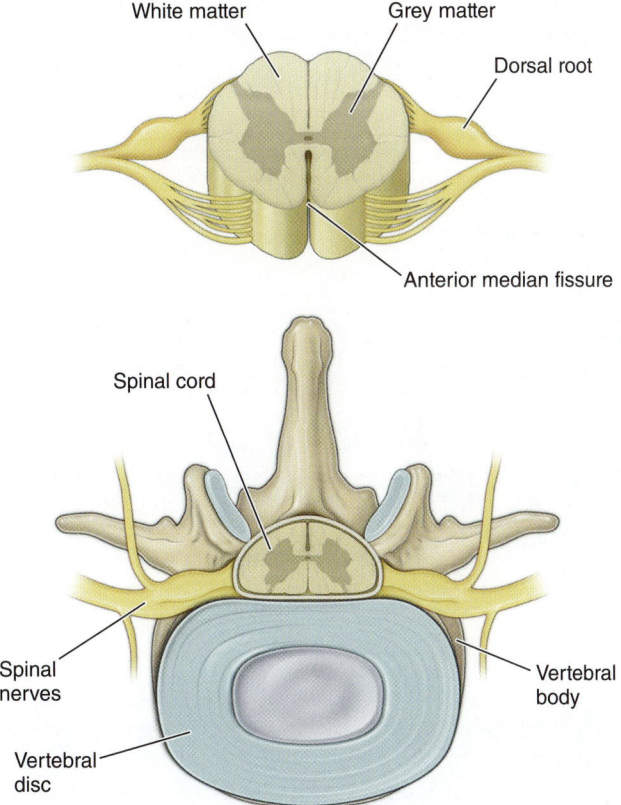

Figure 15-7 Cross section of a vertebra in the spinal cord.

spinal column. The spinal nerves are identified by the region of the vertebral column from which they exit.

Meninges

The brain and spinal cord receive limited protection from three coverings called **meninges** (singular, **meninx**). These coverings are the dura mater, arachnoid, and pia mater (see Fig. 15-8B).

The **dura mater** is the outermost covering of the brain and spinal cord. It is tough, fibrous, and dense and composed primarily of connective tissue. Because of its thickness, this membrane is also called the **pachymeninges**. Beneath the dura mater is a cavity called the **subdural space,** a potential space that doesn't exist unless blood or fluid collects as a result of disease or injury.

The **arachnoid** is the middle covering and, as its name suggests, it has a spider-web appearance. It fits loosely over the underlying structures. A **subarachnoid space** contains **cerebrospinal fluid (CSF),** a colorless fluid that contains proteins, glucose, urea, salts, and some white blood cells. This fluid circulates around the spinal cord and brain and through ventricles located within the inner portion of the brain (see Fig. 15-8A). It provides nutritive substances to the CNS and adds additional protection for the brain and spinal cord by acting as a shock absorber. Normally, CSF is absorbed as rapidly as it is formed, maintaining a constant fluid volume. Any interference with its absorption results in a collection of fluid in the brain, a condition called **hydrocephalus.**

The **pia mater** is the innermost meninx. This membrane directly adheres to the brain and spinal cord. As it passes over the brain, it follows the contours of the gyri and sulci. It contains numerous blood vessels and lymphatics that nourish the underlying tissues. Because of the thinness and delicacy of the arachnoid and pia mater, these two meninges are collectively called the **leptomeninges.**

Peripheral Nervous System

The **peripheral nervous system (PNS)** is composed of all nervous tissue located outside the spinal column and skull. It consists of sensory neurons, which carry impulses from the body to the CNS **(afferent),** and motor neurons, which carry impulses from the brain and spinal cord to

Figure 15-8 Cross section of a human brain with ventricular system. (A) Ventricles of the brain and cerebrospinal fluid (CSF) circulation. (B) Close-up of the meninges and membranes that envelop the brain.

muscles and glands **(efferent)**. The PNS is divided into the somatic nervous system and the autonomic nervous system (see Fig. 15-9). The somatic nervous system is responsible for voluntary muscle movements like walking and talking. The **autonomic nervous system (ANS)** is made up of afferent and efferent neurons that regulate involuntary bodily functions like the heartbeat, digestion, and breathing.

Somatic Nervous System

The somatic nervous system, the part of the PNS associated with voluntary muscle control, is made up of the cranial nerves and the spinal nerves.

Cranial Nerves

The 12 pairs of cranial nerves originate in the brain and emerge through canals or openings in the base of the skull, primarily innervating structures in the head and neck. Each cranial nerve is designated by name and number, each with its own specific function (see Fig. 15-10). Cranial nerves may be sensory, motor, or a mixture of both types of neurons. **Sensory (afferent) nerves** receive impulses from the sense organs, the environment, and the visceral organs and transmit them to the CNS. **Motor (efferent) nerves** conduct impulses from the CNS to muscles and glands. **Mixed nerves** are composed of sensory (afferent) and motor (efferent) neurons. An example of a mixed nerve is the facial nerve. It acts in a motor capacity by transmitting impulses to the facial muscles for smiling or frowning. However, it also acts in a sensory capacity by transmitting taste impulses from the tongue to the brain.

Spinal Nerves

The spinal nerves emerge from the intervertebral spaces in the spinal column and extend to various locations of the body. All 31 pairs of spinal nerves are mixed nerves (see Fig. 15-11). Each pair is identified according to the vertebra from which it exits: cervical, thoracic, lumbar, sacral, and coccygeal. All spinal nerves have two points of attachment to the spinal cord: an anterior (ventral) root and a posterior (dorsal) root. The **anterior root** contains motor fibers, and the **posterior root** contains sensory fibers. These two roots unite to form the spinal nerve, which has afferent and efferent qualities.

Autonomic Nervous System

The ANS is divided into two main branches: the **sympathetic nervous system (SNS)** and **parasympathetic nervous system.** Both branches of the ANS work in concert to maintain physiological balance but often are antagonistic. Ordinarily, what one division stimulates, the other inhibits. The sympathetic division regulates body activities when an immediate action is required in stressful or threatening situations. It increases heart rate, depth of breathing, and muscle strength, preparing the body for a "fight-or-flight" response. Conversely, the parasympathetic division decreases the rate and intensity of these processes and exerts its influence when stressful or threatening situations resolve. It causes a decrease in heart rate, dilation of visceral blood vessels, and an increase in the activity of the digestive tract, preparing the body for "rest-and-digest" responses (see Fig. 15-12).

Figure 15-9 Divisions of the peripheral nervous system.

Ophthalmic

Mandibular

Maxillary

III Oculomotor

VI Abducens

IV Trochlear

V Trigeminal

II Optic

I Olfactory

XII Hypoglossal

VII Facial

Vestibular

Cochlear

VIII Vestibulocochlear

XI Accessory

X Vagus

Afferent (sensory) fibers

Efferent (motor) fibers

IX Glossopharyngeal

Figure 15-10 Cranial nerve distribution.

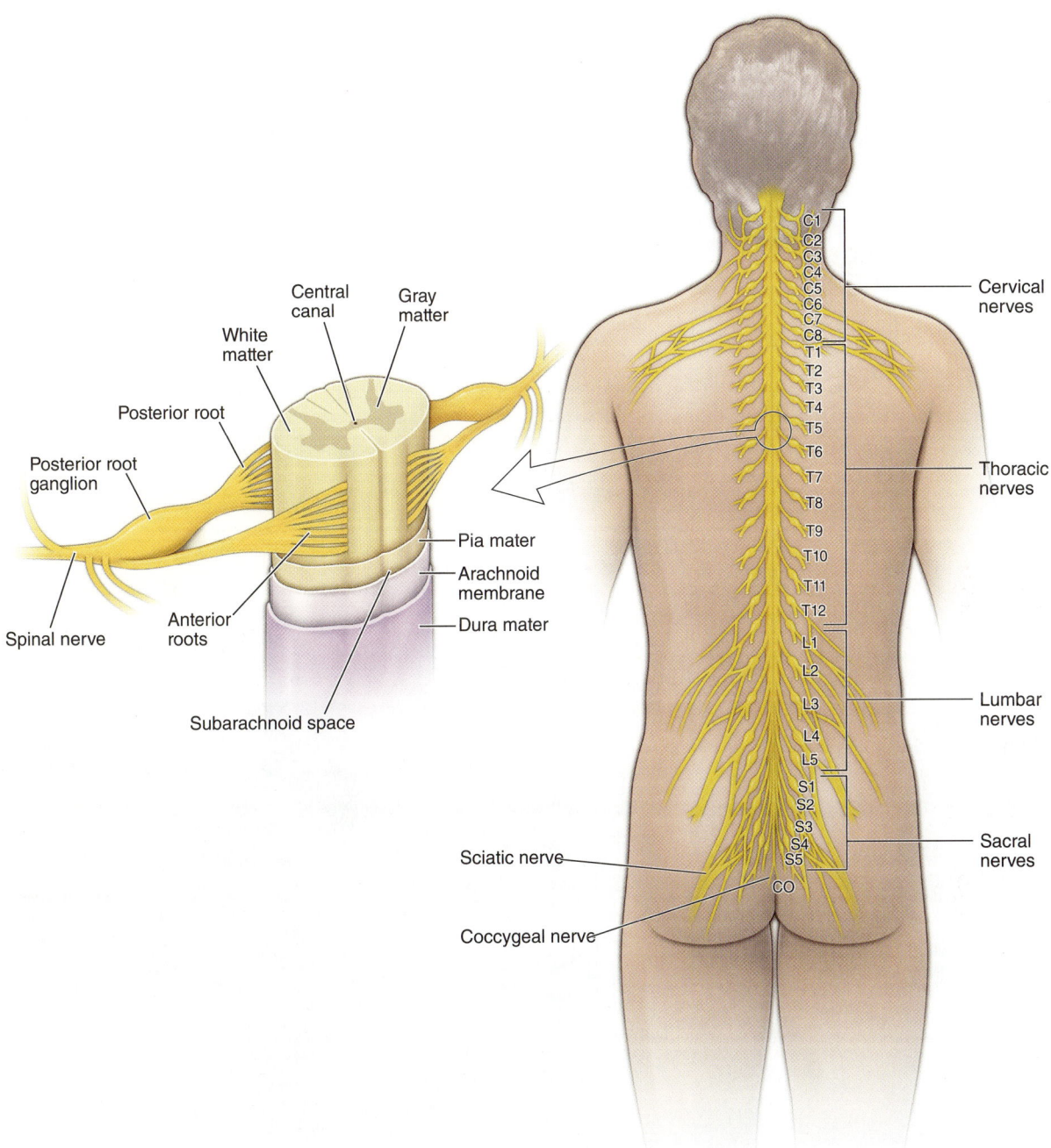

Figure 15-11 Spinal nerves.

Parasympathetic   **Sympathetic**

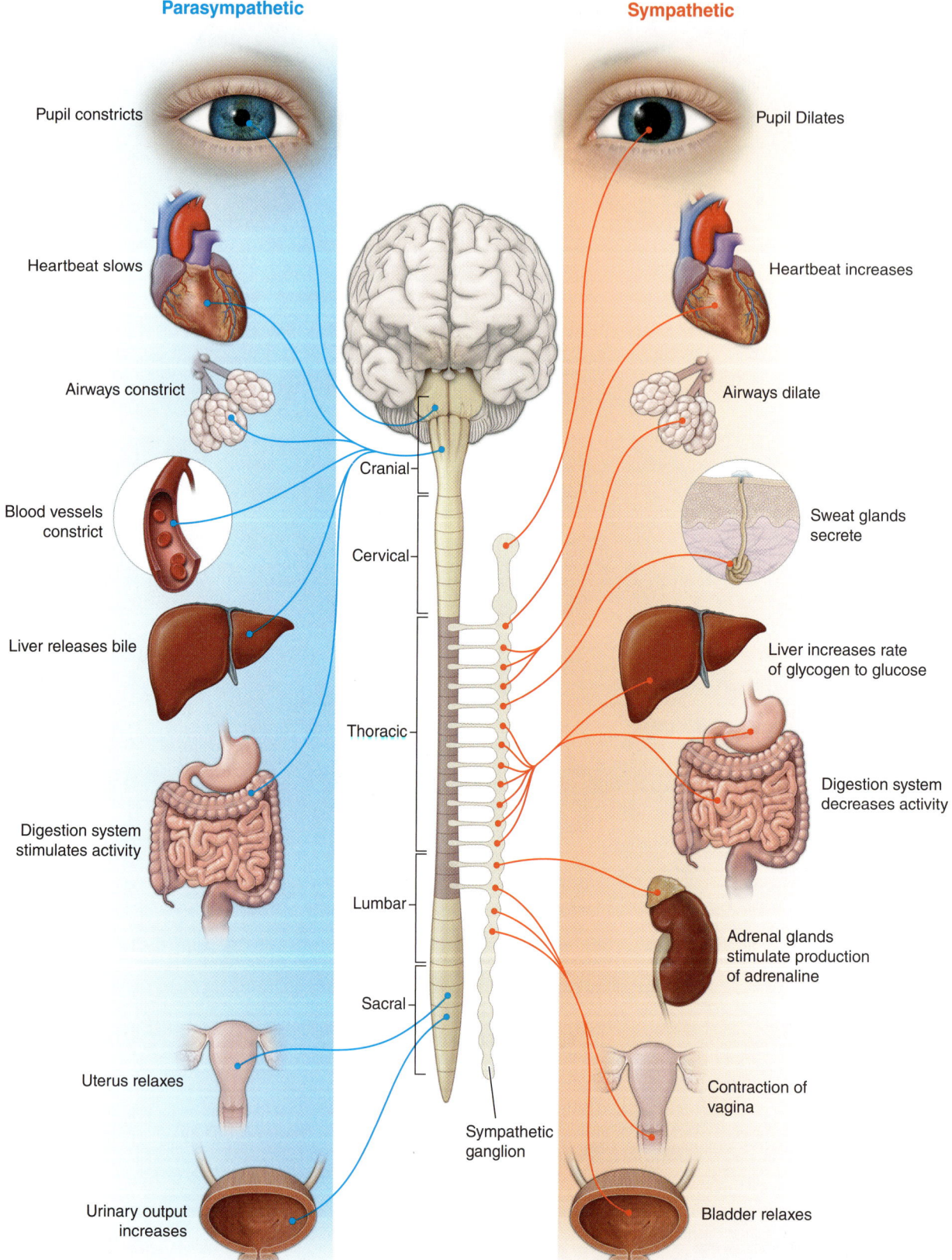

Pupil constricts   Pupil Dilates

Heartbeat slows   Heartbeat increases

Airways constrict   Airways dilate

Blood vessels constrict   Sweat glands secrete

Liver releases bile   Liver increases rate of glycogen to glucose

Digestion system stimulates activity   Digestion system decreases activity

Cranial

Cervical

Thoracic   Adrenal glands stimulate production of adrenaline

Lumbar

Sacral   Contraction of vagina

Uterus relaxes

Sympathetic ganglion

Urinary output increases   Bladder relaxes

Figure 15-12 Autonomic nervous system (ANS). Actions of the parasympathetic and sympathetic nerves.

Anatomy Review: Brain Structures

To review the anatomy of the nervous system, label the illustration using the listed terms.

cerebellum

cerebrum

corpus callosum

diencephalon (interbrain)

frontal lobe

hypothalamus

medulla oblongata

midbrain (mesencephalon)

occipital lobe

parietal lobe

pons

temporal lobe

thalamus

Choroid plexus in third ventricle

Brainstem

Pituitary gland

Spinal cord

 Check your answers by referring to Figure 15–5 on page 555. Review material that you did not answer correctly.

CONNECTING BODY SYSTEMS—NERVOUS SYSTEM

The main function of the nervous system is to identify and respond to internal and external changes in the environment to maintain homeostasis. Specific functional relationships between the nervous system and other body systems are discussed here.

Blood, Lymphatic, and Immune

- The nervous system identifies changes in blood and lymph composition and provides the stimuli to maintain homeostasis.
- The nervous system identifies pathologically altered tissue and assists the immune system in containing injury and promoting healing.

Cardiovascular

- Nervous tissue, especially the conduction system of the heart, transmits a contraction impulse.
- The nervous system identifies pressure changes on vascular walls and responds to regulate blood pressure.

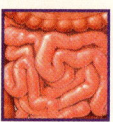

Digestive

- Nervous stimuli of digestive organs regulate digestion, nutrient absorption, and the movement of food through the digestive tract.
- Nerve receptors in the lower colon identify the need to defecate.

Endocrine

- The hypothalamus and pituitary gland secrete hormones that help regulate other endocrine glands throughout the body.

Female Reproductive

- The nervous system transmits the contraction impulses needed for delivery of a fetus.
- The nervous system provides the stimuli needed for lactation.
- The nervous system regulates the hormones needed for the menstrual cycle.

Integumentary

- The sensory nervous system supplies receptors in the skin that respond to environmental stimuli.
- The autonomic nervous system regulates body temperature by controlling shivering and sweating.

Male Reproductive

- The nervous system regulates sexual responses.
- Nervous tissue in reproductive organs provides pleasure responses.
- The nervous system regulates the hormones needed for the production of testosterone and sperm.

Musculoskeletal

- The nervous system provides impulses for contraction, resulting in voluntary and involuntary movement of muscles.
- Autonomic nervous tissue responds to positional changes.

Respiratory

- The nervous system stimulates muscle contractions that create the pressure changes necessary for ventilation.
- The nervous system regulates the rate and depth of breathing.

Urinary

- The nervous system stimulates the thirst reflex when body fluid levels are low.
- The nervous system regulates bladder function.

Medical Word Elements

This section introduces combining forms, suffixes, and prefixes related to the nervous system. Word analyses are also provided. From the information provided, complete the meaning of the medical words in the right-hand column. The first one is completed for you.

Element	Meaning	Word Analysis
Combining Forms		
cerebr/o	cerebrum	**cerebr/o**/tomy (sĕr-ĕ-BRŎT-ō-mē): *incision of the cerebrum* *-tomy:* incision
crani/o	cranium (skull)	**crani/o**/malacia (krā-nē-ō-mă-LĀ-shē-ă): _____ *-malacia:* softening
encephal/o	brain	**encephal/o**/cele (ĕn-SĔF-ă-lō-sēl): _____ *-cele:* hernia, swelling *Encephalocele is a condition in which portions of the brain and meninges protrude through a bony midline defect in the skull.*
gangli/o	ganglion (knot or knotlike mass)	**gangli**/ectomy (găng-glē-ĔK-tō-mē): _____ *-ectomy:* excision, removal *A ganglion is a mass of nerve cell bodies (gray matter) in the peripheral nervous system.*
gli/o	glue; neuroglial tissue	**gli**/oma (glī-Ō-mă): _____ *-oma:* tumor
kinesi/o	movement	brady/**kines**/ia (brăd-ē-kĭ-NĒ-sē-ă): _____ *brady-:* slow *-ia:* condition
lept/o	thin, slender	**lept/o**/mening/o/pathy (lĕp-tō-mĕn-ĭn-GŎP-ă-thē): _____ *-mening/o:* meninges (membranes covering the brain and spinal cord) *-pathy:* disease *The leptomeninges include the pia mater and arachnoid, both of which are thin and delicate in structure, as opposed to the dura mater.*
lex/o	word, phrase	dys/**lex**/ia (dĭs-LĔK-sē-ă): _____ *dys-:* bad; painful; difficult *-ia:* condition *Dyslexia is a difficulty with reading or an inability to read, including the tendency to reverse letters or words when reading or writing.*
mening/o	meninges (membranes covering the brain and spinal cord)	**mening/o**/cele (mĕn-ĬN-gō-sēl): _____ *-cele:* hernia, swelling
meningi/o		**meningi**/oma (mĕn-ĭn-jē-Ō-mă): _____ *-oma:* tumor

Continued

Medical Word Elements—cont'd

Element	Meaning	Word Analysis
ment/o	mind	**ment**/al (mĕnt-ăl): _____ *-al:* pertaining to
phren/o		schiz/o/**phren**/ia (skĭz-ō-FRĔN-ē-ă) _____ *-schiz/o:* split *-ia:* condition
psych/o		**psych**/o/logist: _____ *-logist:* specialist in the study of
myel/o	bone marrow; spinal cord	poli/o/**myel**/itis (pōl-ē-ō-mī-ĕl-Ī-tĭs): _____ *poli/o:* gray; gray matter (of the brain or spinal cord) *-itis:* inflammation
narc/o	stupor; numbness; sleep	**narc**/o/tic (năr-KŎT-ĭk): _____ *-tic:* pertaining to *Narcotics depress the central nervous system, thus relieving pain and producing sleep.*
neur/o	nerve	**neur**/o/lysis (nū-RŎL-ĭs-ĭs): _____ *-lysis:* separation; destruction; loosening *Neurolysis is sometimes performed using cryoablation or radiofrequency techniques to relieve intractable pain as a temporary or permanent measure.*
radicul/o	nerve root	**radicul**/algia (ră-dĭk-ū-LĂL-jē-ă): _____ *-algia:* pain
sthen/o	strength	hyper/**sthen**/ia (hī-pĕr-STHĒ-nē-ă): _____ *hyper-:* excessive, above normal *-ia:* condition *Hypersthenia is characterized by rigid muscles and muscle tension when resting; also called* **hypertonia**
thalam/o	thalamus	**thalam**/o/tomy (thăl-ă-MŎT-ō-mē): _____ *-tomy:* incision *Thalamotomy is performed to treat intractable pain or psychosis.*
thec/o	sheath (usually referring to the meninges)	intra/**thec**/al (ĭn-tră-THĒ-kăl): _____ *intra-:* in, within *-al:* pertaining to
ton/o	tension	dys/**ton**/ia (dĭs-TŌ-nē-ă): _____ *dys-:* bad; painful; difficult *-ia:* condition *Dystonia is characterized by sustained muscle contractions, causing twisting, repetitive movements, or an abnormal posture.*

Medical Word Elements—cont'd

Element	Meaning	Word Analysis
ventricul/o	ventricle (of the heart or brain)	**ventricul**/itis (věn-trĭk-ū-LĪ-tĭs): _____ *-itis:* inflammation

Suffixes

Element	Meaning	Word Analysis
-algesia	pain	an/**algesia** (ăn-ăl-JĒ-zē-ă): _____ *an-:* without, not
-algia		syn/**algia** (sĭn-ĂL-jē-ă): _____ *syn-:* union, together, joined *Synalgia, commonly called* referred pain, *is pain experienced in a part of the body other than the place of pathology. For example, right shoulder pain is commonly associated with gallstones.*
-asthenia	weakness, debility	my/**asthenia** (mī-ăs-THĒ-nē-ă): _____ *my:* muscle
-esthesia	feeling	hyper/**esthesia** (hī-pĕr-ĕs-THĒ-zē-ă): _____ *hyper-:* excessive, above normal *Hyperesthesia involves a marked sensitivity to touch, pain, or other sensory stimuli.*
-kinesia	movement	hyper/**kinesia** (hī-pĕr-kĭ-NĒ-zē-ă): _____ *hyper-:* excessive, above normal
-lepsy	seizure	narc/o/**lepsy** (NĂR-kō-lĕp-sē): _____ *narc/o:* sleep *In narcolepsy, the individual has a sudden and uncontrollable urge to sleep at an inappropriate time, such as when driving.*
-mania	state of mental disorder, frenzy	klept/o/**mania:** (klĕp-tō-MĀN-ē-ă): _____ *klept/o:* to steal
-paresis	partial paralysis	hemi/**paresis** (hĕm-ē-pă-RĒ-sĭs): _____ *hemi-:* one-half *When used alone, the term* paresis *refers to partial paralysis or motor weakness.*
-phasia	speech	a/**phasia** (ă-FĀ-zē-ă): _____ *a-:* without, not
-phobia	fear	acr/o/**phobia** (ăk-rō-FŌ-bē-ă): _____ *acr/o:* extremity *This term refers to the fear of heights.*
-plegia	paralysis	quadri/**plegia** (kwŏd-rĭ-PLĒ-jē-ă): _____ *quadri-:* four

Continued

Medical Word Elements—cont'd

Element	Meaning	Word Analysis
-taxia	order, coordination	a/**taxia** (ă-TĂK-sē-ă): _____ *a-:* without, not **Ataxia** *refers to poor muscle coordination, especially when voluntary movements are attempted.*
-thymia	mind, emotion	dys/**thymia:** (dĭs-THĪ-mē-ă) _____ *dys-:* bad; painful; difficult *This term refers to a chronic form of depression that lasts for at least 2 years; also known as* persistent depressive disorder.
Prefixes		
pachy-	thick	**pachy**/mening/itis (păk-ē-mĕn-ĭn-JĪ-tĭs): _____ *mening:* meninges (membranes covering the brain and spinal cord) *-itis:* inflammation *The dura mater (pachymeninx) is a thick membrane that provides protection for the brain and spinal cord.*
para-	near, beside; beyond	**para**/plegia (păr-ă-PLĒ-jē-ă): _____ *-plegia:* paralysis
syn-	union, together, joined	**syn**/algia (sĭn-ĂL-jē-ă): _____ *-algia:* pain *Nerve pain in a deteriorated hip commonly causes referred pain in a healthy knee.*

Visit the Medical Terminology Systems online resource center at FADavis.com for an audio exercise of the terms in this table. Other activities are also available to reinforce content.

It is time to review medical word elements by completing Learning Activities 15-1 and 15-2.

Disease Focus

Damage to the brain and spinal cord invariably causes signs and symptoms in other parts of the body. Common signs and symptoms for many neurological disorders include headache (HA), insomnia, back or neck pain, weakness, and involuntary movement (**dyskinesia**). Careful observation of the patient during the history and physical examination may provide valuable clues about mental status and cognitive and motor ability.

For diagnosis, treatment, and management of neurological disorders, the medical services of a specialist may be warranted. **Neurology** is the branch of medicine concerned with disorders of the nervous system, including the brain, spinal cord, nerves, and muscles. The physician who specializes in the diagnosis and treatment of nervous system disorders is known as a **neurologist**. **Psychiatry** is the branch of medicine that focuses on the diagnosis, treatment, and prevention of mental, emotional, and behavioral disorders. The physician who specializes in diagnosing and treating these disorders is a **psychiatrist**. Psychiatrists commonly work in association with **clinical psychologists**, professionals with doctoral degrees in psychology who are trained in evaluating human behavior, intelligence, and personality. They provide psychotherapy to help individuals manage symptoms and improve coping skills and perform psychological testing but cannot prescribe medication. Licensed clinical social workers hold a degree in social work with specialized training in mental health. They provide various forms of therapy, often with a focus on connecting clients to community resources and support systems.

Cerebrovascular Disease

Cerebrovascular disease is a group of disorders affecting the vessels that supply blood to the brain. These disorders can lead to various problems including stroke, transient ischemic attack (TIA) or "mini stroke," and vascular dementia. The most common cause of cerebrovascular disease is atherosclerosis. Other causes include blood clots, arterial dissection, and conditions that affect the structure of blood vessels, such as arteriovenous malformations or aneurysms. Symptoms of cerebrovascular disease can vary depending on the type and severity of the condition but may include sudden weakness or numbness, difficulty speaking or understanding speech, sudden severe headache, or loss of balance and coordination. Treatment depends on the underlying cause and may include medication, rehabilitation, and lifestyle changes.

Stroke is the most common type of cerebrovascular disease. When denied oxygen, brain tissue begins to die, and a medical emergency called **stroke, cerebrovascular accident (CVA),** or **"brain attack"** results. The main types of stroke are ischemic stroke and hemorrhagic. Hemorrhagic stroke can be further categorized into intracerebral or subarachnoid hemorrhage. **Ischemic stroke** is the most common, accounting for about 85% of all strokes. The causes of an ischemic stroke are similar to those of a heart attack and include emboli, thrombi, and atherosclerosis that limit blood flow to brain tissue. A common cause of ischemic stroke is atherosclerosis of the arteries of the brain (cerebral) or neck (**carotid**). An **intracerebral hemorrhage** is often associated with conditions such as high blood pressure, blood vessel abnormalities, and use of blood thinning medications and occurs when there is a sudden rupture of an artery within the brain. The bleeding can cause damage to brain cells and increase pressure within the skull, leading to neurological deficits. In a **subarachnoid hemorrhage (SAH),** blood is released into the space between the brain and the tissues that surround the brain. This condition is commonly caused by a ruptured aneurysm and carries significant morbidity and mortality rates.

Depending on the area of the brain affected by the stroke, signs and symptoms include weakness or paralysis in one-half of the body (**hemiparesis, hemiplegia**), speech difficulty (**dysphasia**), lack of muscle coordination (**ataxia**), confusion, and loss of consciousness. A "mini stroke," also called a **transient ischemic attack (TIA),** is a type of stroke in which symptoms resolve within 24 hours and do not cause permanent damage. TIAs require immediate medical attention because they frequently precede a full blown stroke.

Some risk factors for stroke include family history, high blood pressure, diabetes, obesity, smoking, and excessive alcohol use. Managing and controlling these risk factors through lifestyle changes, medication, and regular medical care can help reduce the risk of stroke.

Computed tomography (CT) is the most common scan used to diagnose stroke because it can be performed rapidly and help guide immediate treatment decisions. However, CT scans may not always detect ischemic strokes in the very early stages, so additional imaging with magnetic resonance imaging (MRI) may be necessary. For ischemic strokes, "clot-buster" (**thrombolytic**) medications administered within 3 hours of symptom onset can usually prevent permanent disability. Various other medications and procedures can be used to treat stroke depending on its underlying cause. Treatment for disabilities caused by stroke involves speech, physical, and occupational therapy.

Seizure Disorders

A **seizure disorder**, commonly known as **epilepsy,** is a neurological condition characterized by recurrent seizures, or episodes of abnormal electrical activity in the brain, leading to various symptoms ranging from convulsions and loss of consciousness to subtle momentary lapses in awareness. The abnormal electrical activity in the brain can result from various factors such as brain injuries, congenital anomalies, metabolic disorders, brain tumors, infection, vascular disturbances, and genetic disorders. **Nonepileptic seizures (NES)** are episodes that resemble epileptic seizures but are not caused by abnormal electrical activity in the brain. Instead, they can be triggered by psychological factors, such as stress or trauma, or other medical conditions unrelated to epilepsy, like syncope. When these episodes have a psychological origin, they are referred to as **psychogenic nonepileptic seizures (PNES)**.

There are several types of epileptic seizures, but the two most common forms are partial seizures and generalized seizures. In **partial seizures,** only a portion of the brain is involved. Symptoms may include unusual movements, sensory changes, or unusual emotions. Loss of consciousness may or may not occur, with the episode typically lasting a few seconds to two minutes. In a **generalized seizure,** the entire brain is involved, typically with loss of consciousness. The most common type of generalized seizure is the **tonic-clonic (grand mal) seizure.** In tonic-clonic seizures, the body alternates between excessive muscle tone and rigidity **(tonic)** and jerking muscle contractions **(clonic)** in the extremities. After the seizure, such neurological symptoms as weakness, confusion, HA, and nausea may occur. These symptoms are called a **postictal event,** which commonly lasts for minutes to hours but may last longer with a severe seizure.

Many patients experience a warning signal **(aura)** of an imminent seizure. Auras vary considerably and may include sensory phenomena without a precipitating stimulus, such as a strange taste in the mouth, the sound of a ringing bell, or an inability to react properly to usual situations. Auras provide time for preparation, such as lying down, avoiding staircases, and so forth, to minimize injuries should a grand mal seizure occur.

Diagnosis and evaluation of epilepsies commonly rely on electroencephalography and magnetic source imaging (MSI) to locate the affected area of the brain. Antiepileptic medications help control seizures. Treating PNES typically involves a multidisciplinary team with some common components of psychological therapy, medication, education, and stress and physical health management.

Multiple Sclerosis

Multiple sclerosis (MS) is an autoimmune disease that targets the myelin sheath on the nerves of the CNS. MS causes inflammation, hardening **(sclerosing),** and finally the loss of myelin **(demyelination)** throughout the spinal cord and brain. Myelin deterioration impedes the transmission of electrical impulses from one neuron to another, producing a wide variety of symptoms depending on the location and extent of nerve damage. An MRI shows areas of demyelination, or plaques, as bright spots. Lesions are commonly found in the white matter of the brain, particularly in the periventricular area, the corpus callosum, and the spinal column.

Signs and symptoms of MS include tremors, muscle weakness, bradykinesia, and such visual disturbances as blurred vision, poor contrast, double vision, and eye pain. Other symptoms include bowel and bladder disorders, sexual dysfunction, balance problems, cognitive difficulties, and pain. Many patients require a cane, walker, or wheelchair as the disease progresses. Patients can experience periods of remission when symptoms temporarily disappear, but progressive hardening of myelinated areas leads to other attacks or gradual worsening of symptoms over time without periods of remission. MS generally affects a person's quality of life rather than longevity. Medications and physical therapy can ease or control symptoms, but currently there is no cure for the disease.

Mental Disorders

Mental disorders are syndromes characterized by disturbances in thinking, mood, behavior, or perception that cause significant distress or impairment in daily life. Its forms range from mild to severe. Signs and symptoms can vary widely and can include anxiety, irritability, changes in sleep or eating patterns, hallucinations, mood lability, confused thinking, or prolonged depression. Although many people may experience one or more of these problems from time to time, when any of them are ongoing and affect the ability to meet the demands of daily life, it may be a sign to seek professional evaluation and support from a mental health professional. Causes of mental disorders are often complex and multifaceted, involving a combination of genetic, biological, environmental, and social factors. Left untreated, mental disorders can cause relationship difficulties, work and academic difficulties, social isolation, poverty, and physical health problems.

Research and education have begun to remove some of the stigma attached to psychiatric conditions. Today, mental health disorders are becoming more recognizable and treatable. The *Diagnostic and Statistical Manual of Mental Disorders, Fifth Edition* (DSM-5) is a classification and diagnostic tool that contains standardized criteria for the diagnosis of mental disorders. Family physicians, school psychologists, marriage and family counselors, and even such support groups as grief support and Alcoholics Anonymous (AA) can effectively help in managing psychological problems.

Addiction

Addiction to various substances is currently a significant crisis in the United States affecting millions. According to the Centers for Disease Control (CDC), nearly 50 million people aged 12 or older have had a diagnosed **substance use disorder (SUD)** in the past year. In 2022, over 100,000 drug overdose deaths occurred, driven largely by opioids, particularly synthetic opioids like fentanyl. Of note, addiction does not only refer to substance use; it also includes other compulsive behaviors like gambling, for example.

Addiction is considered both a complex brain disorder and a mental disorder. It is a chronic, relapsing disorder characterized by compulsive behaviors, like drug seeking or gambling, that are continued despite harmful consequences and result in long-lasting negative changes in the brain. Addiction primarily affects the reward system in the brain, overall dysregulating pathways involving dopamine, the neurotransmitter that plays a crucial role in reward, pleasure, motivation, and drive. Addiction also affects areas of the brain involved in learning and memory, judgment, and inhibitory control over behavior. The changes in the brain's structure and function that occur because of addiction explain how the individual develops tolerance and dependence to a substance or behavior. Addiction typically presents as a **comorbidity** with other mental disorders, such as anxiety, depression, or bipolar disorder.

Risk factors for addiction include family history; genetic predisposition; environmental factors such as trauma, brain injury, chronic pain, and social environment; and age of first use. Individuals with mental disorders such as depression, anxiety, attention deficit-hyperactivity disorder (ADHD), or posttraumatic stress disorder (PTSD) are at a higher risk of developing addiction.

Treating addiction is a multifaceted process that often requires a combination of therapies and interventions tailored to the individual. The primary types of addiction treatment include behavioral therapies, medications, and support groups, such as AA and Narcotics Anonymous (NA).

Oncology

Primary CNS tumors originate in the brain (intracranial) or spinal cord, commonly arising from glial cells, meninges, or Schwann cells. **Intracranial tumors** are located within the cranial cavity inside the skull and include both primary and secondary (metastatic) tumors. Primary intracranial tumors are a specific subset of intracranial tumors that originate directly within brain tissue, not spread from other organs. They are classified based on their cell origin, histological characteristics, and whether they are benign or malignant. A major symptom of intracranial tumors is HA, especially upon arising in the morning, during coughing episodes, and upon bending or sudden movement. Occasionally, the optic disc in the back of the eyeball swells **(papilledema)** because of increased intracranial pressure. Personality changes are common and can include mood changes, confusion, and irritability. New onset seizures, nausea, and vomiting can also occur.

Intracranial tumors can arise from any structure within the cranial cavity, including the pituitary and pineal glands, cranial nerves, and the arachnoid and pia mater **(leptomeninges)**. In addition, all of these tissues may be the sites of metastatic spread from primary malignancies that occur outside the nervous system. Secondary (metastatic) tumors of the cranial cavity tend to exhibit growth characteristics similar to those of the primary malignancy but tend to grow more slowly than the parent tumor. Common primary sites include the lung, breast, kidney, and skin (melanoma). Metastatic tumors of the cranial cavity are usually easier to remove and are more common than primary intracranial tumors.

CT scans and MRI help establish a diagnosis but are not definitive. Surgical removal relieves pressure and confirms or rules out malignancy. Even after surgery, most intracranial tumors require radiation therapy as a second line of treatment. Chemotherapy combined with radiation therapy usually provides the best chance for survival and quality of life.

Diseases and Conditions

This section introduces diseases and conditions of the nervous system, along with their meanings and pronunciations. Word analyses for selected terms are also provided.

Term	Definition

agnosia
ăg-NŌ-zē-ă
  a-: without, not
  gnos: knowing
  -ia: condition
	Inability to comprehend auditory, visual, spatial, olfactory, or other sensations, even though the sensory sphere is intact
	The type of agnosia is usually identified by the sense or senses affected, such as visual agnosia. Agnosia is common in parietal lobe tumors.

amyotrophic lateral sclerosis (ALS)
  a-: without, not
  my/o: muscle
  troph: development, nourishment
  -ic: pertaining to
  later: side, to one side
  -al: pertaining to
  scler: hardening; sclera (white of the eye)
  -osis: abnormal condition; increase (used primarily with blood cells)
	Progressive neurodegenerative disease that targets the motor neurons responsible for voluntary muscle movement, ultimately leading to muscle weakness; also known as *Lou Gehrig disease*
	ALS most commonly occurs between 40 to 70 years of age and is typically insidious. The exact cause is not known but genetics and environmental exposure to certain toxins may be linked to the disease. There is no cure, and treatments aim to manage symptoms, maintain quality of life, and slow disease progression.

anencephaly
ăn-ĕn-SĔF-ă-lē
  an-: without, not, loss
  encephal: brain
  -y: noun ending
	Congenital deformity in which some or all of the fetal brain is missing
	In anencephaly, the infant is usually stillborn or dies shortly after birth. This deformity can be detected through amniocentesis or ultrasonography early in pregnancy.

closed head trauma TRAW-mă	Injury to the brain resulting from an external force where the skull remains intact; also known as *closed head injury* *In closed head trauma, the injury site may occur at the impact site, where the brain hits the inside of the skull (coup), or at the rebound site, where the opposite side of the brain strikes the skull (contrecoup).*
coma KŌ-mă	A state of prolonged unconsciousness with an absence of voluntary response to stimuli
concussion kŏn-KŬSH-ŭn	Traumatic brain injury (TBI) caused by a blow, jolt, or bump to the head resulting in the rapid movement of the brain within the skull that can cause temporary or long-term dysfunction *Symptoms of concussion may include HA, temporary loss of consciousness, memory problems, emotional and behavioral changes, dizziness, nausea, vomiting, and blurred vision, but are usually not life threatening. However, they may still have significant short- and long-term effects on cognitive, physical, and emotional health.*
convulsion kŏn-VŬL-shŭn	Any sudden and violent contraction of one or more voluntary muscles in the body, often accompanied by rhythmic movements or jerking, commonly associated with such brain disorders as epilepsy

Diseases and Conditions—cont'd

Term	Definition
dementia dĭ-MĔN-shē-ă *de-:* cessation *ment:* mind *-ia:* condition	Broad term that refers to cognitive deficit, including memory impairment
Alzheimer disease (AD) ĂLTS-hī-mĕr	Type of age-associated dementia caused by various biological and structural changes in the brain including development of lesions called *plaques* that interrupt the passage of electrochemical signals between cells, neurofibrillary tangles that disrupt the transport system inside neurons, neuronal and synaptic loss, and brain atrophy; also called *cerebral degeneration* *AD is the most common form of dementia, accounting for 60% to 80% of cases. Clinical manifestations include memory loss, emotional and behavioral changes, and a decline in cognitive and social skills, eventually leading to death. A combination of medications, lifestyle changes, and supportive therapies can help to manage symptoms, improve quality of life, and slow disease progression; there is currently no cure for AD.*
frontotemporal dementia (FTD)	Dementia that involves degeneration of the frontal and temporal lobes of the brain *Clinical manifestations include changes in personality and behavior, difficulty with language, and impaired executive functioning.*
Lewy body dementia (LBD)	Dementia characterized by the presence of abnormal protein deposits called *Lewy bodies* in the brain cortex, leading to cognitive and motor symptoms *Symptoms include fluctuating cognitive impairment, visual hallucinations, and motor symptoms resembling Parkinson disease–like stiffness and tremors.*
vascular dementia (VaD)	Dementia caused by reduced blood flow to the brain due to strokes or small vessel disease *Clinical features include memory loss, difficulty with planning and organization, mood changes, and motor impairment. Sometimes it presents in a stepwise pattern of decline with periods of stability or mild decline, followed by sudden or abrupt worsening of symptoms after a significant vascular event like stroke or TIA.*
dyslexia dĭs-LĔK-sē-ă *dys-:* bad; painful; difficult *lex:* word, phrase *-ia:* condition	A specific learning disability that affects the person's ability to read, write, and spell, despite adequate intelligence and sensory ability
Guillain-Barré syndrome (GBS) gē-YĂN băr-RĀ	Rare autoimmune condition that attacks the PNS, leading to inflammation and damage to the myelin sheath, resulting in decreased nerve impulses, loss of reflex response, and sudden muscle weakness; also called *infective or idiopathic polyneuritis* *GBS usually follows a gastrointestinal or respiratory infection. In severe cases, the patient may temporarily require respiratory support until the inflammation subsides. GBS often follows an ascending pattern of muscle weakness and paralysis, with symptoms starting in lower extremities and progressing upward toward the trunk and arms.*

Continued

Diseases and Conditions—cont'd

Term	Definition
headache (HA)	Common condition that is characterized by pain in the head or neck region; symptoms vary in intensity and location and are caused by a variety of factors
clusters	Typically intense and occur in cyclical patterns or clusters *Cluster HAs commonly cause intense pain around one eye or one side of the head.*
migraine	Intense, typically one-sided throbbing HAs accompanied by several other symptoms including nausea, vomiting, sensitivity to light and sound, and sometimes aura *Migraines can last from a few hours to several days and have a significant negative effect on daily living.*
tension	The most common type of HA, often described as a mild-to-moderate dull pain or tightness around the forehead, temples, or back of the head and neck *Tension HAs can be caused by stress and muscle tension.*
herpes zoster HĔR-pēz ZŎS-tĕr	Acute inflammatory eruption of highly painful vesicles that develops on one side of the body, often in a stripe pattern that is caused by the same virus that causes chickenpox; also called *shingles* (see Fig. 15-13) *Vaccines can reduce the risk of contracting shingles. Early treatment can shorten the infection or reduce the chance of complications.*

Figure 15-13 Herpes zoster (shingles).

Term	Definition
Huntington chorea HŬNT-ĭng-tŭn kō-RĒ-ă	A hereditary neurodegenerative disorder characterized by quick, involuntary movements, speech disturbances, and mental deterioration; also called *Huntington's disease* *Onset of Huntington chorea commonly occurs between ages 30 and 50. Progression of the disease is generally gradual but leads to severe physical and mental disability over time.*

Diseases and Conditions—cont'd

Term	Definition

hydrocephalus
hī-drō-SĔF-ă-lŭs
   hydr/o: water
   cephal: head
   -us: condition; structure
	Accumulation of cerebrospinal fluid (CSF) in the ventricles of the brain, causing increased intracranial pressure (ICP), thinning of brain tissue, and separation of cranial bones
	The two forms of hydrocephalus are acquired hydrocephalus, which occurs after birth, and congenital hydrocephalus, which occurs during fetal development and is found at birth.

lethargy LĔTH-ăr-jē	Abnormal inactivity or lack of response to normal stimuli *Lethargy can be caused by various medical conditions, lifestyle factors, medications, or psychological issues.*

myasthenia gravis (MG)
mī-ăs-THĒ-nē-ă GRĂV-ĭs
   my: muscle
   -asthenia: weakness, debility
	Chronic, autoimmune neuromuscular disorder caused by disruption in the transmission of signals from nerves to muscles; MG is characterized by weakness and rapid fatigue of the voluntary muscles
	The primary target of the immune system in MG is the acetylcholine receptor on the muscle cell membrane; acetylcholine plays a vital role in muscle contraction (see Fig. 15-14).

Figure 15-14 Myasthenia gravis. (A) Acetylcholine binding to acetylcholine receptor (AChR) sites on muscle to stimulate contraction. (B) Auto-antibodies destroying AChR binding sites and inhibiting the binding of acetylcholine required for muscle contraction.

Continued

Diseases and Conditions—cont'd

Term	Definition
palsy PAWL-zē	Paralysis, usually partial, commonly characterized by weakness and shaking or uncontrolled tremor (see Fig. 15-15)

Figure 15-15 Bell palsy.

Term	Definition
Bell palsy	Facial paralysis caused by a functional disorder of the seventh cranial nerve; also called *facial nerve palsy* *Bell palsy typically affects one side of the face and is commonly associated with herpes simplex virus (HSV-1), but other viruses may be implicated. It is self-limiting and usually resolves spontaneously in 3 to 5 weeks.*
cerebral palsy (CP) sĕ-RĒ-brăl *cerebr:* cerebrum *-al:* pertaining to	Type of paralysis that affects movement and muscle coordination and may affect gross and fine motor skills *CP commonly occurs because of trauma to the brain before or during the birthing process.*
paralysis pă-RĂL-ĭ-sĭs *para-:* near, beside; beyond *-lysis:* separation; destruction; loosening	Loss of voluntary motion in one or more muscle groups with or without loss of sensation *Strokes and spinal cord injuries are the most common causes of paralysis. Strokes usually affect only one side of the body. Spinal cord injuries result in paralysis below the site of the injury (see Fig. 15-16).*

Diseases and Conditions—cont'd

Term	Definition

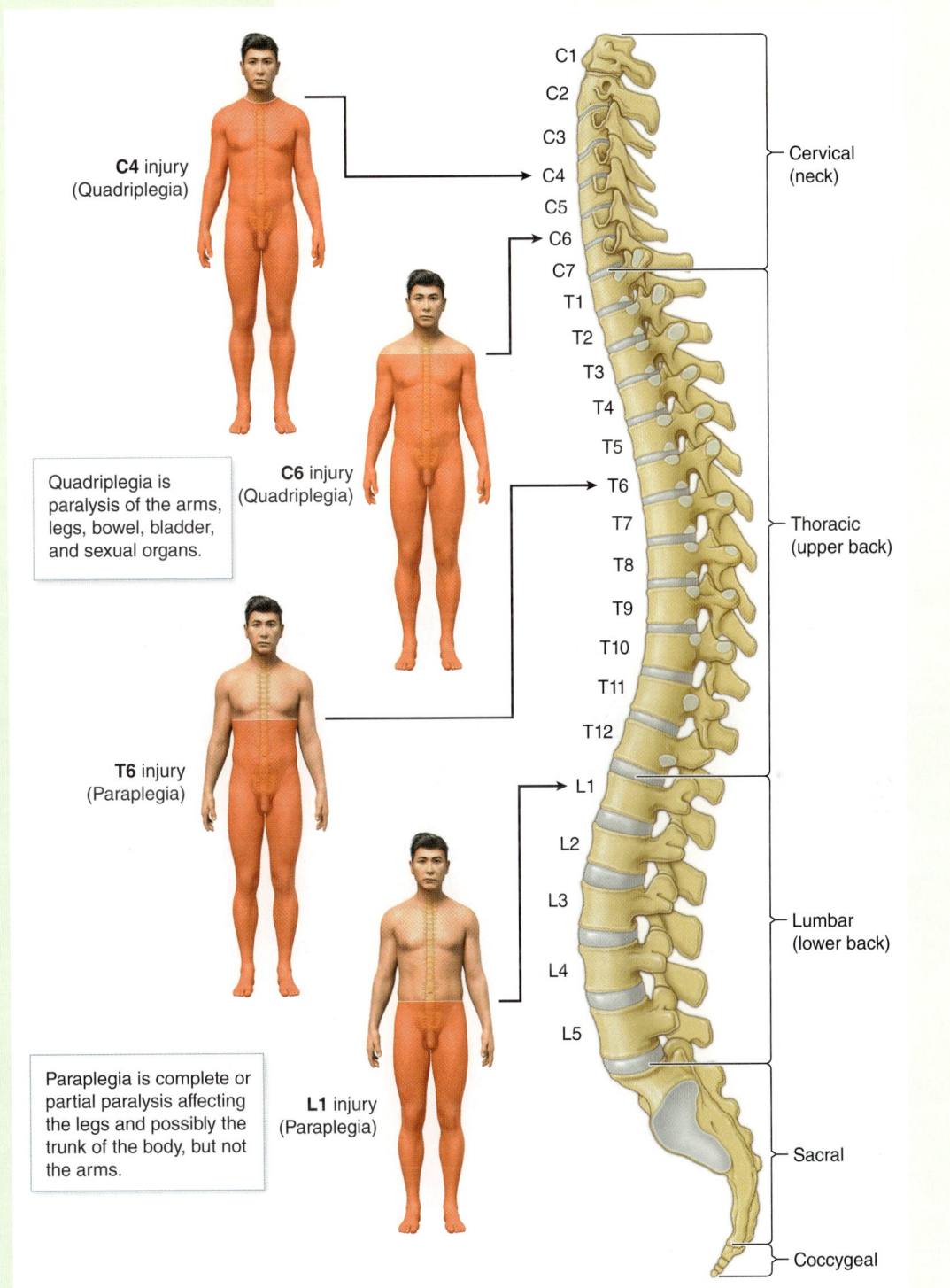

C4 injury
(Quadriplegia)

C6 injury
(Quadriplegia)

T6 injury
(Paraplegia)

L1 injury
(Paraplegia)

Quadriplegia is paralysis of the arms, legs, bowel, bladder, and sexual organs.

Paraplegia is complete or partial paralysis affecting the legs and possibly the trunk of the body, but not the arms.

C1
C2
C3
C4
C5
C6
C7
T1
T2
T3
T4
T5
T6
T7
T8
T9
T10
T11
T12
L1
L2
L3
L4
L5

Cervical (neck)

Thoracic (upper back)

Lumbar (lower back)

Sacral

Coccygeal

Figure 15-16 Spinal cord injuries showing extent of paralysis.

| paresthesia | Sensation of numbness, prickling, tingling, or heightened sensitivity |
| păr-ĕs-THĒ-zē-ă | *Paresthesia can be caused by disorders affecting the CNS such as stroke, TIA, MS, transverse myelitis, and encephalitis.* |

Continued

Diseases and Conditions—cont'd

Term	Definition
Parkinson disease PĂR-kĭn-sŏn	Progressive neurodegenerative disorder characterized by the gradual loss of dopamine producing neurons in certain regions of the brain, leading to impairment in motor function, including tremors, muscular rigidity, postural instability, gait changes, and nonmotor symptoms such as cognitive impairment; also called *paralysis agitans* or *shaking palsy*
poliomyelitis pōl-ē-ō-mī-ĕl-Ī-tĭs *poli/o:* gray; gray matter (of the brain or spinal cord) *myel:* bone marrow; spinal cord *-itis:* inflammation	Inflammation of the gray matter of the spinal cord caused by a virus, commonly resulting in spinal and muscle deformity and paralysis *Polio is preventable with standard vaccinations administered to children.*
radiculopathy ră-dĭk-ū-LŎP-ă-thē *radicul/o:* nerve root *-pathy:* disease	Disorder characterized by pain, weakness, numbness or tingling, that affects one or more nerves at the location where the nerve root exits the spine and commonly the result of a herniated or compressed disk, degenerative changes, arthritis, or bone spurs; also called *radiculitis* *The areas most commonly affected are the neck (cervical radiculopathy) and lower back (lumbar radiculopathy or sciatica). Rest and anti-inflammatory medications are the usual method of treatment.*
Reye syndrome RĪ	Rare but potentially fatal syndrome that causes acute brain swelling and liver damage and is characterized by confusion, hyperventilation, violent behavior, seizures, and possibly coma; also called *acute noninflammatory encephalopathy* and *fatty degenerative liver failure* *Reye syndrome primarily affects children and teenagers recovering from a viral infection, most commonly flu or chickenpox, especially when aspirin products have been used.*
spina bifida SPĪ-nă BĬ-fĭ-dă	Congenital deformity of the neural tube (embryonic structure that becomes the fetal brain and spinal cord), which fails to close during fetal development; also called *neural tube defect* *The most common forms are in Figure 15-17.*

Figure 15-17 Spina bifida.

Diseases and Conditions—cont'd

Term	Definition
meningocele mĕn-ĬN-gō-sēl *mening/o:* meninges (membranes covering the brain and spinal cord) *-cele:* hernia, swelling	Form of spina bifida in which the spinal cord develops properly but the meninges protrude through the spine
myelomeningocele mī-ĕ-lō-mĕn-ĬN-gō-sēl *myel/o:* bone marrow; spinal cord *mening/o:* meninges (membranes covering the brain and spinal cord) *-cele:* hernia, swelling	Most severe form of spina bifida in which the spinal cord and meninges protrude through the spine
occulta ŏ-KŬL-tă	Form of spina bifida in which one or more vertebrae are malformed, and the spinal cord is covered with a layer of skin
syncope SĬN-kō-pē	Brief loss of consciousness and posture caused by a temporary decrease of blood flow to the brain; also called *fainting* *Syncope may be associated with a sudden decrease in blood pressure, a decrease in heart rate, or changes in blood volume or distribution. The person usually regains consciousness and becomes alert right away but may experience a brief period of confusion.*

Mental Disorders

This section introduces mental disorders along with their meanings and pronunciations. Word analyses for selected terms are also provided.

anxiety disorders	A group of mental disorders characterized by excessive and persistent worry or fear that interferes with daily life
generalized anxiety disorder (GAD)	Excessive anxiety occurring more days than not for at least 6 months that is difficult to control and associated with symptoms such as muscle tension, irritability, difficulty concentrating, restlessness, and sleep disturbance
obsessive compulsive disorder (OCD)	Involves persistent, intrusive, and unwanted thoughts, images, or urges and repetitive behaviors or mental acts aimed at preventing or reducing anxiety or distress
posttraumatic stress disorder (PTSD)	Develops after witnessing or experiencing a traumatic event and can include intrusive memories, nightmares, flashbacks, avoidance behaviors, negative alterations in mood and cognition, increased startle response, and hypervigilance
bipolar disorders	Mood disorder characterized by significant mood swings including episodes of depression and mania/hypomania (persistently elevated or irritable mood coupled with decreased need for sleep, increased energy, rapid speech, impulsive or reckless behavior, distractibility, and racing thoughts)

Continued

Diseases and Conditions—cont'd

Term	Definition
depressive disorders	Group of disorders characterized by persistent feelings of sadness and loss of interest in activities (anhedonia) that interfere with daily life
major depressive disorder (MDD)	Persistently low mood and anhedonia that lasts more days than not for at least 2 weeks coupled with other symptoms such as changes in sleep and appetite, low energy, feelings of guilt, difficulties with focus, and thoughts of death
persistent depressive disorder	Chronic low mood lasting for at least 2 years with a constellation of symptoms similar to major depression but less severe; also known as *dysthymia*
feeding and eating disorders	Characterized by persistent disturbances in eating behavior and related thoughts, feelings, and behaviors that significantly affect emotional and physical health and interfere with daily life
anorexia nervosa ăn-ō-RĔK-sē-ă nĕr-VŌS-ă	Extreme food restriction with intense fear of gaining weight and a distorted, poor body image
avoidant/restrictive food intake disorder (ARFID)	Extreme avoidance of particular foods and food groups leading to health concerns such as weight loss or nutritional deficiencies; behavior is not driven by poor body image or desire to lose weight
binge eating disorder	Recurrent episodes of binging (consuming excessive amounts of food in a short period of time with lack of control over eating) not followed by compensatory behavior
bulimia nervosa bū-LĬM-ē-ă nĕr-VŌS-ă	Recurrent episodes of binging followed by compensatory behaviors such as vomiting, use of laxatives, or excessive exercise in an effort to lose weight
neurodevelopmental disorders	Atypical development of the nervous system affecting various aspects of cognition, behavior, and motor functions; these disorders typically develop early in childhood
attention deficit-hyperactivity disorder (ADHD)	Persistent difficulty with several aspects of inattention, hyperactivity, and impulsivity that can include inability to sustain attention, forgetfulness, distractibility, disorganization, difficulties with sitting still, fidgeting, excessive talking, and interrupting
autism spectrum disorder (ASD)	Persistent deficits in social communication and interaction that can include difficulty with social-emotional reciprocity, nonverbal communicative behaviors used for social interaction, and developing and maintaining relationships; symptoms can vary widely in severity and presentation
schizophrenia spectrum disorders skĭz-ō-FRĔN-ē-ă	A category of severe mental disorders characterized by disruptions in thinking, perception, emotional regulation, and behavior, often involving psychosis
delusional disorder dĭh-LOO-zhŭh-nl	Persistently experiencing one or more fixed, false beliefs (delusions) lasting at least 1 month

Diseases and Conditions—cont'd

Term	Definition
schizophrenia skĭz-ō-FRĔN-ē-ă	A severe and chronic disorder involving episodes of psychosis characterized by positive symptoms such as hallucinations, disorganized thinking and behavior, and delusions; negative symptoms including anhedonia, avolition, and affective flattening; and cognitive symptoms such as impaired executive functioning, attention deficits, and memory issues

 It is time to review pathology, diseases, and conditions by completing Learning Activity 15–3.

Diagnostic, Surgical, and Therapeutic Procedures

This section introduces diagnostic, surgical, and therapeutic procedures used to diagnose and treat neurological and mental disorders. Descriptions are provided along with pronunciations and word analyses for selected terms.

Procedure	Description
Diagnostic	
Clinical	
electroencephalography (EEG) ē-lĕk-trō-ĕn-sĕf-ă-LŎG-ră-fē *electr/o:* electricity *encephal/o:* brain *-graphy:* process of recording	Recording of electrical activity in the brain using electrodes placed on the scalp (see Fig. 15-18) *Different wave patterns in the EEG are associated with normal and abnormal waking and sleeping states. They help diagnose such conditions as tumors and infections and help locate seizure focus or areas of inactivity.*

Figure 15-18 Electroencephalography (EEG). A young girl wearing an electrode cap recording electrical activity of the brain. A monitor displays and records the results.

Continued

Diagnostic, Surgical, and Therapeutic Procedures—cont'd

Procedure	Description
electromyography (EMG) ē-lĕk-trō-mī-ŎG-ră-fē *electr/o:* electricity *my/o:* muscle *-graphy:* process of recording	Recording of electrical signals (action potentials) that occur in a muscle when it is at rest and during contraction to assess muscular disease or nerve damage *In an EMG, an electrode inserted into a muscle transmits its electrical activity and displays it on a monitor to assess the health of the muscle and the motor neurons that control it (see Fig. 15-19).* **Figure 15-19** Electromyography (EMG).
lumbar puncture (LP) LŬM-băr PŬNK-chūr	Needle puncture of the spinal cavity to extract cerebral spinal fluid (CSF) for diagnostic purposes, for delivery of therapeutic agents into the spinal canal, or to remove fluid to allow other fluids (such as radiopaque substances) to be injected; also called *spinal puncture* and *spinal tap* (see Fig. 15-20) L3 vertebra L4 vertebra Subarachnoid space containing cerebrospinal fluid **Figure 15-20** Lumbar puncture (LP).
nerve conduction velocity (NCV) NĔRV kŏn-DŬK-shŭn vĕ-LŎ-sĭ-tē	Test that measures the speed at which impulses travel through a nerve *In NCV, one electrode stimulates a nerve while other electrodes placed over different areas of the nerve record an electrical signal (action potential) as it travels through the nerve. This test helps diagnose and assess severity of nerve damage or dysfunction in muscular and neurological disorders that affect the PNS.*

Diagnostic, Surgical, and Therapeutic Procedures—cont'd

Procedure	Description
Laboratory	
cerebrospinal fluid (CSF) analysis sĕr-ē-brō-SPĪ-năl *cerebr/o:* cerebrum *spin:* spine *-al:* pertaining to	Laboratory test to examine a sample of the fluid surrounding the brain and spinal cord that helps diagnose disorders of the CNS, including viral and bacterial infections, tumors, and hemorrhage
Imaging	
computed tomography angiography (CTA, CT angiography) kŏm-PŪ-tĕd tō-MŎG-ră-fē ăn-jē-ŎG-ră-fē *tom/o:* to cut *-graphy:* process of recording *angi/o:* vessel (usually blood or lymph) *-graphy:* process of recording	Radiographic image of the interior of a vessel in combination with a CT scan to produce high-resolution, three-dimensional images of blood vessels *CTA identifies blocked blood vessels, aneurysms, vascular malformations, and buildup of plaque in a blood vessel. It also aids in differentiating hemorrhagic stroke and ischemic stroke.*
discography dĭs-KŎG-ră-fē	A specialized diagnostic tool using a CT scan or x-ray to visualize and evaluate intervertebral disks in the spine after injection of a contrast medium into the disk of interest
echoencephalography (EEG) ĕk-ō-ĕn-sĕf-ă-LŎG-ră-fē *echo-:* repeated sound *encephal/o:* brain *-graphy:* process of recording	Ultrasound technique used to study intracranial structures of the brain and diagnose conditions that cause a shift in the midline structures of the brain *EEG is a bedside procedure that is especially useful in detecting hemorrhage and hydrocephalus in children less than 2 years of age and infants in the neonatal unit but has largely been replaced by CT for older children and adults.*
magnetic source imaging (MSI)	Noninvasive neuroimaging technique to pinpoint the specific location where seizure activity originates and enable custom surgical treatment for tumor and epileptic tissue resection *MSI is medically necessary for presurgical evaluation of persons with epilepsy to identify and localize areas of epileptic activity.*
myelography mī-ĕ-LŎG-ră-fē *myel/o:* bone marrow; spinal cord *-graphy:* process of recording	Radiographic examination to detect pathology of the spinal cord, spinal canal, and nerve roots, including the location of a spinal cord injury, cysts, and tumors after injection of a contrast medium
positron emission tomography (PET) PŎZ-ĭ-trŏn ē-MĬSH-ŭn tō-MŎG-ră-fē	CT that records the positrons (positively charged particles) emitted from a radiopharmaceutical and produces a cross-sectional image of metabolic activity of body tissues to determine the presence of disease *PET is particularly useful in scanning the brain and nervous system to diagnose disorders that involve abnormal tissue metabolism, such as schizophrenia, brain tumors, epilepsy, stroke, and AD, in addition to cardiac and pulmonary disorders.*
Surgical	
cryosurgery krī-ō-SĔR-jĕr-ē	Technique that exposes abnormal tissue to extreme cold to destroy it *Cryosurgery is sometimes used to destroy malignant tumors of the brain.*

Continued

Diagnostic, Surgical, and Therapeutic Procedures—cont'd

Procedure	Description
thalamotomy thăl-ă-MŎT-ō-mē *thalam/o:* thalamus *-tomy:* incision	Localized destruction of the thalamus to treat movement disorders such as Parkinson disease, essential tremor, and dystonia ***Thalamotomy is generally associated with a low risk of neurological deficits or changes in personality.***
tractotomy trăk-TŎT-ō-mē	Transection of a nerve tract in the brainstem or spinal cord ***Tractotomy is sometimes used to relieve intractable pain.***
trephination trĕf-ĭn-Ā-shŭn	Technique that cuts a circular opening into the skull to reveal brain tissue or decrease intracranial pressure
ventriculoperitoneal shunting vĕn-trĭk-ū-lō-pĕr-ĭ-tō-NĒ-ăl SHŬNT-ĭng *ventricul/o:* ventricle *peritone:* peritoneum *-al:* pertaining to	Relieves intracranial pressure due to hydrocephalus by diverting (shunting) excess cerebrospinal fluid from the brain ventricles into the peritoneal or thoracic cavity (see Fig. 15-21)

Figure 15-21 Ventriculoperitoneal shunt.

Diagnostic, Surgical, and Therapeutic Procedures—cont'd

Procedure	Description
Therapeutic	
Botox	Involves the use of botulinum toxin injections to manage various neurological disorders; works by blocking release of acetylcholine (Ach), resulting in muscle relaxation *Botox injections can be used for migraine prevention, muscle spasticity, and cervical dystonia.*
electroconvulsive therapy (ECT)	Medical treatment most commonly used in patients with treatment resistant depression, severe symptomatology such as suicidal thoughts or psychosis, or bipolar disorder; it involves a brief electrical stimulation of the brain while the patient is under anesthesia *ECT is known to cause changes in brain chemistry that can quickly reverse symptoms of certain mental disorders. Common side effects include HA, memory loss, and confusion, but these are usually short term.*

intravenous (IV) tissue plasminogen activator (tPA)
  intra-: in, within
  ven: vein
  -ous: pertaining to
	Treatment for ischemic stroke using tPA, a potent clot-busting drug, injected directly into a vein
	
	IV tPA helps treat ischemic stroke but must be given as early as possible, ideally within the first 3 hours of stroke onset, during which treatment is most effective. Knowing the symptoms of stroke and calling 911 are essential for effectively treating the patient.

ketamine therapy KĔT- ă-mēn	Traditionally used as an anesthetic but can be used in low doses for treatment-resistant depression, anxiety, and chronic pain; works on the brain's glutamate system and promotes synaptic growth and brain neuroplasticity *Ketamine can be administered intravenously, orally, or intranasally under close medical supervision in an outpatient setting. Treatment works rapidly, often within hours to days.*
low-level laser therapy (LLLT)	Use of low-level lasers or light-emitting diodes (LEDs) to deliver light to the body's tissues; cells absorb the light, which leads to various therapeutic effects including nerve regeneration, wound healing, reduction of inflammation, and pain relief *This is a noninvasive treatment that can be used in the outpatient setting. It has shown to have positive benefits in treating neurological conditions such as peripheral neuropathy, MS, migraines, recovery from stroke, and pain associated with trigeminal neuralgia.*
plasmapheresis plăz-mă-fĕr-Ē-sĭs	Extracorporeal procedure used to treat a variety of medical conditions by removing plasma from the bloodstream and replacing it with donor plasma or plasma substitutes *Plasmapheresis helps treat such autoimmune diseases as multiple sclerosis, Guillain-Barré syndrome, and myasthenia gravis.*

Continued

Diagnostic, Surgical, and Therapeutic Procedures—cont'd

Procedure	Description
psychotherapy *psych/o:* mind *-therapy:* treatment	Treatment method to help with a variety of mental disorders provided by a trained mental health professional to improve emotional wellness, enhance coping skills, foster self-esteem, and promote healthy behavior change; also referred to as *talk therapy* *Evidence-based psychotherapies have been scientifically tested and found to be effective for several mental health disorders. Some common types include cognitive behavioral therapy (CBT), interpersonal therapy (ITP), exposure therapy, acceptance and commitment therapy (ACT), motivational interviewing (MI), and behavioral activation (BA).*
stereotactic radiosurgery (SRS) stĕr-ē-ō-TĂK-tĭk rā-dē-ō-SŬR-jĕr-ē	Procedure that uses three-dimensional imaging (stereotactic) along with high doses of highly focused radiation to destroy tumors and other abnormal growths in the brain, spinal column, and other body sites with minimal exposure to surrounding healthy tissue *Because of its accuracy and precision, the principles used in SRS are now being applied to treat various body tumors with a procedure called* **stereotactic body radiotherapy (SBRT).**
transcranial magnetic stimulation (TMS) trănz-KRĀ-nē-ăl *trans-:* across, through *crani/o:* cranium (skull) *-al:* pertaining to	TMS is a noninvasive technique used to stimulate nerve cells in the brain using magnetic fields, primarily used in the treatment of MDD that has not responded to medication and psychotherapy *TMS targets areas of the brain involved with mood regulation, like the prefrontal cortex. Treatment sessions are typically daily for several weeks and last about 20 to 40 minutes. It is generally well tolerated.*

Pharmacology

Neurological agents help relieve or eliminate pain, suppress seizures, control tremors, and reduce muscle rigidity (see Table 15-2). Anesthetics can produce a complete or partial loss of feeling with or without loss of consciousness and are used for procedures like surgery. Psychotropic agents modulate neurotransmitter activity in the brain to treat mental disorders. These medications are used as mood stabilizers, anxiolytics, antidepressants, antipsychotics, and to treat symptoms of ADHD and narcolepsy. Hypnotics, a class of drugs used as sedatives, depress CNS function to relieve agitation and induce sleep.

TABLE 15-2 Drugs Used to Treat Neurological and Psychiatric Disorders

This table lists common drug classifications used to treat neurological and psychiatric disorders, along with their therapeutic actions and selected generic and trade names.

Classification	Therapeutic Action	Generic and Trade Names
Neurological		
anesthetics ăn-ĕs-THĔT-ĭks	Produce partial or complete loss of sensation, with or without loss of consciousness *Forms of anesthetics include general, local, and nerve block.*	
general	Act upon the brain to produce complete loss of feeling with loss of consciousness *General anesthetics affect all areas of the body, including the brain. Because they suppress all reflexes, including coughing and swallowing, breathing tubes are usually required during their administration.*	**propofol** PRŎ-pō-fŏl *Diprivan*
local	Act upon nerves or nerve tracts to affect only a local area *Local anesthetics are injected directly into the area involved in the local surgery. Patients may remain fully alert unless additional medications to induce sleep are given.*	**procaine** PRŌ-kān *Novocain* **lidocaine** LĪ-dō-kān *Xylocaine*
nerve block	Blocks pain from the area supplied by that nerve *A nerve block is a type of regional anesthetic usually used for procedures on the arms, legs, hands, feet, and face.*	**levobupivacaine** lĕv-ō-bū-PĪ-vă-kān *Chirocaine*
anticonvulsants ăn-tĭ-kŏn-VŬL-sănts	Stabilize neuronal excitability and inhibit abnormal electrical activity in the brain by altering electrical transmission along neurons or altering the chemical composition of neurotransmitters; also called *antiepileptics* *Many anticonvulsants are used as mood stabilizers or for treatment of neuropathic pain syndromes.*	**carbamazepine** kăr-bă-MĂZ-ĕ-pēn *Tegretol* **valproate** văl-PRŌ-āt *Depacon* **phenytoin** FĔN-ĭ-tō-ĭn *Dilantin*
antiparkinsonian agents ăn-tĭ-păr-kĭn-SŌN-ē-ăn	Control tremors and muscle rigidity associated with Parkinson disease by increasing dopamine in the regions of the brain crucial for movement control and coordination	**levodopa** lē-vō-DŌ-pă *L-Dopa, Larodopa* **levodopa/carbidopa** kăr-bĭ-DŌ-pă *Sinemet, Sinemet CR*

(continued)

TABLE 15-2 Drugs Used to Treat Neurological and Psychiatric Disorders—cont'd

Classification	Therapeutic Action	Generic and Trade Names
Psychiatric		
antianxiety agents ăn-tĭ-ăng-ZĪ-ĕ-tē	Interact at distinct receptor sites in the limbic and cortical system to decrease anxiety	**alprazolam** ăl-PRĀ-zō-lăm *Xanax* **buspirone** bū-SPĪ-rōn *Buspar*
antidepressants ăn-tĭ-dē-PRĔS-săntz	Treat multiple symptoms of depression by modulating levels of specific neurotransmitters in the brain such as serotonin, norepinephrine, and dopamine *Antidepressants fall under different classifications, and some are also used to treat various anxiety disorders and pain.*	**citalopram** sī-TĂL-ō-prăm *Celexa* **fluoxetine** floo-ŎK-sĕ-tēn *Prozac* **venlafaxine** VĔN-lă-fĕx-ēn *Effexor*
antipsychotics ăn-tĭ-sī-KŎT-ĭks	Treat psychosis, paranoia, and schizophrenia by altering chemicals in the brain, including the limbic system, which controls emotions	**clozapine** CLŌ-ză-pēn *Clozaril* **risperidone** rĭs-PĔR-ĭ-dōn *Risperdal*
hypnotics hĭp-NŎT-ĭks	Depress central nervous system (CNS) functions, promote sedation and sleep, and relieve agitation, anxiousness, and restlessness	**eszopiclone** ĕs-ZŌ-plĭ-kōn *Lunesta* *Restoril* **zolpidem** ZŌL-pĭ-dĕm *Ambien*
partial opioid agonist-antagonist	Primarily used in the treatment of opioid dependence and addiction; also used to treat moderate to severe pain	**buprenorphine/naloxone** BŪ-prĕ-nŏr-fēn/nă-LŎK-sōn *Suboxone* **Nalbuphine** NĂL-bŭ-fēn *Nubain*
stimulants STĬM-ū-lăntz	Reduce impulsive behavior, improve attention and executive function by influencing the level and activity of certain neurotransmitters in areas of the brain that promote wakefulness, alertness, and cognition *Stimulants have a calming effect on people with attention deficit-hyperactiviy disorder (ADHD) and can also be used to treat narcolepsy.*	**dextroamphetamine** dĕks-trō-ăm-FĔT-ă-mēn *Dexedrine* **methylphenidate** mĕth-ĭl-FĔN-ĭ-dāt *Ritalin*

Abbreviations

This section introduces abbreviations related to the nervous system, along with their meanings.

Abbreviation	Meaning	Abbreviation	Meaning
AA	Alcoholics Anonymous	DA	dopamine
ACh	acetylcholine	DSM5	*Diagnostic and Statistical Manual of Mental Disorders, Fifth Edition*
AChR	acetylcholine receptor	ECT	electroconvulsive therapy
ACT	acceptance and commitment therapy	EEG	electroencephalography; echoencephalography
AD	Alzheimer disease	EMG	electromyography
ADHD	attention deficit-hyperactivity disorder	5-HT	5-hydroxytryptamine (serotonin)
ALS	amyotrophic lateral sclerosis	FTD	frontotemporal dementia
ANS	autonomic nervous system	GABA	gamma-aminobutyric acid
ARFID	avoidant/restrictive food intake disorder	GAD	generalized anxiety disorder
ASD	autism spectrum disorder; atrial septal defect	GBS	Guillain-Barré syndrome; gallbladder series (x-ray studies)
BA	behavioral activation	HA	headache
CBT	cognitive behavioral therapy	HSV	herpes simplex virus
CDC	Centers for Disease Control	ICP	intracranial pressure
CNS	central nervous system	IPT	interpersonal therapy
CP	cerebral palsy	IV	intravenous
CSF	cerebrospinal fluid	LBD	Lewy body dementia
CT	computed tomography	LLLT	low-level laser therapy
CTA	computed tomography angiography	LP	lumbar puncture
CVA	cerebrovascular accident	MDD	major depressive disorder

Continued

Abbreviation	Meaning	Abbreviation	Meaning
MG	myasthenia gravis	**PNS**	peripheral nervous system
MI	motivational interviewing, myocardial infarction	**PTSD**	posttraumatic stress disorder
MRI	magnetic resonance imaging	**SAH**	subarachnoid hemorrhage
MS	multiple sclerosis; mental status; musculoskeletal; mitral stenosis	**SBRT**	stereotactic body radiotherapy
MSE	mental status examination	**SNS**	sympathetic nervous system
MSI	magnetic source imaging	**SRS**	stereotactic radiosurgery
NA	Narcotics Anonymous	**SUD**	substance use disorder
NCV	nerve conduction velocity	**TBI**	traumatic brain injury
NE	norepinephrine	**TIA**	transient ischemic attack
NES	nonepileptic seizures	**TMS**	transcranial magnetic stimulation
PET	positron emission tomography	**tPA**	tissue plasminogen activator
PNES	psychogenic nonepileptic seizures	**VaD**	vascular dementia

It is time to review procedures, pharmacology, and abbreviations by completing Learning Activity 15–4.

LEARNING ACTIVITIES

The activities that follow provide a review of the nervous system terms introduced in this chapter. Complete each activity and review your answers to evaluate your understanding of the chapter.

Visit the Medical Language Laboratory at medicallanguagelab.com. Use it to enhance your study and reinforcement of this chapter with the flash card activity. We recommend that you complete the flash card activity before starting Learning Activities 15-1 and 15-2.

Learning Activity 15-1
Medical Word Elements

Use the listed elements to build medical words. You may use elements more than once.

Combining Forms		Suffixes		Prefixes	
cerebr/o	myel/o	-al	-lepsy	hyper-	quadri-
encephal/o	narc/o	-algia	-oma	intra-	uni-
gangli/o	neur/o	-asthenia	-pathy		
kinesi/o	radicul/o	-cele	-plegia		
later/o	thec/o	-ectomy	-rrhaphy		
mening/o	ventricul/o	-itis	-stomy		
my/o		-kinesia	-therapy		

1. forming an opening (mouth) in the ventricle _____
2. tumor of a nerve _____
3. pain in a nerve root _____
4. excision of a ganglion _____
5. seizure of sleep _____
6. pertaining to one side _____
7. inflammation of the meninges _____
8. paralysis of four (extremities) _____
9. movement that is excessive _____
10. weakness or debility of muscles _____
11. disease of the cerebrum _____
12. pertaining to within the sheath _____
13. hernia(tion) or swelling of the brain _____
14. treatment (using) movement _____
15. suture of the spinal cord _____

 Check your answers in Appendix A. Review any material that you did not answer correctly.

Correct Answers _____ X 6.67 = _____ % Score

Learning Activity 15-2
Building Medical Words

Use *encephal/o* (brain) to build words that mean:

1. disease of the brain _____
2. herniation of the brain _____
3. radiography of the brain _____

Use *cerebr/o* (cerebrum) to build words that mean:

4. disease of the cerebrum _____
5. inflammation of the cerebrum _____

Use *crani/o* (cranium [skull]) to build words that mean:

6. herniation (through the) cranium _____
7. instrument for measuring the skull _____

Use *neur/o* (nerve) to build words that mean:

8. pain in a nerve _____
9. specialist in the study of the nervous system _____
10. crushing a nerve _____

Use *myel/o* (bone marrow; spinal cord) to build words that mean:

11. herniation of the spinal cord _____
12. paralysis of the spinal cord _____

Use *psych/o* (mind) to build words that mean:

13. pertaining to the mind _____
14. abnormal condition of the mind _____

Use the suffix *-kinesia* (movement) to build words that mean:

15. movement that is slow _____
16. painful or difficult movement _____

Use the suffix *-plegia* (paralysis) to build words that mean:

17. paralysis of one-half (of the body) _____
18. paralysis of four (limbs) _____

Use the suffix *-phasia* (speech) to build words that mean:

19. difficult speech _____

20. lacking or without speech _____

Build surgical terms that mean:

21. destruction of a nerve _____

22. incision of the skull _____

23. surgical repair of the skull _____

24. suture of a nerve _____

25. incision of the brain _____

✓ *Check your answers in Appendix A. Review material that you did not answer correctly.*

Correct Answers _____ X 4 = _____ % Score

Learning Activity 15-3
Diseases and Conditions

Match the terms with the definitions in the numbered list.

ALS	bipolar	dementia	multiple sclerosis	radiculopathy
Alzheimer	clonic	epilepsies	myelomeningocele	schizophrenia
anhedonia	cluster headache	Guillain-Barré	paraplegia	shingles
anorexia nervosa	concussion	hemiparesis	Parkinson	spina bifida
ataxia	convulsion	ischemic	poliomyelitis	TIA

1. weakness in one-half of the body _____

2. cognitive deficit, including memory impairment _____

3. disease associated with formation of small plaques in the cerebral cortex _____

4. lack of pleasure _____

5. phase of a grand mal seizure characterized by uncontrolled jerking of the body _____

6. autoimmune syndrome that causes acute inflammation of peripheral nerves _____

7. defective muscle coordination _____

8. mood disorder with episodes of depression and mania or hypomania _____

9. chronic or recurring seizure disorders _____

10. stroke caused by narrowing of the carotid arteries _____

11. disease caused by the same organism that causes chickenpox in children _____

12. disease of the nerve root associated with the spinal cord _____

13. paralysis of the lower portion of the trunk and both legs _____

14. disease that causes inflammation of the gray matter of the spinal cord _____

15. sudden, violent contraction of one or more voluntary muscles _____

16. most severe form of spina bifida, where the spinal cord and meninges protrude through the spine _____

17. characterized by positive symptoms such as hallucinations, disorganized thinking and behavior, and delusions _____

18. disease characterized by head nodding, bradykinesia, tremors, and shuffling gait _____

19. disease characterized by demyelination in the spinal cord and brain _____

20. loss of consciousness caused by trauma to the head _____

21. usually causes intense pain around one eye or one side of the head _____

22. intense fear of gaining weight and extreme food restriction with a distorted, poor body image _____

23. progressive neurodegenerative disease that targets the motor neurons responsible for voluntary muscle movement _____

24. type of stroke in which symptoms resolve within 24 hours and do not cause permanent damage _____

25. congenital deformity of the neural tube, which fails to close during fetal development _____

✔ *Check your answers in Appendix A. Review any material that you did not answer correctly.*

Correct Answers _____ X 4 = _____ % Score

Learning Activity 15-4

Procedures, Pharmacology, and Abbreviations

Match the terms with the definitions in the numbered list.

antipsychotics	EMG	myelography
CP	general anesthetics	NCV
CSF analysis	hypnotics	stimulants
ECT	ketamine	TIA
EEG	lumbar puncture	trephination

1. alternative therapy used for treatment resistant depression, anxiety, and pain that works on the glutamate system of the brain _____

2. radiological examination of the spinal canal, nerve roots, and spinal cord _____

3. treat psychosis, paranoia, and schizophrenia by modulating neurotransmitters in the brain _____

4. short electrical stimulation of the brain while under anesthesia to treat severe depression _____

5. act upon the brain to produce complete loss of feeling with loss of consciousness _____

6. diagnostic test that records electrical activity in the brain to detect neurological conditions _____

7. treat attention deficit-hyperactivity disorder and narcolepsy _____

8. type of paralysis affecting movement that commonly occurs from brain trauma during the birthing process _____

9. stroke with symptoms that resolve in about 24 hours _____

10. laboratory analysis used to diagnose infections, tumors, and intracranial hemorrhage _____

11. tests the speed at which impulses travel through a nerve _____

12. recording of electrical signals when a muscle is at rest and during contraction to assess nerve damage _____

13. procedure to extract spinal fluid for diagnostic purposes, to introduce anesthetic agents, or to remove fluid _____

14. agents that depress central nervous system functions, promote sedation and sleep, and relieve agitation, anxiousness, and restlessness _____

15. incision of a circular opening into the skull to reveal brain tissue and decrease intracranial pressure _____

Check your answers in Appendix A. Review any material that you did not answer correctly.

Correct Answers _____ X 6.67 = _____ % Score

DOCUMENTING HEALTH-CARE ACTIVITIES

This section provides practical application activities in the form of exercises to help develop skills in documenting patient care. First read the medical report, then complete the activities and exercises that follow.

Documenting Health-Care Activity 15-1
Chart Note: Medication Management Follow-Up

Patient: Mozzy Garcia   **Date:** May 12, 20XX

CC: 24-year-old single, unemployed male with a history of anxiety is presenting today for medication management follow up. He was last seen on 4/1/xx when no changes were made to his medication regimen of sertraline 100 mg PO daily. Today, he presents with the chief complaint of depression.

SUBJECTIVE: Patient reports that he has been experiencing depressed mood for the last 2 months without apparent trigger. He notes anhedonia, low appetite, low energy, and poor focus. He has been experiencing initial insomnia and hypersomnia; he typically sleeps 12 hours per night. Denies suicidal thoughts, intentions, and plans. No history of suicide attempts. He has hope and his family, cat, and friends are protective. Anxiety levels are manageable overall. Sometimes he gets anxious about performing daily chores and he will feel overwhelmed, tense, and irritable. Denies hypomania/mania. Denies homicidal thoughts, intentions, and plans. Denies hallucinations and paranoia. He is not active in therapy. Denies any substance use including alcohol, marijuana, nicotine, and caffeine. Patient first started sertraline several years ago and has largely had a positive response; he takes it daily. Denies side effects.

Review of Systems:
Recent increase in thyroid medication dose. Otherwise, ROS is negative.

MENTAL STATUS EXAMINATION

APPEARANCE: Well-appearing male, good eye contact and engagement, nasal piercing, facial hair, no abnormal involuntary movements.

MOOD: Dysphoric.

AFFECT: Restricted.

SPEECH: Fluent English speaker, speech of normal rate and volume.

THOUGHT PROCESS: Linear, logical, goal directed.

THOUGHT CONTENT: Primarily symptom and stressor focused, no suicidal or homicidal thoughts, intentions, or plans. No delusions or obsessions.

PERCEPTION: Denies hallucinations, does not appear to be attending to any internal stimuli.

INTELLECT: No evidence for impaired intellectual functioning.

INSIGHT/JUDGEMENT: Both fair.

RISK ASSESSMENT:
Overall, patient does not present as an imminent risk of harm to himself or others. He is low risk for suicide and stable for outpatient care.

DSM-5 DIAGNOSIS:
1. MDE, single episode, moderate.
2. Unspecified anxiety disorder.

PLAN:

Psychoeducation: diagnoses, treatment options/alternatives and risks and benefits of treatment discussed.

Therapy: None currently.

Medications: Increase sertraline to 150 mg PO daily.

Safety: Safety plan, calling 911, and reporting to closest ER reviewed. Patient voiced understanding and consented to the treatment plan.

Follow Up: 6 weeks.

Ruby S. Abbott, D.O.
Ruby S. Abbott, D.O.

Terminology

The terms listed in the table that follows are taken from *Chart Note: Medication Management Follow Up*. Use a medical dictionary such as *Taber's Cyclopedic Medical Dictionary*, the appendices of this book, or other resources to define each term. Then review the pronunciation for each term and practice by reading the medical record aloud.

Term	Definition
anhedonia ĂN-hĕ-dō-nē-ă	
delusions dĭh-LOO-zhŭnz	
dysphoric dĭs-FŎR-ē-ă	
hallucinations hă-loo-sĭ-NĀ-shŭnz	
hypersomnia hī-pĕr-SŎM-nē-ă	
insomnia ĭn-SŎM-nē-ă	
internal stimuli ĭn-TĔR-năl STĬM- ū-lī	
mania MĀ-nē-ă	
MDE	
PO	
sertraline SĔR-tră-lēn	

Visit the Medical Terminology Systems online resource center at FADavis. com to practice pronunciation and reinforce the meanings of the terms in this medical report.

Critical Thinking

Review *Chart Note: Medication Management Follow-Up* to answer the questions.

1. What are some of the symptoms of depression the patient is experiencing?

_____

_____

_____

2. How long has the patient been experiencing symptoms of depression?

_____

_____

_____

3. What other psychiatric disorder has the patient experienced?

_____

_____

_____

4. What are some of the reasons the patient would be considered low risk for suicide?

_____

_____

_____

5. What medication is being used to treat the patient's symptoms?

_____

_____

_____

6. What medical condition could be contributing to the patient's depression symptoms?

_____

_____

_____

Consultation Report: Acute-Onset Paraplegia

Physician Center

2422 Rodeo Drive ■ ■ **Sun City, USA 12345** ■ ■ **(555)788–2427**

CONSULTATION

Jacobs, Elaine   August 15, 20xx

CHIEF COMPLAINT: Low back pain and lower extremity weakness

HISTORY OF PRESENT ILLNESS: This is a 41-year-old, right-handed white female with a history of low back pain for the past 15–20 years after falling at work. She has had four subsequent lumbar surgeries, with the most recent on 7/20/xx. She was admitted to the hospital for pain management. The patient had a subarachnoid catheter placed at the T10-11 level for pain control on 7/28/xx. This was followed by trials of clonidine for hypertension and methadone for pain management; however, bladder retention was noted after clonidine administration. The catheter was removed, and the patient noted subacute onset of paresis, paresthesia, and pain in the legs approximately 2 1/2–3 hours later. We were consulted for a neurological assessment of the lower extremity weakness.

IMPRESSION: Patient has symptoms of acute-onset paraplegia. Differential diagnoses include a subarachnoid hemorrhage, epidural abscess, and transverse myelitis.

PLAN: Patient will be placed on IV steroids. Consult physical therapy for clearance to use compression stockings for lymphedema and potential manipulation of that region. Documentation of spinal fluid will be obtained under fluoroscopy. Glucose and blood pressure must be monitored carefully.

Jake S. Domer, MD
Jake S. Domer, MD

JSD:st

Terminology

The terms listed in the table that follows are taken from *Consultation Report: Acute-Onset Paraplegia.* Use a medical dictionary such as *Taber's Cyclopedic Medical Dictionary*, the appendices of this book, or other resources to define each term. Then review the pronunciation for each term and practice by reading the medical record aloud.

Term	Definition
abscess ĂB-sĕs	
acute ă-KŪT	
epidural ĕp-ĭ-DOO-răl	
fluoroscopy floo-or-ŎS-kō-pē	
lumbar LŬM-băr	
lymphedema lĭmf-ĕ-DĒ-mă	
myelitis mī-ĕ-LĪ-tĭs	
paraplegia păr-ă-PLĒ-jē-ă	
paresthesia păr-ĕs-THĒ-zē-ă	
subarachnoid sŭb-ă-RĂK-noyd	
T10–11	

Visit the Medical Terminology Systems online resource center at FADavis.com to practice pronunciation and reinforce the meanings of the terms in this medical report.

Critical Thinking

Review Consultation Report: Acute-Onset Paraplegia to answer the questions.

1. What was the original cause of the patient's current problems, and what treatments were provided?

_____

_____

_____

2. Why was the patient admitted to the hospital?

_____

_____

_____

3. What medications did the patient receive, and why was each given?

_____

_____

_____

4. What was the cause of bladder retention?

_____

_____

_____

5. What occurred after the catheter was removed?

_____

_____

_____

6. What three disorders were listed in the differential diagnosis?

_____

_____

_____

Constructing Chart Notes

To construct chart notes, replace the italicized and boldfaced terms in each of the two case studies with one of the listed medical terms.

bradykinesia	*neuralgia*	*Parkinson disease*
bradyphasia	*neuropathy*	*sciatica*
dysphagia	*osteophyte*	*tremor*
herniation		

Mr. K, a 58-year-old male, works at a local newspaper. For most of his life, he has been tying and lifting bundles of papers and placing them in trucks for delivery throughout the city. He complains of (1) **nerve pain** of the lower back and, when standing, (2) **pain that radiates down the nerve** of his right leg, causing his foot to "tingle." The results of an MRI show a (3) **protrusion** of the disc at the L3–L4, compressing the nerve. The MRI also reveals a small (4) **bone spur** impinging on the same nerve. A nerve conduction velocity will be ordered to assess (5) **nerve disease**.

1. _____
2. _____
3. _____
4. _____
5. _____

Mr. M is an 82-year-old man who was brought to our office by his daughter. She expresses concern because her father frequently has a "far-away stare," and his left hand has developed a noticeable (6) **shake.** His (7) **slow speech** and "word slurring" make it difficult for her to understand and respond to him, causing him further frustration. The daughter notes that her father has (8) **slow movement** and (9) **difficulty in swallowing,** often gagging on his food. The results of a complete medical history, examination, and full neurological workup indicate that this gentleman is suffering from (10) **shaking palsy**. The plan is to begin treatment with levodopa.

6. _____
7. _____
8. _____
9. _____
10. _____

✔ *Check your answers in Appendix A. Review any material that you did not answer correctly.*

Correct Answers _____ X 10 = _____ % Score

Special Senses

Chapter Outline

Objectives

Upon completion of this chapter, you will be able to:

- Locate and describe the structures of the eye and ear.
- Describe the functional relationship between the eyes and the ears and other body systems.
- Pronounce, spell, and build words related to the special senses.
- Describe diseases, conditions, and procedures related to the special senses.
- Explain pharmacology related to the treatment of eye and ear disorders.
- Demonstrate your knowledge of this chapter by completing the learning and documenting health-care activities.

Anatomy and Physiology

General sensations perceived by the body include touch, pressure, pain, and temperature. These sensations are not identified with any specific site of the body. Specific sensations include smell, taste, vision, hearing, and equilibrium (balance). Each specific sensation is connected to a specific organ or structure in the body. This chapter presents information on the sense of vision provided by the eye and the senses of hearing and equilibrium provided by the ear.

Anatomy and Physiology Key Terms

This section introduces important terms associated with the special senses, along with their definitions and pronunciations. Word analyses for selected terms are also provided. Pronounce the term and place a check mark in the box after you do so.

Term	Definition
accommodation ☐ ă-kŏm-ō-DĀ-shŭn	Adjustment of the eye for various distances so that images focus on the retina of the eye
acuity ☐ ă-KŪ ĭ-tē	Clearness or sharpness of a sensory function
adnexa ☐ ăd-NĔK-să	Tissues or structures in the body adjacent to or near a related structure *The adnexa of the eye include the extraocular muscles, orbits, eyelids, conjunctiva, and lacrimal apparatus.*
humor	Any fluid or semifluid of the body
labyrinth ☐ LĂB-ĭ-rĭnth	Series of intricate communicating passages *The labyrinth of the ear includes the cochlea, semicircular canals, and vestibule.*
opaque ☐ ō-PĂK	Substance or surface that neither transmits nor allows the passage of light
perilymph ☐ PĔR-ĭ-lĭmf	Fluid that very closely resembles spinal fluid but is found in the cochlea
photopigment ☐ fō-tō-PĬG-mĕnt	Light-sensitive pigment in the retinal cones and rods that absorbs light and initiates the visual process; also called *visual pigment*
refractive ☐ rĕ-FRĂK-tĭv	Ability to bend light rays as they pass from one medium to another
stereopsis ☐ stĕr-ē-ŎP-sĭs	Depth perception provided by visual information derived from two eyes located in slightly different positions so that each produces its own unique view of an object

Pronunciation Help	Long Sound	ā — rate	ē — rebirth	ī — isle	ō — over	ū — unite
	Short Sound	ă — apple	ĕ — ever	ĭ — it	ŏ — not	ŭ — cut

Eye

The eye is a globe-shaped organ composed of three distinct tunics, or layers: the fibrous tunic, the vascular tunic, and the sensory tunic (see Fig. 16-1).

Fibrous Tunic

The outermost layer of the eyeball, the **fibrous tunic,** serves as a protective coat for the more sensitive structures beneath. It includes the (1) **sclera,** (2) **cornea,** and (3) **conjunctiva.** The sclera, or "white of the eye," provides strength, shape, and structure to the eye. As the sclera passes in front of the eye, it bulges forward to become the cornea. Rather than being **opaque,** the cornea is transparent, allowing light to enter the interior of the eye. The cornea is one of the few body structures that does not contain capillaries and must rely on eye fluids for nourishment. The conjunctiva covers the outer surface of the eye and lines the eyelids.

Vascular Tunic

The middle layer of the eyeball, the **vascular tunic,** is also known as the **uvea.** The uvea consists of the choroid, iris, and ciliary body. The (4) **choroid** provides the blood supply for the entire eye. It contains pigmented cells that prevent extraneous light from entering the inside of the eye. An opening in the choroid allows the optic nerve to enter the inside of the eyeball. The anterior portion of the choroid contains two modified structures, the (5) **iris** and the (6**) ciliary body.** The iris is a colored, contractile membrane with a perforated center called the (7) **pupil.** The iris regulates the amount of light passing through the pupil to the interior of the eye. As environmental light increases, the pupil constricts; as light decreases, the pupil dilates. The ciliary body is a circular muscle that produces aqueous **humor.** The ciliary body is attached to a capsular bag that holds the (8) **lens** between the (9) **suspensory ligaments.** As the ciliary muscle contracts and relaxes, it alters the shape of the lens, making it thicker or thinner. These changes in shape allow the eye to focus on an image, a process called **accommodation (Acc).**

Figure 16-1 Eye structures.

Sensory Tunic

The innermost **sensory tunic** is the delicate, double-layered (10) **retina.** It consists of a thin, outer **pigmented layer** lying over the choroid and a thick, inner **nervous layer,** or visual portion. The retina is responsible for the reception and transmission of visual impulses to the brain. It has two types of visual receptors: rods and cones. **Rods** function in dim light and produce black-and-white vision. **Cones** function in bright light and produce color vision. In the central portion of the retina is a highly sensitive structure called the **macula.** In the center of the macula is the (11) **fovea.** When the eye focuses on an object, light rays from that object are directed to the fovea. Because the fovea is composed of only cones that lie very close to each other, it provides the greatest **acuity** for color vision.

Rods and cones contain a chemical called **photopigment,** or **visual pigment.** As light strikes the photopigment, a chemical change occurs that stimulates rods and cones. The chemical changes produce impulses that are transmitted through the (12) **optic nerve** to the brain, where they are interpreted as vision. The optic nerve and blood vessels of the eye enter at the (13) **optic disc.** Its center is referred to as the **blind spot** because the area has neither rods nor cones for vision.

One of two major fluids **(humors)** of the eye is **aqueous humor.** It is found in the (14) **posterior chamber** and (15) **anterior chamber** of the anterior portion of the eye and provides nourishment for the lens and the cornea. The ciliary body continually produces aqueous humor, which drains from the eye through a small opening called the (16) **canal of Schlemm.** If aqueous humor fails to drain from the eye at the rate at which it is produced, a condition called **glaucoma** results. The second major humor of the eye is **vitreous humor,** a jellylike substance that fills the interior of the eye, the (17) **vitreous chamber.** The vitreous humor, lens, and aqueous humor are the **refractive** structures of the eye, focusing light rays sharply on the retina. If any one of these structures does not function properly, vision is impaired.

Adnexa

The **adnexa** of the eye include all supporting structures of the eye globe. Six extraocular muscles control the movement of the eye: the superior, inferior, lateral, and medial rectus muscles and the superior and inferior oblique muscles. These muscles coordinate the eyes so that they move in a synchronized manner. In normal vision, each eye views an image from a somewhat different vantage point, thus transmitting a slightly different image to the brain. The result is binocular perception of depth or three-dimensional space, a phenomenon known as **stereopsis.**

Two movable folds of skin constitute the eyelids, each with eyelashes that are highly sensitive to touch, thus providing a warning that triggers a blink reflex when dust or other irritants are near the eye (see Fig. 16-2). The (1) **conjunctiva** lines the inner surface of the eyelids and the sclera.

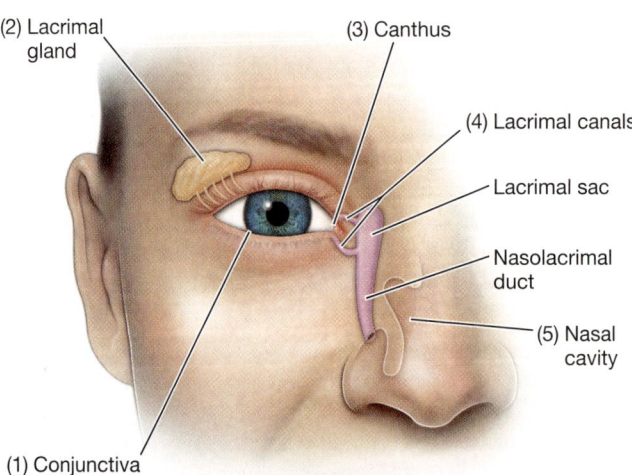

Figure 16-2 Lacrimal apparatus.

It lubricates the eye by producing mucus and tears, although a smaller volume than the tears associated with the **lacrimal apparatus.** Lying superior and to the outer edge of each eye are the (2) **lacrimal glands,** which produce tears that bathe and lubricate the eyes. The tears collect at the inner edges of the eyes, the (3) **canthi** (singular, **canthus**), and pass through pinpoint openings, the (4) **lacrimal canals,** to the mucous membranes that line the inside of the (5) **nasal cavity.**

Ear

The ear is the sense receptor organ for two senses: hearing and equilibrium. Hearing is a function of the cochlea. Equilibrium is a function of the semicircular canals and vestibule.

Hearing

The ear consists of three major sections: the outer ear, or **external ear;** the middle ear, or **tympanic cavity;** and the inner ear, or **labyrinth** (see Fig. 16-3). The external ear conducts sound waves through air; the middle ear, through bone; and the inner ear, through fluid. This series of transmissions ultimately generates impulses that are sent to the brain and interpreted as sound.

An (1) **auricle** (or pinna) collects waves traveling through air and channels them to the (2) **external auditory canal,** also called the **ear canal.** The ear canal is a slender tube lined with glands that produce a waxy secretion called **cerumen.** Its stickiness traps tiny foreign particles and prevents them from entering the deeper areas of the canal. The (3) **tympanic membrane** (also called the **tympanum** or **eardrum**) is a flat, membranous structure drawn over the end of the ear canal. Sound waves entering the ear canal strike against the tympanic membrane, causing it to vibrate. These vibrations cause movement of the three smallest bones of the body, collectively called the **ossicles.** These tiny articulating bones, the (4) **malleus** (or **hammer**), the (5) **incus** (or **anvil**), and the (6) **stapes** (or **stirrups**), are located within the tympanic cavity and form a connection between the tympanic membrane and the (7) **cochlea,** the first structure of the inner ear. The cochlea is a snail-shaped structure filled with a fluid called **perilymph**. Its inner surfaces are lined with a highly sensitive hearing structure called the **organ of Corti,** which contains

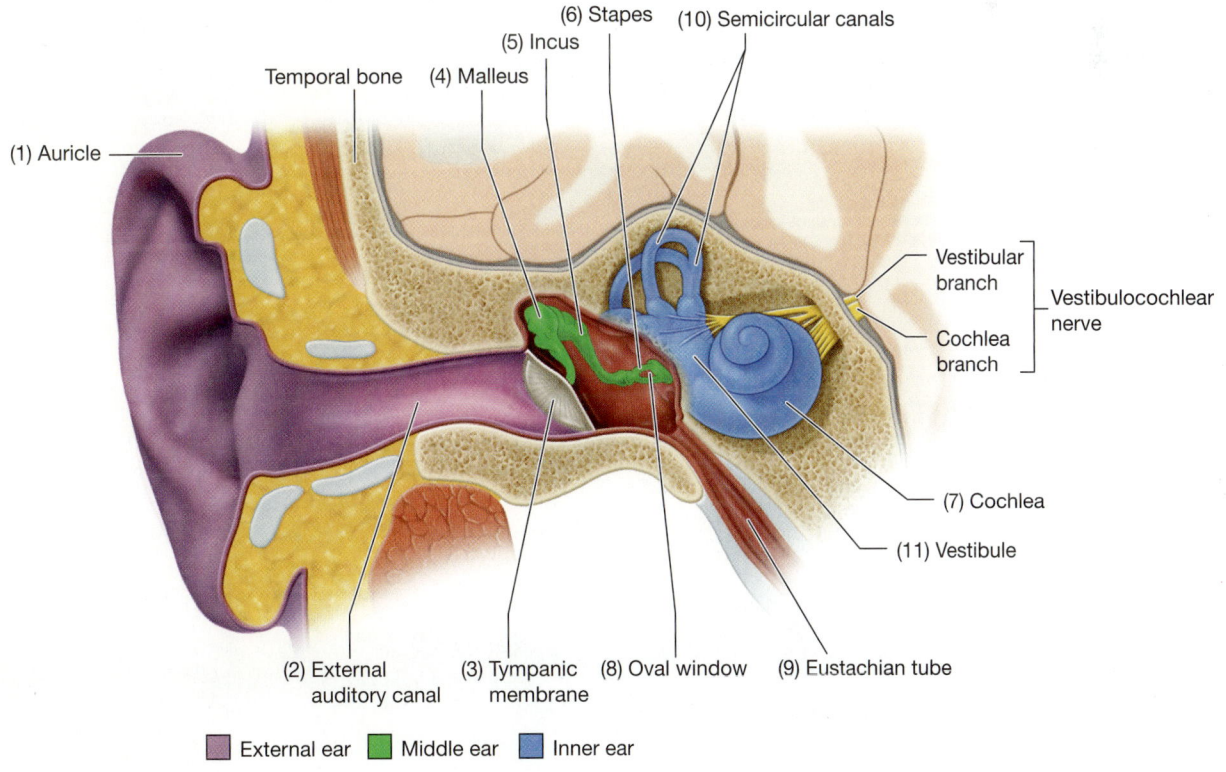

Figure 16-3 Ear structures.

tiny nerve endings called **hair cells.** A membrane-covered opening on the external surface of the cochlea called the (8) **oval window** provides a place for attachment of the stapes. The movement of the ossicles in the middle ear causes the stapes to exert a gentle pumping action against the oval window. The pumping action forces the perilymph to disturb the hair cells, generating impulses that are transmitted to the brain by way of the auditory nerve, where they are interpreted as sound. The (9) **eustachian tube** connects the middle ear to the pharynx. It equalizes pressure on the outer and inner surfaces of the eardrum. When there is an inequality of pressure on either side of the membrane, a deliberate swallow will commonly restore equality.

Equilibrium

The inner ear consists of a system of fluid-filled tubes and sacs and the nerves that connect these structures to the brain. Because of its mazelike design, it is referred to as the **labyrinth.** The labyrinth, which rests inside the skull bones, includes not only the cochlear system (the organ devoted to hearing) but also the vestibular system, which is devoted to the control of equilibrium (balance) and eye movements. The vestibular system contains the (10) **semicircular canals** and the (11) **vestibule.** The vestibule joins the cochlea and the semicircular canals. Many complex structures located in this maze are responsible for maintaining balance.

Anatomy Review: Eye

To review the anatomy of the eye, label the illustration using the listed terms.

anterior chamber	*cornea*	*optic disc*	*retina*
canal of Schlemm	*fovea*	*optic nerve*	*sclera*
choroid	*iris*	*posterior chamber*	*suspensory ligaments*
ciliary body	*lens*	*pupil*	*vitreous chamber*
conjunctiva			

Retinal artery and vein

Inferior rectus muscle

Check your answers by referring to Figure 16–1 on page 607. Review material that you did not answer correctly.

Anatomy Review: Ear

To review the anatomy of the ear, label the illustration using the listed terms.

auricle	*incus*	*stapes*
cochlea	*malleus*	*tympanic membrane*
eustachian tube	*oval window*	*vestibule*
external auditory canal	*semicircular canals*	

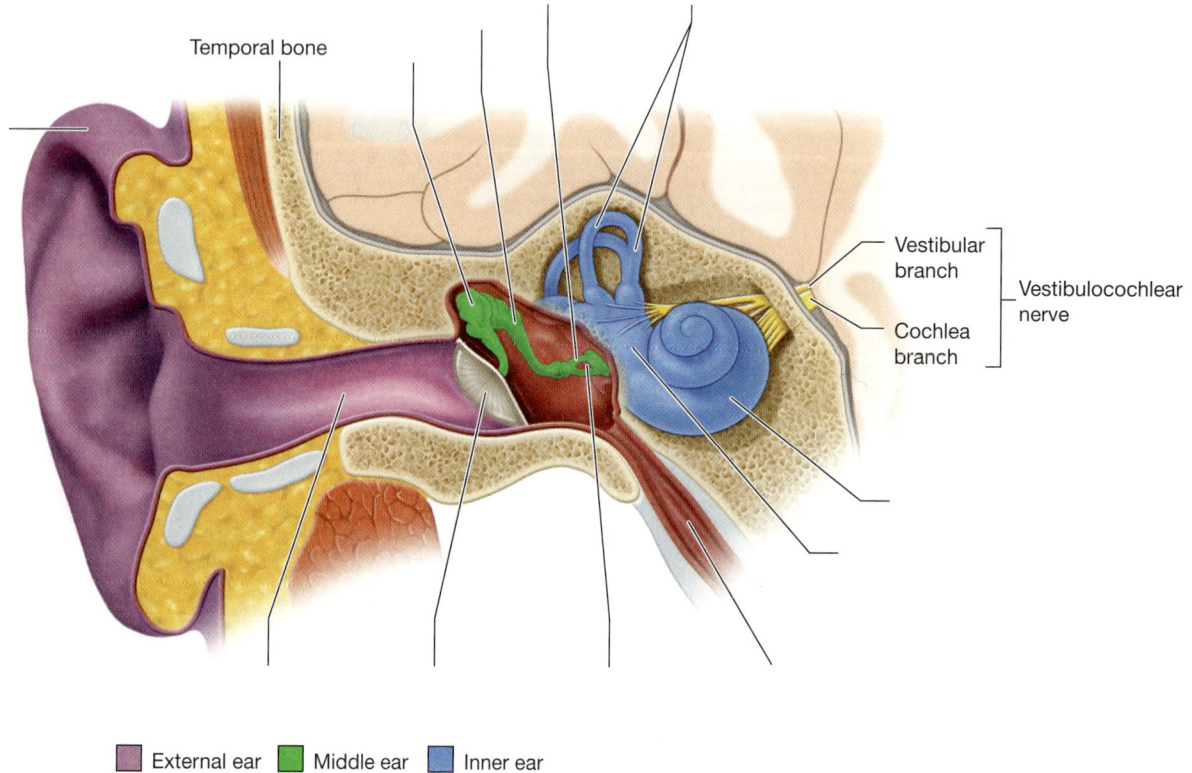

☐ External ear ☐ Middle ear ☐ Inner ear

 Check your answers by referring to Figure 16-3 on page 609. Review material that you did not answer correctly.

Medical Word Elements

This section introduces combining forms, suffixes, and prefixes related to the special senses. Word analyses are also provided. From the information provided, complete the meaning of the medical words in the right–hand column. The first one is completed for you.

Element	Meaning	Word Analysis
Combining Forms		
Eye		
ambly/o	dull, dim	**ambly**/opia (ăm-blē-Ō-pē-ă): *dimness of vision* *-opia:* vision *In amblyopia, visual stimulation through the optic nerve of one eye (lazy eye) is impaired, thus resulting in poor or dim vision.*
aque/o	water	**aque**/ous (Ā-kwē-ŭs): _____ *-ous:* pertaining to
blephar/o	eyelid	**blephar/o**/ptosis (blĕf-ă-rō-TŌ-sĭs): _____ *-ptosis:* prolapse, downward displacement
choroid/o	choroid	**choroid/o**/pathy (kō-roy-DŎP-ă-thē): _____ *-pathy:* disease
conjunctiv/o	conjunctiva	**conjunctiv**/al (kŏn-jŭnk-TĪ-văl): _____ *-al:* pertaining to
core/o	pupil	**core/o**/meter (kō-rē-ŎM-ĕ-tĕr): _____ *-meter:* instrument for measuring
pupill/o		**pupill/o**/graphy (pū-pĭ-LŎG-ră-fē): _____ *-graphy:* process of recording
corne/o	cornea	**corne**/al (KOR-nē-ăl): _____ *-al:* pertaining to
cycl/o	ciliary body of the eye; circular; cycle	**cycl/o**/plegia (sī-klō-PLĒ-jē-ă): _____ *-plegia:* paralysis
dacry/o	tear; lacrimal apparatus (duct, sac, or gland)	**dacry**/oma (dăk-rē-Ō-mă): _____ *-oma:* tumor
lacrim/o		**lacrim/o**/tomy (lăk-rĭ-MŎT-ō-mē): _____ *-tomy:* incision
dacryocyst/o	lacrimal sac	**dacryocyst/o**/ptosis (dăk-rē-ō-sĭs-tŏp-TŌ-sĭs): _____ *-ptosis:* prolapse, downward displacement

Continued

Medical Word Elements—cont'd

Element	Meaning	Word Analysis
glauc/o	gray	**glauc/**oma (glaw-KŌ-mă): _____ *-oma:* tumor *If not treated, glaucoma results in increased intraocular pressure (IOP) that destroys the retina and optic nerve.*
goni/o	angle	**goni/o/**scopy (gŏ-nē-ŎS-kŏ-pē): _____ *-scopy:* visual examination *Gonioscopy helps differentiate the two forms of glaucoma (open- and closed-angle).*
irid/o	iris	**irid/o/**plegia (ĭr-ĭd-ō-PLĒ-jē-ă): _____ *-plegia:* paralysis
kerat/o	horny tissue; hard; cornea	**kerat/o/**tomy (kĕr-ă-TŎT-ō-mē): _____ *-tomy:* incision
ocul/o	eye	**ocul/o/**myc/osis (ŏk-ū-lō-mī-KŌ-sĭs): _____ *myc:* fungus *-osis:* abnormal condition; increase (used primarily with blood cells)
ophthalm/o		**opthalm/o/**logist (ŏf-thăl-MŎL-ō-jĭst): _____ *-logist:* specialist in the study of *Ophthalmologists are physicians who specialize in the medical and surgical management of diseases and disorders of the eyes.*
opt/o	eye, vision	**opt/o/**metry (ŏp-TŎM-ě-trē): _____ *-metry:* act of measuring *Optometry is the health-care field focused on assessing eye health and vision, identifying vision issues, prescribing corrective lenses or therapy, and detecting specific eye diseases or conditions.*
optic/o		**optic/**al (ŎP-tĭ-kăl): _____ *-al:* pertaining to
phac/o	lens	**phac/o/**cele (FĀK-ō-sēl): _____ *-cele:* hernia, swelling *The usual cause of phacocele is blunt trauma to the eye.*
phot/o	light	**phot/o/**phobia (fō-tō-FŌ-bē-ă): _____ *-phobia:* fear *Intolerance to light is associated with people with light-colored eyes and those who suffer from migraines or glaucoma. Some medications also cause a marked intolerance to light.*
presby/o	old age	**presby/**opia (prěz-bē-Ō-pē-ă): _____ *-opia:* vision *Presbyopia is the loss of accommodation caused by weakening of the ciliary muscles as a result of the aging process.*

Medical Word Elements—cont'd

Element	Meaning	Word Analysis
retin/o	retina	**retin**/osis (rĕt-ĭ-NŌ-sĭs): _____ *-osis:* abnormal condition; increase (used primarily with blood cells) *Retinosis includes any degenerative process of the retina not associated with inflammation.*
scler/o	hardening; sclera (white of eye)	**scler/o**/malacia (sklĕ-rō-mă-LĀ-shē-ă): _____ *-malacia:* softening
scot/o	darkness	**scot**/oma (skō-TŌ-mă): _____ *-oma:* tumor *Scotoma is an area of diminished vision in the visual field.*
vitr/o	vitreous body (of the eye)	**vitr**/ectomy (vĭ-TRĔK-tō-mē): _____ *-ectomy:* excision, removal *The removal of the vitreous body allows surgical procedures that would otherwise be impossible, including repair of macular holes and tears in the retina.*
Ear		
audi/o	hearing	**audi/o**/meter (aw-dē-ŎM-ĕ-tĕr): _____ *-meter:* instrument for measuring
labyrinth/o	labyrinth (inner ear)	**labyrinth/o**/tomy (lăb-ĭ-rĭn-THŎT-ō-mē): _____ *-tomy:* incision
mastoid/o	mastoid process	**mastoid**/ectomy (măs-toyd-ĔK-tō-mē): _____ *-ectomy:* excision, removal

ot/o	ear	**ot/o**/py/o/rrhea (ō-tō-pī-ō-RĒ-ă): _____
		  py/o: pus
		  -rrhea: discharge, flow

salping/o	tubes (usually fallopian or eustachian [auditory] tubes)	**salping/o**/pharyng/eal: (săl-pĭng-gō-fă-RĬN-jē-ăl): _____
		  -al: pertaining to
		  pharyng: pharynx

staped/o	stapes	**staped**/ectomy (stā-pĕ-DĔK-tō-mē): _____ *-ectomy:* excision, removal *Stapedectomy is performed to improve hearing, especially in cases of otosclerosis.*
tympan/o	tympanic membrane (eardrum)	**tympan/o**/stomy (tĭm-pă-NŎS-tō-mē): _____ *-stomy:* forming an opening (mouth) *Tympanostomy is usually performed to insert small pressure-equalizing (PE) tubes through the tympanum.*

Continued

Medical Word Elements—cont'd

Element	Meaning	Word Analysis
myring/o		**myring/o**/myc/osis (mĭr-ĭn-gō-mī-KŌ-sĭs): _____ *myc:* fungus *-osis:* abnormal condition; increase (used primarily with blood cells)

Suffixes

Element	Meaning	Word Analysis
-acusia	hearing	an/**acusia** (ăn-ă-KŪ-sē-ă): _____ *an-:* without, not
-cusis		presby/**cusis** (prĕz-bĭ-KŪ-sĭs): _____ *presby:* old age *Presbycusis generally occurs in both ears and primarily affects perception of high-pitched tones.*
-opia	vision	dipl/**opia** (dĭp-LŌ-pē-ă): _____ *dipl-:* double, twofold
-opsia		heter/**opsia** (hĕt-ĕr-ŎP-sē-ă): _____ *heter-:* different
-tropia	turning	eso/**tropia** (ĕs-ō-TRŌ-pē-ă): _____ *eso-:* inward *Esotropia is also called* convergent strabismus *or* crossed eyes.

Prefixes

Element	Meaning	Word Analysis
exo-	outside, outward	**exo**/tropia (ĕks-ō-TRŌ-pē-ă): _____ *-tropia:* turning *Exotropia is also called* divergent strabismus.
hyper-	excessive, above normal	**hyper**/opia (hī-pĕr-Ō-pē-ă): _____ *-opia:* vision

Visit the Medical Terminology Systems online resource center at FADavis.com for an audio exercise of the terms in this table. Other activities are also available to reinforce content.

It is time to review medical word elements by completing Learning Activities 16-1 and 16-2.

Disease Focus

Common signs and symptoms of eye disorders include a decrease in visual acuity, headaches, and pain in the eye or adnexa. However, many disorders of the eye are serious but asymptomatic; therefore, regular eye checkups are necessary. For diagnosis, treatment, and management of visual disorders, the medical services of a specialist may be warranted. **Ophthalmology** is the medical specialty concerned with disorders of the eye. The physician who treats these disorders is called an **ophthalmologist.** Optometrists work with ophthalmologists in a medical practice or practice independently. **Optometrists** are not medical doctors but are doctors of optometry (OD). They diagnose vision problems and eye diseases, prescribe eyeglasses and contact lenses, and prescribe drugs to treat eye disorders. Although they cannot perform surgery, they commonly provide preoperative and postoperative care.

Common signs and symptoms of ear disorders include hearing impairment, ringing in the ears, pain or drainage from the ears, loss of balance, dizziness, and nausea. For diagnosis, treatment, and management of hearing disorders, the medical services of a specialist may be warranted. **Otolar-yngology** is the medical specialty concerned with disorders of the ear, nose, and throat (ENT). The physician who treats these disorders is called an **otolaryngologist**. Many otolaryngologists employ audiologists. The **audiologist** specializes in nonmedical management of the auditory and balance systems. Using various testing strategies (such as hearing tests, otoacoustic emission measurements, and electrophysiologic tests), the audiologist aims to determine whether a person can hear within the normal range and, if not, which portions of hearing (high, middle, or low frequencies) are affected and to what degree. If there is a hearing loss or vestibular abnormality, an audiologist may recommend a hearing aid, cochlear implant, or surgery or provide an appropriate medical referral.

Eye Disorders

Common eye disorders include glaucoma and macular degeneration.

Glaucoma

Glaucoma is characterized by increased intraocular pressure (IOP) caused by failure of aqueous humor to drain from the eye through a thin duct called the **canal of Schlemm** (see Fig. 16-4). The increased pressure leads to optic nerve damage and vision loss. Glaucoma may occur as a

Figure 16-4 Glaucoma. Circulation of the aqueous humor builds up in the anterior chamber of the eye, resulting in increased intraocular pressure (IOP) that damages the optic nerve.

primary or congenital disease or secondary to other causes, such as injury, infection, surgery, or prolonged topical corticosteroid use. Primary glaucoma can be chronic or acute. The **chronic form** is also called **open-angle glaucoma**. The **acute form** is called **angle-closure glaucoma**. Chronic glaucoma may produce no symptoms except gradual loss of peripheral vision over a period of years. Headaches, blurred vision, and dull pain in the eye may also be present. During an ophthalmoscopic examination, cupping of the optic discs is visible. However, acute glaucoma causes extreme ocular pain, blurred vision, redness of the eye, and dilation of the pupil. Nausea and vomiting may also occur. If untreated, acute glaucoma causes complete and permanent blindness within 2 to 5 days.

The more common and chronic form of glaucoma is open-angle glaucoma, which is progressive and often asymptomatic in the early stages. The trabecular function becomes compromised and leads to a buildup of aqueous humor over time, causing a slow rise in IOP. Treatment for open-angle glaucoma includes medications that cause the pupils to constrict **(miotics),** which permits aqueous humor to escape from the eye, thereby relieving IOP. If miotics are ineffective, **trabeculoplasty** or **selective laser trabeculoplasty** (SLT) may be performed.

The rarer form of glaucoma is angle-closure glaucoma, where the anterior chamber angle suddenly becomes closed or blocked, leading to a rapid increase in IOP. This acute form of glaucoma presents with sudden onset of severe pain, headache, nausea, vomiting, blurred vision, and seeing halos around lights. It is a medical emergency and requires immediate intervention to relieve IOP and prevent optic nerve damage and vision loss. Treatment consists of medications and **laser peripheral iridotomy** (LPI) or surgical **iridectomy**.

Macular Degeneration

Macular degeneration is a deterioration of the macula, the most sensitive portion of the retina. The macula is responsible for central, or "straight-ahead" vision, required for reading, driving, detail work, and recognizing faces (see Fig. 16-5). Although deterioration of the macula is associated with toxic effects of some drugs, the most common type is **age-related macular**

Normal macula   Macular degeneration

Normal vision   Central vision loss

Figure 16-5 Macular degeneration.

degeneration (ARMD, AMD). ARMD is a leading cause of vision loss in the United States in those over 60 years of age. The disease is unpredictable and progresses differently in each individual.

Two forms of ARMD have been identified: wet and dry. The less common but more severe form is **wet ARMD,** which affects about 10% of those afflicted with the disease. New blood vessels form under the macula that leak and destroy the vision cells, leading to severe loss of central vision and permanent visual impairment. If identified in its early stages, scheduled injections with antineogenic drugs directly into the vitreous can halt the progression of vision loss. Other treatment includes using a laser beam to destroy the newly forming blood vessels. However, the treatment may not be permanent.

The more common form of macular degeneration is **dry ARMD.** Patients with dry ARMD are encouraged to see their ophthalmologist frequently and perform a simple at-home test (**Amsler grid**) that detects changes in vision that could indicate disease progression.

Ear Disorders

Common ear disorders include otitis media and otosclerosis.

Otitis Media

Otitis media (OM) is an inflammation of the middle ear. This infection may be caused by a virus or bacterium. However, the most common culprit is *Streptococcus pneumoniae.* OM is found most commonly in infants and young children, especially in the presence of an upper respiratory infection (URI). Symptoms may include earache and draining of pus from the ear (**otopyorrhea**). In its most severe form, OM may lead to infection of the mastoid process (**mastoiditis**) or inflammation of brain tissue near the middle ear (**otoencephalitis**). Recurrent episodes of OM may cause scarring of the tympanic membrane, leading to hearing loss. Treatment consists of bedrest, medications to relieve pain (**analgesics**), and antibiotics. Occasionally, an incision of the eardrum (**myringotomy, tympanotomy**) may be necessary to relieve pressure and promote drainage.

Otosclerosis

Otosclerosis is a disorder characterized by an abnormal stiffness (**ankylosis**) and immobilization of bones of the middle ear that causes hearing loss. The ossicle most commonly affected is the stapes, the bone that attaches to the oval window of the cochlea. The formation of a spongy growth at the footplate of the stapes decreases its ability to move the oval window, resulting in hearing loss. Occasionally, the patient perceives a ringing sound (**tinnitus**) within the ear and experiences dizziness and a progressive loss of hearing, especially of low tones. Development of otosclerosis is typically tied to genetic factors; if one or both parents have the disorder, the child is at high risk for developing the disease. Surgical correction involves removing part of the stapes (**stapedectomy** or, more commonly, **stapedotomy**) and implanting a prosthetic device that allows sound waves to pass to the inner ear. The procedure requires only a local anesthetic and usually lasts only 45 minutes. Hearing is immediately restored.

Oncology

Oncological disorders can occur in almost any structure of the eye or ear as a primary malignancy or spread from other areas of the body to the eye or ear via metastasis.

Eye

Two major **neoplastic diseases** account for more than 90% of all primary intraocular diseases: **retinoblastoma,** found primarily in children, and **melanoma,** found primarily in adults. Most retinoblastomas tend to be familial. The cell involved is the retinal neuron. Vision is impaired, and in about 30% of patients, the disease is found in both eyes (**bilateral**).

Melanoma may occur in the orbit, the bony cavity of the eyeball, the iris, or the ciliary body, but it arises most commonly in the pigmented cells of the choroid. The disease is usually asymptomatic until there is a hemorrhage into the anterior chamber. Accurate diagnosis is by an ophthalmologist and a retina vitreous specialist utilizing specialized scans and instrumentation to detect a fleshy mass on the iris. When malignancy occurs in the choroid, it usually appears as a brown or gray mushroom-shaped lesion.

Treatment for retinoblastoma usually involves the removal of the affected eye(s) **(enucleation),** followed by radiation. Melanoma in which the lesion is on the iris requires iridectomy. For melanoma of the choroid, enucleation is necessary. Many eye tumors are noninvasive and are not necessarily life threatening.

Ear

Malignant and nonmalignant tumors can arise in the external ear, the canal, or the middle ear. Malignant tumors of the ear include basal cell carcinoma and squamous cell tumors.

The most common ear malignancy is **basal cell carcinoma,** which usually occurs on the top of the pinna as the result of sun exposure. It is found more commonly in elderly patients or those with fair skin. Small, craterlike ulcers form as the disease progresses. Basal cell carcinoma does not readily metastasize. However, failure to treat it in a timely manner may result in the need for extensive surgery to remove the tumor.

Squamous cell carcinoma, on the other hand, is much more invasive. However, it is a very rare type of ear tumor. In appearance, it closely resembles basal cell carcinoma, and biopsy is required to make a definitive diagnosis. Squamous cell carcinoma grows more slowly than basal cell carcinoma; however, because of its tendency to metastasize to the surrounding nodes and the nodes of the neck, it must be removed. Surgery combined with radiation therapy is the most effective treatment for squamous cell carcinoma.

Diseases and Conditions

This section introduces diseases and conditions of the eye and ear, along with their meanings and pronunciations. Word analyses for selected terms are also provided.

Term	Definition
Eye	

achromatopsia
 ă-krō-mă-TŎP-sē-ă
   a-: without, not
   chromat: color
   -opsia: vision
	Severe congenital deficiency in color perception; also called *complete color blindness*

Diseases and Conditions—cont'd

Term	Definition
ametropia ă-mĕ-TRŌ-pē-ă *a-:* without, not *metr:* uterus (womb) measure *-opia:* vision	Failure of light rays to focus sharply on the retina as a result of a defect in the lens, cornea, or shape of the eyeball; also called *error of refraction* (see Fig. 16-6)

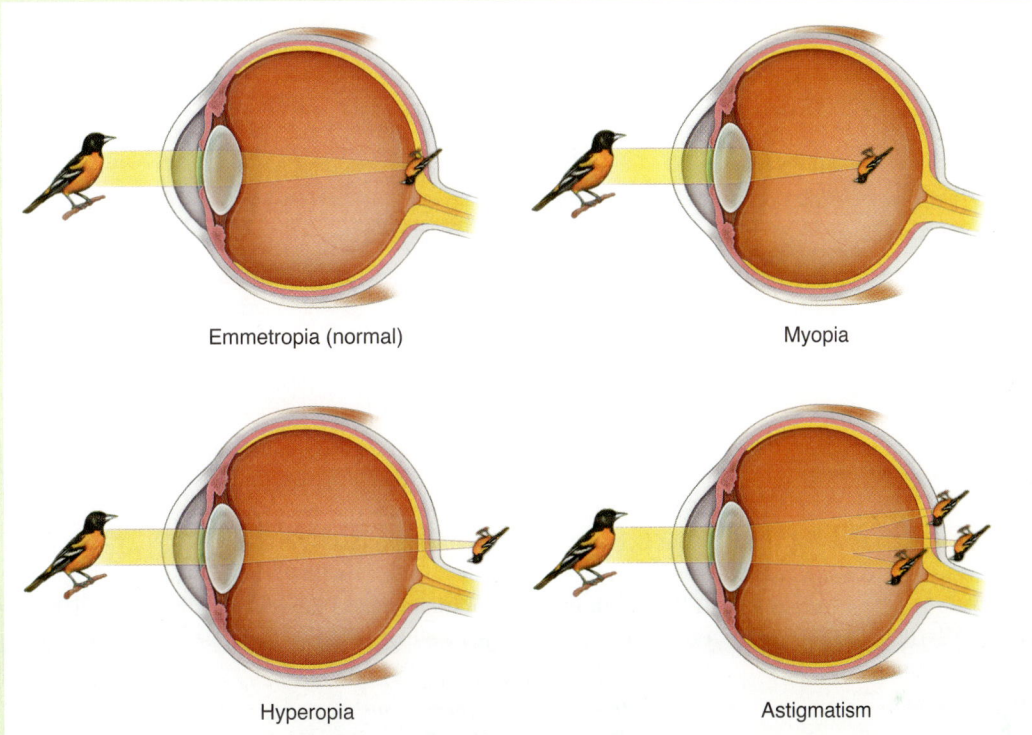

Emmetropia (normal)   Myopia

Hyperopia   Astigmatism

Figure 16-6 Ametropia.

astigmatism (Ast) ă-STĬG-mă-tĭzm	Distorted vision resulting from a defective curvature of the cornea or lens causing light rays to diffuse over a large area of the retina rather than being sharply focused *Correction for Ast requires the use of lenses that alter the way light enters the eyes.*
hyperopia hī-pĕr-Ō-pē-ă *hyper-:* excessive, above normal *-opia:* vision	Visual defect in which the eyeball is too short, and the image falls behind the retina; also called *farsightedness* *Correction of hyperopia requires the use of biconvex lenses.*
myopia mī-Ō-pē-ă	Visual defect in which the eyeball is too long, and the image falls in front of the retina; also called *nearsightedness* *Correction of myopia requires the use of biconcave lenses.*

Continued

Diseases and Conditions—cont'd

Term	Definition
cataract KĂT-ă-răkt	Opacity that forms on the lens and impairs vision, caused by proteins that slowly build up over time (see Fig. 16-7) *Most cataracts are age related. Surgical treatment to remove the clouded lens and replace it with an artificial intraocular lens (IOL) is one of the safest and most effective surgeries performed in medicine.*

Figure 16-7 Cataract development in the right eye.

Term	Definition
chalazion kă-LĀ-zē-ōn	Small, hard tumor developing on the eyelid, somewhat similar to a sebaceous cyst; also called *meibomian cyst*
conjunctivitis kŏn-jŭnk-tĭ-VĪ-tĭs *conjunctiv:* conjunctiva *–itis:* inflammation	Inflammation of the conjunctiva and inner eyelids with vascular congestion; also called *pinkeye* (see Fig. 16-8) *Causes of conjunctiva include irritants, an allergy, and viral, bacterial, or fungal infections. The viral form of conjunctivitis is highly contagious. Avoiding contact with others and careful hand washing help control the spread.*

Figure 16-8 Conjunctivitis.

Term	Definition
diabetic retinopathy rĕt-ĭn-ŎP-ă-thē *retin/o:* retina *–pathy:* disease	Chronic condition of the retina marked by formation of new, fragile blood vessels (**neovascularization**), microaneurysms, and hemorrhages in the retina caused by uncontrolled diabetes that progresses from mild to severe

Diseases and Conditions—cont'd

Term	Definition
nonproliferative diabetic retinopathy (NPDR)	Mild stage of diabetic retinopathy characterized by microaneurysms in the blood vessels of the retina with possible mild vision changes that are often asymptomatic
proliferative diabetic retinopathy (PDR)	Severe stage of diabetic retinopathy characterized by neovascularization, vitreous hemorrhage, fluid leaking from the blood vessels leading to the formation of hard exudates, and macular edema *Untreated PDR leads to significant vision loss, including severe and sudden vision changes if bleeding occurs, and the risk of blindness (see Fig. 16-9).*

Normal Retina   **Diabetic** Retina

Figure 16-9 Proliferative diabetic retinopathy (PDR) compared with the normal retina. Note the progression of damage to the retina caused by the abnormalities in the formation of pathological blood vessels.

Term	Definition
drusen DROO-zĕn	Small yellowish deposits composed of retinal pigment cells that develop under the retina and are associated with an increased risk of developing age-related macular degeneration (ARMD)
ectropion ĕk-TRŌ-pē-ŏn	Eversion, or outward turning, of the edge of the lower eyelid, causing it to pull away from the eye, generally associated with aging and weakness of the small muscles around the eyelid
entropion ĕn-TRŌ-pē-ŏn	Inversion, or inward turning, of the edge of the lower eyelid, commonly causing friction as the eyelashes and outer eyelid rub against the surface of the eye
epiphora ĕ-PĬF-ō-ră	Abnormal overflow of tears *Epiphora is often caused by tear duct obstruction, allergies, dry eyes, eye infections and inflammation, or exposure to environmental irritants like smoke, wind, and pollution.*
floaters	Particles of cellular debris in the vitreous humor that cast shadows on the retina; also known as *vitreous floaters* *Floaters often occur normally and then disappear but may be an indication of a retinal tear or detachment, especially when accompanied by flashes of light (photopsia).*

Continued

Diseases and Conditions—cont'd

Term	Definition
hordeolum hor-DĒ-ō-lŭm	Localized, circumscribed, inflammatory swelling of one of the several sebaceous glands of the eyelid; also called *stye* (see Fig. 16-10) *Hordeola are commonly caused by a bacterial infection.* **Figure 16-10** Hordeolum or sty.
metamorphopsia mĕt-ă-mor-FŎP-sē-ă *meta-:* change; beyond *morph:* form, shape, structure *-opsia:* vision	Visual distortion of objects *Metamorphopsia is commonly associated with errors of refraction, retinal disease, choroiditis, detachment of the retina, and tumors of the retina or choroid.*
nyctalopia nĭk-tă-LŌ-pē-ă *nyctal:* night *-opia:* vision	Impaired vision in dim light; also called *night blindness* *Common causes of nyctalopia include cataracts, vitamin A deficiency, certain medications, and hereditary causes.*
nystagmus nĭs-TĂG-mŭs	Type of involuntary eye movements that appear jerky and may reduce vision or be associated with other, more serious conditions that limit vision
papilledema păp-ĭl-ĕ-DĒ-mă	Swelling and hyperemia of the optic disc, usually associated with increased intracranial pressure; also called *choked disc*
photophobia fō-tō-FŌ-bē-ă *phot/o:* light *-phobia:* fear	Unusual intolerance of and sensitivity to light *Photophobia commonly occurs in such diseases as meningitis, inflammation of the eyes, measles, and rubella.*
retinal detachment RĔT-ĭ-năl *retin:* retina *-al:* pertaining to	Separation of the retina from the choroid, which disrupts vision and results in blindness if not repaired *Retinal detachment may follow trauma, choroidal hemorrhages, or tumors and may be associated with diabetes mellitus.*

Diseases and Conditions—cont'd

Term	Definition
strabismus stră-BĬZ-mŭs	Misalignment of the eyes so that they do not focus on the same object at the same time, sending two different images to the brain; also called *heterotropia* or *tropia* *The two most common forms of strabismus are esotropia (ST) and exotropia (XT) (Fig. 16–11).*

Figure 16-11 Types of strabismus. (A) Exotropia, where the affected eye turns outward. (B) Esotropia, where the affected eye turns inward.

Term	Definition
trachoma tră-KŌ-mă	Chronic, contagious form of conjunctivitis that typically leads to blindness

Ear

Term	Definition
acoustic neuroma ă-KOOS-tĭk nū-RŌ-mă *acous:* hearing *-tic:* pertaining to *neur:* nerve *-oma:* tumor	Benign tumor that develops from the eighth cranial nerve or vestibulo-cochlear nerve (responsible for hearing and balance) that grows within the auditory canal, resulting in progressive hearing loss, headache, facial numbness, dizziness, and an unsteady gait *The prognosis for acoustic neuroma is generally good, especially when the tumor is detected early and medically managed. However, treatment can sometimes result in complications, such as hearing loss, balance issues, or facial nerve damage.*
cholesteatoma KŌ-lē-stē-ă-tō-mă	Benign tumor in the middle ear composed of cholesterol and epithelial cells that is most often caused by chronic OM *Cholesteatoma grows slowly and over time enlarges and erodes the bones of the middle ear and skull, leading to hearing loss, dizziness, and infection.*
hearing loss	Loss in the ability to hear
anacusis ăn-ă-KŪ-sĭs *an-:* without, not *-acusis:* hearing	Complete deafness *Anacusis may be unilateral or bilateral.*
conductive kŏn-DŬK-tĭv	Hearing loss resulting from any condition that prevents sound wave transmission from the external ear to the cochlea *Conductive hearing loss may result from wax obstructing the external auditory canal, inflammation of the middle ear, ankylosis of the ear bones, or fixation of the footplate of the stirrup.*

Continued

Diseases and Conditions—cont'd

Term	Definition
noise-induced (NIHL)	Hearing loss that results from exposure to very loud sounds *Working with noisy machinery, listening to loud music, or discharging rifles, guns, or explosives may cause NIHL.*
prebyacusis prĕz-bē-ă-KŪ-sĭs *presby:* old age *-acusis:* hearing	Hearing loss resulting from old age *Patients with presbyacusis are generally able to hear low tones but lose the ability to hear higher tones. This type of hearing loss is irreversible.*
sensorineural sĕn-sō-rē-NŪ-răl *sensori:* to feel *neur:* nerve *-al:* pertaining to	Hearing loss caused by damage to the cochlea or the auditory nerve
labyrinthitis lăb-ĭ-rĭn-THĪ-tĭs *labyrinth:* labyrinth (inner ear) *-itis:* inflammation	Inflammation of the inner ear that usually results from an acute viral disease, such as mumps, measles, or influenza *Labyrinthitis may lead to sudden incapacitating vertigo, nausea, and various degrees of hearing loss.*
Ménière disease mĕn-ē-ĀR	Increased fluid pressure of the endolymphatic system that leads to progressive loss of hearing; also called *endolymphatic/labyrinthine hydrops* *Ménière disease is characterized by vertigo, sensorineural hearing loss, and tinnitus.*
otitis externa ō-TĪ-tĭs ĕks-TĚR-nă *ot:* ear *-itis:* inflammation	Infection of the external auditory canal *Common causes of otitis externa include exposure to water when swimming (swimmer's ear), bacterial or fungal infections, seborrhea, eczema, and chronic conditions such as allergies.*
tinnitus tĭn-Ī-tŭs	Perception of ringing, hissing, or other sounds in the ears or head when no external sound is present *Tinnitus may be caused by a blow to the head, ingestion of large doses of aspirin, anemia, noise exposure, stress, impacted wax, hypertension, and certain types of medications and tumors.*
vertigo VĚR-tĭ-gō	Sensation of a spinning motion of oneself or of the surroundings *Vertigo usually results from damage to inner ear structures associated with balance and equilibrium.*

⊕ *It is time to review pathology, diseases, and conditions by completing Learning Activity 16-3.*

Diagnostic, Surgical, and Therapeutic Procedures

This section introduces diagnostic, surgical, and therapeutic procedures used to diagnose and treat eye and ear disorders. Descriptions are provided, along with pronunciations and word analyses for selected terms.

Procedure	Description
Diagnostic	
Clinical	
Eye	
electronystagmography (ENG) ē-lĕk-trō-nĭs-tăg-MŎG-ră-fē	Method of assessing and recording eye movements by measuring the electrical activity of the extraocular muscles *In ENG, electrodes are placed above, below, and to the side of each eye. A ground electrode is placed on the forehead. The electrodes record eye movement relative to the position of the ground electrode.*
gonioscopy gō-nē-ŎS-kō-pē *goni/o:* angle *-scopy:* visual examination	Examination of the angle of the anterior chamber of the eye to determine ocular motility and rotation and diagnose and manage glaucoma
ophthalmodynamometry ŏf-thăl-mō-dī-nă-MŎM-ĕ-trē	Measurement of the blood pressure of the retinal vessels *Ophthalmodynamometry helps in assessing the ocular circulation and provides valuable information about the blood flow to the eye, particularly in cases of suspected ocular or systemic vascular diseases such as carotid artery disease and glaucoma.*
ophthalmoscopy ŏf-thăl-MŎS-kō-pē *ophthalm/o:* eye *-scopy:* visual examination	Visual examination of the interior of the eye using a handheld instrument called an *ophthalmoscope*, which has various adjustable lenses for magnification and a light source to illuminate the interior of the eye *Ophthalmoscopy helps detect eye disorders and other disorders that cause changes in the eye.*
retinoscopy rĕt-ĭn-ŎS-kō-pē *retin/o:* retina *-scopy:* visual examination	Evaluation of refractive errors of the eye by projecting a light into the eyes and determining the movement of reflected light rays *Retinoscopy is especially important in determining errors of refraction in babies and small children who cannot be refracted by traditional methods.*
slit-lamp examination (SLE)	Stereoscopic magnified view of the anterior eye structures in detail, which includes the cornea, lens, iris, sclera, and vitreous humor *The application of fluorescein dye during a SLE makes it easier to detect and remove foreign bodies and treat infection, corneal ulcers, and abrasions.*

Continued

Diagnostic, Surgical, and Therapeutic Procedures—cont'd

Procedure	Description
tonometry tŏn-ŎM-ĕ-trē *ton/o:* tension *-metry:* act of measuring	Evaluation of intraocular pressure by measuring the resistance of the eyeball to indentation by an applied force *Tonometry is a standard eye test to detect glaucoma and part of most routine ophthalmic examinations. The applanation method of tonometry uses a sensor to depress the cornea and is the most accurate method of tonometry (see Fig. 16-12).*

Figure 16-12 Tonometry for glaucoma detection.

Diagnostic, Surgical, and Therapeutic Procedures—cont'd

Procedure	Description
visual acuity (VA) test ă-KŪ-ĭ-tē	Part of an eye examination that determines the smallest letters that can be read on a standardized chart, called a *Snellen chart,* at a distance of 20 feet; results are commonly expressed as a fraction (see Fig. 16-13) *The top number refers to the distance from the chart, and the bottom number indicates the distance at which a person with normal eyesight can read the same line. For example, 20/40 indicates that the patient correctly read letters at 20 feet that can be read by a person with normal vision at 40 feet.* Figure 16-13 Snellen chart with letters

Ear

Procedure	Description
audiometry aw-dē-ŎM-ĕ-trē *audi/o:* hearing *-metry:* act of measuring	Measurement of hearing acuity at differing soundwave frequencies and volumes to detect the various types of hearing impairment *Each ear is assessed independently. The patient signals an ability to hear a sound by raising a hand or finger.*
caloric stimulation test	Test that uses different water temperatures to assess the vestibular portion of the nerve of the inner ear (acoustic nerve) to determine whether nerve damage is the cause of vertigo *In the caloric stimulation test, cold and warm water are separately introduced into each ear while electrodes placed around the eye record nystagmus. Eyes move in a predictable pattern when the water is introduced, except with acoustic nerve damage.*
otoscopy ō-TŎS-kō-pē *ot/o:* ear *-scopy:* visual examination	Visual examination of the external auditory canal and the tympanic membrane using an otoscope

Continued

Diagnostic, Surgical, and Therapeutic Procedures—cont'd

Procedure	Description
pneumatic nŭ-MĂT-ĭk	Otoscopic procedure that assesses the ability of the tympanic membrane to move in response to a change in air pressure *In pneumatic otoscopy, a tight seal is created in the ear canal, and then a very slight positive pressure and then a negative pressure are applied by squeezing and releasing a rubber bulb attached to the pneumatic otoscope. The fluctuation in air pressure causes movement of a normal tympanic membrane.*
tuning fork tests	Hearing tests using a vibrating tuning fork to determine type of hearing loss *Conductive hearing loss involves impairment of middle ear structures (malleus, incus, and stapes). Sensorineural hearing loss involves impairment of the inner ear, auditory nerve, or brain.*
Rinne RĬN-nē	Tuning fork test that evaluates unilateral hearing loss by comparing sound through bone conduction (BC) versus air conduction (AC); also called *air and bone conduction hearing test* *In the Rinne test, the physician places a vibrating fork against the mastoid bone (bone conduction) and in front of the auditory meatus (air conduction). In a normal test, AC provides longer and louder sound perception than does BC (see Fig. 16-14).*

Figure 16-14 Rinne test. (A) Bone conduction. (B) Air conduction. (From Simplified 7ed, p. 556, Fig. 11-15.)

Procedure	Description
Weber	Tuning fork test that determines whether hearing loss occurs in the middle ear (conductive hearing loss) or in the auditory nerves or hair cells of the inner ear (sensorineural); also called *conductive and sensorineural hearing loss test* *In the Weber test, a vibrating tuning fork placed on the center of the forehead directs sound to each ear simultaneously. If sound perception is equal in both ears, hearing is normal.*

Imaging

Procedure	Description
dacryocystography dăk-rē-ō-sĭs-TŎG-ră-fē *dacryocyst/o:* lacrimal sac *-graphy:* process of recording	Radiographic imaging procedure of the nasolacrimal (tear) glands and ducts *Dacryocystography is performed for excessive tearing (epiphora) to determine the cause of hypersecretion of the lacrimal gland or obstruction in the lacrimal passages.*

Diagnostic, Surgical, and Therapeutic Procedures—cont'd

Procedure	Description
fluorescein angiography floo-RĔS-ēn ăn-jē-ŎG-ră-fē *angio:* vessel (usually blood or lymph) *-graphy:* process of recording	Evaluation of blood vessels and their leakage in and beneath the retina after injection of fluorescein dye, which circulates while photographs of the vessels within the eye are obtained *Fluorescein angiography facilitates the in vivo study of retinal blood flow circulation and is particularly useful in the management of diabetic retinopathy and macular degeneration, two leading causes of blindness.*

Surgical

Eye

Procedure	Description
blepharoplasty BLĔF-ă-rō-plăs-tē *blephar/o:* eyelid *-plasty:* surgical repair	Cosmetic surgery that removes fatty tissue above and below the eyes that commonly forms as a result of the aging process or excessive exposure to the sun
cyclodialysis sī-klō-dī-ĂL-ĭ-sĭs *cycl/o:* ciliary body of the eye; circular, cycle *dia:* through, across *-lysis:* separation; destruction; loosening	Formation of an opening between the anterior chamber and the suprachoroidal space for the draining of aqueous humor in glaucoma
enucleation ē-nū-klē-Ā-shŭn	Removal of the eyeball from the orbit *Enucleation is performed to treat cancer of the eye when the tumor is large and fills most of the structure.*
evisceration ē-vĭs-ĕr-Ā-shŭn	Removal of the contents of the eye while leaving the sclera and cornea intact *Evisceration is performed when the blind eye is painful or unsightly. The eye muscles are left intact, and a thin prosthesis called a **cover shell** is fitted over the sclera and cornea.*
keratoplasty kĕr-ă-tō-PLĂS-tē	Surgical procedure in which a damaged or diseased cornea is replaced with a donor cornea; also known as a *corneal transplant* *Keratoplasty is performed to restore vision that cannot be corrected by other means, such as glasses, contact lenses, or medication.*
LASIK surgery	Procedure using a specialized laser passed through a temporary flap made in the cornea to reshape underlying corneal tissue *This procedure corrects farsightedness, nearsightedness, and astigmatism. Unfortunately, not all patients are candidates for LASIK surgery. LASIK is the acronym for laser-assisted in situ keratomileusis.*

Continued

Diagnostic, Surgical, and Therapeutic Procedures—cont'd

Procedure	Description
phacoemulsification with lens implant fă-kō-ē-mŭl-sĭ-fĭ-KĀ-shŭn	Ultrasonic destruction and removal of cataracts and replacement with a new, clear artificial lens (see Fig. 16-15) *The surgery usually takes less than 15 minutes, and the patient goes home about 2 hours postsurgery.*

Artificial lens

Lens capsule

Cataract removal

Artificial lens insertion

Figure 16-15 Phacoemulsification for cataract removal.

Procedure	Description
retinopexy rĕt-ĭ-nō-PĔK-sē *retin/o:* retina *-pexy:* fixation (of an organ)	Surgery performed to repair a retinal tear or detached retina
scleral buckle	Surgery to repair a retinal detachment by placement of a flexible silicon band around the sclera that gently pushes the wall of the eye against the detached retina *This procedure helps to reattach the retina to its proper position and prevents further detachment. It can significantly improve or preserve vision if performed in a timely manner.*
sclerostomy sklĕ-RŎS-tō-mē *scler/o:* hardening; sclera (white of the eye) *-stomy:* forming an opening (mouth)	Surgical formation of an opening in the sclera *Sclerostomy is commonly performed on the anterior chamber in conjunction with surgery for glaucoma for relief of pressure.*
vitrectomy vĭ-TRĔK-tō-mē *vitr:* vitreous body (of the eye) *-ectomy:* excision, removal	Removal of the vitreous humor and replacement with a clear solution *Vitrectomy is a common yet critical procedure for managing diabetic retinopathy, tears and holes in the macula, and other age-related eye conditions.*
Ear	
cochlear implant insertion KŎK-lē-ăr ĬM-plănt *cochle:* cochlea *-ar:* pertaining to	Placement of an artificial hearing device that produces hearing sensations by electrically stimulating nerves inside the inner ear *The cochlear implant provides a sense of sound for those with severe to profound hearing loss, giving these individuals a better quality of life.*

Diagnostic, Surgical, and Therapeutic Procedures—cont'd

Procedure	Description
otoplasty Ō-tō-plăs-tē *ot/o:* ear *-plasty:* surgical repair	Corrective surgery for a deformed or excessively large or small pinna *Otoplasty is also performed to rebuild new ears for those who lost them through burns or other trauma and for those who were born without them.*
pressure-equalizing (PE) tube placement	Insertion of tubes through the tympanic membrane, commonly used to treat chronic otitis media; also called *tympanostomy tubes* or *ventilation tubes* *PE tubes remain in the ear for several months and then fall out on their own or are removed surgically (see Fig. 16-16).*

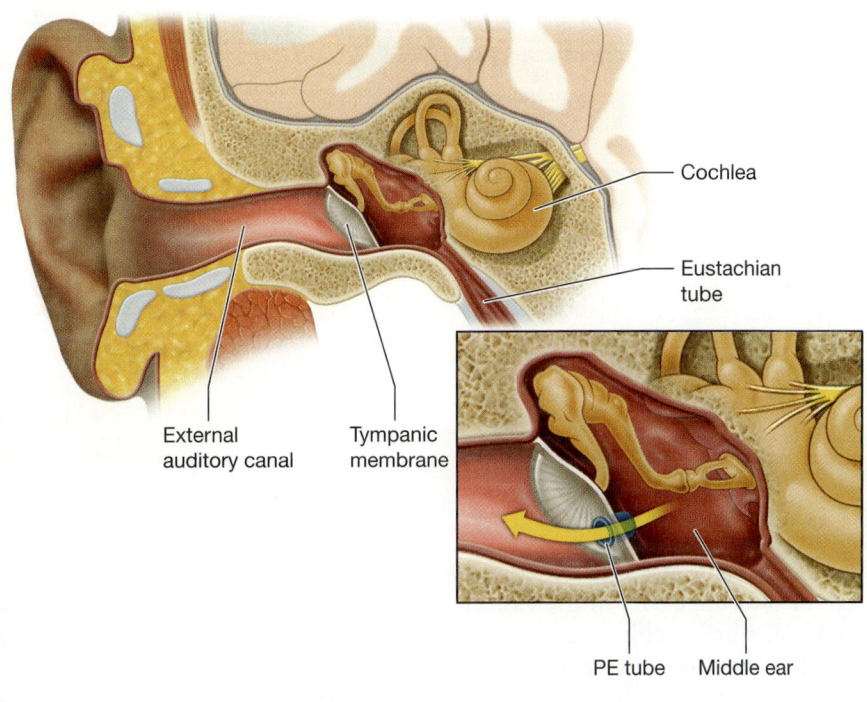

Figure 16-16 Placement of a pressure-equalizing tube.

Procedure	Description
tympanoplasty tĭm-păn-ō-PLĂS-tē *tympan/o:* tympanic membrane (eardrum) *-plasty:* surgical repair	Reconstruction of the eardrum, commonly to repair perforation; also called *myringoplasty* *Connective tissue located beneath the skin directly behind the ear is used for the tympanic graft.*

Therapeutic

Eye

Amsler grid test	Simple eye test used by the patient at home to detect any changes in vision that could indicate disease progression *The Amsler grid looks like a piece of graph paper that the patient stares at to see if the lines suddenly become blurry or distorted. These occurrences are reported to the doctor at an office visit follow-up to check vision further. This test is particularly useful for monitoring changes in vision in patients with macular degeneration and diabetic retinopathy.*

Continued

Diagnostic, Surgical, and Therapeutic Procedures—cont'd

Procedure	Description
eye refraction test rĕ-FRĂK-shŭn	Visual acuity test to determine the prescription for eyeglasses or contact lenses if required *In an eye refraction test, the patient looks through a device called a phoropter and reads letters or symbols on a wall chart using lenses of differing strengths until vision is corrected to be as close to normal as possible.*
retinal photocoagulation rĕ-tin-ŭl fō-tō-kō-ăg-ū-LĀ-shŭn *retin:* retina *-al:* pertaining to	Technique that uses light energy in the form of a laser beam to seal or cauterize retinal tissue; also called *laser photocoagulation* *Retinal photocoagulation is a widely used technique for treating various retinal disorders, including diabetic retinopathy, retinal ischemia, microvascular abnormalities in macular degeneration, adhesions, retinal breaks, and detachment of the retina.*
Ear	
ear irrigation	Flushing of the ear canal with water or saline to dislodge foreign bodies or impacted cerumen (earwax)
hearing aids	Electronic devices that are worn to correct hearing loss *There is a wide range of devices available with improved technology that are less noticeable than those from a decade ago.*

Pharmacology

Disorders of the eyes and ears are commonly treated with instillation of drops onto the surface of the eye or into the cavity of the ear. The eyes and ears are typically irrigated with liquid solution to remove foreign objects and provide topical application of medications. Pharmacological agents used to treat eye disorders include antibiotics for bacterial eye infections, beta blockers and carbonic anhydrase inhibitors for glaucoma, and ophthalmic decongestants and moisturizers for irritated eyes. Mydriatics and miotics are used not only to treat eye disorders but also to dilate (mydriatics) and contract (miotics) the pupil during eye examinations. Ear medications include antiemetics to relieve the nausea associated with inner ear infections, products to loosen and remove wax buildup in the ear canal, and local anesthetics to relieve the pain associated with ear infections (see Table 16-1).

TABLE 16-1 Drugs Used to Treat Eye and Ear Disorders

This table lists common drug classifications used to treat eye and ear disorders, their therapeutic actions, and selected generic and trade names.

Classification	Therapeutic Action	Generic and Trade Names
Eye		
antiangiogenics, angiogenesis inhibitors	Inhibits the growth of new blood vessels *Used in the treatment of wet macular degeneration.* *Antiangiogenics block the formation of new blood vessels that support tumor growth and are used to prevent the growth of cancer.*	**bevacizumab** běv-ă-CĬZ- ū-măb *Avastin*
antibiotics, ophthalmic ăn-tĭ-bī-ŎT-ĭks, ŏf-THĂL-mĭk	Inhibit growth of microorganisms that infect the eye *Ophthalmic antibiotics are dispensed as topical ointments and solutions to treat various bacterial eye infections, such as conjunctivitis (pinkeye).*	**tobramycin** TŌ-bră-mī-sĭn *Tobrex* **ciprofloxacin** sĭp-rō-FLŎX-ă-sĭn *Ciloxan*
antiglaucoma agents ăn-tĭ-glaw-KŌ-mă	Increase aqueous humor outflow or decrease its production, resulting in decreased intraocular pressure *Combinations of antiglaucoma drugs that work by different mechanisms are commonly used.*	**timolol** TĪ-mō-lŏl *Betimol* **dorzolamide** dor-ZŌ-lă-mīd *Trusopt* **latanoprost** lă-TĂN-ă-prŏst *Xalatan*
anti-inflammatory, ophthalmics ăn-tĭ-ĭn-FLĂM-ă-tō-rē, ŏf-THĂL-mĭks	Reduce inflammation after corneal injury or ophthalmic surgery or in chronic inflammatory eye conditions	**prednisolone** Prěd-NĬS-ō-lōn *Pred-Forte* **ketorolac** kē-TOR-ō-lăk *Acular*
artificial tears	Soothe eyes that are dry because of environmental irritants and allergens *Artificial tears generally contain multiple ingredients and are administered topically.*	**cellulose derivatives** SĔL-ū-lōs *Refresh Tears* **glycerin, propylene glycol** GLĬ-sěr-ĭn, PRŌ-pĭl-ēn GLĪ-cŏl *Moisture Eyes*
miotics mī-ŎT-ĭks	Cause the pupil to constrict *Miotics are used to treat glaucoma.*	**pilocarpine** P Ī-l ō-căr-pēn *Pilocar, Vuity*

(continued)

TABLE 16-1 Drugs Used to Treat Eye and Ear Disorders—cont'd

Classification	Therapeutic Action	Generic and Trade Names
mydriatics mĭd-rē-ĂT-ĭks	Disrupt parasympathetic nerve supply to the eye or stimulate the sympathetic nervous system, causing the pupil to dilate *Mydriatics commonly help dilate the pupil to treat inflammatory conditions or in preparation for internal examinations of the eye.*	**atropine sulfate** ĂT-rō-pēn SŬL-fāt *Atriposol, Atreza*
decongestants, ophthalmic dē-kŏn-JĔST-ănts, ŏf-THĂL-mĭk	Constrict the small arterioles of the eye, decreasing redness and relieving conjunctival congestion *Ophthalmic decongestants are over-the-counter products that temporarily relieve the itching and minor irritation commonly associated with allergy.*	**tetrahydrozoline** tĕt-ră-hī-DRŌZ-ō-lēn *Murine, Visine*
Ear		
antiemetics ăn-tĭ-ĕ-MĔT-ĭks	Treat and prevent nausea, vomiting, dizziness, and vertigo by reducing the sensitivity of the inner ear to motion or inhibiting stimuli from reaching the part of the brain that triggers nausea and vomiting *Antiemetics are commonly used to treat vertigo.*	**meclizine** MĔK-lĭ-zēn *Antivert, Bonine*
otic analgesics Ō-tĭk ăn-ăl-JĒ-zĭks	Provide temporary relief from pain and inflammation associated with otic disorders *Otic analgesics may be prescribed for OM and otitis externa. Some otic analgesics are also wax emulsifiers.*	**antipyrine and benzocaine** ăn-tĭ-PĪ-rēn, BĔN-zō-kān *Auroguard, Dolotic*
vertigo and motion sickness	Decrease sensitivity of the inner ear to motion and prevent nerve impulses in the inner ear from reaching the vomiting center of the brain	**meclizine** MĔk-lĭ-zīn *Antivert, Dramamine*
wax emulsifiers ē-MŬL-sĭ-fī-ĕrz	Loosen and help remove impacted cerumen (ear wax) *Excessive wax may be washed out, vacuumed out, or removed using special instruments.*	**carbamide peroxide** KĂR-bă-mīd pĕr-ŎK-sīd *Debrox Drops, Murine Ear Drops*

Abbreviations

This section introduces abbreviations related to the eye and ear, along with their meanings.

Abbreviation	Meaning	Abbreviation	Meaning
Eye			
Acc	accommodation	OD	doctor of optometry
ARMD, AMD	age-related macular degeneration	PDR	proliferative diabetic retinopathy
Ast	astigmatism	SLE	slit-lamp examination; systemic lupus erythematosus
ENG	electronystagmography	SLT	selective laser trabeculoplasty
IOL	intraocular lens	ST	esotropia
IOP	intraocular pressure	VA	visual acuity
LASIK	laser-assisted in situ keratomileusis	VF	visual field
LPI	laser peripheral iridotomy	XT	exotropia
NPDR	nonproliferative diabetic retinopathy		
Ear			
AC	air conduction	OM	otitis media
BC	bone conduction	PE	pressure-equalizing (tube); physical examination; pulmonary embolism
ENT	ears, nose, and throat	URI	upper respiratory infection
NIHL	noise-induced hearing loss		

It is time to review procedures, pharmacology, and abbreviations by completing Learning Activity 16–4.

LEARNING ACTIVITIES

The activities that follow provide review of the special senses terms introduced in this chapter. Complete each activity and review your answers to evaluate your understanding of the chapter.

Visit the Medical Language Laboratory at medicallanguagelab.com. Use it to enhance your study and reinforcement of this chapter with the flash card activity. We recommend that you complete the flash card activity before starting Learning Activities 16-1 and 16-2.

Learning Activity 16-1
Medical Word Elements

Use the listed elements to build medical words. You may use the elements more than once.

Combining Forms		Suffixes		Prefixes	
ambly/o	myring/o	-acusia	-osis	an-	intra-
audi/o	ocul/o	-ar	-plasty	dipl-	
blephar/o	ot/o	-cele	-ptosis		
goni/o	phac/o	-itis	-rrhea		
kerat/o	presby/o	-meter	-tomy		
labyrinth/o	scler/o	-opia			
mastoid/o					

1. dimness of vision _____

2. herniation of the lens _____

3. double vision _____

4. downward displacement of the eyelid _____

5. instrument for measuring the (iridocorneal) angle _____

6. pertaining to within the eye _____

7. incision of the cornea _____

8. discharge from the ear _____

9. instrument for measuring hearing _____

10. total deafness _____

11. inflammation of the labyrinth of the inner ear _____

12. abnormal condition of hardening of (bones of) the ear _____

13. inflammation of the mastoid _____

14. surgical repair of the eardrum _____

15. (poor) hearing (associated with) old age _____

✓ *Check your answers in Appendix A. Review any material that you did not answer correctly.*

Correct Answers _____ X 6.67 = _____ % Score

Learning Activity 16-2
Building Medical Words

Use *ophthalm/o* (eye) to build words that mean

1. paralysis of the eye _____
2. study of the eye _____

Use *pupill/o* (pupil) to build a word that means

3. examination of the pupil _____

Use *kerat/o* (cornea) to build words that mean

4. softening of the cornea _____
5. instrument for measuring the cornea _____

Use *scler/o* (sclera) to build words that mean

6. inflammation of the sclera _____
7. softening of the sclera _____

Use *irid/o* (iris) to build words that mean

8. paralysis of the iris _____
9. herniation of the iris _____

Use *retin/o* (retina) to build words that mean

10. disease of the retina _____
11. inflammation of the retina _____

Use *blephar/o* (eyelid) to build words that mean

12. paralysis of the eyelid _____
13. prolapse of the eyelid _____

Use *ot/o* (ear) to build a word that means

14. flow of pus from the ear _____

Use *audi/o* (hearing) to build a word that means

15. instrument for measuring hearing _____

Use *myring/o* (tympanic membrane [eardrum]) to build a word that means

16. instrument for cutting the eardrum _____

Use the suffix *-opia* (vision) to build words that mean

17. dim or dull vision _____

18. excessive (farsighted) vision _____

Use the suffix *-acusis* (hearing) to build words that mean

19. without hearing _____

20. excessive (sensitivity to) hearing _____

Build surgical words that mean

21. removal of the stapes _____

22. incision of the labyrinth _____

23. removal of the mastoid process _____

24. surgical repair of the eardrum _____

25. incision of the cornea _____

✓ *Check your answers in Appendix A. Review material that you did not answer correctly.*

Correct Answers _____ X 4 = _____ % Score

Learning Activity 16-3
Diseases and Conditions

Match the terms with the definitions in the numbered list.

achromatopsia	drusen	nyctalopia	presbyacusis
amblyopia	exotropia	otitis externa	retinoblastoma
anacusis	hordeolum	otitis media	sensorineural
cataract	neovascular	otoencephalitis	tinnitus
chalazion	nonproliferative	otosclerosis	vertigo

1. opacity that forms on the lens and impairs vision _____
2. severe congenital form of color blindness _____
3. impaired vision in dim light _____
4. impaired hearing resulting from old age _____
5. complete deafness _____
6. infection of the external auditory canal _____
7. ankylosis of the middle ear bones resulting in hearing loss _____
8. middle ear infection commonly found in infants and children _____
9. diabetic retinopathy characterized by microaneurysms in the blood vessels of the retina with possible mild vision changes _____
10. hearing loss caused by damage to the cochlea or the auditory nerve _____
11. localized, circumscribed inflammatory swelling of a sebaceous gland of the eyelid; stye _____
12. inflammation of the brain tissue near the middle ear _____
13. wet form of macular degeneration _____
14. feeling of dizziness or spinning _____
15. outward deviation of the eye _____
16. small, yellowish deposits that develop on the retina and are associated with macular degeneration _____
17. tumor of the eyelid similar to a sebaceous cyst _____
18. "lazy-eye" syndrome _____
19. neoplastic disease of the eye found primarily in children _____
20. perception of ringing in the ears with no external stimuli _____

✔ *Check your answers in Appendix A. Review any material that you did not answer correctly.*

Correct Answers _____ X 5 = _____ % Score

Learning Activity 16-4

Procedures, Pharmacology, and Abbreviations

Match the terms with the definitions in the numbered list.

caloric stimulation	*gonioscopy*	*ophthalmic decongestants*	*tonometry*
cochlear implant	*keratoplasty*	*ophthalmoscopy*	*visual acuity*
enucleation	*LPI*	*PDR*	*vitrectomy*
evisceration	*miotics*	*PE*	*wax emulsifiers*
fluorescein angiography	*mydriatics*	*ST*	*XT*

1. test that uses different temperatures to assess the vestibular portion of the nerve _____

2. visual examination of the interior of the eye _____

3. artificial device that produces hearing sensations by electrically stimulating nerves inside the inner ear _____

4. assesses blood vessels and retinal circulation using a colored dye while photographs are taken _____

5. severe stage of diabetic retinopathy characterized by neovascularization, vitreous hemorrhage, and leaky blood vessels _____

6. agents that dilate the pupils in preparation for internal eye examinations _____

7. measurement of the intraocular pressure for detecting glaucoma _____

8. test that determines the smallest letters that can be read on a standardized chart _____

9. removal of the contents of the eyeball, leaving the sclera and cornea _____

10. cause the pupils to constrict _____

11. loosen and help remove impacted cerumen _____

12. removal of the entire eyeball from its orbit _____

13. esotropia _____

14. constrict small arterioles of the eye to decrease redness and conjunctival congestion _____

15. exotropia _____

16. visual examination of the angle of the anterior chamber of the eye _____

17. surgical procedure in which a damaged or diseased cornea is replaced with a donor cornea _____

18. laser treatment for open-angle glaucoma _____

19. type of tube inserted in the eardrum to treat chronic otitis media _____

20. removal of the vitreous humor followed by replacement with a clear solution _____

Check your answers in Appendix A. Review any material that you did not answer correctly.

Correct Answers _____ X 5 = _____ % Score

DOCUMENTING HEALTH-CARE ACTIVITIES

This section provides practical application activities in the form of exercises to help develop skills in documenting patient care. First read the medical report, then complete the activities and exercises that follow.

Documenting Health-Care Activity 16-1
Operative Report: Retained Foreign Bodies

Physicians Day Surgery

1514 Ninth Avenue ■ ■ Sun City, USA 12345 ■ ■ (555) 936–1933

OPERATIVE REPORT

Date:	5/13/xx		Surgeon:	Richard Roake, MD
Patient:	Hirsch, Annie		Patient ID#:	33328

PREOPERATIVE DIAGNOSIS: Foreign body, ears.

POSTOPERATIVE DIAGNOSIS: Foreign body, ears.

OPERATIVE INDICATIONS: Patient is a 9-year-old girl who presents with bilateral retained tympanostomy tubes. The tubes had been placed for more than 2½ years.

ANESTHESIA: General.

COMPLICATIONS: None.

OPERATIVE FINDINGS: Retained tympanostomy tubes, bilateral.

PROCEDURE: Removal of foreign bodies from ears with placement of paper patches.

INFORMED CONSENT: The risks and alternatives were explained to the mother, and she consented to the surgery.

In the supine position under satisfactory general anesthesia via mask, the patient was draped in a routine fashion.

The operating microscope was used to inspect the right ear. A previously placed tympanostomy tube was found to be in position and was surrounded with hard cerumen. The cerumen and the tube were removed, resulting in a very large perforation. The edges of the perforation were freshened sharply with a pick, and a paper patch was applied.

Patient tolerated the surgery very well and was sent to recovery in stable condition.

Richard Roake, MD
Richard Roake, MD

rk:bg

D: 5–13–20xx

T: 5–13–20xx

Terminology

The terms listed in the table that follows are taken from *Operative Report: Retained Foreign Bodies*. Use a medical dictionary such as *Taber's Cyclopedic Medical Dictionary*, the appendices of this book, or other resources to define each term. Then review the pronunciation for each term and practice by reading the medical record aloud.

Term	Definition
bilateral bī-LĂT-ĕr-ăl	
cerumen sĕ-ROO-mĕn	
perforation pĕr-fō-RĀ-shŭn	
supine sū-PĪN	
tympanostomy tĭm-pă-NŎS-tō-mē	

Visit the Medical Terminology Systems online resource center at FADavis.com to practice pronunciation and reinforce the meanings of the terms in this medical report.

Critical Thinking

Review *Operative Report: Retained Foreign Bodies* to answer the questions.

1. Did the surgery involve one or both ears?

_____

_____

_____

2. What was the nature of the foreign body in the patient's ears?

_____

_____

_____

3. What ear structure was involved?

_____

_____

_____

4. What instrument was used to locate the tubes?

_____

_____

_____

5. What was the material in which the tubes were embedded?

_____

_____

_____

6. What occurred when the cerumen and tubes were removed?

_____

_____

_____

7. How was the perforation treated?

_____

_____

_____

Documenting Health-Care Activity 16-2

Operative Report: Phacoemulsification and Lens Implant

Physicians Day Surgery

1514 Ninth Avenue ■ ■ Sun City, USA 12345 ■ ■ (555) 936–1933

OPERATIVE REPORT

Date:	5/14/xx	Surgeon:	Lewis Sloope, MD
Patient:	Deetrick, Douglas	Patient ID#:	33422

PREOPERATIVE DIAGNOSIS: Right eye cataract.

POSTOPERATIVE DIAGNOSIS: Right eye cataract.

OPERATION: Phacoemulsification, right eye, with posterior chamber lens implantation.

COMPLICATIONS: None.

PROCEDURE: This 68-year-old male was brought to the operating suite on 8/4/xx as an outpatient. Intravenous anesthesia and retrobulbar block to the right eye were administered. The right eye was prepped in the usual manner. A blepharostat was inserted, and a surgical microscope was positioned. Conjunctival peritomy was performed. Using a keratome, the anterior chamber was entered at the 12 o'clock position. A capsulorrhexis was performed. The cataract was removed by phacoemulsification.

After confirming the 20.5 diopters on the package, the implant was easily inserted into the capsular bag. The wound was observed and shown to be fluid tight. The incision required no sutures. TobraDex ointment was applied, and a sterile patch was taped into place.

Patient was monitored until stable. Postoperative care was reviewed, and patient was released with instructions to return to the office the following day.

Lewis Sloope, MD
Lewis Sloope, MD

rk:bg

D: 5–14–20xx

T: 5–14–20xx

Terminology

The terms listed in the table that follows are taken from *Operative Report: Phacoemulsifica-tion and Lens Implant.* Use a medical dictionary such as *Taber's Cyclopedic Medical Dictionary,* the appendices of this book, or other resources to define each term. Then review the pronunciation for each term and practice by reading the medical record aloud.

Term	Definition
blepharostat BLĔF-ă-rō-stăt	
capsulorrhexis kăp-sū-lō-RĔK-sĭs	
cataract KĂT-ă-răkt	
conjunctival kŏn-jŭnk-TĪ-văl	
diopter dī-ŎP-tĕr	
keratome KĔR-ă-tōm	
peritomy pĕr-ĬT-ō-mē	
phacoemulsification fă-kō-ē-mŭl-sĭ-fĭ-KĀ-shŭn	
posterior chamber pŏs-TĒR-ē-or CHĂM-bĕr	
retrobulbar block rĕt-rō-BŬL-băr	
TobraDex TŌ-bră-dĕks	

Visit the Medical Terminology Systems online resource center at FADavis. com to practice pronunciation and reinforce the meanings of the terms in this medical report.

Critical Thinking

Review *Operative Report: Phacoemulsification and Lens Implant* to answer the questions.

1. What technique was used to destroy the cataract?

   _____

   _____

   _____

2. In what portion of the eye was the implant placed?

   _____

   _____

   _____

3. What anesthetics were used for surgery?

   _____

   _____

   _____

4. What was the function of the blepharostat?

   _____

   _____

   _____

5. What is a keratome?

   _____

   _____

   _____

6. Where was the implant inserted?

   _____

   _____

   _____

Constructing Chart Notes

To construct chart notes, replace the italicized and boldfaced terms in each of the two case studies with one of the listed medical terms.

antiglaucoma agents	otalgia	pharyngalgia
asymptomatic	otorrhea	tinnitus
gonioscopy	pediatrician	tonometry
hyperopia		

Mrs. B is an established patient and presents for her annual eye examination. Although she had (1) *no symptoms* in 20xx, the results of the (2) *pressure measurement* of the eyes were above normal. For the last 3 years, she was effectively managed with (3) *medications that decrease intraocular pressure.* The patient now complains of losing side vision. Results of her eye refraction show there have been no changes in her (4) *farsightedness.* A (5) *visual examination of the angle* of the anterior chamber of the eyes indicates bilateral open-angle glaucoma that will require surgery. The plan is to schedule Mrs. B for trabeculoplasty using a low-level laser.

1. _____
2. _____
3. _____
4. _____
5. _____

Johnny K. was seen at this clinic by Dr. Roberts, a (6) *specialist in children's disorders.* His mother said that for the past 3 days he has complained of an (7) *earache,* (8) *a sore throat,* and (9) *ringing in the ears.* Earlier today, his mother noted an (10) *ear discharge* from the left ear. Upon examination, a perforated eardrum was clearly evident in the left ear. The right eardrum was intact. His tonsillar area showed evidence of strep throat, which was confirmed with a rapid strep test. The patient will begin a regimen of erythromycin with follow-up in 10 days.

6. _____
7. _____
8. _____
9. _____
10. _____

Check your answers in Appendix A. Review any material that you did not answer correctly.

Correct Answers _____ X 10 = _____ % Score

Answer Key

Chapter 1—Basic Elements of a Medical Word

Learning Activity 1-1
Understanding Medical Word Elements

1. word root *or* root, combining form, suffix, and prefix
2. arthr
3. False—A combining vowel is usually an "o."
4. True
5. True
6. True
7. False—To define a medical word, first define the suffix or the end of the word. Second, define the first part of the word. Third, define the middle of the word.

8. True
9. splen/o
10. hyster/o
11. enter/o
12. neur/o
13. ot/o
14. dermat/o
15. immun/o

Learning Activity 1-2
Identifying Word Roots and Combining Forms

1. nephritis
2. arthrodesis
3. cutane/ous
4. dentist
5. gastrectomy
6. chondritis
7. hepatoma
8. muscular

9. gastric
10. osteoma
11. erythr
12. hepat/o
13. arthr
14. oste/o/arthr
15. cholangi/o

Learning Activity 1-3
Understanding Pronunciations

1. macron
2. breve
3. long
4. short
5. k

6. n
7. is
8. eye
9. second
10. separate

Learning Activity 1-4
Identifying Suffixes and Prefixes

1. -tomy
2. -scope
3. -itis
4. -ic
5. -cyte

6. an-
7. pre-
8. intra-
9. para-
10. poly-

Defining Medical Words

Term	Definition
1. gastritis	inflammation of the stomach
2. nephritis	inflammation of the kidney(s)
3. gastrectomy	excision of the stomach
4. osteoma	tumor of bone
5. hepatoma	tumor of the liver
6. hepatitis	inflammation of the liver

Term	Rule	Summary of the Rule
7. arthr/itis	1	Word root (WR) links a suffix that begins with a vowel.
8. scler/osis	1	WR links a suffix that begins with a vowel.
9. arthr/o/centesis	2	Combining form (CF) links a suffix that begins with a consonant.
10. colon/o/scope	2	CF links a suffix that begins with a consonant.
11. chondr/itis	1	WR links a suffix that begins with a vowel.
12. chondr/oma	1	WR links a suffix that begins with a vowel.
13. oste/o/chondr/	3, 1	CF links multiple roots to each other. This rule holds true even if the next WR begins with a vowel.
14. muscul/ar	1	WR links a suffix that begins with a vowel.
15. oste/o/arthr/itis	3, 1	CF links multiple roots to each other. This rule holds true even if the next WR begins with a vowel. WR links a suffix that begins with a vowel.

Building Medical Words

1. splenectomy
2. appendectomy
3. pancreatectomy
4. cholecystectomy
5. nephrectomy
6. gastrectomy
7. splenitis
8. hepatitis
9. pancreatitis
10. cholecystitis
11. colitis
12. otitis
13. hepatomegaly
14. splenomegaly
15. gastromegaly

Chapter 2—Suffixes

Learning Activity 2-1
Building Surgical Words

1. episiotomy
2. colectomy
3. arthrocentesis
4. myorrhaphy
5. colostomy
6. osteotome
7. tympanotomy
8. tracheostomy
9. thrombolysis
10. lithotomy
11. hemorrhoidectomy
12. colostomy
13. osteoclasis
14. osteotome
15. arthrocentesis
16. lithotomy
17. mastectomy
18. tympanotomy
19. tracheostomy
20. splenectomy

Learning Activity 2-2
Building More Surgical Words

1. arthrodesis
2. rhinoplasty
3. tenoplasty
4. myorrhaphy
5. mastopexy
6. cystorrhaphy
7. osteoclasis
8. neurotripsy
9. enterolysis
10. lithotripsy
11. rhinoplasty
12. arthrocentesis
13. blepharorrhaphy
14. mastopexy
15. cystorrhaphy
16. tenoplasty
17. appendectomy
18. lithotripsy
19. enterolysis
20. neurotripsy

Learning Activity 2-3
Selecting a Surgical Suffix

1. colostomy
2. arthrocentesis
3. splenectomy
4. lithotripsy
5. dermatome
6. tracheostomy
7. lithotomy
8. mastectomy
9. neurolysis
10. thyroidotomy
11. mastopexy
12. colectomy
13. gastrorrhaphy
14. hysteropexy
15. rhinoplasty
16. arthrodesis
17. osteoclasis
18. hemorrhoidectomy
19. myorrhaphy
20. tympanotomy

Learning Activity 2-4
Selecting Diagnostic, Pathological, and Related Suffixes

1. hepatotoxic
2. neuralgia
3. leukemia
4. dermatosis
5. nephromegaly
6. otorrhea
7. blepharospasm
8. hysterorrhexis
9. cystocele
10. hyperemesis
11. myopathy
12. osteomalacia
13. bronchiectasis
14. osteopenia
15. cardiograph

Learning Activity 2-5
Building Pathological and Related Words

1. neuropathy
2. cholelith
3. carcinogenesis *or* carcinogen
4. osteomalacia
5. hemophobia
6. neuroma
7. hepatocele
8. bronchiectasis
9. dermatosis
10. chondromalacia
11. blepharoptosis
12. arteriosclerosis
13. cephalodynia
14. blepharospasm
15. hepatomegaly

Learning Activity 2-6
Selecting Adjective, Noun, and Diminutive Suffixes

1. aquatic
2. bacterial
3. gastric *or* gastral
4. axillary
5. cardiac *or* cardial
6. membranous
7. spinal *or* spinous
8. mania
9. psychiatry
10. sigmoidoscopy
11. alcoholism
12. allergist
13. internist
14. arteriole
15. venule

Forming Plural Words

Singular	Plural	Rule
1. diagnosis	diagnoses	Drop *is* and add *es*.
2. testis	testes	Drop *is* and add *es*.
3. vertebra	vertebrae	Retain *a* and add *e*.
4. keratosis	keratoses	Drop *is* and add *es*.
5. prognosis	prognoses	Drop *is* and add *es*.
6. spermatozoon	spermatozoa	Drop *on* and add *a*.
7. appendix	appendices	Drop *ix* and add *ices*.
8. coccus	cocci	Drop *us* and add *i*.
9. ganglion	ganglia	Drop *on* and add *a*.
10. bronchus	bronchi	Drop *us* and add *i*.
11. thrombus	thrombi	Drop *us* and add *i*.
12. septum	septa	Drop *um* and add *a*.
13. bacterium	bacteria	Drop *um* and add *a*.
14. fornix	fornices	Drop *ix* and add *ices*.
15. nevus	nevi	Drop *us* and add *i*.

Chapter 3—Prefixes

Identifying and Defining Prefixes

Word	Definition of Prefix
1. inter/dental	between
2. hypo/dermic	under, below, deficient
3. ab/duction	from, away from
4. multi/gravida	many, much

Word	Definition of Prefix
5. sub/lingual	under, below
6. quadri/plegia	four
7. anti/bacterial	against
8. tri/ceps	three
9. an/esthesia	without, not
10. intra/muscular	in, within
11. supra/pelvic	above, excessive, superior
12. bi/lateral	two
13. trans/vaginal	across, through
14. brady/cardia	slow
15. tachy/pnea	rapid
16. dys/tocia	bad, painful, difficult
17. eu/pnea	good, normal
18. hetero/graft	different
19. ultra/sonic	excess, beyond
20. circum/renal	around

Learning Activity 3-2

Matching Prefixes of Position, Number and Measurement, and Direction

1. retroversion
2. hypodermic
3. adduction
4. subnasal
5. postoperative
6. intercostal
7. epigastric
8. periodontal
9. diplopia
10. monotherapy
11. suprarenal
12. hemiplegia
13. circumrenal
14. macrocyte
15. polyphobia

Learning Activity 3-3
Matching Other Prefixes

1. dyspepsia
2. heterograft
3. bradypnea
4. hypercalcemia
5. bradycardia
6. anticonvulsant
7. amastia
8. infracostal
9. eupnea
10. paranasal
11. tachycardia
12. contraception
13. homograft
14. dystocia
15. homeoplasia

Chapter 4—Body Structure

Learning Activity 4-1
Matching Body Structures and Directional Terms

1. h. ventral cavity that contains digestive, repro-ductive, and excretory structures
2. d. away from the midsagittal plane of the body
3. j. part of the spine known as the *neck*
4. b. tailbone
5. k. movement toward the median plane
6. f. turning outward
7. l. away from the head; toward the tail or lower part of a structure
8. i. turning inward or inside out
9. n. part of the spine known as the *loin*
10. a. pertaining to the sole of the foot
11. o. near the back of the body
12. e. lying horizontal with face downward
13. g. nearer to the center (trunk of the body)
14. m. pertaining to outer wall of a body cavity
15. c. ventral cavity that contains heart, lungs, and associated structures

Learning Activity 4-2
Basic Word Elements

1. melan/o
2. dist/o
3. -ar
4. anter/o
5. leuk/o
6. cyan/o
7. xanth/o
8. dors/o
9. poli/o
10. peri-
11. later/o
12. caud/o
13. tom/o
14. ultra-
15. ventr/o
16. super-
17. hist/o
18. proxim/o
19. -graphy
20. endo-

Building Basic Terms

1. anterior
2. cephalad
3. dorsal
4. ventral
5. cirrhosis
6. erythrocyte
7. melanoma
8. radiologist
9. epigastric
10. hypogastric
11. chromic
12. mycosis
13. visceral
14. albinism
15. spinal

Building Medical Words

1. cytologist
2. cytology
3. erythrocyte
4. leukocyte
5. melanocyte
6. ventral
7. proximal
8. medial
9. distal
10. lateral
11. fluoroscopy
12. endoscopy
13. cytology
14. gastrology
15. histology

Diseases and Conditions

1. febrile
2. diagnosis
3. adhesion
4. gangrene
5. hernia
6. peritonitis
7. septicemia
8. suppuration
9. prognosis
10. inflammation
11. jaundice
12. symptom
13. edema
14. melanoma
15. perforation

Learning Activity 4-6
Procedures and Abbreviations

1. robotic surgery
2. curettage
3. CBC
4. ablation
5. endoscopy
6. fluoroscopy
7. US
8. electrocautery
9. C&S
10. MRI
11. anastomosis
12. nuclear scan
13. palpation
14. I&D
15. computed tomography

Documenting Health-Care Activity 4-1 (Critical Thinking)
Emergency Room Report: Spider Bite

1. What was the presenting problem?

The patient had a spider bite on his left thigh for several weeks.

2. How did the lesion affect the patient's leg movement?

His leg movement was not affected and he has full range of motion of the leg.

3. What procedure was performed on the affected area?

Incision and drainage (I&D).

4. What finding by the doctor led to performing this procedure?

The fluctuant mass with loculated fluid, an abscess, led to the I&D by the doctor.

5. Why was a culture performed on the wound?

A culture was performed to isolate and identify the bacteria causing the infection and to make sure the prescribed antibiotic would be effective in treating the infection.

6. What medication was prescribed to treat the infection?

Bactrim DS, in the morning and at bedtime for 10 days.

Documenting Health-Care Activity 4-2 (Critical Thinking)
Radiology Report: Injury of Left Wrist, Elbow, and Humerus

1. Where are the fractures located?

Distal shafts of the radius and ulna.

2. What caused the soft tissue deformity?

A fracture caused deformity to the surrounding soft tissue.

3. Did the radiologist take any side views of the left elbow?

The radiologist obtained a single view of the left elbow in the lateral projection.

4. In the AP view of the humerus, what structure was also visualized?

A portion of the elbow.

5. What findings are causes of concern for the radiologist?

Lucency through the distal humerus on the AP view along its medial aspect and elevation of the anterior and posterior fat pads.

Chapter 5—Integumentary System

Learning Activity 5-1
Medical Word Elements

1. intradermal
2. melanocyte
3. pediculosis
4. heterograft
5. hyperhidrosis
6. melanoma
7. hypodermic
8. dermatoplasty
9. lipocyte
10. pyoderma
11. dermatologist
12. xeroderma
13. anhidrosis
14. homograft
15. ichthyosis
16. scleroderma
17. mycosis
18. seborrhea
19. trichopathy
20. keratosis

Learning Activity 5-2
Building Medical Words

1. adipoma *or* lipoma
2. adipocele *or* lipocele
3. adipoid *or* lipoid
4. adipocyte *or* lipocyte
5. dermatitis
6. dermatomycosis
7. onychoma
8. onychomalacia
9. onychosis
10. onychomycosis
11. onychocryptosis
12. onychopathy
13. scleroderma
14. sclerosis
15. dermatology
16. dermatologist
17. adipectomy *or* lipectomy
18. onychectomy
19. autograft
20. dermatoplasty *or* dermoplasty

Learning Activity 5-4
Matching Burn and Oncology Terms

1. i. spread of cancer from primary site to other parts of the body
2. e. no evidence of primary tumor
3. h. cancerous; may be life-threatening
4. g. burn that heals without scar formation
5. f. determines degree of abnormal cancer cells compared with normal
6. a. develops from keratinizing epidermal cells
7. b. noncancerous
8. j. primary tumor size, small with minimal invasion
9. c. no evidence of metastasis
10. d. extensive damage to underlying connective tissue

Diseases and Conditions

1. comedo
2. pallor
3. eczema
4. Bowen disease
5. psoriasis
6. pediculosis
7. vitiligo
8. tinea
9. scabies
10. impetigo
11. urticaria
12. chloasma
13. ecchymosis
14. petechiae
15. alopecia
16. abscess
17. erythema
18. eschar
19. pruritus
20. verruca

Procedures, Pharmacology, and Abbreviations

1. Mohs
2. fulguration
3. corticosteroids
4. debridement
5. parasiticides
6. keratolytics
7. intradermal test
8. BCC
9. ung
10. xenograft
11. antifungals
12. IMP
13. antihistamines
14. dermabrasion
15. patch test

Pathology Report: Skin Lesion

1. In the specimen section, what does "skin on dorsum left wrist" mean?

Skin was obtained from the back, or posterior, surface of the left wrist.

2. What was the inflammatory infiltrate?

Lymphocytic inflammatory infiltrate in the papillary dermis.

3. What was the pathologist's diagnosis for the left forearm?

Nodular and infiltrating basal cell carcinoma near the elbow.

4. Provide a brief description of Bowen disease, the pathologist's diagnosis for the left wrist.

Bowen disease is a form of intraepidermal carcinoma (squamous cell) characterized by reddish-brown scaly or crusted lesions that resemble a patch of psoriasis or dermatitis.

Documenting Health-Care Activity 5-2 (Critical Thinking)
Patient Referral Letter: Onychomycosis

1. What pertinent disorders were identified in the past medical history?

History of hypertension and breast cancer.

2. What pertinent surgery was identified in the past surgical history?

Mastectomy.

3. Did the doctor identify any problems in the vascular system or nervous system?

Vascular and neurological systems were intact.

4. What was the significant finding in the laboratory results?

Alkaline phosphatase was elevated.

5. What treatment did the doctor use for the onychomycosis?

Debridement and medication or Sporanox PulsePak.

6. What did the doctor recommend regarding the abnormal laboratory finding?

The doctor recommended a repeat of the liver enzymes in approximately 4 weeks.

Documenting Health-Care Activity 5-3
Constructing Chart Notes

1. erythematous
2. pruritic
3. dermatologist
4. metastasize
5. Mohs surgery
6. asymptomatic
7. biopsy
8. oncologist
9. lymphadenectomy
10. chemotherapy

Chapter 6—Digestive System

Learning Activity 6-1
Medical Word Elements

1. gingivoplasty
2. colonoscopy
3. hepatitis
4. hypogastric
5. dyspepsia
6. sialolith
7. stomatopathy
8. perianal
9. jejunorrhaphy
10. pharyngitis
11. esophagoscope
12. anorexia
13. hematemesis
14. dental
15. dysphagia

Learning Activity 6-2
Building Medical Words

1. esophagodynia *or* esophagalgia
2. esophagospasm
3. esophagostenosis
4. gastroplasty
5. gastrodynia *or* gastralgia
6. gastropathy
7. jejunectomy
8. duodenal
9. ileostomy
10. jejunoileal
11. enteritis
12. enteropathy
13. enterocolitis
14. colitis
15. colorectal
16. coloptosis
17. colopathy
18. proctostenosis *or* rectostenosis
19. rectocele *or* proctocele
20. proctoplegia *or* proctoparalysis
21. cholecystectomy
22. cholelithiasis
23. hepatoma
24. hepatomegaly
25. pancreatitis

Learning Activity 6-3
Building Surgical Words

1. gingivectomy
2. glossectomy
3. esophagoplasty
4. gastrectomy
5. gastrojejunostomy
6. esophagectomy
7. gastroenterocolostomy
8. enteroplasty
9. enteropexy
10. choledochorrhaphy
11. abdominocentesis
12. cholelithotripsy
13. hernioplasty
14. hemorrhoidectomy
15. enterotome
16. colostomy
17. hepatopexy
18. proctoplasty *or* rectoplasty
19. cholecystectomy
20. choledochoplasty

Learning Activity 6-4
Diseases and Conditions

1. volvulus
2. dysphagia
3. hemorrhoids
4. halitosis
5. anorexia
6. melena
7. cirrhosis
8. cachexia
9. obstipation
10. borborygmus
11. ascites
12. Crohn disease
13. steatorrhea
14. leukoplakia
15. flatus
16. halitosis
17. fistula
18. obstipation
19. intussusception
20. hiatal hernia

Learning Activity 6-5

Procedures, Pharmacology, and Abbreviations

1. MRCP
2. VSG
3. IBS
4. antispasmodics
5. paracentesis
6. lower GI series
7. gastroscopy
8. antiemetics
9. intubation
10. anastomosis
11. stool guaiac
12. endoscopy
13. laxatives
14. antacids
15. stool culture
16. liver function tests
17. GERD
18. PUD
19. proctosigmoidoscopy
20. upper GI series

Documenting Health-Care Activity 6-1 (Critical Thinking)

Chart Note: GI Evaluation

1. Referring to Figure 6-4, describe the location of the gallbladder in relation to the liver.

Posterior and inferior portion of the right lobe of the liver.

2. Why did the patient undergo the cholecystectomy?

To treat cholecystitis and cholelithiasis.

3. What were the patient's prior surgeries?

Tonsillectomy, appendectomy, and cholecystectomy.

4. How does the patient's most recent postoperative episode of discomfort (pain) differ from the initial pain she described?

The continuous, deep right-sided pain took on a crescendo pattern and then a decrescendo pattern. Initially, it was intermittent and sharp epigastric pain.

5. What finding in the physical examination is a possible symptom of a SBO?

The high-pitched bowel sounds heard by the doctor during abdominal auscultation could indicate an obstruction.

Documenting Health-Care Activity 6-2 (Critical Thinking)

Operative Report: Esophagogastroduodenoscopy With Biopsy

1. What caused the hematemesis?

Etiology was unknown. Inflammation of the stomach and duodenum was noted.

2. What procedures were carried out to determine the cause of bleeding?

During x-ray tomography using the videoendoscope, biopsies were taken of the stomach and duodenum. It was also noted that the patient previously had esophageal varices.

3. How much blood did the patient lose during the procedure?

None.

4. Were there any ulcerations or erosions found during the exploratory procedure that might account for the bleeding?

No.

5. What type of sedation was used during the procedure?

Demerol and Versed administered intravenously.

6. What did the doctors find when they examined the stomach and duodenum?

Diffuse, punctate erythema.

Constructing Chart Notes

1. dysphagia
2. dyspepsia
3. gastric reflux
4. antacids
5. hiatal hernia

6. anorexia
7. nausea
8. sclerae
9. jaundice
10. hepatomegaly

Chapter 7—Respiratory System

Learning Activity 7-1
Medical Word Elements

1. pleurocentesis
2. bronchoscope
3. tonsillectomy
4. bradypnea
5. dysphonia
6. cyanosis
7. hypoxia
8. anosmia

9. septoplasty
10. sinusotomy
11. hypercapnia
12. eupnea
13. bronchiectasis
14. stethoscope
15. pneumonia

Learning Activity 7-2
Building Medical Words

1. rhinorrhea
2. rhinitis
3. laryngoscopy
4. laryngitis
5. laryngostenosis
6. bronchiectasis
7. bronchogenic
8. bronchospasm
9. pneumothorax
10. pneumoconiosis

11. pulmonologist
12. bronchopulmonary
13. dyspnea
14. bradypnea
15. tachypnea
16. apnea
17. tracheostomy
18. thoracocentesis *or* thoracentesis
19. lobectomy
20. septoplasty

Learning Activity 7-3
Diseases and Conditions

1. atelectasis
2. empyema
3. rhonchus
4. hypoxia
5. COVID-19
6. COPD
7. hypoxemia
8. cystic fibrosis
9. influenza
10. emphysema
11. hemoptysis
12. epistaxis
13. pulmonary edema
14. pulmonary embolism
15. deviated septum
16. coryza
17. OSA
18. pleurisy
19. consolidation
20. pertussis

Learning Activity 7-4
Procedures, Pharmacology, and Abbreviations

1. sputum culture
2. polysomnography
3. CXR
4. antral lavage
5. antihistamine
6. antitussive
7. sweat test
8. oximetry
9. thoracentesis
10. aerosol therapy
11. decongestant
12. Mantoux test
13. ABGs
14. expectorant
15. throat culture
16. pulmonary function tests
17. HBOT
18. septoplasty
19. pneumonectomy
20. CPAP

Documenting Health-Care Activity 7-1 (Critical Thinking)
SOAP Note: Respiratory Evaluation

1. What symptom caused the patient to seek medical help?

Shortness of breath.

2. What was the patient's previous history?

Difficult breathing, high blood pressure, chronic obstructive pulmonary disease, and peripheral vascular disease.

3. What were the abnormal findings of the physical examination?

Bilateral wheezes and rhonchi heard anteriorly and posteriorly.

4. What changes were noted from the previous film?

Interstitial vascular congestion with possible superimposed inflammatory change and some pleural reactive change.

5. What are the present assessments?

Acute exacerbation of chronic obstructive pulmonary disease, heart failure, hypertension, and peripheral vascular disease.

6. What new diagnosis was made that did not appear in the previous medical history?

Heart failure.

Documenting Health-Care Activity 7-2 (Critical Thinking)
SOAP Note: Chronic Interstitial Lung Disease

1. When did the patient notice dyspnea?

With activity.

2. Other than the respiratory system, what other body systems are identified in the history of present illness?

Cardiovascular, urinary, and nervous systems.

3. What were the findings regarding the neck?

Supple and no evidence of thyromegaly or adenomegaly.

4. What abnormal lung sounds were heard on auscultation?

Basilar crackles without wheezing or rhonchi.

5. What appears to be the likely cause of the chronic interstitial lung disease?

Combination of pulmonary fibrosis and heart failure.

6. What did the cardiac examination reveal?

Trace of edema without clubbing or murmur.

Documenting Health-Care Activity 7-3
Constructing Chart Notes

1. dyspnea
2. coryza
3. deviated nasal septum
4. septoplasty
5. T&A
6. myalgia
7. cephalodynia
8. sinusitis
9. pharyngitis
10. antitussive

Chapter 8—Cardiovascular System

Learning Activity 8-1
Medical Word Elements

1. bradycardia
2. atheroma
3. stenosis
4. ventricular
5. transseptal
6. phlebectasis
7. aortogram
8. valvuloplasty
9. sclerosis
10. sclerotherapy
11. thrombolysis
12. arrhythmia
13. periarterial
14. cardiomegaly
15. aneurysmectomy

Learning Activity 8-2
Building Medical Words

1. atheroma
2. atherosclerosis
3. phlebitis
4. phlebothrombosis
5. venule
6. venospasm
7. cardiologist
8. cardiorrhexis
9. cardiomyopathy
10. cardiomegaly
11. angioplasty
12. angioma
13. thrombogenesis
14. thrombosis
15. aortostenosis
16. aortography
17. cardiocentesis
18. arteriorrhaphy
19. embolectomy
20. thrombolysis

Learning Activity 8-3
Diseases and Conditions

1. infarction
2. angina
3. insufficiency
4. tachycardia
5. syncope
6. bruit
7. CHF
8. palpitation
9. fibrillation
10. aneurysm
11. embolism
12. arrhythmia
13. regurgitation
14. diaphoresis
15. arteriosclerosis
16. hypertension
17. hyperlipidemia
18. coarctation
19. hyperlipidemia
20. heart block

Learning Activity 8-4
Procedures, Pharmacology, and Abbreviations

1. Holter monitor test
2. ECHO
3. PTT
4. nitrates
5. statins
6. diuretics
7. troponin
8. Doppler
9. stress test
10. defibrillation
11. cardioversion
12. ECG
13. ICD
14. stent placement
15. anticoagulants
16. sclerotherapy
17. CABG
18. endarterectomy
19. PTCA
20. LDL

Documenting Health-Care Activity 8-1 (Critical Thinking)

Chart Note: Acute Myocardial Infarction

1. How long had the patient experienced chest pain before she was seen in the hospital?

Approximately 2 hours

2. Did the patient have a previous history of chest pain?

Yes.

3. Initially, what medications were administered to stabilize the patient?

Streptokinase and heparin.

4. What two laboratory tests will be used to evaluate the patient?

Partial thromboplastin time and cardiac enzymes.

5. During the current admission, what part of the heart was damaged?

The lateral front side of the heart (anterior of the heart).

6. Was the location of damage to the heart for this admission the same as that for the initial MI?

No, in the earlier admission, the damage was to the lower part of the heart.

Documenting Health-Care Activity 8-2 (Critical Thinking)

Operative Report: SOAP Note: Deep Venous Thrombosis

1. What were the findings on the ultrasound of the right leg?

Acute thrombosis of the right popliteal veins and a thrombus in one of the tibial veins in the calf.

2. How was the DVT initially treated?

Lovenox and eventually warfarin.

3. What is causing the continued weightbearing difficulty on the right foot?

Weightbearing difficulty is most likely due to his right foot stress fracture.

4. What is the risk factor for DVT in this patient?

Immobilization.

5. What are the recommendations for follow-up?

Continue anticoagulation with warfarin for 3 to 6 months, follow-up popliteal ultrasound, and knee-high support stocking.

Documenting Health-Care Activity 8-3

Constructing Chart Notes

1. angina pectoris
2. diaphoresis
3. palpitations
4. hypertension
5. edema
6. myocardial infarction
7. ischemia
8. angioplasty
9. catheter
10. stent

Chapter 9—Blood, Lymphatic, and Immune Systems

Learning Activity 9-1
Medical Word Elements

1. lymphadenopathy
2. thymectomy
3. splenomegaly
4. thrombosis
5. morphology
6. sideropenia
7. hypochromic
8. microcytic
9. lymphangioma
10. erythroblast
11. hemolysis
12. nuclear
13. adenoma
14. agranular
15. hemopoiesis

Learning Activity 9-2
Building Medical Words

1. thrombosis
2. thrombolysis
3. erythrocytosis
4. leukocytosis
5. lymphocytosis
6. reticulocytosis
7. leukopenia *or* leukocytopenia
8. erythropenia *or* erythrocytopenia
9. thrombocytopenia *or* thrombopenia
10. lymphocytopenia
11. hemopoiesis *or* hematopoiesis
12. leukopoiesis *or* leukocytopoiesis
13. thrombocytopoiesis
14. immunologist
15. immunology
16. tonsillectomy
17. thymectomy
18. lymphadenectomy
19. splenotomy
20. splenopexy

Learning Activity 9-3
Diseases and Conditions

1. hemoglobinopathy
2. lymphedema
3. SLE
4. aplastic
5. anaphylaxis
6. opportunistic
7. Hodgkin disease
8. sensitization
9. erythropenia
10. multiple myeloma
11. mononucleosis
12. sepsis
13. myelogenous
14. Kaposi sarcoma
15. sickle cell
16. thrombocytopenia
17. hemolytic
18. urticaria
19. hemophilia
20. graft rejection

Learning Activity 9-4
Procedures, Pharmacology, and Abbreviations

1. PT
2. lymphangiography
3. monospot
4. anticoagulants
5. WBC
6. homologous
7. ANA
8. lymphoscintigraphy

9. plasmapheresis
10. DIC
11. autologous
12. antimicrobials
13. RBC
14. thrombolytics
15. transfusion

Documenting Health-Care Activity 9-1 (Critical Thinking)
Discharge Summary: Sickle Cell Crisis

1. What blood product was administered to the patient?

Two units of packed red blood cells.

2. Why was this blood product given to the patient?

The patient was anemic as a result of sickle cell anemia.

3. What medications were given for pain relief?

Vicodin and morphine.

4. Why was a CT scan performed on the patient?

To determine the cause of abdominal pain.

5. What were the three findings of the CT scan?

Ileus in the small bowel, dilated small bowel loops, and abnormal enhancement pattern in the kidney.

6. Why should the patient see his PCP?

To follow up on the renal abnormality.

Documenting Health-Care Activity 9-2 (Critical Thinking)
Discharge Summary: PCP and HIV

1. How do you think the patient acquired the HIV infection?

From her husband, who died of HIV.

2. What four disorders in the medical history are significant for HIV?

Several episodes of diarrhea, sinusitis, thrush, and vaginal candidiasis.

3. What was the x-ray finding?

Diffuse lower lobe infiltrates.

4. What antibiotic was prescribed for the pneumonia?

Bactrim.

5. What two procedures are going to be performed to confirm the diagnosis of *Pneumocystis* pneumonia?

Bronchoscopy and alveolar lavage.

Documenting Health-Care Activity 9-3
Constructing Chart Notes

1. lymphadenopathy
2. splenomegaly
3. leukocytosis
4. erythropenia
5. hematologist

6. hemophilia
7. ecchymoses
8. arthralgia
9. hemarthrosis
10. hemostasis

Chapter 10—Musculoskeletal System

Learning Activity 10-1
Medical Word Elements

1. atrophy
2. leiomyoma
3. brachialgia
4. patellar
5. chondromalacia
6. arthrodesis
7. ankylosis
8. craniotome
9. osteoporosis
10. arthritis
11. lumbar
12. dystrophy
13. synovitis
14. syndactylism
15. arthrocentesis
16. dactylitis
17. osteoclast
18. cephalalgia
19. chondroma
20. fascioplasty

Learning Activity 10-2
Building Medical Words

1. osteocytes
2. osteosarcoma
3. osteoarthropathy
4. osteogenesis
5. cervicalgia, cervicodynia
6. cervicobrachial
7. cervicofacial
8. myeloma
9. myelosarcoma
10. myelocyte
11. myeloid
12. suprasternal
13. sternoid
14. chondroblast
15. arthrotomy
16. osteoarthritis
17. pelvimeter
18. myospasm
19. myasthenia
20. myorrhexis
21. phalangectomy
22. thoracotomy
23. vertebrectomy
24. arthrodesis
25. myoplasty

Learning Activity 10-3
Diseases and Conditions

1. subluxation
2. rickets
3. spondylolisthesis
4. claudication
5. muscular dystrophy
6. talipes
7. sequestrum
8. myasthenia gravis
9. carpal tunnel
10. ganglion cyst
11. hypotonia
12. Ewing
13. greenstick fracture
14. kyphosis
15. osteoporosis
16. scoliosis
17. chondrosarcoma
18. comminuted fracture
19. spondylitis
20. gout
21. bunion
22. pyogenic
23. necrosis
24. ankylosis
25. phantom limb

Learning Activity 10-4
Procedures, Pharmacology, and Abbreviations

1. calcium supplements
2. OREF
3. vertebroplasty
4. foraminotomy
5. ACL
6. myelography
7. ORIF
8. DXA scan
9. CTS
10. laminectomy
11. arthrography
12. arthrodesis
13. amputation
14. THA
15. NSAIDs
16. arthroscopy
17. sequestrectomy
18. bone scintigraphy
19. relaxants
20. closed reduction

Documenting Health-Care Activity 10-1 (Critical Thinking)

Operative Report: Right Knee Arthroscopy and Medial Meniscectomy

1. Describe the meniscus and identify its location.

The meniscus is the curved, fibrous cartilage in the knees and other joints.

2. What is the probable cause of the tear in the patient's meniscus?

The continuous pressure on the knees from jogging on a hard surface, such as pavement.

3. What does normal ACL and PCL refer to in the report?

The anterior and posterior cruciate ligaments appeared to be normal.

4. Explain the McMurray sign test.

Rotation of the tibia on the femur is used to determine injury to meniscal structures. An audible click during manipulation of the tibia with the leg flexed is an indication that the meniscus has been injured.

5. Why was the surgery performed even though the Lachman and McMurray tests were negative (normal)?

The medial compartment of the knee showed an inferior surface posterior and midmedial meniscal tear that was flipped up on top of itself. The surgeon resected the tear, and the remaining meniscus was contoured back to a stable rim.

Documenting Health-Care Activity 10-2 (Critical Thinking)

Emergency Department Report: Oblique Spiral Fracture of Left Tibia

1. What findings on physical examination showed limited range of motion?

Physical examination revealed limited range of motion with dorsiflexion and plantarflexion of the left ankle.

2. What medication was the patient taking for pain, and did it provide relief?

Ibuprofen was taken and provided minimal pain relief with 7/10 pain.

3. What were the findings of the x-rays?

AP and lateral views of the left tibia-fibula demonstrate oblique spiral fracture of the distal tibial diaphysis with minimal displacement.

4. How was the injured site stabilized?

Patient fitted with a splint with soft cast.

5. Under what conditions should the patient seek medical help?

Patient is to return to the ER if he notices any throbbing, numbness, tingling, loss of sensation, or capillary refill that is not relieved by removing or loosening the splint.

Documenting Health-Care Activity 10-3

Constructing Chart Notes

1. comminuted
2. clavicle
3. open fracture
4. femur
5. orthopedist
6. osteopenia
7. kyphosis
8. spondylalgia
9. osteoporosis
10. pathological fractures

Chapter 11—Urinary System

Learning Activity 11-1
Medical Word Elements

1. cystogram
2. nephrocele
3. pyeloplasty
4. anuria
5. glomerulopathy
6. cystoscopy
7. dialysis
8. hematuria
9. oliguria
10. ureterectasis
11. meatotome
12. azotemia
13. lithogenesis
14. lithotripsy
15. nephropathy

Learning Activity 11-2
Building Medical Words

1. nephromegaly
2. nephropyosis *or* pyonephrosis
3. nephrolith
4. pyelonephritis
5. pyelopathy
6. ureterectasis *or* ureterectasia
7. ureterolith
8. ureteralgia *or* ureterodynia
9. cystitis
10. cystoscope
11. cystocele
12. vesicocele
13. vesicourethral
14. urethrostenosis
15. urethroplasty
16. urology
17. uropathy
18. dysuria
19. hematuria
20. proteinuria
21. ureteroplasty
22. cystectomy
23. urethrorrhaphy
24. pyelostomy
25. cystopexy

Learning Activity 11-3
Diseases and Conditions

1. urgency
2. fistula
3. diuresis
4. anuria
5. azotemia
6. hydronephrosis
7. urolithiasis
8. interstitial cystitis
9. colic
10. pyelonephritis
11. cystocele
12. incontinence
13. polycystic
14. neurogenic bladder
15. nephropyosis
16. nephrotic syndrome
17. enuresis
18. reflux
19. Wilms tumor
20. nephrolithiasis

Procedures, Pharmacology, and Abbreviations

1. CT urogram
2. electromyography
3. creatinine clearance
4. RCC
5. C&S
6. diuretics
7. stent placement
8. ESWL
9. peritoneal
10. renal nuclear scan
11. hemodialysis
12. nephrostomy
13. bladder US
14. potassium
15. UA

Documenting Health-Care Activity 11-1 (Critical Thinking)
Operative Report: Cystoscopy With Cystolithotripsy

1. What were the findings from the resectoscopy?

The prostate and bladder appeared normal, but there was a left ureterocele.

2. What were the name and size of the urethral sound used in the procedure?

#26 French Van Buren.

3. What is the function of the urethral sound?

To dilate the urethra.

4. In what direction was the ureterocele incised?

Longitudinally.

5. Was fulguration required? Why or why not?

Fulguration was not required because there was no bleeding.

Documenting Health-Care Activity 11-2 (Critical Thinking)
Operative Report: Extracorporeal Shock-Wave Lithotripsy

1. What previous procedures were performed on the patient?

ESWL and double-J stent placement.

2. Why is the current procedure being performed?

To fragment the remaining calculus and remove the double-J stent.

3. What imaging technique was used for positioning the patient to ensure that the shock waves would strike the calculus?

Fluoroscopy.

4. In what position was the patient placed in the cystoscopy suite?

Dorsal lithotomy.

5. How was the double-J stent removed?

Through a cystoscope it was removed with grasping forceps as the scope was withdrawn.

Documenting Health-Care Activity 11-3
Constructing Chart Notes

1. hematuria
2. pyuria
3. ureterolithiasis
4. pyelectasis
5. lithotripsy
6. oliguria
7. hypertension
8. proteinuria
9. glomerulonephritis
10. prognosis

Chapter 12—Female Reproductive System

Learning Activity 12-1
Medical Word Elements

1. salpingoplasty
2. prenatal
3. dystocia
4. hysterorrhexis
5. oophorectomy
6. cervicitis
7. amniocentesis
8. perineorrhaphy
9. colposcopy
10. primigravida
11. pseudocyesis
12. hemosalpinx
13. multipara
14. menarche
15. galactopoiesis

Learning Activity 12-2
Building Medical Words

1. gynecology
2. gynecologist
3. cervicovaginitis
4. cervicovesical
5. colposcope
6. colposcopy
7. vaginitis
8. vaginocele
9. hysteromyoma
10. hysteropathy
11. hysterosalpingography
12. mastopexy
13. mastectomy
14. uterocele
15. uterocervical
16. uterovesical
17. oophoroma
18. oophorosalpingitis
19. salpingocele
20. salpingography
21. oophoropexy *or* ovariopexy
22. hystero-oophorectomy
23. episiorrhaphy *or* perineorrhaphy
24. hysterosalpingo-oophorectomy
25. amniocentesis

Learning Activity 12-3
Diseases and Conditions

1. oligomenorrhea
2. primipara
3. gestation
4. sterility
5. retroversion
6. fibrocystic disease
7. dystocia
8. condylomata
9. Down syndrome
10. endometriosis
11. dyspareunia
12. metrorrhagia
13. menarche
14. fibroids
15. pyosalpinx
16. breech
17. eclampsia
18. choriocarcinoma
19. candidiasis
20. primigravida

Learning Activity 12-4
Procedures, Pharmacology, and Abbreviations

1. lumpectomy
2. DBT
3. amniocentesis
4. antifungals
5. PCOS
6. cordocentesis
7. cerclage
8. tubal ligation
9. cryosurgery
10. laparoscopy
11. episiotomy
12. PID
13. chorionic villus sampling
14. estrogens
15. oxytocins
16. OCPs
17. IUD
18. FNA
19. Pap test
20. prostaglandins

Documenting Health-Care Activity 12-1 (Critical Thinking)
SOAP Note: Primary Herpes 1 Infection

1. Did the patient have any discharge? If so, describe it.

Yes, a brownish discharge.

2. What type of discomfort did the patient experience around the vulvar area?

She was experiencing severe itching (pruritus), fever, and blisters.

3. Has the patient been taking her oral contraceptive pills regularly?

Yes.

4. Where was the viral culture obtained?

Ulcerlike lesion on the right labia.

5. Even though the patient's partner used a condom, how do you think the patient became infected with herpes?

She probably got infected from the cold sore when having oral-genital sex.

Documenting Health-Care Activity 12-2 (Critical Thinking)
Preoperative Consultation: Menometrorrhagia

1. How many pregnancies did this woman have? How many viable infants did she deliver?

Two pregnancies and one viable birth.

2. What is a therapeutic abortion?

An abortion performed when the pregnancy endangers the mother's mental or physical health or when the fetus has a known condition incompatible with life.

3. Why did the physician propose to perform a hysterectomy?

The patient desired definitive treatment for menometrorrhagia and had declined palliative treatment.

4. What are the advantages of laparoscopic surgery?

Advantages of laparoscopic surgery include lower risk of infection, less scarring, faster recovery, reduced blood loss, improved outcomes, and enhanced visualization.

5. Did the surgeon plan to remove one or both ovaries and fallopian tubes?

The surgeon planned to perform a bilateral (pertaining to two sides) salpingo-oophorectomy.

6. What is the purpose of the Premarin?

The ovaries, which produce estrogen, were removed. The Premarin will provide hormone replacement therapy of estrogen.

Documenting Health-Care Activity 12-3
Constructing Chart Notes

1. gravida 3, para 3
2. metrorrhagia
3. menorrhagia
4. dysmenorrhea
5. uterine fibroids
6. nullipara
7. menarche
8. menopause
9. mammography
10. needle biopsy

Chapter 13—Male Reproductive System

Learning Activity 13-1
Medical Word Elements

1. oligospermia
2. varicocele
3. epididymectomy
4. genitourinary
5. gonadectomy
6. anorchism
7. prostatomegaly
8. scrotoplasty
9. epispadias
10. vesiculography
11. balanitis
12. androgen
13. dysuria
14. vasectomy
15. hypogonadism

Learning Activity 13-2
Building Medical Words

1. orchidectomy
2. orchidoptosis
3. balanorrhea
4. balanocele
5. spermatocyte
6. spermatoblast
7. spermatocele
8. prostatocystitis
9. prostatorrhea
10. prostatomegaly
11. prostatolith
12. hypospadias
13. hyperspadias
14. vesiculitis
15. vesiculography
16. gonadopathy
17. gonadotropin
18. vasectomy
19. scrotoplasty
20. cryotherapy

Learning Activity 13-3

Diseases and Conditions

1. gynecomastia
2. herpes
3. cryptorchidism
4. anorchidism
5. phimosis
6. Peyronie disease
7. varicocele
8. testicular torsion
9. condyloma
10. hypospadias
11. balanitis
12. priapism
13. hyperplasia
14. hydrocele
15. sterility
16. epididymitis
17. chlamydia
18. chancre
19. BPH
20. leukorrhea

Learning Activity 13-4

Procedures, Pharmacology, and Abbreviations

1. TUMT
2. holmium
3. TSE
4. brachytherapy
5. RALP
6. semen analysis
7. androgens
8. scrotal
9. cryosurgery
10. vasectomy
11. urethroplasty
12. vasovasostomy
13. antiandrogens
14. TURP
15. PSA
16. antivirals
17. orchiopexy
18. circumcision
19. HPV
20. BPH

Documenting Health-Care Activity 13-1 (Critical Thinking)

Consultation Report: Benign Prostatic Hyperplasia

1. What is the reason for the present admission?

Left inguinal hernia repair and right ventral hernia repair.

2. What occurred when the physician removed the Foley catheter?

The patient complained of dysuria, frequency, and a feeling of incomplete emptying with weak stream.

3. What did the patient's previous history indicate regarding these symptoms?

He had a history of urinary hesitancy, weak stream, and voiding every 2 to 3 hours.

4. Why was it difficult to assess for bladder distention?

The incision lies over the bladder area.

5. Was there a definitive diagnosis identified in the impression?

The impression indicates questionable urine retention.

6. What procedure will the physician perform if the patient has difficulty voiding?

The doctor will catheterize the patient.

Documenting Health-Care Activity 13-2 (Critical Thinking)
Chart Note: Acute Epididymitis

1. What were the complaints of the patient?

Severe left-sided groin pain, scrotal pain, and urethritis.

2. What procedure did the physician perform regarding the urethral discharge?

The discharge was expressed upon compression of the glans, and swabs were obtained for testing.

3. What information does the chart note provide regarding the left testicle?

Moderate pain and tenderness, which is alleviated with elevation of the testicles.

4. How does the chart note describe the left epididymis?

Palpable, with significant induration and tenderness.

5. What did the rectal examination reveal?

Mild prostatic hyperplasia and tenderness.

Documenting Health-Care Activity 13-3
Constructing Chart Notes

1. leukorrhea
2. dysuria
3. pruritus
4. orchialgia
5. meatus
6. PSA
7. digital rectal examination
8. prostatomegaly
9. asymptomatic
10. benign

Chapter 14—Endocrine System

Learning Activity 14-1
Medical Word Elements

1. thymoma
2. pancreatitis
3. polydipsia
4. glycogenesis
5. endocrine
6. adipsia
7. exocrine
8. hyperglycemia
9. thymolysis
10. thyromegaly
11. adrenalitis
12. hypocalcemia
13. hyperkalemia
14. acromegaly
15. toxicologist

Learning Activity 14-2
Building Medical Words

1. thymoma
2. thymomegaly
3. thymotomy
4. hyperkalemia
5. hypokalemia
6. hyperglycemia
7. hypoglycemia
8. glycogenesis
9. pancreatitis
10. pancreatolysis
11. pancreatopathy
12. thyroiditis
13. thyromegaly
14. parathyroidectomy
15. adrenalectomy

Learning Activity 14-3
Diseases and Conditions

1. acromegaly
2. myxedema
3. diuresis
4. hirsutism
5. cretinism
6. thyroid storm
7. Addison disease
8. exophthalmic goiter
9. hyperkalemia
10. pheochromocytoma
11. type 1
12. hyponatremia
13. glycosuria
14. Cushing syndrome
15. type 2

Learning Activity 14-4
Procedures, Pharmacology, and Abbreviations

1. FBS
2. RAIU
3. corticosteroids
4. GH
5. thyroid scan
6. parathyroidectomy
7. DKA
8. DI
9. GLP-1 agonists
10. TED
11. T_4
12. CGM
13. GTT
14. antithyroids
15. transsphenoidal
16. T_3
17. TFT
18. exophthalmometry
19. total calcium test
20. insulin

Documenting Health-Care Activity 14-1 (Critical Thinking)
Consultation Note: Hyperparathyroidism

1. What is an adenoma?

Benign tumor of a gland.

2. What does the physician suspect caused the patient's hyperparathyroidism?

Possible parathyroid adenoma.

3. What type of laboratory findings revealed parathyroid disease?

Elevated calcium level.

4. What is hypercalciuria?

Excessive amount of calcium in the urine.

5. If the patient smoked 548 packs of cigarettes per year, how many packs did she smoke in an average day?

Approximately 1.5 packs per day (365 days per year/548 packs = 1.5).

Documenting Health-Care Activity 14-2 (Critical Thinking)
SOAP Note: Diabetes Mellitus

1. How long has this patient been experiencing voracious eating?

For the past 10 days.

2. Was the patient's obesity a result of overeating or a metabolic imbalance?

No, it was due to overeating.

3. Why did the doctor experience difficulty in examining the patient's abdomen?

Because she was obese.

4. Was the patient's blood glucose above or below normal on admission?

Above normal.

5. What is the reference range for fasting blood glucose?

The reference range for fasting blood glucose is 70 to 110 mg/dL.

Documenting Health-Care Activity 14-3
Constructing Chart Notes

1. polydipsia
2. polyuria
3. polyphagia
4. hyperglycemia
5. glycosuria
6. lethargy
7. constipation
8. bradycardia
9. hypopnea
10. triiodothyronine and thyroxine

Chapter 15—Nervous System

Learning Activity 15-1
Medical Word Elements

1. ventriculostomy
2. neuroma
3. radiculalgia
4. gangliectomy
5. narcolepsy
6. unilateral
7. meningitis
8. quadriplegia
9. hyperkinesia
10. myasthenia
11. cerebropathy
12. intrathecal
13. encephalocele
14. kinesiotherapy
15. myelorrhaphy

Learning Activity 15-2
Building Medical Words

1. encephalopathy
2. encephalocele
3. encephalography
4. cerebropathy
5. cerebritis
6. craniocele
7. craniometer
8. neuralgia *or* neurodynia
9. neurologist
10. neurotripsy
11. myelocele
12. myeloplegia
13. psychotic *or* psychic
14. psychosis
15. bradykinesia
16. dyskinesia
17. hemiplegia
18. quadriplegia
19. dysphasia
20. aphasia
21. neurolysis
22. craniotomy
23. cranioplasty
24. neurorrhaphy
25. encephalotomy

Learning Activity 15-3
Diseases and Conditions

1. hemiparesis
2. dementia
3. Alzheimer
4. anhedonia
5. clonic
6. Guillain-Barré
7. ataxia
8. bipolar
9. epilepsies
10. ischemic
11. shingles
12. radiculopathy
13. paraplegia
14. poliomyelitis
15. convulsion
16. myelomeningocele
17. schizophrenia
18. Parkinson
19. multiple sclerosis
20. concussion
21. cluster headache
22. anorexia nervosa
23. ALS
24. TIA
25. spina bifida

Learning Activity 15-4
Procedures, Pharmacology, and Abbreviations

1. ketamine
2. myelography
3. antipsychotics
4. ECT
5. general anesthetics
6. EEG
7. stimulants
8. CP
9. TIA
10. CSF analysis
11. NCV
12. EMG
13. lumbar puncture
14. hypnotics
15. trephination

Documenting Health-Care Activity 15-1 (Critical Thinking)
Chart Note: Medication Management Follow-Up

1. What are some of the symptoms of depression the patient is experiencing?

Anhedonia, low appetite, low energy, poor focus, initial insomnia, hypersomnia.

2. How long has the patient been experiencing symptoms of depression?

Two months.

3. What other psychiatric disorder has the patient experienced?

Anxiety disorder.

4. What are some of the reasons the patient would be considered low risk for suicide?

No suicidal thoughts, no substance use, he has hope; his family, cat, and friends are protective.

5. What medication is being used to treat the patient's symptoms?

Sertraline.

6. What medical condition could be contributing to the patient's depression symptoms?

Hypothyroidism.

Documenting Health-Care Activity 15-2 (Critical Thinking)
Consultation Report: Acute-Onset Paraplegia

1. What was the original cause of the patient's current problems, and what treatments were provided?

Fall at work about 15 to 20 years ago and four subsequent lumbar surgeries.

2. Why was the patient admitted to the hospital?

Pain management.

3. What medications did the patient receive, and why was each given?

Clonidine for hypertension and methadone for pain.

4. What was the cause of bladder retention?

Administration of clonidine.

5. What occurred after the catheter was removed?

Subacute onset of paresis, paresthesias, and pain in the legs, approximately 2.5 to 3 hours later.

6. What three disorders were listed in the differential diagnosis?

Subarachnoid hemorrhage, epidural abscess, and transverse myelitis.

Constructing Chart Notes

1. neuralgia
2. sciatica
3. herniation
4. osteophyte
5. neuropathy

6. tremor
7. bradyphasia
8. bradykinesia
9. dysphagia
10. Parkinson disease

Chapter 16—Special Senses

Learning Activity 16-1
Medical Word Elements

1. amblyopia
2. phacocele
3. diplopia
4. blepharoptosis
5. goniometer
6. intraocular
7. keratotomy
8. otorrhea

9. audiometer
10. anacusia
11. labyrinthitis
12. otosclerosis
13. mastoiditis
14. myringoplasty
15. presbyacusia

Learning Activity 16-2
Building Medical Words

1. ophthalmoplegia *or* ophthalmoparalysis
2. ophthalmology
3. pupilloscopy
4. keratomalacia
5. keratometer
6. scleritis
7. scleromalacia
8. iridoplegia *or* iridoparalysis
9. iridocele
10. retinopathy
11. retinitis
12. blepharoplegia
13. blepharoptosis
14. otopyorrhea

15. audiometer
16. myringotome
17. amblyopia
18. hyperopia
19. anacusis
20. hyperacusis
21. stapedectomy
22. labyrinthotomy
23. mastoidectomy
24. myringoplasty *or* tympanoplasty
25. keratotomy

Learning Activity 16-3
Diseases and Conditions

1. cataract
2. achromatopsia
3. nyctalopia
4. presbycusis
5. anacusis
6. otitis externa
7. otosclerosis
8. otitis media
9. nonproliferative
10. sensorineural
11. hordeolum
12. otoencephalitis
13. neovascular
14. vertigo
15. exotropia
16. drusen
17. chalazion
18. amblyopia
19. retinoblastoma
20. tinnitus

Learning Activity 16-4
Procedures, Pharmacology, and Abbreviations

1. caloric stimulation
2. ophthalmoscopy
3. cochlear implant
4. fluorescein angiography
5. PDR
6. mydriatics
7. tonometry
8. visual acuity
9. evisceration
10. miotics
11. wax emulsifiers
12. enucleation
13. ST
14. ophthalmic decongestants
15. XT
16. gonioscopy
17. keratoplasty
18. LPI
19. PE
20. vitrectomy

Documenting Health-Care Activity 16-1 (Critical Thinking)
Operative Report: Retained Foreign Bodies

1. Did the surgery involve one or both ears?

It was bilateral, involving both ears.

2. What was the nature of the foreign body in the patient's ears?

Retained tympanostomy tubes

3. What ear structure was involved?

Eardrum, or tympanum.

4. What instrument was used to locate the tubes?

Operating microscope.

5. What was the material in which the tubes were embedded?

Earwax, or cerumen.

6. What occurred when the cerumen and tubes were removed?

It resulted in a large perforation.

7. How was the perforation treated?

The edges were freshened sharply with a pick, and a paper patch was applied.

Documenting Health-Care Activity 16-2 (Critical Thinking)
Operative Report: Phacoemulsification and Lens Implant

1. What technique was used to destroy the cataract?

Phacoemulsification, an ultrasound technique.

2. In what portion of the eye was the implant placed?

Posterior chamber.

3. What anesthetics were used for surgery?

Intravenous and retrobulbar block.

4. What was the function of the blepharostat?

To separate the eyelids during surgery.

5. What is a keratome?

A knife used to incise the cornea.

6. Where was the implant inserted?

In the capsular bag.

Documenting Health-Care Activity 16-3
Constructing Chart Notes

1. asymptomatic
2. tonometry
3. antiglaucoma agents
4. hyperopia
5. gonioscopy
6. pediatrician
7. otalgia
8. pharyngalgia
9. tinnitus
10. otorrhea

Common Abbreviations and Symbols

Common Abbreviations

This table lists common abbreviations used in health care and related fields, along with their meanings.*

Abbreviation	Meaning	Abbreviation	Meaning
A		AM, a.m.	in the morning or before noon
A, B, AB, O	blood types in ABO blood group	AML	acute myelogenic leukemia
		ANA	antinuclear antibody
A&P	auscultation and percussion	ANS	autonomic nervous system
AA	Alcoholics Anonymous	AOM	acute otitis media
AAA	abdominal aortic aneurysm	AP	anteroposterior
AB	abortion	APC	antigen-presenting cell
AB, Ab, ab	antibody; abortion	APTT	activated partial thromboplastin time
ABC	aspiration biopsy cytology	ARDS	acute respiratory distress syndrome
ABG	arterial blood gas(es)	ARF	acute renal failure
AC	air conduction	ARFID	avoidant/restrictive food intake disorder
Acc	accommodation	ARMD, AMD	age-related macular degeneration
ACch	acetylcholine	AS	aortic stenosis
ACE	angiotensin-converting enzyme (inhibitor)	ASD	atrial septal defect; autism spectrum disorder
AChR	acetylcholine receptor	ASHD	arteriosclerotic heart disease
ACL	anterior cruciate ligament	AST	angiotensin sensitivity test; aspartate aminotransferase
ACS	acute coronary syndrome	Ast	astigmatism
ACT	acceptance and commitment therapy	ATN	acute tubular necrosis
ACTH	adrenocorticotropic hormone	AV	atrioventricular; arteriovenous
AD	Alzheimer disease	*B*	
ad lib.	as desired	Ba	barium
ADD	attention deficit disorder	BA	behavioral activation
ADH	antidiuretic hormone (vasopressin)	baso	basophil (type of white blood cell)
ADHD	attention deficit-hyperactivity disorder	BBB	bundle branch block
		BC	bone conduction
ADLs	activities of daily living	BCC	basal cell carcinoma
ADT	androgen deprivation therapy	BE	barium enema; below the elbow
AE	above the elbow	BEAM	brain electrical activity mapping
AED	automatic external defibrillator; automatic external device	BK	below the knee
		BKA	below-knee amputation
		BM	bowel movement
AFB	acid-fast bacillus (TB organism)	BMD	bone mineral density
		BMI	body mass index
AFib	atrial fibrillation	BMR	basal metabolic rate
AGN	acute glomerulonephritis	BMT	bone marrow transplant
AI	artificial insemination	BNO	bladder neck obstruction
AICD	automatic implantable cardioverter defibrillator	BP	blood pressure
		BPH	benign prostatic hyperplasia; benign prostatic hypertrophy
AIDS	acquired immunodeficiency syndrome, acquired immune deficiency syndrome	BPM, bpm	beats per minute
		BRCA	breast cancer
AK	above the knee	BS	blood sugar
ALL	acute lymphocytic leukemia	BSE	breast self-examination
ALS	amyotrophic lateral sclerosis	BUN	blood urea nitrogen
ALT	alanine aminotransferase	Bx, bx	biopsy

Abbreviation	Meaning	Abbreviation	Meaning
C		CPK	creatine phosphokinase (cardiac enzyme released into the bloodstream after a heart attack)
c/o	complains of, complaints		
C&S	culture and sensitivity	CPR	cardiopulmonary resuscitation
C1, C2, and so on	first cervical vertebra, second cervical vertebra, and so on	CRF	chronic renal failure
		CRRT	continuous renal replacement therapy
CA	cancer; chronological age; cardiac arrest	C-section, CS	cesarean section
		CSA	central sleep apnea
Ca	calcium; cancer	CSF	cerebrospinal fluid
CABG	coronary artery bypass graft	CT	computed tomography
CAD	coronary artery disease	CTA	computed tomography angiography
CAH	chronic active hepatitis; congenital adrenal hyperplasia	CTS	carpal tunnel syndrome
		CV	cardiovascular
CAT	computed axial tomography	CVA	cerebrovascular accident
Cath	catheterization	CVD	cardiovascular disease
CBC	complete blood count	CVS	chorionic villus sampling
CBT	cognitive behavioral therapy	CWP	childbirth without pain
CC	cardiac catheterization; chief complaint	CXR	chest x-ray, chest radiograph
		cysto	cystoscopy
CCU	coronary care unit	*D*	
CDC	Centers for Disease Control		
CDH	congenital dislocation of the hip	D	diopter (lens strength)
		DA	dopamine
CF	cystic fibrosis	D&C	dilation and curettage
CGM	continuous glucose monitor	DBT	digital breast tomosynthesis
CHB	complete heart block	DCS	decompression sickness
CHD	coronary heart disease	Decub.	decubitus (lying down)
chemo	chemotherapy	D.O.	doctor of osteopathy
CHF	congestive heart failure	D.P.M.	doctor of podiatric medicine
Chol	cholesterol	Derm	dermatology
CIS	carcinoma in situ	DES	diffuse esophageal spasm; drug-eluting stent
CK	creatine kinase (cardiac enzyme); conductive keratoplasty	DEXA, DXA	dual energy x-ray absorptiometry
		DI	diabetes insipidus; diagnostic imaging
CK-MB	creatine kinase MB	DIC	disseminated intravascular coagulation
CLL	chronic lymphocytic leukemia	diff	differential count (white blood cells)
cm	centimeter (1/100 of a meter)	DJD	degenerative joint disease
CML	chronic myelogenous leukemia	DKA	diabetic ketoacidosis
		DM	diabetes mellitus
CNB	core needle biopsy	DMARDs	disease-modifying antirheumatic drugs
CNS	central nervous system	DNA	deoxyribonucleic acid
CO	coccygeal nerves	DOE	dyspnea on exertion
CO_2	carbon dioxide	DPI	dry powder inhaler
COLD	chronic obstructive lung disease	DPT	diphtheria, pertussis, tetanus
		DRE	digital rectal examination
COPD	chronic obstructive pulmonary disease	DSA	digital subtraction angiography
		DSM-5	Diagnostic and Statistical Manual of Mental Disorders, Fifth Edition
COVID-19	coronavirus disease 2019		
CP	cerebral palsy	DTR	deep tendon reflex
CPAP	continuous positive airway pressure	DUB	dysfunctional uterine bleeding
		DVT	deep vein thrombosis; deep venous thrombosis
CPD	cephalopelvic disproportion	Dx	diagnosis

Continued

Abbreviation	Meaning	Abbreviation	Meaning
E		**FTD**	frontotemporal dementia
EBR	external beam radiation	**FTND**	full-term normal delivery
EBRT	external beam radiotherapy	**FVC**	forced vital capacity
EBT	external beam therapy	**Fx**	fracture
EBV	Epstein-Barr virus	**G**	
ECCE	extracapsular cataract extraction	**G**	gravida (pregnant)
ECG	electrocardiogram; electrocardiography	**GABA**	gamma-aminobutyric acid
ECHO	echocardiogram; echocardiography; echoencephalogram; echoencephalography	**GB**	gallbladder
		GBP	gastric bypass
		GBS	gallbladder series (x-ray studies); Guillain-Barré syndrome
ECRB	extensor carpi radialis brevis (muscle or tendon)	**GC**	gonococcus (*Neisseria gonorrhoeae*)
ECT	electroconvulsive therapy	**GER**	gastroesophageal reflux
ED	erectile dysfunction; emergency department	**GERD**	gastroesophageal reflux disease
		GH	growth hormone
EEG	electroencephalography	**GI**	gastrointestinal
EF	ejection fraction	**GISTs**	gastrointestinal stromal tumors
EGD	esophagogastroduodenoscopy	**GTT**	glucose tolerance test
EKG	electrocardiogram; electrocardiography	**GU**	genitourinary
		GVHD	graft-versus-host disease
ELT	endovenous laser ablation; endoluminal laser ablation	**GVHR**	graft-versus-host reaction
		GYN	gynecology
Em	emmetropia	**H**	
EMG	electromyography	**H₂O**	water
ENG	electronystagmography	**HA**	headache
ENT	ears, nose, and throat	**HAV**	hepatitis A virus
EOM	extraocular movement	**Hb, Hgb**	hemoglobin
eos	eosinophil (type of white blood cell)	**HBOT**	hyperbaric oxygen therapy
		HBV	hepatitis B virus
EPS	electrophysiology studies	**HCG**	human chorionic gonadotropin
ESR	erythrocyte sedimentation rate	**HCl**	hydrochloric acid
		HCT	helical computed tomography; hematocrit
ESRD	end-stage renal disease	**Hct**	hematocrit
ESWL	extracorporeal shock-wave lithotripsy	**HCV**	hepatitis C virus
		HD	hemodialysis; hip disarticulation; hearing distance
ETT	exercise tolerance test	**HDL**	high-density lipoprotein
EUS	endoscopic ultrasonography	**HDN**	hemolytic disease of the newborn
F		**HDV**	hepatitis D virus
		HEV	hepatitis E virus
5-HT	5-hydroxytryptamine (serotonin)	**HF**	heart failure
		Hg	mercury
FBS	fasting blood sugar	**HHV-8**	human herpes virus 8
FECG, FEKG	fetal electrocardiogram	**HIV**	human immunodeficiency virus
FH	family history	**HMD**	hyaline membrane disease
FHR	fetal heart rate	**HNP**	herniated nucleus pulposus (herniated disk)
FHT	fetal heart tone		
FNA	fine needle aspiration	**HoLEP**	holmium laser enucleation of the prostate
FS	frozen section	**HP**	hemipelvectomy
FSH	follicle-stimulating hormone	**HPV**	human papillomavirus

Abbreviation	Meaning	Abbreviation	Meaning
HRT	hormone replacement therapy	**L**	
HSG	hysterosalpingography	L1, L2, and so on	first lumbar vertebra, second lumbar vertebra, and so on
HSV	herpes simplex virus	LA	left atrium
HSV-2	herpes simplex virus type 2	LASIK	laser-assisted in situ keratomileusis
HTN	hypertension	LAT, lat	lateral
Hx	history	LBBB	left bundle branch block
I, J		LBD	Lewy body dementia
I&D	incision and drainage	LBW	low birth weight
IBD	irritable bowel disease	LD	lactate dehydrogenase; lactic acid dehydrogenase (cardiac enzyme)
IBS	irritable bowel syndrome	LDH	lactate dehydrogenase
IC	interstitial cystitis	LDL	low-density lipoprotein
ICD	implantable cardioverter-defibrillator	LES	lower esophageal sphincter
ICP	intracranial pressure	LFT	liver function test
ICU	intensive care unit	LH	luteinizing hormone
ID	intradermal	LLLT	low-level laser therapy
IDDM	insulin-dependent diabetes mellitus	LLQ	left lower quadrant
Igs	immunoglobulins	LMP	last menstrual period
IM	intramuscular; infectious mononucleosis	LOC	loss of consciousness
		LP	lumbar puncture
IMP	impression (synonymous with *diagnosis*)	LPI	laser peripheral iridotomy
		LPR	laryngopharyngeal reflux
INR	international normalized ratio	LS	lumbosacral spine
IOL	intraocular lens	LSO	left salpingo-oophorectomy
IOP	intraocular pressure	lt	left
IPPB	intermittent positive-pressure breathing	LUQ	left upper quadrant
		LV	left ventricle
IPT	interpersonal therapy	lymphos	lymphocytes
IRDS	infant respiratory distress syndrome	**M**	
IS	intracostal space	MD	major depression, doctor of medicine
IUD	intrauterine device	M.D.	doctor of medicine
IUGR	intrauterine growth rate; intrauterine growth retardation	MDD	major depressive disorder
		MDI	metered-dose inhaler
IV	intravenous	MEG	magnetoencephalography
IVC	intravenous cholangiogram; intravenous cholangiography	MG	myasthenia gravis
		mg	milligram (1/1,000 of a gram)
IVF	in vitro fertilization	mg/dl, mg/dL	milligram per deciliter
IVF-ET	in vitro fertilization and embryo transfer	MI	myocardial infarction, motivational interviewing
IVP	intravenous pyelogram; intravenous pyelography	mix astig	mixed astigmatism
		mL	milliliter (1/1,000 of a liter)
K		mm	millimeter (1/1,000 of a meter)
K	potassium (an electrolyte)	MM	multiple myeloma
KD	knee disarticulation	mm Hg	millimeters of mercury
KS	Kaposi sarcoma	MNL	mononuclear leukocytes
KUB	kidney, ureter, bladder	MPI	myocardial perfusion imaging
		MR	mitral regurgitation
		MRA	magnetic resonance angiogram; magnetic resonance angiography

Continued

Abbreviation	Meaning	Abbreviation	Meaning
MRCP	magnetic resonance cholangiopancreatography	OREF	open reduction external fixation
MRI	magnetic resonance imaging	ORIF	open reduction internal fixation
MS	musculoskeletal; multiple sclerosis; mental status; mitral stenosis	ORTH, ortho	orthopedics
		OSA	obstructive sleep apnea
MSE	mental status examination	**P**	
MSH	melanocyte-stimulating hormone	P	phosphorus; pulse
MUGA	multiple-gated acquisition (scan)	p̄	after
MVP	mitral valve prolapse	PA	posteroanterior; pernicious anemia; pulmonary artery
myop	myopia (nearsightedness)	PAC	premature atrial contraction
N		PAD	peripheral artery disease
Na	sodium (an electrolyte)	Pap	Papanicolaou (test)
NA	Narcotics Anonymous	para 1, 2, 3, and so on	unipara, bipara, tripara, and so on (number of viable births)
NB	newborn	PAT	paroxysmal atrial tachycardia
NCLC	nonsmall cell lung cancer	PBI	protein-bound iodine
NCV	nerve conduction velocity	PCL	posterior cruciate ligament
NE	norepinephrine	PCNL	percutaneous nephrolithotomy
NES	nonepileptic seizures	PCO_2	partial pressure of carbon dioxide
NETs	neuroendocrine tumors	PCOS	polycystic ovarian syndrome
NF	neurofibromatosis	PCP	*Pneumocystis* pneumonia; primary care physician
NG	nasogastric	PCTA	percutaneous transluminal coronary angioplasty
NIDDM	non–insulin-dependent diabetes mellitus	PCV	packed cell volume
NIHL	noise-induced hearing loss	PDR	proliferative diabetic retinopathy
NK cell	natural killer cell	PDT	photodynamic therapy
NMT	nebulized mist treatment	PE	physical examination; pulmonary embolism; pressure-equalizing (tube)
NPDR	nonproliferative diabetic retinopathy	PERRLA	pupils equal, round, and reactive to light and accommodation
NPH	neutral protamine Hagedorn (insulin)	PET	positron emission tomography
NRDS	neonatal respiratory distress syndrome	PFT	pulmonary function tests
NSAIDs	nonsteroidal anti-inflammatory drugs	PGH	pituitary growth hormone
		pH	symbol for degree of acidity or alkalinity
NSCLC	nonsmall cell lung cancer	PID	pelvic inflammatory disease
NSR	normal sinus rhythm	PIH	pregnancy-induced hypertension
O		PKD	polycystic kidney disease
O_2	oxygen	PMH	past medical history
OB	obstetrics	PMI	point of maximum impulse
OCG	oral cholecystography	PMN	polymorphonuclear
OCPs	oral contraceptive pills	PMNL, poly	polymorphonuclear leukocyte
OD	overdose	PMP	previous menstrual period
O.D.	doctor of optometry	PMS	premenstrual syndrome
OM	otitis media	PND	paroxysmal nocturnal dyspnea
OP	outpatient; operative procedure	PNES	psychogenic nonepileptic seizures
		PNS	peripheral nervous system
		PO_2	partial pressure of oxygen
		post	posterior
		PPD	purified protein derivative

Abbreviation	Meaning	Abbreviation	Meaning
PPV	pars plana vitrectomy	**S**	
PRL	prolactin	S1, S2, and so on	first sacral vertebra, second sacral vertebra, and so on
PSA	prostate-specific antigen		
PSMA	prostate-specific membrane antigen (PET scan)	SA, S-A	sinoatrial
		SAB	spontaneous abortion
PT	prothrombin time, physical therapy	SAH	subarachnoid hemorrhage
		SaO$_2$	arterial oxygen saturation
pt	patient	SBO	small bowel obstruction
PTCA	percutaneous transluminal coronary angioplasty	SBRT	stereotactic body radiotherapy
		SCLC	small cell lung cancer
PTH	parathyroid hormone (also called parathormone)	SD	shoulder disarticulation
		segs	segmented neutrophils
PTSD	post-traumatic stress disorder	SERMs	selective estrogen receptor modulators
PTT	partial thromboplastin time	SICS	small incision cataract surgery
PUBS	percutaneous umbilical blood sampling	SIDS	sudden infant death syndrome
		SLE	systemic lupus erythematosus; slit-lamp examination
PUD	peptic ulcer disease		
PVC	premature ventricular contraction	SLNB	sentinel lymph node biopsy
		SLT	selective laser trabeculoplasty
PVD	peripheral vascular disease	SNS	sympathetic nervous system
PVP	photoselective vaporization of the prostate	SOB	shortness of breath
		sono	sonogram
Q		sp. gr.	specific gravity
qEEG	quantitative electroencephalography	SPECT	single-photon emission computed tomography
		ST	esotropia
R		stat., STAT	immediately
R/O	rule out	STD	sexually transmitted disease
RA	right atrium; rheumatoid arthritis	STI	sexually transmitted infection
		SUD	substance use disorder
RAI	radioactive iodine	Sx	symptom
RAIU	radioactive iodine uptake	**T**	
RALP	robotic-assisted laparoscopic prostatectomy	T&A	tonsillectomy and adenoidectomy
		T1, T2, and so on	first thoracic vertebra, second thoracic vertebra, and so on
RBC, rbc	red blood cell		
RCC	renal cell carcinoma	T$_3$	triiodothyronine (thyroid hormone)
RD	respiratory distress	T$_4$	thyroxine (thyroid hormone)
RDS	respiratory distress syndrome	TAH	total abdominal hysterectomy
RF	rheumatoid factor; radio frequency	TB	tuberculosis
		TBI	traumatic brain injury
RGB	Roux-en-Y gastric bypass	TED	thyroid eye disease
RHD	rheumatic heart disease	TFT	thyroid function test
RIRS	retrograde intrarenal surgery	TG	triglycerides
RK	radial keratotomy	THA	total hip arthroplasty
RLQ	right lower quadrant	ther	therapy
ROM	range of motion	THR	total hip replacement
RP	retrograde pyelogram; retrograde pyelography	ThuLEP	thulium fiber laser enucleation of the prostate
RSO	right salpingo-oophorectomy	TIA	transient ischemic attack
rt	right	TKA	total knee arthroplasty
RUQ	right upper quadrant	TKR	total knee replacement
RV	residual volume; right ventricle		

Continued

Abbreviation	Meaning	Abbreviation	Meaning
TMS	transcranial magnetic stimulation	UP	ureteropelvic
tPA	tissue plasminogen activator	UPP	uvulopalatopharyngoplasty
TPR	temperature, pulse, and respiration	URI	upper respiratory infection
		URS	ureteroscopy
TRAM	transverse rectus abdominis muscle (flap)	US	ultrasound; ultrasonography
		UTI	urinary tract infection
TRUS	transrectal ultrasound	**V**	
TSE	testicular self-examination	VA	visual acuity
TSH	thyroid-stimulating hormone	VaD	vascular dementia
		VC	vital capacity
TUMT	transurethral microwave thermotherapy	VCUG	voiding cystourethrography
		VD	venereal disease
TURBT	transurethral resection of bladder tumor	VF	visual field
		VSD	ventricular septal defect
TURP	transurethral resection of the prostate	VSG	vertical sleeve gastrectomy
		VT	ventricular tachycardia
TVH	total vaginal hysterectomy	VUR	vesicoureteral reflux
Tx	treatment	**W**	
U		WBC, wbc	white blood cell
		WD	well developed
U&L, U/L	upper and lower	WN	well nourished
UA	urinalysis	WNL	within normal limits
UC	ulcerative colitis; uterine contractions	**X, Y, Z**	
UGI	upper gastrointestinal	XP, XDP	xeroderma pigmentosum
UGIS	upper gastrointestinal series	XT	exotropia
ung	ointment		

*For a listing of discontinued, or "do not use," abbreviations, see Appendix H.

Symbols

This table lists common symbols used in health care and related fields, along with their meanings.

Abbreviation	Meaning	Abbreviation	Meaning
@	at	Ø	no
aa	of each	#	number; following a number, pounds
'	foot	÷	divided by
"	inch	/	divided by
Δ	change; heat	×	multiplied by; magnification
	prescription, treatment, therapy	=	equals
		≈	approximately equal
→	to, in the direction of	°	degree
↑	increase(d), up	%	percent
↓	decrease(d), down	♀	female
+	plus, positive	♂	male
−	minus, negative		
±	plus or minus; either positive or negative; indefinite		

Glossary of Medical Word Elements

Medical Word Elements

Element	Meaning
A	
a-	without, not
-a	noun ending
ab-	from, away from
abdomin/o	abdomen
abort/o	to miscarry
-ac	pertaining to
acid/o	acid
acous/o	hearing
acr/o	extremity
acromi/o	acromion (projection of the scapula)
-acusia	hearing
-acusis	hearing
-ad	toward
ad-	toward
aden/o	gland
adenoid/o	adenoids
adip/o	fat
adren/o	adrenal glands
adrenal/o	adrenal glands
aer/o	air
af-	toward
agglutin/o	clumping, gluing
agora-	marketplace
-al	pertaining to
albin/o	white
albumin/o	albumin (protein)
-algesia	pain
-algia	pain
allo-	other, differing from the normal
alveol/o	alveolus; air sac
ambly/o	dull, dim
amni/o	amnion (amniotic sac)
an-	without, not
an/o	anus
ana-	against; up; back
andr/o	male
aneurysm/o	aneurysm (widened blood vessel)
angi/o	vessel (usually blood or lymph)
angin/o	choking pain
aniso-	unequal, dissimilar
ankyl/o	stiffness; bent, crooked
ante-	before, in front of
anter/o	anterior, front
anthrac/o	coal, coal dust
anti-	against
aort/o	aorta
append/o	appendix
appendic/o	appendix

Element	Meaning
aque/o	water
-ar	pertaining to
-arche	beginning
arteri/o	artery
arteriol/o	arteriole
arthr/o	joint
-ary	pertaining to
asbest/o	asbestos
-asthenia	weakness, debility
astr/o	star
-ate	having the form of, possessing
atel/o	incomplete; imperfect
ather/o	fatty plaque
-ation	process (of)
atri/o	atrium
audi/o	hearing
audit/o	hearing
aur/o	ear
auricul/o	ear
auto-	self, own
ax/o	axis, axon
azot/o	nitrogenous compounds
B	
bacteri/o	bacteria (singular, bacterium)
balan/o	glans penis
bas/o	base (alkaline, opposite of acid)
bi-	two
bi/o	life
bil/i	bile, gall
-blast	embryonic cell
blast/o	embryonic cell
blephar/o	eyelid
brachi/o	arm
brachy-	short
brady-	slow
bronch/o	bronchus (plural, bronchi)
bronchi/o	bronchus (plural, bronchi)
bronchiol/o	bronchiole
bucc/o	cheek
C	
calc/o	calcium
calcane/o	calcaneum (heel bone)
-capnia	carbon dioxide (CO_2)
carcin/o	cancer
cardi/o	heart
-cardia	heart condition
carp/o	carpus (wrist bones)
cata-	down

Medical Word Elements—cont'd

Element	Meaning	Element	Meaning
caud/o	tail	corp/o	body
		corpor/o	body
cauter/o	heat, burn	cortic/o	cortex
cec/o	cecum	cost/o	ribs
-cele	hernia, swelling	crani/o	cranium (skull)
-centesis	surgical puncture	crin/o	secrete
cephal/o	head	-crine	secrete
-ceps	head	cruci/o	cross
-ception	conceiving	cry/o	cold
cerebell/o	cerebellum	crypt/o	hidden
cerebr/o	cerebrum	culd/o	cul-de-sac
cervic/o	neck; cervix uteri (neck of uterus)	-cusia	hearing
chalic/o	limestone	-cusis	hearing
cheil/o	lip	cutane/o	skin
chem/o	chemical; drug	cyan/o	blue
chlor/o	green	cycl/o	ciliary body of the eye; circular; cycle
chol/e	bile, gall	-cyesis	pregnancy
cholangi/o	bile vessel	cyst/o	bladder
cholecyst/o	gallbladder	cyt/o	cell
choledoch/o	bile duct	-cyte	cell
chondr/o	cartilage		
chori/o	chorion	**D**	
choroid/o	choroid		
chrom/o	color	dacry/o	tear; lacrimal apparatus (duct, sac, or gland)
chromat/o	color	dacryocyst/o	lacrimal sac
-cide	killing	dactyl/o	fingers; toes
circum-	around	de-	cessation
cirrh/o	yellow	dendr/o	tree
-cision	a cutting	dent/o	teeth
-clasia	to break; surgical fracture	derm/o	skin
-clasis	to break; surgical fracture	-derma	skin
-clast	to break; surgical fracture	dermat/o	skin
clavicul/o	clavicle (collar bone)	-desis	binding, fixation (of a bone or joint)
-clysis	irrigation, washing	di-	double
coccyg/o	coccyx (tailbone)	dia-	through, across
cochle/o	cochlea	dipl-	double
col/o	colon	dipl/o	double
colon/o	colon	dips/o	thirst
colp/o	vagina	-dipsia	thirst
condyl/o	condyle	dist/o	far, farthest
coni/o	dust	dors/o	back (of the body)
conjunctiv/o	conjunctiva	duct/o	to lead; carry
-continence	to hold back	-duction	act of leading, bringing, conducting
contra-	against, opposite	duoden/o	duodenum (first part of the small intestine)
cor/o	pupil		
core/o	pupil	dur/o	dura mater; hard
corne/o	cornea	-dynia	pain
coron/o	heart	dys-	bad; painful; difficult

Continued

Medical Word Elements—cont'd

Element	Meaning	Element	Meaning
E		**G**	
-eal	pertaining to	galact/o	milk
ec-	out, out from	gangli/o	ganglion (knot or knotlike mass)
echo-	repeated sound	gastr/o	stomach
-ectasis	dilation, expansion	-gen	forming, producing, origin
ecto-	outside, outward	gen/o	forming, producing, origin
-ectomy	excision, removal	-genesis	forming, producing, origin
-edema	swelling	genit/o	genitalia
ef-	away from	gest/o	pregnancy
electr/o	electricity	gingiv/o	gum(s)
-ema	state of; condition	glauc/o	gray
embol/o	embolus (plug)	gli/o	glue; neuroglial tissue
-emesis	vomiting	-glia	glue; neuroglial tissue
-emia	blood condition	-globin	protein
emphys/o	to inflate	glomerul/o	glomerulus
en-	in, within	gloss/o	tongue
encephal/o	brain	glott/o	glottis
end-	in, within	gluc/o	sugar, sweetness
endo-	in, within	glucos/o	sugar, sweetness
enter/o	intestine (usually small intestine)	glyc/o	sugar, sweetness
eosin/o	dawn (rose colored)	glycos/o	sugar, sweetness
epi-	above, upon	gnos/o	knowing
epididym/o	epididymis	-gnosis	knowing
epiglott/o	epiglottis	gon/o	seed (ovum or spermatozoon)
episi/o	vulva	gonad/o	gonads, sex glands
erythem/o	red	goni/o	angle
erythemat/o	red	-grade	to go
erythr/o	red	-graft	transplantation
eschar/o	scab	-gram	record, writing
-esis	condition	granul/o	granule
eso-	inward	-graph	instrument for recording
esophag/o	esophagus	-graphy	process of recording
esthes/o	feeling	-gravida	pregnant woman
-esthesia	feeling	gyn/o	woman, female
eti/o	cause	gynec/o	woman, female
eu-	good; normal	**H**	
ex-	out, out from		
exo-	outside, outward	hallucin/o	hallucination
extra-	outside	hedon/o	pleasure
F		hem/o	blood
		hemangi/o	blood vessel
faci/o	face	hemat/o	blood
fasci/o	band, fascia (fibrous membrane supporting and separating muscles)	hemi-	one half
		hepat/o	liver
femor/o	femur (thigh bone)	hetero-	different
-ferent	to carry	hidr/o	sweat
fibr/o	fiber, fibrous tissue	hist/o	tissue
fibul/o	fibula (smaller bone of the lower leg)	histi/o	tissue
fluor/o	luminous, fluorescence	home/o	same, alike

Medical Word Elements—cont'd

Element	Meaning	Element	Meaning
homeo-	same, alike	-ist	specialist
homo-	same	-isy	state of; condition
humer/o	humerus (upper arm bone)	-itic	pertaining to
hydr/o	water	-itis	inflammation
hyp-	under, below, deficient	-ive	pertaining to
hyper-	excessive, above normal	-ization	process (of)
hypn/o	sleep	**J, K**	
hypo-	under, below, deficient	jaund/o	yellow
hyster/o	uterus (womb)	jejun/o	jejunum (second part of the small intestine)
I		kal/i	potassium (an electrolyte)
-ia	condition	kary/o	nucleus
-iac	pertaining to	kerat/o	horny tissue; hard; cornea
-iasis	abnormal condition (produced by something specified)	kern/o	kernel (nucleus)
iatr/o	medicine; treatment	ket/o	ketone bodies (acids and acetones)
-iatry	physician; treatment	keton/o	ketone bodies (acids and acetones)
-ic	pertaining to	kinesi/o	movement
-ical	pertaining to	-kinesia	movement
-ice	noun ending	kinet/o	movement
ichthy/o	dry, scaly	klept/o	to steal
-ician	specialist	kyph/o	humpback
-icle	small, minute	**L**	
-icterus	jaundice	labi/o	lip
idi/o	unknown, peculiar	labyrinth/o	labyrinth (inner ear)
-ile	pertaining to	lacrim/o	tear; lacrimal apparatus (duct, sac, or gland)
ile/o	ileum (third part of the small intestine)	lact/o	milk
ili/o	ilium (lateral, flaring portion of the hip bone)	-lalia	speech, babble
im-	not	lamin/o	lamina (part of the vertebral arch)
immun/o	immune, immunity, safe	lapar/o	abdomen
in-	in, not	laryng/o	larynx (voice box)
-ine	pertaining to	later/o	side, to one side
infer/o	lower, below	lei/o	smooth
infra-	below, under	leiomy/o	smooth (visceral) muscle
inguin/o	groin	-lepsy	seizure
insulin/o	insulin	lept/o	thin, slender
inter-	between	leuk/o	white
intra-	in, within	lex/o	word, phrase
-ion	the act of	lingu/o	tongue
-ior	pertaining to	lip/o	fat
irid/o	iris	lipid/o	fat
-is	noun ending	-listhesis	slipping
isch/o	to hold back; block	-lith	stone, calculus
ischi/o	ischium (lower portion of the hip bone)	lith/o	stone, calculus
-ism	condition	lob/o	lobe
iso-	same, equal	log/o	study of
		-logist	specialist in the study of

Continued

Medical Word Elements—cont'd

Element	Meaning	Element	Meaning
-logy	study of	my/o	muscle
lord/o	curve, swayback	myc/o	fungus (plural, fungi)
-lucent	to shine; clear	mydr/o	widen, enlarge
lumb/o	loins (lower back)	myel/o	bone marrow; spinal cord
lymph/o	lymph	myos/o	muscle
lymphaden/o	lymph gland (node)	myring/o	tympanic membrane (eardrum)
lymphangi/o	lymph vessel	myx/o	mucus
-lysis	separation; destruction; loosening	**N**	
M		narc/o	stupor; numbness; sleep
macro-	large	nas/o	nose
mal-	bad	nat/o	birth
-malacia	softening	natr/o	sodium (an electrolyte)
mamm/o	breast	necr/o	death, necrosis
-mania	state of mental disorder, frenzy	neo-	new
mast/o	breast	nephr/o	kidney
mastoid/o	mastoid process	neur/o	nerve
maxill/o	maxilla (upper jaw bone)	neutr/o	neutral; neither
meat/o	opening, meatus	nid/o	nest
medi-	middle	noct/o	night
medi/o	middle	nucle/o	nucleus
mediastin/o	mediastinum	nulli-	none
medull/o	medulla	nyctal/o	night
mega-	enlargement	**O**	
megal/o	enlargement	obstetr/o	pregnancy; childbirth
-megaly	enlargement	ocul/o	eye
melan/o	black	odont/o	teeth
men/o	menses, menstruation	-oid	resembling
mening/o	meninges (membranes covering the brain and spinal cord)	-ole	small, minute
		olig/o	scanty
meningi/o	meninges (membranes covering the brain and spinal cord)	-oma	tumor
		omphal/o	navel (umbilicus)
menstr/o	monthly discharge of blood	onc/o	tumor
ment/o	mind	onych/o	nail
meso-	middle	oophor/o	ovary
meta-	change, beyond	-opaque	obscure
metacarp/o	metacarpus (hand bones)	ophthalm/o	eye
metatars/o	metatarsus (foot bones)	-opia	vision
-meter	instrument for measuring	-opsia	vision
metr/o	uterus (womb); measure	-opsy	view of
metri/o	uterus (womb)	opt/o	eye, vision
-metry	act of measuring	optic/o	eye, vision
micr/o	small	or/o	mouth
micro-	small	orch/o	testis (plural, testes)
mono-	one	orchi/o	testis (plural, testes)
morph/o	form, shape, structure	orchid/o	testis (plural, testes)
muc/o	mucus	-orexia	appetite
multi-	many, much	orth/o	straight
muscul/o	muscle	-ory	pertaining to
mut/a	genetic change		

Medical Word Elements—cont'd

Element	Meaning	Element	Meaning
-ose	pertaining to; sugar	-phil	attraction for
-osis	abnormal condition; increase (used primarily with blood cells)	phil/o	attraction for
		-philia	attraction for
-osmia	smell	phim/o	muzzle
oste/o	bone	phleb/o	vein
ot/o	ear	-phobia	fear
-ous	pertaining to	-phonia	voice
ovari/o	ovary	-phoresis	carrying, transmission
ox/i	oxygen	-phoria	feeling (mental state)
ox/o	oxygen	phot/o	light
-oxia	oxygen	phren/o	diaphragm; mind
P		-phylaxis	protection
		physi/o	physical function
pachy-	thick	-physis	growth
palat/o	palate (roof of the mouth)	pil/o	hair
pan-	all	pituitar/o	pituitary gland
pancreat/o	pancreas	-plakia	plaque
-para	to bear (offspring)	plas/o	formation, growth
para-	near, beside; beyond	-plasia	formation, growth
parathyroid/o	parathyroid glands	-plasm	formation, growth
-paresis	partial paralysis	-plasty	surgical repair
patell/o	patella (kneecap)	-plegia	paralysis
path/o	disease	pleur/o	pleura
-pathy	disease	-plexy	stroke
pector/o	chest	-pnea	breathing
ped/i	foot; child	pneum/o	air; lung
ped/o	foot; child	pneumon/o	air; lung
pedicul/o	lice	pod/o	foot
pelv/i	pelvis	-poiesis	formation, production
pelv/o	pelvis	poikil/o	varied, irregular
pen/o	penis	poli/o	gray; gray matter (of the brain or spinal cord)
-penia	decrease, deficiency		
-pepsia	digestion	poly	many, much
per-	through	polyp/o	small growth
peri-	around	-porosis	porous
perine/o	perineum (area between the scrotum [or vulva in the female] and anus)	post-	after, behind
		poster/o	back (of the body), behind, posterior
		-potence	power
peritone/o	peritoneum	-prandial	meal
-pexy	fixation (of an organ)	pre-	before, in front of
phac/o	lens	presby/o	old age
phag/o	swallowing, eating	primi-	first
-phage	swallowing, eating	pro-	before, in front of
-phagia	swallowing, eating	proct/o	anus, rectum
phalang/o	phalanges (bones of the fingers and toes)	prostat/o	prostate gland
		proxim/o	near, nearest
pharmaceutic/o	drug, medicine	pseudo-	false
pharyng/o	pharynx (throat)	psych/o	mind
-phasia	speech	-ptosis	prolapse, downward displacement
phe/o	dusky, dark		

Continued

Medical Word Elements—cont'd

Element	Meaning	Element	Meaning
ptyal/o	saliva	-scopy	visual examination
-ptysis	spitting	scot/o	darkness
pub/o	pubis (anterior part of the pelvic bone)	seb/o	sebum, sebaceous
		semi-	one-half
pulmon/o	lung	semin/i	semen; seed
pupill/o	pupil	semin/o	semen; seed
py/o	pus	sept/o	septum
pyel/o	renal pelvis	sequestr/o	separation
pylor/o	pylorus	ser/o	serum
pyr/o	fire	sial/o	saliva, salivary gland
Q, R		sider/o	iron
		sigmoid/o	sigmoid colon
quadri-	four	silic/o	flint
rachi/o	spine	sin/o	sinus, cavity
radi/o	radiation, x-ray; radius (lower arm bone on the thumb side)	sinus/o	sinus, cavity
		-sis	state of; condition
radicul/o	nerve root	-social	society
rect/o	rectum	somat/o	body
ren/o	kidney	somn/o	sleep
reticul/o	net, mesh	son/o	sound
retin/o	retina	-spadias	slit, fissure
retro-	backward, behind	-spasm	involuntary contraction, twitching
rhabd/o	rod shaped (striated)	sperm/i	spermatozoa, sperm cells
rhabdomy/o	rod-shaped (striated) muscle	sperm/o	spermatozoa, sperm cells
rhin/o	nose	spermat/o	spermatozoa, sperm cells
rhytid/o	wrinkle	sphygm/o	pulse
roentgen/o	x-rays	-sphyxia	pulse
-rrhage	bursting forth (of)	spin/o	spine
-rrhagia	bursting forth (of)	spir/o	breathe
rrhaphy	suture	splen/o	spleen
-rrhea	discharge, flow	spondyl/o	vertebrae (backbone)
-rrhexis	rupture	squam/o	scale
-rrhythm/o	rhythm	staped/o	stapes
rube/o	red	-stasis	standing still
S		steat/o	fat
		sten/o	narrowing, stricture
sacr/o	sacrum	-stenosis	narrowing, stricture
salping/o	tube (usually the fallopian or eustachian [auditory] tube)	stern/o	sternum (breastbone)
		steth/o	chest
-salpinx	tube (usually the fallopian or eustachian [auditory] tube)	sthen/o	strength
		stigmat/o	point, mark
sarc/o	flesh (connective tissue)	stomat/o	mouth
-sarcoma	malignant tumor of connective tissue	-stomy	forming an opening (mouth)
scapul/o	scapula (shoulder blade)	sub-	under, below
-schisis	a splitting	sudor/o	sweat
schiz/o	split	super-	upper, above
scler/o	hardening; sclera (white of the eye)	super/o	upper, above
scoli/o	crooked, bent	supra-	above; excessive; superior
scop/o	to view	sym-	union, together, joined
-scope	instrument for examining		

Medical Word Elements—cont'd

Element	Meaning	Element	Meaning
syn-	union, together, joined	tubercul/o	a little swelling
synapt/o	synapsis, point of contact	tympan/o	tympanic membrane (eardrum)
synov/o	synovial membrane, synovial fluid	**U**	
T		-ula	small, minute
tachy-	rapid	-ule	small, minute
tax/o	order, coordination	uln/o	ulna (lower arm bone on the opposite side of the thumb)
-taxia	order, coordination	ultra-	excess, beyond
tele/o	distant	-um	structure, thing
ten/o	tendon	umbilic/o	umbilicus, navel
tend/o	tendon	ungu/o	nail
tendin/o	tendon	uni-	one
-tension	to stretch	ur/o	urine, urinary tract
test/o	testis (plural, testes)	ureter/o	ureter
thalam/o	thalamus	urethr/o	urethra
thalass/o	sea	-uria	urine
thec/o	sheath (usually referring to the meninges)	urin/o	urine, urinary tract
thel/o	nipple	-us	condition; structure
therapeut/o	treatment	uter/o	uterus (womb)
-therapy	treatment	uvul/o	uvula
therm/o	heat	**V, W**	
thorac/o	chest	vagin/o	vagina
-thorax	chest	valv/o	valve
thromb/o	blood clot	valvul/o	valve
thym/o	thymus gland	varic/o	dilated vein
-thymia	mind; emotion	vas/o	vessel; vas deferens; duct
thyr/o	thyroid gland	vascul/o	vessel (usually blood or lymph)
thyroid/o	thyroid gland	ven/o	vein
tibi/o	tibia (larger bone of the lower leg)	ventr/o	belly, belly side
-tic	pertaining to	ventricul/o	ventricle (of the heart or brain)
-tocia	childbirth, labor	-verse	to turn
tom/o	to cut	-version	turning
-tome	instrument to cut	vertebr/o	vertebrae (backbone)
-tomy	incision	vesic/o	bladder
ton/o	tension	vesicul/o	seminal vesicle
tonsill/o	tonsils	vest/o	clothes
tox/o	poison	viscer/o	internal organs
-toxic	pertaining to poison	vitr/o	vitreous body (of the eye)
toxic/o	poison	vitre/o	glassy
trabecul/o	trabecula (supporting bundles of fibers)	vol/o	volume
trache/o	trachea (windpipe)	voyeur/o	to see
trans-	across, through	vulv/o	vulva
tri-	three	**X, Y, Z**	
trich/o	hair	xanth/o	yellow
trigon/o	trigone (triangular region at the base of the bladder)	xen/o	foreign, strange
		xer/o	dry
-tripsy	crushing	xiph/o	sword
-trophy	development, nourishment	-y	condition; process
-tropia	turning		
-tropin	stimulate		

English Terms

Meaning	Element	Meaning	Element
A		**B**	
abdomen	abdomin/o, lapar/o	back (of the body)	dors/o
abnormal condition (produced by something specified)	-iasis	back (of the body), behind, posterior	poster/o
		backward, behind	retro-
abnormal condition; increase (used primarily with blood cells)	-osis	bacteria (singular, bacterium)	bacteri/o
		bad	mal-
above, upon	epi-	bad; painful; difficult	dys-
above; excessive; superior	supra-	band, fascia (fibrous membrane supporting and separating muscles)	fasci/o
acid	acid/o		
acromion (projection of the scapula)	acromi/o		
		base (alkaline, opposite of acid)	bas/o
across, through	trans-	before, in front of	ante-, pre-, pro-
act of leading, bringing, conducting	-duction	beginning	-arche
		belly, belly side	ventr/o
act of measuring	-metry	below, under	infra-
adenoids	adenoid/o	between	inter-
adrenal glands	adren/o, adrenal/o	bile duct	choledoch/o
after, behind	post-	bile vessel	cholangi/o
against	anti-	bile, gall	bil/i, chol/e
against, opposite	contra-	binding, fixation (of a bone or joint)	-desis
against; up; back	ana-		
air	aer/o	birth	nat/o
air; lung	pneum/o, pneumon/o	black	melan/o
albumin (protein)	albumin/o	bladder	cyst/o, vesic/o
all	pan-	blood	hem/o, hemat/o
alveolus; air sac	alveol/o	blood clot	thromb/o
amnion (amniotic sac)	amni/o	blood condition	-emia
aneurysm (widened blood vessel)	aneurysm/o	blood vessel	hemangi/o
		blue	cyan/o
angle	goni/o	body	corp/o, corpor/o, somat/o
anterior, front	anter/o		
anus	an/o	bone	oste/o
anus, rectum	proct/o	bone marrow; spinal cord	myel/o
aorta	aort/o	brain	encephal/o
appendix	append/o, appendic/o	breast	mamm/o, mast/o
appetite	-orexia	breathe	spir/o
arm	brachi/o	breathing	-pnea
around	circum-, peri-	bronchiole	bronchiol/o
arteriole	arteriol/o	bronchus (plural, bronchi)	bronch/o, bronchi/o
artery	arteri/o	bursting forth (of)	-rrhage, -rrhagia
asbestos	asbest/o		
atrium	atri/o	**C**	
attraction for	-phil, phil/o, -philia	calcaneum (heel bone)	calcane/o
away from	ef-	calcium	calc/o
axis, axon	ax/o		

English Terms—cont'd

Meaning	Element	Meaning	Element
cancer	carcin/o	death, necrosis	necr/o
carbon dioxide (CO_2)	-capnia	decrease, deficiency	-penia
carpus (wrist bones)	carp/o	deficiency, under, below	hyp-, hyp/o
carrying, transmission	-phoresis	development, nourishment	-trophy
cartilage	chondr/o	diaphragm; mind	phren/o
cause	eti/o	different	hetero-
cecum	cec/o	digestion	-pepsia
cell	cyt/o, -cyte	dilated vein	varic/o
cerebellum	cerebell/o	dilation, expansion	-ectasis
cerebrum	cerebr/o	discharge, flow	-rrhea
cessation	de-	disease	path/o, -pathy
change, beyond	meta-	distant	tele/o
cheek	bucc/o	double	di-, dipl-, dipl/o
chemical; drug	chem/o	down	cata-
chest	pector/o, steth/o, thorac/o, -thorax	drug, medicine	pharmaceutic/o
		dry	xer/o
childbirth, labor	-tocia	dry, scaly	ichthy/o
choking pain	angin/o	dull, dim	ambly/o
chorion	chori/o	duodenum (first part of the small intestine)	duoden/o
choroid	choroid/o		
ciliary body of the eye; circular; cycle	cycl/o	dura mater; hard	dur/o
		dusky, dark	phe/o
clavicle (collar bone)	clavicul/o	dust	coni/o
clothes	vest/o	**E**	
clumping, gluing	agglutin/o		
coal, coal dust	anthrac/o	ear	aur/o, auricul/o, ot/o
coccyx (tailbone)	coccyg/o	electricity	electr/o
cochlea	cochle/o	embolus (plug)	embol/o
cold	cry/o	embryonic cell	-blast, blast/o
colon	col/o, colon/o	enlargement	mega-, megal/o, -megaly
color	chrom/o, chromat/o		
conceiving	-ception	epididymis	epididym/o
condition	-esis, -ia, -ism	epiglottis	epiglott/o
condition; process	-y	esophagus	esophag/o
condition; structure	-us	excess, beyond	ultra-
condyle	condyl/o	excessive, above normal	hyper-
conjunctiva	conjunctiv/o	excision, removal	-ectomy
cornea	corne/o	extremity	acr/o
cortex	cortic/o	eye	ocul/o, ophthalm/o
cranium (skull)	crani/o	eye, vision	opt/o, optic/o
crooked, bent	scoli/o	eyelid	blephar/o
cross	cruci/o	**F**	
crushing	-tripsy		
cul-de-sac	culd/o	face	faci/o
curve, swayback	lord/o	false	pseudo-
cutting	-cision	far, farthest	dist/o
D		fat	adip/o, lip/o, lipid/o, steat/o
darkness	scot/o	fatty plaque	ather/o
dawn (rose colored)	eosin/o	fear	-phobia

Continued

English Terms—cont'd

Meaning	Element	Meaning	Element
feeling	esthes/o, -esthesia	hardening; sclera (white of the eye)	scler/o
feeling (mental state)	-phoria		
femur (thigh bone)	femor/o	having the form of, possessing	-ate
fiber, fibrous tissue	fibr/o		
fibula (smaller bone of the lower leg)	fibul/o	head	cephal/o, -ceps
		hearing	acous/o, -acusia, -acusis, audi/o, audit/o, -cusia, -cusis
fingers; toes	dactyl/o		
fire	pyr/o		
first	primi-	heart	cardi/o, coron/o
fixation (of an organ)	-pexy	heart condition	-cardia
flesh (connective tissue)	sarc/o	heat	therm/o
flint	silic/o	heat, burn	cauter/o
foot	pod/o	hernia, swelling	-cele
foot; child	ped/i, ped/o	hidden	crypt/o
foreign, strange	xen/o	horny tissue; hard; cornea	kerat/o
form, shape, structure	morph/o	humerus (upper arm bone)	humer/o
formation, growth	plas/o, -plasia, -plasm	humpback	kyph/o
formation, production	-poiesis		
forming an opening (mouth)	-stomy	**I**	
forming, producing, origin	-gen, gen/o, -genesis	ileum (third part of the small intestine)	ile/o
four	quadri-	ilium (lateral, flaring portion of the hip bone)	ili/o
from, away from	ab-		
fungus (plural, fungi)	myc/o	immune, immunity, safe	immun/o
		in, not	in-
G		in, within	en-, end-, endo-, intra-
gallbladder	cholecyst/o	incision	-tomy
ganglion (knot or knotlike mass)	gangli/o	incomplete; imperfect	atel/o
		inflammation	-itis
genetic change	mut/a	instrument for examining	-scope
genitalia	genit/o	instrument for measuring	-meter
gland	aden/o	instrument for recording	-graph
glans penis	balan/o	instrument to cut	-tome
glassy	vitre/o	insulin	insulin/o
glomerulus	glomerul/o	internal organs	viscer/o
glottis	glott/o	intestine (usually small intestine)	enter/o
glue; neuroglial tissue	gli/o, -glia		
gonads, sex glands	gonad/o	involuntary contraction, twitching	-spasm
good; normal	eu-		
granule	granul/o	inward	eso-
gray	glauc/o	iris	irid/o
gray; gray matter (of the brain or spinal cord)	poli/o	iron	sider/o
		irrigation, washing	-clysis
green	chlor/o	ischium (lower portion of the hip bone)	ischi/o
groin	inguin/o		
growth	-physis	**J, K**	
gum(s)	gingiv/o		
		jaundice	-icterus
H		jejunum (second part of the small intestine)	jejun/o
hair	pil/o, trich/o		
hallucination	hallucin/o	joint	arthr/o

English Terms—cont'd

Meaning	Element	Meaning	Element
kernel (nucleus)	kern/o	milk	galact/o, lact/o
ketone bodies (acids and acetones)	ket/o, keton/o	milk	lact/o
		mind	ment/o, psych/o
kidney	nephr/o, ren/o	mind; emotion	-thymia
killing	-cide	monthly discharge of blood	menstr/o
knowing	gnos/o, -gnosis	mouth	or/o, stomat/o
L		movement	kinesi/o, -kinesia, kinet/o
labyrinth (inner ear)	labyrinth/o	mucus	muc/o, myx/o
lacrimal sac	dacryocyst/o	muscle	muscul/o, my/o, myos/o
lamina (part of the vertebral arch)	lamin/o	muzzle	phim/o
large	macro-	**N**	
larynx (voice box)	laryng/o	nail	onych/o, ungu/o
lens	phac/o	narrowing, stricture	sten/o, -stenosis
lice	pedicul/o	navel (umbilicus)	omphal/o
life	bi/o	near, beside; beyond	para-
light	phot/o	near, nearest	proxim/o
limestone	chalic/o	neck; cervix uteri (neck of uterus)	cervic/o
lip	cheil/o, labi/o		
little swelling	tubercul/o	nerve	neur/o
liver	hepat/o	nerve root	radicul/o
lobe	lob/o	nest	nid/o
loins (lower back)	lumb/o	net, mesh	reticul/o
lower, below	infer/o	neutral; neither	neutr/o
luminous, fluorescence	fluor/o	new	neo-
lung	pulmon/o	night	noct/o, nyctal/o
lymph	lymph/o	nipple	thel/o
lymph gland (node)	lymphaden/o	nitrogenous compounds	azot/o
lymph vessel	lymphangi/o	none	nulli-
M		nose	nas/o, rhin/o
male	andr/o	not	im-
malignant tumor of connective tissue	-sarcoma	noun ending	-a, -ice, -is
		nucleus	kary/o, nucle/o
many, much	multi-, poly	**O**	
marketplace	agora-	obscure	-opaque
mastoid process	mastoid/o	old age	presby/o
maxilla (upper jaw bone)	maxill/o	one	mono-, uni-
meal	-prandial	one half	hemi-, semi-
mediastinum	mediastin/o	opening, meatus	meat/o
medicine	iatr/o	order, coordination	tax/o, -taxia
medulla	medull/o	other, differing from the normal	allo-
meninges (membranes covering the brain and spinal cord)	mening/o, meningi/o		
		out, out from	ec-, ex-
menses, menstruation	men/o	outside	extra-
metacarpus (hand bones)	metacarp/o	outside, outward	ecto-, exo-
metatarsus (foot bones)	metatars/o	ovary	oophor/o, ovari/o
middle	medi-, medi/o, meso-	oxygen	ox/i, ox/o, -oxia

Continued

English Terms—cont'd

Meaning	Element	Meaning	Element
P		**Q, R**	
pain	-algesia, -algia, -dynia	radiation, x-ray; radius (lower arm bone on the thumb side)	radi/o
palate (roof of the mouth)	palat/o		
pancreas	pancreat/o		
paralysis	-plegia	rapid	tachy-
parathyroid glands	parathyroid/o	record, writing	-gram
partial paralysis	-paresis	rectum	rect/o
patella (kneecap)	patell/o	red	erythem/o,
pelvis	pelv/i, pelv/o		erythemat/o,
penis	pen/o		erythr/o, rube/o
perineum (area between the scrotum [or vulva in the female] and anus)	perine/o	renal pelvis	pyel/o
		repeated sound	echo-
		resembling	-oid
peritoneum	peritone/o	retina	retin/o
pertaining to	-ac, -al, -ar, -ary, -eal, -iac, -ic, -ical, -ile, -ine, -ior, -itic, -ive, -ory, -ous, -tic	rhythm	-rrhythm/o
		ribs	cost/o
		rod shaped (striated)	rhabd/o
		rod-shaped (striated) muscle	rhabdomy/o
pertaining to poison	-toxic		
pertaining to sugar	-ose	rupture	-rrhexis
phalanges (bones of the fingers and toes)	phalang/o	**S**	
pharynx (throat)	pharyng/o	sacrum	sacr/o
physical function	physi/o	saliva	ptyal/o
physician; treatment	iatr/o, -iatry	saliva, salivary gland	sial/o
pituitary gland	pituitar/o	same	homo-
plaque	-plakia	same, alike	home/o, homeo-
pleasure	hedon/o	same, equal	iso-
pleura	pleur/o	scab	eschar/o
point, mark	stigmat/o	scale	squam/o
poison	tox/o, toxic/o	scanty	olig/o
porous	-porosis	scapula (shoulder blade)	scapul/o
potassium (an electrolyte)	kal/i	sea	thalass/o
power	-potence	sebum, sebaceous	seb/o
pregnancy	-cyesis, gest/o	secrete	crin/o, -crine
pregnancy; childbirth	obstetr/o	seed (ovum or spermatozoon)	gon/o
pregnant woman	-gravida		
process (of)	-ation, -ization	seizure	-lepsy
process of recording	-graphy	self, own	auto-
prolapse, downward displacement	-ptosis	semen; seed	semin/o, semin/i
		seminal vesicle	vesicul/o
prostate gland	prostat/o	separation	sequestr/o
protection	-phylaxis	separation; destruction; loosening	-lysis
protein	-globin		
pubis (anterior part of the pelvic bone)	pub/o	septum	sept/o
		serum	ser/o
pulse	sphygm/o, -sphyxia	sheath (usually referring to the meninges)	thec/o
pupil	cor/o, core/o, pupill/o		
pus	py/o	short	brachy-
pylorus	pylor/o	side, to one side	later/o

English Terms—cont'd

Meaning	Element	Meaning	Element
sigmoid colon	sigmoid/o	suture	-rrhaphy
sinus, cavity	sin/o, sinus/o	swallowing, eating	phag/o, -phage, -phagia
skin	cutane/o, derm/o, derma, dermat/o	sweat	hidr/o, sudor/o
sleep	hypn/o, somn/o	swelling	-edema
slipping	-listhesis	swelling (little)	tubercul/o
slit, fissure	-spadias	sword	xiph/o
slow	brady-	synapsis, point of contact	synapt/o
small	micr/o, micro-	synovial membrane, synovial fluid	synov/o
small growth	polyp/o		
small, minute	-icle, -ole, -ula, -ule	**T**	
smell	-osmia		
smooth	lei/o	tail	caud/o
smooth muscle (visceral)	leiomy/o	tear; lacrimal apparatus (duct, sac, or gland)	dacry/o, lacrim/o
society	-social		
sodium (an electrolyte)	natr/o	teeth	dent/o, odont/o
softening	-malacia	tendon	ten/o, tend/o, tendin/o
sound	son/o	tension	ton/o
specialist	-ician, -ist	testis (plural, testes)	orch/o, orchi/o, orchid/o, test/o
specialist in the study of	-logist		
speech	-phasia	thalamus	thalam/o
speech, babble	-lalia	the act of	-ion
spermatozoa, sperm cells	sperm/i, sperm/o, spermat/o	thick	pachy-
		thin, slender	lept/o
spine	rachi/o, spin/o	thirst	dips/o, -dipsia
spitting	-ptysis	three	tri-
spleen	splen/o	through	per-
split	schiz/o	through, across	dia-
splitting	-schisis	thymus gland	thym/o
standing still	-stasis	thyroid gland	thyr/o, thyroid/o
stapes	staped/o	tibia (larger bone of the lower leg)	tibi/o
star	astr/o		
state of mental disorder, frenzy	-mania	tissue	hist/o, histi/o
		to bear (offspring)	-para
state of; condition	-ema, -isy, -sis	to break; surgical fracture	-clasia, -clasis, -clast
sternum (breastbone)	stern/o	to carry	-ferent
stiffness; bent, crooked	ankyl/o	to cut	tom/o
stimulate	-tropin	to go	-grade
stomach	gastr/o	to hold back	-continence
stone, calculus	-lith, lith/o	to hold back; block	isch/o
straight	orth/o	to inflate	emphys/o
strength	sthen/o	to lead; carry	duct/o
stroke	-plexy	to miscarry	abort/o
structure, thing	-um	to one side; side	later/o
study of	log/o, -logy	to pull	ill/o
stupor; numbness; sleep	narc/o	to see	voyeur/o
sugar, sweetness	gluc/o, glucos/o, glyc/o, glycos/o	to shine; clear	-lucent
		to steal	klept/o
surgical puncture	-centesis	to stretch	-tension
surgical repair	-plasty	to turn	-verse

Continued

English Terms—cont'd

Meaning	Element	Meaning	Element
to view	scop/o	uterus (womb)	hyster/o, metri/o, uter/o
toes, fingers	dactyl/o		
tongue	gloss/o, lingu/o	uterus (womb); measure	metr/o
tonsils	tonsill/o	uvula	uvul/o
toward	-ad, ad-, af-	**V**	
trabecula (supporting bundles of fibers)	trabecul/o	vagina	colp/o, vagin/o
trachea (windpipe)	trache/o	valve	valv/o, valvul/o
transplantation	-graft	varied, irregular	poikil/o
treatment	therapeut/o, -therapy, iatr/o	vein	phleb/o, ven/o
		ventricle (of the heart or brain)	ventricul/o
tree	dendr/o		
trigone (triangular region at the base of the bladder)	trigon/o	vertebrae (backbone)	spondyl/o, vertebr/o
tube (usually the fallopian or eustachian [auditory] tube)	salping/o, -salpinx	vessel (usually blood or lymph)	angi/o, vascul/o
		vessel; vas deferens; duct	vas/o
		view of	-opsy
tumor	-oma, onc/o	vision	-opia, -opsia
turning	-tropia, -version	visual examination	-scopy
two	bi-	vitreous body (of the eye)	vitr/o
tympanic membrane (eardrum)	myring/o, tympan/o	voice	-phonia
		volume	vol/o
U		vomiting	-emesis
		vulva	episi/o, vulv/o
ulna (lower arm bone on the opposite side of the thumb)	uln/o	**W, X, Y, Z**	
umbilicus, navel	umbilic/o	water	aque/o, hydr/o
under, below	sub-	weakness, debility	-asthenia
under, below, deficient	hyp-, hyp/o, hypo-	white	albin/o, leuk/o
unequal, dissimilar	aniso-	widen, enlarge	mydr/o
union, together, joined	sym-, syn-	without, not	a-, an-
unknown, peculiar	idi/o	woman, female	gyn/o, gynec/o
upper, above	super-, super/o	word, phrase	lex/o
ureter	ureter/o	wrinkle	rhytid/o
urethra	urethr/o	x-rays	roentgen/o
urine	-uria	yellow	cirrh/o, jaund/o, xanth/o
urine, urinary tract	ur/o, urin/o		

Index of Genetic Disorders

Index of Clinical, Laboratory, and Imaging Procedures

Clinical

Laboratory

Imaging

Index of Pharmacology

Index of Oncological Terms

Index of Discontinued Abbreviations and Eponyms

Discontinued Abbreviations

The Joint Commission (JC) and the Institute for Safe Medication Practices (ISMP) report that the following abbreviations are commonly misinterpreted and have resulted in harmful medical errors. Both organizations and health-care systems have compiled comprehensive "Do Not Use" and error prone lists (available on their websites) for health-care providers.

To prevent harmful medical errors from occurring, both organizations recommend discontinuance of those abbreviations. Instead, the abbreviations should be written out. Nevertheless, some of the abbreviations on the "Do Not Use" list are still used by health-care providers. This table lists these abbreviations, along with their meanings.

Abbreviation	Meaning	Abbreviation	Meaning
Medication and Therapy Time Schedule		qPM	every evening
a.c.	before meals	tid, t.i.d.	three times a day
bid, b.i.d.	twice a day	*Other Related Abbreviations*	
hs	half strength	AD	right ear
h.s.	at bedtime	AS	left ear
NPO, n.p.o.	nothing by mouth	AU	both ears
p.c.	after meals	cc	cubic centimeter, same as mL (1/1,000 of
p.o.	by mouth		a liter; use *mL* for milliliters or write out
p.r.n.	as required		the meaning)
q2h	every 2 hours	dc, DC, D/C	discharge; discontinue
Q.D., QD,	every day	IU	International Unit
q.d., qd		OD	right eye
q.h.	every hour	OS	left eye
q.i.d.	four times a day	OU	both eyes
Q.O.D.,	every other day	subcu, sub q,	subcutaneous (injection)
QOD, q.o.d.,		Sub-Q, subQ	
qod		U, u	unit
qAM	every morning	UD	use as directed

Discontinued Eponyms

The *International Classification of Diseases,* 10th edition, Clinical Modification (ICD-10-CM) contains the use of eponyms when assigning certain codes for diagnoses and procedures. However, all surgical eponyms have been removed from the *International Classification of Diseases,* 10th edition, Procedure Coding System (ICD-10-PCS). In their place are root terms that describe the objective of the procedure and other parameters to assign proper codes. The ICD-10-PCS procedural codes are more specific and clinically accurate, and they have a more logical structure than the previous coding systems. There are still some diagnostic eponyms in ICD-10-PCS, but most have been replaced with constructed terms that identify the diseases or conditions. This table lists common eponyms, along with ICD-10-PCS constructed words and where each eponym appears in this textbook.

While a comprehensive list of all discontinued eponyms and their replacements in ICD-11 is not readily available, the general trend is toward adopting descriptive terms that clearly convey the nature of the disease. For detailed information on specific conditions and their current terminology, consulting the official ICD-11 reference guide or database is recommended.

It's important to note that the transition from ICD-10 to ICD-11 involves numerous updates beyond the renaming of diseases, including structural changes and the addition of new categories to better reflect contemporary medical knowledge and practices.

Eponyms	ICD-10-PCS Constructed Word*	Systems, 9th Edition
Addison disease	corticoadrenal insufficiency	Chapter 14, Endocrine System
Alzheimer disease	cerebral degeneration	Chapter 15, Nervous System
Bell palsy	facial nerve palsy	Chapter 15, Nervous System
Bowen disease	carcinoma in situ of skin	Chapter 5, Integumentary System
Colles fracture	fracture of lower end of radius	Chapter 10, Musculoskeletal System
Crohn disease	regional enteritis	Chapter 6, Digestive System
Cushing syndrome	adrenal hyperplasia resulting from excess adrenocorticotropic hormone (ACTH)	Chapter 14, Endocrine System
Down syndrome	trisomy 21	Chapter 12, Female Reproductive System
Graves disease	autoimmune hyperthyroidism	Chapter 14, Endocrine System
Guillain-Barré syndrome	infective or idiopathic polyneuritis	Chapter 15, Nervous System
Heberden nodes	generalized osteoarthrosis of hand	Chapter 10, Musculoskeletal System
Hodgkin disease	classical Hodgkin lymphoma	Chapter 9, Blood, Lymphatic, and Immune Systems
Huntington chorea	neurodegenerative genetic disorder	Chapter 15, Nervous System
Kaposi sarcoma	malignant neoplasm of soft tissue	Chapter 9, Blood, Lymphatic, and Immune Systems
Ménière disease	endolymphatic/labyrinthine hydrops	Chapter 16, Special Senses
Paget disease	osteitis deformans	Chapter 10, Musculoskeletal System
Parkinson disease	paralysis agitans	Chapter 15, Nervous System
Reye syndrome	acute noninflammatory encephalopathy and fatty degenerative liver failure	Chapter 15, Nervous System
Wilms tumor	Nephroblastoma	Chapter 11, Urinary System
Surgical/Dx Procedures		
Doppler ultrasonography	ultrasonography using sound pitch	Chapter 8, Cardiovascular System
Mohs	micrographic surgery	Chapter 5, Integumentary System
Rinne tuning fork test	air and bone conduction hearing test	Chapter 16, Special Senses
Roux-en-Y gastric bypass (RGB)	gastric bypass with gastroenterostomy	Chapter 6, Digestive System
Weber tuning fork test	conductive and sensorineural hearing loss test	Chapter 16, Special Senses

*The compliance date for implementation of ICD-10-CM/PCS was October 1, 2015, for all entities covered by the Health Insurance Portability and Accountability Act (HIPAA).

Index

Page numbers followed by f, b, and t indicate figures, boxes, and tables on the corresponding pages.